T0396986

Lecture Notes in Electrical Engineering

Volume 269

For further volumes:
http://www.springer.com/series/7818

Shaozi Li · Qun Jin · Xiaohong Jiang
James J. (Jong Hyuk) Park
Editors

Frontier and Future Development of Information Technology in Medicine and Education

ITME 2013

Volume 1

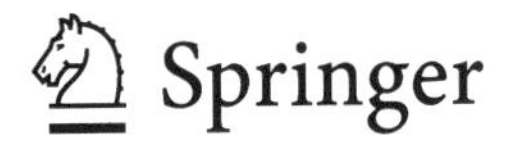

Editors
Shaozi Li
Cognitive Science
Xiamen University
Xiamen
People's Republic of China

Xiaohong Jiang
School of Systems Information Science
Future University Hakodate
Hakodate, Hokkaido
Japan

Qun Jin
Networked Information Systems Lab,
Human Informatics and Cognitive Sciences
Waseda University
Waseda
Japan

James J. (Jong Hyuk) Park
Department of Computer Science and Engineering
Seoul National Universityof Science and Technology (SeoulTech)
Seoul
Korea, Republic of South Korea

ISSN 1876-1100 ISSN 1876-1119 (electronic)
ISBN 978-94-007-7617-3 ISBN 978-94-007-7618-0 (eBook)
DOI 10.1007/978-94-007-7618-0
Springer Dordrecht Heidelberg New York London

Library of Congress Control Number: 2013948373

Printed on acid-free paper

Springer is part of Springer Science+Business Media (www.springer.com)

Message from the ITME 2013 General Chairs

ITME 2013 is the 5th International Symposium on IT in Medicine and Education. This conference took place in July 19–21, 2013, in Xining, China. The aim of the ITME 2013 was to provide an international symposium for scientific research on IT in Medicine and Education. It was organized by Qinghai University, Future University Hakodate, Xiamen University, Shandong Normal University. ITME 2013 is the next event in a series of highly successful international symposia on IT in Medicine and Education, ITME-12 (Hokkaido, Japan, August 2012), ITME-11 (Guangzhou, China, December 2011), ITME-09 (Jinan, China, August 2009), ITME-08 (Xiamen, China, December 2008).

The papers included in the proceedings cover the following topics: IT Application in Medicine Education, Medical Image Processing and compression, e-Health and e-Hospital, Tele-medicine and Tele-surgery, Standard in Health Informatics and cross-language solution, Computer-Aided Diagnostic (CAD), Health informatics education, Biomechanics, modeling and computing, Digital Virtual Organ and Clinic Application, Three Dimension Reconstruction for Medical Imaging, Hospital Management Informatization, Construction of Medical Database, Medical Knowledge Mining, IT and Biomedicine, IT and Clinical Medicine, IT and Laboratory Medicine, IT and Preclinical Medicine, IT and Medical Informatics, Architecture of Educational Information Systems, Building and Sharing Digital Education Resources on the Internet, Collaborative Learning/Training, Computer Aided Teaching and Campus Network Construction, Curriculum Design and Development for Open/Distance Education, Digital Library, e-Learning Pedagogical Strategies, Ethical and Social Issues in Using IT in Education, Innovative Software and Hardware Systems for Education and Training, Issues on University Office Automation and Education Administration Management Systems, Learning Management Information Systems, Managed Learning Environments, Multimedia and Hypermedia Applications and Knowledge Management in Education, Pedagogical Issues on Open/Distance Education, Plagiarism Issues on Open/Distance Education, Security and Privacy issues with e-learning, Software Agents and Applications in Education. Accepted and presented papers highlight new trends and challenges of Medicine and Education. The presenters showed how new research could lead to novel and innovative applications. We hope you will find these results useful and inspiring for your future research.

We would like to express our sincere thanks to Steering Chair: Zongkai Lin (Institute of Computing Technology, Chinese Academy of Sciences, China). Our special thanks go to the Program Chairs: Shaozi Li (Xiamen University, China), Ying Dai (Iwate Prefectural University, Japan), Osamu Takahashi (Future University Hakodate, Japan), Dongqing Xie (Guangzhou University, China), Jianming Yong (University of Southern Queensland, Australia), all program committee members, and all the additional reviewers for their valuable efforts in the review process, which helped us to guarantee the highest quality of the selected papers for the conference.

We cordially thank all the authors for their valuable contributions and the other participants of this conference. The conference would not have been possible without their support. Thanks are also due to the many experts who contributed to making the event a success.

June 2013

Yongnian Liu
Xiaohong Jiang
James J. (Jong Hyuk) Park
Qun Jin
Hong Liu

Message from the ITME 2013 Program Chairs

Welcome to the 5th International Symposium on IT in Medicine and Education (ITME 2013), which will be held on July 19–21, 2013, in Xining, China. ITME 2013 will be the most comprehensive conference focused on the IT in Medicine and Education. ITME 2013 will provide an opportunity for academic and industry professionals to discuss the recent progress in the area of Medicine and Education. In addition, the conference will publish high-quality papers which are closely related to the various theories and practical applications on IT in Medicine and Education. Furthermore, we expect that the conference and its publications will be a trigger for further related research and technology improvements in these important subjects.

For ITME 2013, we received many paper submissions, after a rigorous peer review process; only very outstanding papers will be accepted for the ITME 2013 proceedings, published by Springer. All submitted papers have undergone blind reviews by at least two reviewers from the technical program committee, which consists of leading researchers around the globe. Without their hard work, achieving such a high-quality proceeding would not have been possible. We take this opportunity to thank them for their great support and cooperation. We would like to sincerely thank the following keynote speakers who kindly accepted our invitations, and, in this way, helped to meet the objectives of the conference: Prof. Qun Jin, Department of Human Informatics and Cognitive Sciences, Waseda University, Japan, Prof. Yun Yang, Swinburne University of Technology, Melbourne, Australia, Prof. Qinghua Zheng, Department of Computer Science and Technology, Xi'an Jiaotong University, China. We also would like to thank all of you for your participation in our conference, and also thank all the authors, reviewers, and organizing committee members.

Thank you and enjoy the conference!

Shaozi Li, China
Ying Dai, Japan
Osamu Takahashi, Japan
Dongqing Xie, China
Jianming Yong, Australia

Organization

General Conference Chairs

Prof. Yongnian Liu (QHU, China)
Prof. Xiaohong Jiang (FUN, Hakodate, Japan)
Prof. James J. (Jong Hyuk) Park, Seoul National University of Science and Technology, Korea
Prof. Qun Jin (Waseda, Japan)
Prof. Hong Liu (SDNU, China)

General Conference Co-Chairs

Prof. Yu Jianshe (GZHU, China)
Prof. Ramana Reddy (WVU, USA)
Dr. Bin Hu (UCE Birmingham, UK)
Prof. Dingfang Chen (WHUT, China)
Prof. Junzhong Gu (ECNU, China)

Program Committee Chairs

Prof. Shaozi Li (XMU, China)
Prof. Ying Dai (Iwate Prefecture University, Japan)
Prof. Osamu Takahashi (FUN, Hakodate, Japan)
Prof. Dongqing Xie (GZHU, China)
Dr. Jianming Yong (USQ, Australia)

Organizing Committee Chairs

Prof. Mengrong Xie (QHU, China)
Prof. Gaoping Wang (HAUT, China)

Dr. Jiatuo Xu (SHUTCM, Shanghai, China)
Prof. Zhimin Yang (Shandong University)

Local Arrangement Co-Chairs

Prof. Jing Zhao (QHU, China)
Prof. Peng Chen (QHU, China)

Publication Chairs

Prof. Hwa Young Jeong, Kyung Hee University, Korea
Dr. Min Jiang (XMU, Xiamen, China)

Program Committee

Ahmed Meddahi, Institute Mines-Telecom/TELECOM Lille1, France
Ahmed Shawish, Ain Shams University, Egypt
Alexander Pasko, Bournemouth University, UK
Angela Guercio, Kent State University
Bob Apduhan, Kyushu Sangyo University, Japan
Cai Guorong, Jimei University, China
Cao Donglin, Xiamen University, China
Changqin Huang, Southern China Normal University, China
Chaozhen Guo, Fuzhou University, China
Chensheng Wang, Beijing University of Posts and Telecommunications, China
Chuanqun Jiang, Shanghai Second Polytechnic University, China
Cui Lizhen, Shandong University, China
Cuixia Ma, Institute of Software Chinese Academy of Sciences, China
Feng Li, Jiangsu University, China
Fuhua Oscar Lin, Athabasca University, Canada
Hiroyuki Mituhara, Tokushima University, Japan
Hongji Yang, De Montfort University, UK
Hsin-Chang Yang, National University of Kaohsiung, Taiwan
Hsin-Chang Yang, National University of Kaohsiung, Taiwan
I-Hsien Ting, National University of Kaohsiung, Taiwan
Jens Herder, University of Applied Sciences, Germany
Jian Chen, Waseda University, Japan
Jianhua Zhao, Southern China Normal University, China
Jianming Yong, University of Southern Queensland, Australia
Jiehan Zhou, University of Oulu, Finland

Jungang Han, Xi'an University of Posts and Telecommunications, China
Junqing Yu, Huazhong University of Science and Technology, China
Kamen Kanev, Shizuoka University, Japan
Kiss Gabor, Obuda University, Hungary
Lei Yu, The PLA Information Engineering University, China
Li Xueqing, Shandong University, China
Luhong Diao, Beijing University of Technology, China
Masaaki Shirase, Future University Hakodate, Japan
Masashi Toda, Future University, Japan
Mohamed Mostafa Zayed, Taibah University, KSA
Mohammad Tariqul Islam, Multimedia University, Malaysia
Mohd Nazri Ismail, Universiti Kuala Lumpur, Malaysia
Neil Y. Yen, University of Aizu, Japan
Osamu Takahashi, Future University Hakodate, Japan
Paolo Maresca, University Federico II, Italy
Pierpaolo Di Bitonto, University of Bari, Italy
Ping Jiang, University of Hull, UK
Qiang Gao, Beihang University, China
Qianping Wang, China University of Mining and Technology, China
Qingguo Zhou, Lanzhou University, China
Qinghua Zheng, Xi'an Jiao Tong University, China
Rita Francese, University of Salerno, Italy
Roman Y. Shtykh, Waseda University, Japan
Rongrong Ji, Columbia University, USA
Shaohua Teng, Guangdong University of Technology, China
Shufen Liu, Jilin University, China
Su Songzhi, Xiamen University, China
Tianhong Luo, Chongqing Jiaotong University, China
Tim Arndt, Cleveland State University, USA
Tongsheng Chen, Comprehensive Information Corporation, Taiwan
Wei Song, Minzu University of China, Tsinghua University, China
Wenan Tan, Shanghai Second Polytechnic University, China
Wenhua Huang, Southern Medical University, China
Xiaokang Zhou, Waseda University, Japan
Xiaopeng Sun, Liaoning Normal University, China
Xiaosu Zhan, Beijing University of Posts and Telecommunications, China
Xinheng Wang, Swansea University, UK
Xiufen Fu, Guangdong University of Technology, China
Yaowei Bai, Shanghai Second Polytechnic University, China
Yingguang Li, Nanjing University of Aeronautics and Astronautics, China
Yinglong Wang, Shandong Academy of Sciences, China
Yinsheng Li, Fudan University, China
Yiwei Cao, IMC AG, Germany
Yong Tang, South China Normal University, China
Yoshitaka Nakamura, Future University Hakodate, Japan

Yuichi Fujino, Future University, Japan
Yujie Liu, China University of Petroleum, China
Zhang Zili, Southwestern University, China
Zhao Junlan, Inner Mongolia Finance and Economics College, China
Zhaoliang Jiang, Shandong University, China
Zhendong Niu, Beijing Institute of Technology, China
Zhenhua Duan, Xidian University, China
Zhongwei Xu, Shandong University at Weihai, China
Zonghua Zhang, Institute Mines-Telecom/TELECOM Lille1, France
Zongmin Li, China University of Petroleum, China
Zongpu Jia, Henan Polytechnic University, China

Contents

Volume 1

Volume 2

Volume 3

Volume 4

Chapter 1
The Anti-Apoptotic Effect of Transgenic Akt1 Gene on Cultured New-Born Rats Cardiomyocytes Mediated by Ultrasound/ Microbubbles Destruction

Dongye Li, Xueyou Jiang, Tongda Xu, Jiantao Song, Hong zhu and Yuanyuan Luo

Abstract The purpose of this study was to transfect exogenous Akt1 to 293FT cells and cultured new-born rats cardiomyocytes respectively for exploring the feasibility and safety of the new method. In addition, the protective effects on cultured cardiomyocytes suffering from ischemia/reperfusion injury (I/R inury) of the transgenic Akt1 gene mediated by ultrasound-induced microbubble destruction (US/MB) were also observed. 293FT cells and cardiomyocytes were divided into four groups, group A: only pEGFPC1- Akt1; group B: MB + pEGFPC1-Akt1; group C: US + pEGFPC1-Akt1; group D: US + MB + pEGFPC1-Akt1. The results showed that microbubble alone could not deliver exogenous genes to target cells without ultrasound, but the latter could without the help of microbubble, ultrasound with simultaneous microbubble could enhance the transfection rate significantly. Ultrasound frequency 1.7 MHz, mechanical index (MI) 1.5, irradiation time 2 min, MB volume concentration 15 %. According to the above ultrasound parameters, Akt1 gene was transfected to cultured cardiomyocytes and then allowed them to suffer from I/R injury, our results showed that the transgenic Akt1 gene was expressed and had significant anti-apoptotic effect. The results suggested that US/MB was a promising gene delivery system for gene therapy in heart diseases.

Keywords Ultrasound · Microbubble · Gene transfection · Akt · Cardiomyocyte

D. Li (✉) · T. Xu · H. zhu · Y. Luo
Department of Cardiology, Institute of Cardiovascular Diseases, the Affiliated Hospital of Xuzhou Medical College, Xuzhou 221002, China
e-mail: ldy@xzmc.edu.cn

X. Jiang
Department of Cardiology of Second Hospital of NanJing, Nanjing 210000, China

J. Song
Department of Cardiology, the Affiliated Hospital of Shandong Medical University, Ji-nan 250001, China

S. Li et al. (eds.), *Frontier and Future Development of Information Technology in Medicine and Education*, Lecture Notes in Electrical Engineering 269,
DOI: 10.1007/978-94-007-7618-0_1,

1.1 Introduction

With evolving knowledge in molecular and cellular cardiology, gene therapy has been investigated in animal models and even in clinical studies in the field of ischemic heart disease. Up to date, vectors of cardiac gene therapy are still limited by their own disadvantages. Viral vectors were used widely in gene therapy because of their high transfection efficiency. However, they are limited by immunogenic properties as well as the difficulty and expense of preparing large amounts of pure virus needed in vivo. The traditional non-viral vectors such as naked DNA and liposome are also not ideal tools due to their low transfection efficiency [1]. Recently, ultrasound-induced microbubble destruction (US/MB) has been used as a new technique for gene delivery. Isao et al. [2] reported that US/MB could enable myocardial HGF gene transfer with systemic administration of naked plasmid. So US/MB may be an useful tool for gene delivery.

Akt is a Ser/Thr protein and is activated by several cardioprotective ligand-receptor systems, such as insulin, insulin-like growth factor (IGF-1). The activated Akt exert a powerful cardioprotective effects [3]. Matsui et al. used adenoviral vectors to transfer Akt to the rats myocardium and found Akt activation reduced infarct size and the number of apoptotic cells [4]. In our previous study, we also found exogenous Akt mediated by liposome promote cardiomyocyte survival significantly. Akt may represent an important target for therapy in ischemic heart disease.

In the present study, the aim was to investigate the feasibility and safety of Akt1 gene transfection mediated by US/MB and the effects of exogenous Akt1 gene on cardiomyocytes after ischemia/reperfusion injury (I/R injury) in vitro.

1.2 Materials and Methods

1.2.1 Plasmid Preparations

The plasmid pEGFPC1- Akt1 were kindly gifted from professor Downward (Institute of Signal Transfection in London). The plasmid DNA was propagated from DH5 α cultures and purified with kits (Promega company) according to the company protocol. DNA concentration was determined by ultraviolet spectrophotometry.

1.2.2 Animals and Cell Preparations

New-born Sprague–Dawley (SD) rats between 1 and 3 days despite gender were used for the study. Cardiomyocytes of new-born SD rats were isolated by enzyme digestion and were purified by means of differential attachment technique and Brdu inhibition.

1.2.3 Microbubbles

SonoVue (Bracco, Italy) is lipid-shelled US contrast agent composed of millions of microbubbles filled with sulfur hexafluoride gas that are 2.5–6.0 μm in average diameter, and 90 % of which are smaller than 6.0 μm. Microbubbles were prepared according to the manufacturer's instructions. The SonoVue powder was dissolved in 0.9 % saline and then added plasmid DNA immediately making the plasmid DNA concentration to 100 μg/ml and incubated for 30 min under 4 °C before it was used for transfection.

1.2.4 Transfect Akt1 Gene Mediated by US/MB

293FT cells and cardiomyocytes were divided into four groups respectively, group A: only pEGFPC1-Akt1; group B: MB + pEGFPC1-Akt1; group C: US + pEGFPC1-Akt1; group D: US + MB + pEGFPC1-Akt1. Cells in each group were divided into five culture dishes respectively in order to detect the transfection rate and cell death. The transfection parameter was set as follow: the distance between US probe and the bottom of dishes was 1 cm; US frequence was 1.7 MHz; mechanical index (MI) was 1.5; irradiation time was 2 min. The cell death rate was determined 6 h after transfection and the GFP transgene expression was detected 48 h after transfection.

1.2.5 Optimum of Parameter About Cardiomyocytes

According to previous study, the transfection rate of 293FT cells was almost higher than that of cardiomyocytes. In order to ameliorate the transfection rate, different experimental conditions were tried. (1) According to different MI, cells were assigned to three groups: group A, MI 0.5; group B, MI 1.0; group C, MI 1.5. (2) Cells were divided into four groups and given four different irradiation times: group A, 1 min; group B, 2 min; group C, 3 min; group D, 4 min. (3) After choosing the optimal MI and irradiation time, four different microbubbles volume concentration: 10; 15; 20 and 25 % were tried. The transfection rate was assessed by observing the expression of GFP gene under fluorescent microscope.

1.2.6 Make Cardiomyocytes Ischemic/Reperfusion Models

Using the determined optimal transfection parameters, plasmid encoding Akt1 gene and enhanced GFP were transfected to the cultured cardiomyocytes.

In addition, some groups were also set as control: (a) without any plasmid (b) plasmid alone as control, (c) plasmid plus US/MB plus LY294002 (PI3 K/Akt inhibitor), (d) plasmid plus US/MB. 48 h after transfection, cells in each group would undergo I/R injury. At the end of reperfusion, the cell apoptotic rate was detected by Hoechst kit and the expression of Akt1 protein was detected by Western blot.

1.2.7 Detect Akt1 Protein Expression by Western Blot

Cardiomyocytes transfected with PBS, plasmid, plasmid plus Akt inhibitor or plasmid plus microbubbles were cultured with 10 % FBS DMED in normal conditions for 48 h, and then subjected to I/R injury in vitro. After that, cells proteins were isolated for Western blot analysis. Briefly, cardiomyocytes were lysed at 4 °C in lysis buffer, and equal amounts of protein were subjected to SDS-PAGE. Standard Western blot analysis was conducted using Akt1 antibody (1:1000, cell signaling). Anti-β-actin antibody was used as control (1:3000, Zhongshan).

1.2.8 Statistical Analysis

Data are expressed as means and standard deviations and analyzed by SPSS16.0 statistics software. The difference in each group was analyzed by one-way ANOVA and t test. There was statistical significance when $P < 0.05$.

1.3 Results

1.3.1 US/MB Significantly Improved Gene Transfection Efficiency

Cardiomyocytes were successfully isolated and 90 % of them beating with the rate of 40–120 bpm. The rate of survival and the purity of cardiomyocytes were both about 95 % (Fig. 1.1). The expression of GFP was not observed in 293FT cells which were added plasmid alone (group A), whereas plasmid plus microbubbles without ultrasound did not enhance transfection rate neither (group B). In 293FT cells of group C and group D, GFP expression were observed and the transfection rate were 4.26, 34.56 % respectively. The expression of GFP in each group of cardiomyocytes was similar to that in 293FT cells. But the transfection rate of cardiomyocytes in group C and group D was lower than that in 293FT cells, 2.81

Fig. 1.1 Cardiomyocytes of new-born S–D rats cultured in 10 % FBS DMEM on day 6. The Brdu was added into medium to inhibit fibroblast proliferation. The rate of survival and the purity of cardiomyocytes were both about 95 % (×200)

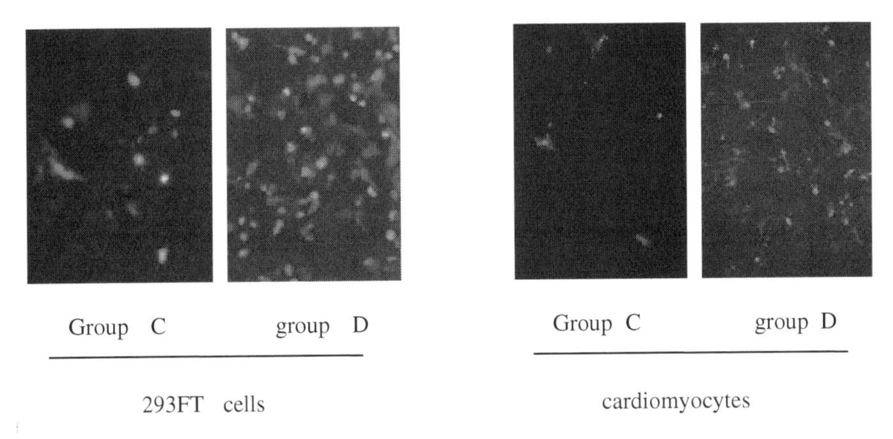

Fig. 1.2 The results of GFP expression in 293FT cells and cardiomyocytes. Grpup C: plasmid + ultrasound. Group D: plasmid + US/MB. No GFP expression was seen in group A or group B in the two kinds of cells (×200)

and 12.90 % respectively. There was significant difference in transfection rate between group C and group D of both 293FT cells and cardiomyocytes ($P < 0.05$). Ultrasound plus microbubbles could significantly improve the transfection rate of cells. As for the cell death rate, it was higher in group D than that in group C both in 293FT cells and cardiomyocytes ($P < 0.05$; Fig. 1.2, Table 1.1).

Table 1.1 The transfection rate and death rate of 293FT cells and cardiomyocytes in the four groups respectively. Dates are present as ($\overline{X} \pm S$) %

Group	293FT cells		Cardiomyocytes	
	Transfection rate	Death rate	Transfection rate	Death rate
A	0	3.29 ± 0.49	0	2.16 ± 0.30
B	0	3.35 ± 0.62	0	2.27 ± 0.37
C	4.26 ± 0.69#	4.66 ± 0.78 #	2.81 ± 0.39#	2.66 ± 0.40
D	34.56 ± 1.66#▲	7.85 ± 0.71#▲	12.90 ± 0.67#▲	5.32 ± 0.45#

Note: # $P < 0.05$ versus group A; ▲$P < 0.05$ versus group C

1.3.2 The Optimal Parameter About Cardiomyocytes

The transfection rate was positively related with MI, irradiation time and MB concentration, with increasing of the above three parameters, the cell death rate also increased. Consideration of the balance of two sides, such optimal parameters were determined: ultrasound frequency 1.7 MHz, MI 1.5, irradiation time 2 min, MB volume concentration 15 % (Table 1.2).

Table 1.2 The results of the transfection rate and death rate of cultured cardiomyocytes under different ultrasound parameters (MI, irradiation time) and different MB concentration. Data are present as ($\overline{X} \pm S$) %

	Transfection	Rate death rate
MI[a]		
A (0.5)	8.28 ± 0.63	4.43 ± 0.44
B (1.0)	11.18 ± 0.76#	4.69 ± 0.61
C (1.5)	12.90 ± 0.67#★	5.32 ± 0.45#
Irradiation time[b]		
A (1 min)	10.66 ± 0.73	4.02 ± 0.59
B (2 min)	12.90 ± 0.67#	5.32 ± 0.45#
C (3 min)	13.02 ± 0.74#	5.55 ± 0.47#
D (4 min)	13.20 ± 0.69#	6.47 ± 0.61#★▲
MB concentration[c]		
A (10 %)	9.35 ± 0.60	3.50 ± 0.42
B (15 %)	12.77 ± 0.79#	3.71 ± 0.34
C (20 %)	12.90 ± 0.67#	5.26 ± 0.49#★
D (25 %)	13.49 ± 0.84#	8.95 ± 1.24#★▲

[a] # $P < 0.05$ versus A; ★$P < 0.05$ versus B

[b] The MI 1.5 was adopted to determine the optimal irradiation time. # $P < 0.05$ versus A; ★$P < 0.05$ versus B; ▲$P < 0.05$ versus C

[c] The MI 1.5 and irradiation time 2 min was adopted to determine the optimal irradiation time. # $P < 0.05$ versus A; ★$P < 0.05$ versus B; ▲$P < 0.05$ versus C

1.3.3 *Effect of Exogenous Akt1 Gene on Cardiomyocytes Mediated by US/MB*

Apoptotic cardiomyocytes could be observed in each group due to I/R injury, but the apoptosis rate of group D was the lowest among all groups. The circumstance in group C was properly opposite. There was no significant difference in the apoptosis rate between group A and group B (Fig. 1.3, Table 1.3).

The protein expression of Akt1 was observed obviously in each group, but it was higher in group C and D than that in group A and B. There was no significant difference between group A and B, also no difference between group C and D (Fig. 1.4).

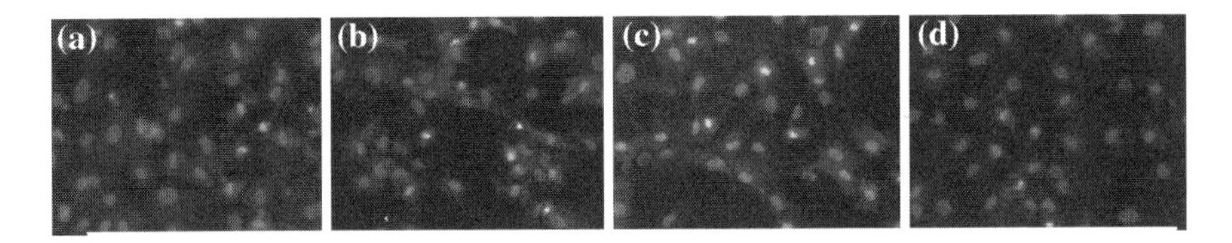

Fig. 1.3 The results of apoptotic rate in the four groups of cardiomyocytes subjected to I/R injury. **a**: control group, **b**: only plasmid encoding Akt1, **c**: Akt inhibitor, d: transfected Akt1 mediated by US/MB. Apoptotic cells were detected by Hoechst kit, normal cells were dyed light blue and apoptotic cells were dyed sapphirine by Hoechst (×200)

Table 1.3 The apoptotic rate of cultured cardiomyocytes after I/R injury

Group	Apoptotic rate
a	12.80 ± 0.42
b	12.45 ± 0.67
c	13.89 ± 0.69#★
d	8.81 ± 0.57#★▲

Fig. 1.4 The Akt1 protein expression in the four groups of cardiomyocytes subjected to I/R injury

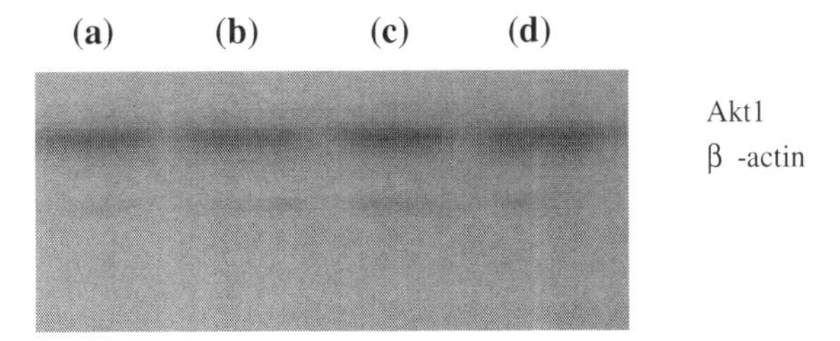

1.4 Discussion

In recent years, with the development of microbubbles which was not merely regarded as ultrasound contrast agents, it could be used as a vector for delivering drugs or genes [5]. This study was designed to explore the feasibility and safety of Akt1 gene transfection mediated by US combined with microbubbles.

Microbubbles have specific acoustic properties that make them useful for delivering genes to cultured cells and even to tissues in vivo. When they are exposed to high pressure (MI $>$ 1.0), microbubbles will be destructed due to forced expansion and compression of bubbles. Several studies have shown that destruction of microbubbles leads to permeability of cells, the genes or drugs will release from microbubbles to the cells [6, 7].

In 2005, a report published on Radiology compare with three microbubble contrast agents (Optison, SonoVue, and levovist) for their effects on gene delivering in conjunction with ultrasound [8]. Findings had shown that enhanced gene transfer with additional ultrasound was achieved only with SonoVue. SonoVue is a widely used contrast agent composed of millions of microbubbles filled with sulfur hexafluoride gas, it is relatively stable in solutions. In the present study, we have observed that microbubbles alone without ultrasound could not improve transgene expression, GFP expression was not observed under conditions: plasmid alone or plasmid plus microbubbles with the use of ultrasound. Recently, the effect of ultrasound alone has been shown to increase cell permeability [9], our study also indicated that the expression of exogenous gene was enhanced by ultrasound without microbubbles, but the transfection rate was very low.

Although the exact mechanism by which microbubbles increase cell permeability remains to be clarified, delivery of genes with microbubbles is a promising technique, however, side effects of microbubbles destruction on cells deserve our attention. In theory, microbubbles exposed to ultrasound could cause mechanical stress to act on cells and consequently lead to cell injury [10]. In the present study, we found that with increasing of MI and irradiation, the transfection rate increased, but the apoptosis rate also increased. So, in order to get maximal transfection rate and minimal adverse effects, the optimal combination of several ultrasound parameters must be set no matter in any experimental testing.

Fischer et al. has investigated transfer plasmid CAX-enhanced GFP to neuron cells origin from different tissues mediated by several tools (ultrasound, liposome or FuGene6) and found that the transfection rate was vary from the different source of cells [11]. The result of recent study showed that transfection efficiency of the recombinant expression plasmid pEGFP-C1/RB94 into human retinoblastoma cells was increased using ultrasound-targeted microbubble destruction, with liposome as the positive control [12]. Our data indicated the transfection rate of 293FT cells was much higher than that of cardiomyocytes. This may due to the characteristics of the two types of cells. Generally speaking, cardiomyocytes were terminal differentiation cells and were not prone to accepted exogenous genes, whereas 293FT cells were very active in proliferation.

The Ser/Thr kinase Akt is a 57KD protein which has powerful effects to promote cells survival. Ischemic preconditioning (IPC) is a very useful method to reduce I/R injury and its protective mechanisms were very complicated and were not elucidated fully until now, but several studies indicated the activation of Akt signaling pathway was implicated in the process of IPC recently [13]. Matsui et al. transfected exogenous Akt to the heart which subjected to transient ischemia and found exogenous Akt could also exert a powerful cardioprotective effect. According to the results of the above experiments, Akt especially Akt1 which expressed abundantly in heart is probably a therapeutic target for ischemic heart disease in future.

In the present study, we adopted the relative new gene delivery system of microbubbles in combination with ultrasound to transfect cardiomyocytes with exogenous Akt1. Despite of the low transfection rate, it would be a promising gene delivery tool with the development of ultrasound technique and the contrast agent.

References

1. Oliver JM, Hugo AK, Raffi B (2007) Targeting the heart with gene therapy-optimized gene delivery methods. Cardiovasc Res 73:453–462
2. Isao K, Koji O, Akira O et al (2004) Using ultrasonic microbubble destruction transfer: the first demonstration of myocardial transfer of a "functional" gene. Treatment of acute myocardial infarction by hepatocyte growth factor gene. J Am Coll Cardiol 44:644–653
3. Kulik G, Klippel A, Weber MJ (1997) Antiapoptotic signalling by the IGF-I receptor, phosphatidylinositol 3-kinase, and Akt. Mol Cell Biol 17:1595–1606
4. Takashi M, Jingzang T, Federica M et al (2001) Akt Activation preserves cardiac function and prevents injury after transient cardiac ischemia in vivo. Circulation 104:330–335
5. Sirsi SR, Borden MA (2012) Advances in ultrasound mediated gene therapy using microbubble contrast agents. Theranostics 2:1208–1222
6. Price RJ, Kaul S (2002) Contrast ultrasound targeted drug and gene delivery: an update on a new therapeutic modality. J Cardiovasc Pharmacol Ther 73:171–180
7. Staub D, Partovi S, Imfeld S et al (2013) Novel applications of contrast-enhanced ultrasound imaging in vascular medicine. Vasa 42:17–31
8. Wan Xinghua, Liang Hai-Dong, Dong Baowei et al (2005) Gene transfer with microbubble ultrasound and plasmid DNA into skeletal muscle of mice: comparison between commercially available microbubble. Radiology 237:224–229
9. Lawrie A, Brisken AF, Francis SE et al (1999) Ultrasound enhances reporter gene expression after transfection of vascular cells in vitro. Circulation 99:2617–2620
10. Unnikrishnan S, Klibanov AL (2012) Microbubbles as ultrasound contrast agents for molecular imaging: preparation and application. Am J Roentgenol 199:292–299
11. Fischer AJ, Stanke JJ, Omar G et al (2006) Ultrasound- mediated gene transfer into neuronal cells. J Biotechnol 122:393–411
12. Zheng MM, Zhou XY, Wang LP et al (2012) Experimental research of RB94 gene transfection into retinoblastoma cells using ultrasound-targeted microbubble destruction. Ultrasound Med Biol 38:1058–1066
13. Derek JH, Mihaela MM, Derek MY (2004) Cross-talk between the survival kinases during early reperfusion: its contribution to ischemic preconditioning. Cardiovasc Res 63:305–312

Chapter 2
Logic Operation in Spiking Neural P System with Chain Structure

Jing Luan and Xi-yu Liu

Abstract In this paper, a new P system called spiking neural P system with chain structure (SNPC, for short) has been proposed, which combines spiking neural P system (SNP, for short) with discrete Morse theory, that is to say, neural membrane cells in spiking neural P system are set on chain by discrete gradient vector path, building a SNP system with chain structure. Compared with original SNP system, the structural design of SNPC system is simpler, showing stronger parallelism, and avoiding the time-consuming phenomenon caused by the random selection of membranes in computational process of P system. The logic operation in SNPC system has been completed, compared with the implemented method in traditional P system, the efficiency of the algorithm significantly improved, showing the advantage of SNPC system.

Keywords Membrane computing · Spiking neural P system · Discrete Morse theory · Logic operation

2.1 Introduction

Natural computing is a field trying to simulate nature in the process of calculation. Membrane computing is a new branch of natural computing, which focuses natural computing at the cellular level and belongs to a kind of molecular computing.

J. Luan (✉) · X. Liu
School of Management Science and Engineering, Shandong Normal University, Jinan 250014, China
e-mail: kaluanjing@163.com

X. Liu
e-mail: sdxyliu@163.com

S. Li et al. (eds.), *Frontier and Future Development of Information Technology in Medicine and Education*, Lecture Notes in Electrical Engineering 269,
DOI: 10.1007/978-94-007-7618-0_2,

It regards the whole membrane as a computing unit, abstracting the chemical reactions and material flow at the cellular level as the calculating process [1]. This computing model was proposed by Paun, Romanian Academy of Sciences, in 1998, due to its maximum parallelism and well distributed manner, showing strong computational completeness and efficiency, and has aroused widespread concern and research.

According to different organizations of cells which inspire the different computing models, P systems can be classified to three main types as follows: (i) Cell-like P systems inspired from living cells; (ii) Tissue-like P systems inspired from tissues; (iii) Neural-like P systems inspired from neural systems. In this paper, we will use a class of neural-like P systems which is called spiking neural P systems (SNP systems, for short). Inspired from the biological phenomenon that neurons cooperate in the brain by exchanging spikes via synapses, Păun et al. developed the SNP systems in 2006 [4]. Similar to neural-like P systems, these systems have the network structure.

SNP system on chain is a new membrane structure, not network structure but chain structure, linking traditional membrane according to certain rules and forming a chain structure. The chain structure makes the process of membrane computing not to select next reacting membrane at random, but to react in accordance with the order of the membrane in the chain in successive. Avoid the time-consuming phenomenon resulted from randomness greatly and improve the computational efficiency of the SNP system. In this paper, based on the discrete Morse theory forming the SNP system with chain structure(SNPC, for short), the discrete gradient vector path is the standard to link the membranes, that is to say, along the discrete gradient vector path of the discrete Morse theory to form membrane structure. Morse theory had been proposed for a long time, and it is a useful tool in differential topology, used for investigating the topology of smooth manifolds, particularly for computer graphics, being the focus of the study. In the end of last century, Forman extended several aspects of the fundamental tool to discrete structures, providing an effective tool to describe the topology of the discrete objects, and made a big contribute to theory and applied mathematics. Its combinatorial aspect allows computation completely independent of a geometric realization, greatly enriching its range of applications. The literature [2] has proved the possibility of solving optimization problems with discrete Morse theory, showing the computational efficiency and power. The SNPC system, which combines SNP system with discrete Morse theory, enhances the computational power and efficiency of membrane system.

The maximum parallelism of P system makes the fulfillment of logic operation possible, and reduces the computational complexity greatly. Literature [3] has proved the possibility of performing the logic operation of the P system, and provided effective method to complete the logic operation, which is easier compared with the implementation in the general computer architecture. In this paper, we propose a new method with SNPC system to fulfill the basic logic operation (AND 、OR 、NOT), the efficiency of the algorithm being improved.

In the paper, in the Sect. 2.2, SNP system is introduced briefly. Then the improved SNP system, that is to say, the SNP system with chain structure and skin membrane is given in the Sect. 2.3, and the formal presentation and rules are described. In the Sect. 2.4, the method with SNPC system to solve the basic logic operations (AND, OR, NOT) is given. And then the summary and outlook of the SNPC system are introduced.

2.2 Spiking Neural P System

2.2.1 Preliminary of SNP

SNP system is a new computing device in the field of membrane computing. This new P system is proposed in 2006 by Ionescu et al. for the first time, which simulates the biological phenomena of collaborative of the neurons through synapses and processing spike [4].

Unlike the P system proposed before, SNP system has its own unique composition and operation mode: its basic calculating unit is neuron, and is indicated by the nodes in the directed graph commonly, the arc between nodes indicating synaptic. There is a certain number of a in each neuron, which represents spike. The rules in the SNP system are mainly two, that is to say, firing rules and forgotten rules. The firing rules make neuron send information to other neurons with spikes, and then other neurons can receive these spikes after a certain period of time. The forgotten rules are used to eliminate a certain number of spikes in the neurons.

There are two main calculation modes in SNP system, generating and accepting modes. In the generating mode, the membrane system is regarded as a generator, due to not need to input characters to the system. For the accepting mode, in contrast to the generating mode, the SNP system can omit the output neurons, and the data read from the environment through the input neurons [5].

2.2.2 The Structure of SNP

In fact, SNP system is a special kind of Tissue-like and Neural-like P system, which can be obtained by simulating the function of spike neurons. There are some common definitions and symbols of SNP system. For the alphabet V, V^* is the collection of all finite strings on the V, where λ denotes the empty string. V^+ denote all non-empty finite string of V. If $V = \{a\}$ (here call V single-letter collection), $\{a\}^*$, $\{a\}^+$ are respectively abbreviated as a^*, a^+.

The regular expression over the alphabet V is defined as followed:

(1) λ and $a \in V$ are regular expression;
(2) if E_1 and E_2 are regular expressions over V, then $E_1 + E_2$, E_1E_2 and E_1^* are regular expressions over V;

(3) nothing else is a regular expression over V.

A language L over V is a set of strings over V, with each regular expression E, we associate a language L(E), defined as followed:

(1) $L(\lambda) = \{\lambda\}$, and for each a∈V, $L(a) = \{a\}$;
(2) for any expression E_1, E_2 over V, $L(E_1 \cup E_2) = L(E_1) \cup L(E_2)$, $L(E_1 E_2) = L(E_1) L(E_2)$, $L(E_1{}^{+}) = L(E_1)^{+}$.
A spiking neural P system of degree $m \geq 1$ is a construct of the form $\Pi = (O, \sigma_1, \ldots, \sigma_m, syn, in, out)$, where

(i) $O = \{a\}$is the singleton alphabet (a is called spike);
(ii) $\sigma_1, \ldots, \sigma_m$ are neurons, of the form $\sigma_i = (n_i, R_i)$, $1 \leq i \leq m$, where:

(1) $n_i \geq 0$ is the initial number of spikes contained by the neuron σ_i;
(2) R_i is a finite set of rules of the following two forms:
(i) firing rules: $E/a^c \rightarrow a^p$; $d, c \geq 1, p \geq 1, d \geq 0$, where E is a regular expression over a, d is the delay time, that is, the interval between using the rule and releasing the spike, and $c \geq p$;
(ii) forgetting rules: $E'/a^s \rightarrow \lambda$, $s \geq 1$, where E′ is a regular expression over a, with the restriction that, for Ri in type i) each rule $E/a^c \rightarrow a^p$; d, satisfies $L(E) \cap L(E') = \varphi$;
(3) syn $\{1, 2, \ldots, m\} \times \{1, 2, \ldots, m\}$indicates the synapses between neurons, for any $1 \leq i \leq m$, there is $(i, i) \notin$ syn;
(4) in, out $\in\{1, 2, \ldots, m\}$indicate that the input and output neuron.

2.3 Spiking Neural P Chain System with Skin

P chain system is a new model of P system, which constructs membrane on the chain structure by some rules, getting P system with chain structure. Its outstanding advantage is that the communication between membranes is not at random, but in accordance with the order of the membrane in the chain in successive, successfully avoiding the time-consuming phenomenon caused by the random. In this paper, the rules of constructing the membrane structure we choose are combined with the discrete Morse theory, forming the membrane system over the discrete gradient vector path, that is to say, each cell on the discrete gradient vector path represents a membrane, and part or all of the path are considered as a membrane system. The discrete gradient vector path is a path satisfied:

(1) simplices $a_0^{(p)}, \beta_0^{(P+1)}, a_1^{(p)}, \beta_1^{(P+1)}, \ldots, \beta_r^{(P+1)}, a_{r+1}^{(p)}$, such that for each i = 0, …, r, $\{a_r, \beta_r\} \in V$ and $\beta_i \succ a_{i+1} \neq a_i$,
(2) if $r \geq 0$ and $a_0 = a_{r+1}$, such a path is a nontrivial closed path,

(3) a discrete vector field V on M is a collection of pairs $\{a^{(p)}, \beta^{(P+1)}\}$ of simplicies of M with $a \prec \beta$ such that each simplex is in at most one pair of V,
(4) a discrete vector field V is the gradient vector field of a discrete Morse function if and only if there are no nontrivial closed V-paths.

The chain structure spiking neural P system with skin is a kind of enrichment and expansion of P chain system and SNP system. It simulates the transmitting spike function of neurons and owns a chain structure. The SNPC system with skin of degree m ≥ 1 is a construct of the form:

$\Pi = (O, \sigma_0, \sigma_1, ..., \sigma_m$, syn, in, out),

Where:

(1) O = {a}is the singleton alphabet (a is called spike);
(2) $\sigma_0, \sigma_1, ..., \sigma_m$ are m + 1 neurons; 0 ≤ i ≤ m, σ_0 representing skin membrane, $\sigma_1, ..., \sigma_m$ are m cells abstracting from discrete gradient vector path, satisfied $\sigma_0 \prec \sigma_1 \prec \ldots \prec \sigma_m$. Neurons σ_i is the form of $\sigma_i = (n_i, R_i)$, where:
(1) $n_i \geq 0$ is the initial number of spikes contained by the neuron σ_i;
(2) R_i is a finite set of rules of the following two forms:
(i) $C/a^c \rightarrow a^p$; d, c ≥ 1, p ≥ 1, d ≥ 0, where C is the constraint condition of the rule, d is the delay time, that is, the interval between using the rule and releasing the spike, and c ≥ p;
(ii) forgetting rules: $C'/a^s \rightarrow \lambda$, s ≥ 1, where C′ is the constraint condition of the rule, with the restriction that, for R_i in type (i) each rule $C/a^c \rightarrow a^p$; d, satisfies $C \cap C' = \varphi$;
(3) syn = {0, 1, 2, …, m} indicates the link relationship between neurons, for any 1 ≤ i ≤ m, there is $\sigma_0 \prec \sigma_1 \prec \ldots \prec \sigma_m$;
(4) in, out ∈{1, 2, …, m} indicate that the input and output neuron.

The rules (i) are used as followed: When restrain C is met, if there are k spikes in neuron σ_i and k ≥ c, the rule $C/a^c \rightarrow a^p$; d can be inspired in neuron σ_i. When this rule is used in neuron σ_i, it will consume c spikes (remaining k-c spikes); at the same time, generate p spikes after d unit time, and immediately sent p spikes to its follow-up neuron. What's more, during the time from using this rule to transmission the generating spikes, the neuron is closed, that is, don't receive any spikes. If the neuron fires the rule $C/a^c \rightarrow a^p$; d, d ≥ 1 at the t step, the neuron is closed during the step t, t + 1,…,t + d − 1. When a neuron is closed, all the rules over it can't be used, only if the neuron is open, the rules over it can be inspired. If a neuron sends spikes to a closed neuron, the closed neuron can't receive the spikes, and these spikes will disappear naturally. For the output neuron, it can send spikes to the environment.

The rules (ii) are used as followed: When restrain C′is met, if there are k′ spikes in neuron σ_i and k′ ≥ s, the forgetting rule $C'/a^s \rightarrow \lambda$ can be inspired in neuron σ_i, and all the firing rules over the neuron can't be used. When this rule is used in neuron σ_i, it will consume s spikes, but don't generate new spikes.

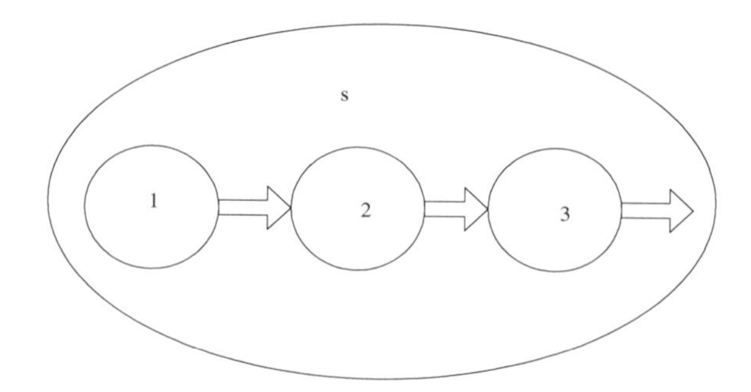

Fig. 2.1 The SNPC system with skin

The diagram of SNPC system with skin as shown in Fig. 2.1.

In Fig. 2.1, there are four membranes, and the outmost membrane is the skin, whose two main functions is that, receive the objects from chain structure membrane system and send the objects to the chain structure membrane system followed a certain rules, and whose existence makes the communication between the nonadjacent neurons be possible. There are three membranes in the chain structure membrane system, where membrane 1 is the input membrane, whose objects can be generated by the reaction in the membrane, or can be from the skin membrane, and membrane 3 is the output membrane, whose objects are sent to the skin or environment directly.

2.4 Logic Operation in SNPC

The logic operation is the basic operations of other complex logic processes, and literature [3] has proved the possibility of completion logic operation in P system. In this paper, based on that, we prove the feasibility of SNPC system to perform basic logic operations. When performing Logic operation by SNPC system, we assume that there are enough spikes in environment can be sent into the system by input membrane (the first membrane), and use spike a 、 a´ and null string λ to represent TRUE or FALSE.

2.4.1 Logic NOT

Logic NOT operation meets $\neg T = F, \neg F = T$, here in SNPC system, using spiking a or anti-spike a´ representing TRUE or FALSE and they are opponent. The application NOT operation in SNPC system, the membrane system required design as followed:

Π(Not) = (O, σ_0, σ_1, σ_2, syn, in, out)

Where:

$$O = \{a,\ a'\};$$
$$\sigma_1 = \{n_1,\ R_1\},\ \sigma_2 = \{n_2,\ R_2\};$$
$$n_1 = \{0|\varphi\},\ n_2 = \{2|\ a'\};\ R_1 = \{\ a \rightarrow a\},\ R_2 = \{\{\ a'a \rightarrow \lambda;\ a' \rightarrow a'\}\};$$

in = 1, out = 2.

Here, rules R_2 are chained rules, and it is applied as followed which refers to the literature [7]: There is a chained rules R_2 which contains two vectors of rules. In the membrane, if the first rule of chained rules R is applied, then in the next step the rest of the rules from R will be applied in order in consecutive steps. However, if a rule from an already started vector of chained rules R can't be applied, then the execution of R is dropped, that is, for the current application of R, the remaining rules are not executed anymore.

As shown in Fig. 2.2, there are three membranes, a skin and two chain structure membranes. In membrane σ_1, whose function is sending objects a to the system, there are one rules a → a. In the whole P system, when all rules which can be inspired are applied once, we call it one step. In other words, in each step, all rules which can be applied have to be applied to all possible objects. In the aspect of a representing TRUE, then a´ is FALSE, at the beginning, in membrane σ_1, when there is spike a from environment to membrane 1, rules a → a will be executed. Then import a (TRUE) to membrane σ_2, then chained rule $R_2 = \{\{a'a \rightarrow \lambda;\ a' \rightarrow a'\}\}$ will be inspired, consuming one a´ due to rule a´a → λ and producing one a´ due to rule a´ → a´, and send a´ (FALSE) out as the output. Else if a represents FALSE, and a´ is TRUE, sending a (FALSE) into membrane σ_2, will export a´ (TRUE) as the output. The SNPC system completes the function of logic NOT operation.

2.4.2 Logic AND

Logic AND operation meets $F \wedge F = F, F \wedge T = F, T \wedge T = T$, using spiking a representing TRUE and anti-spike a´ representing FALSE or the opponent case,

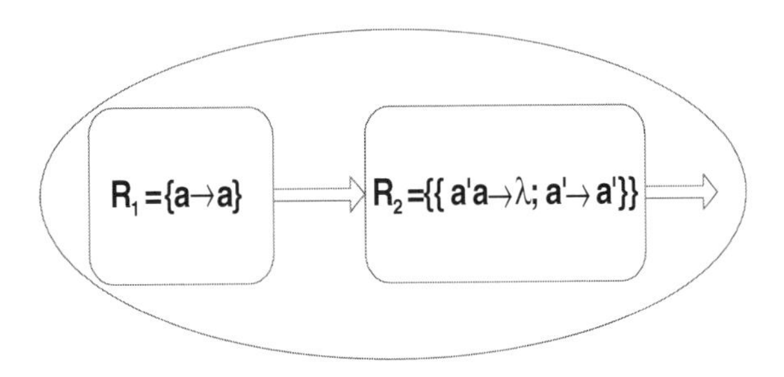

Fig. 2.2 SNPC for logic NOT operation

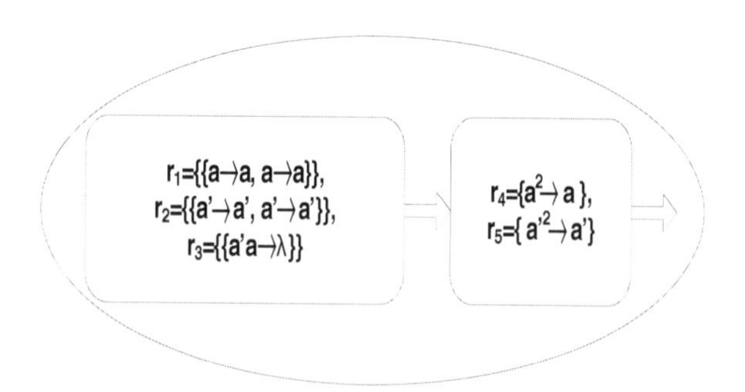

Fig. 2.3 SNPC for logic AND Operation

and λ here representing FALSE. The application AND operation in SNPC system, the membrane system required design as followed:

Π(AND) = (O, σ_0, σ_1, σ_2, …, σm, syn, in, out)

Where:

$$O = \{a, a'\};$$

$$\sigma_1 = \{n_1,\ R_1\},\ \sigma_2 = \{n_2,\ R_2\};\ R_1 = \{r_1,\ r_2,\ r_3\},\ R_2 = \{r_1,\ r_2\};$$

$$r_1 = \{\{a \to a,\ a \to a\}\},\ r_2 = \{\{a' \to a',\ a' \to a'\}\},\ r_3 = \{\{a'a \to \lambda\}\};$$

$$r_4 = \{a^2 \to a\},\ r_5 = \left\{a'^2 \to a'\right\};$$

in = 1, out = 2.

Here, rules r_1, r_2, r_3 are chained rules too. As shown in Fig. 2.3, there are three membranes, a skin and two chain structure membranes. In membrane σ_1, whose function is receiving the objects from environment and sending them to the system, if receive two objects a (TRUE), and chained rule r_2 is selected and executed, meaning that double a (TRUE) into membrane σ_2, then rule $a^2 \to a$ will be inspired, and send a (TRUE) out as the output. If receive two objects a´ (FALSE), and chained rule r_1 is inspired and applied, sending double a´ (FALSE) to membrane σ_2, then rule $a'^2 \to a'$ will be inspired, and send a´ (FALSE) out as the output. If receive an objects a (TRUE) and an object a´ (FALSE), rule r_3 will be executed and export null to membrane σ_2. Then the whole system will not have the output, as agreed λ representing FALSE. The SNPC complete the function of logic AND operation.

2.4.3 Logic OR

Logic OR operation meets $F \vee F = F, F \vee T = T, T \vee T = T$, using spiking a representing TRUE and anti-spike a´ representing FALSE or the opponent case. And further instructions, λ represents TRUE. The application OR operation in SNPC system, the membrane system required design as followed:

Π (OR) = (O, σ_0,σ_1,σ_2, …,σm, syn, in, out),

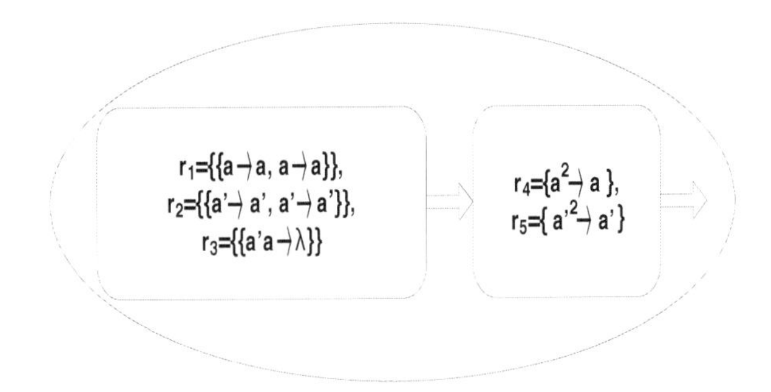

Fig. 2.4 SNPC for logic OR Operation

Where,

$$\begin{aligned}
&O = \{a, a'\};\\
&\sigma_1 = \{n_1,\ R_1\},\ \sigma_2 = \{n_2,\ R_2\};\ R_1 = \{r_1, r_2, r_3\},\ R_2 = \{r_1, r_2\};\\
&r_1 = \{a \to a, a \to a\},\ r_2 = \{a' \to a', a' \to a'\},\ r_3 = \{a'a \to \lambda\};\\
&r_4 = \{a^2 \to a\},\ r_5 = \left\{a'^2 \to a'\right\};
\end{aligned}$$

in = 1, out = 2.

Here, rules r_1, r_2, r_3 are chained rules too. As shown in Fig. 2.4, there are three membranes, a skin and two chain structure membranes. In membrane σ_1, whose function is receiving the objects from environment and sending them to the system, if receive two objects a (TRUE), and chained rule r_2 is selected and executed, meaning that double a (TRUE) into membrane σ_2, then rule $a^2 \to a$ will be inspired, and send a (TRUE) out as the output. If receive two objects a´ (FALSE), and chained rule r1 is inspired and applied, sending double a´ (FALSE) to membrane σ_2, then rule $a'^2 \to a'$ will be inspired, and send a´ (FALSE) out as the output. If receive an object a (TRUE) and an object a´ (FALSE), rule r_3 will be executed and export null to membrane σ_2. Then the whole system will not have the output, as agreed λ representing TRUE. The SNPC complete the function of logic OR operation.

2.5 Conclusion

The membrane computing simulates the natural process of biological systems, and all the theoretical foundation based on the theory and practice of biochemistry. From the above inference process, we can see a high parallelism and distribution of computing capacity of SNPC system. Compared with method in literature [3], the method to solve basic logic operations (AND、OR、NOT) proposed in this paper is more efficient, in which the design of membrane system is simpler, and the time complexity to achieve the operation has also been further improved (with the linear time, but the efficiency of SNPC system is higher). Because a lot of computational problems are based on these basic logic operations, the results of this paper can be used as the basis of the more complex applications.

SNPC system is a new P system, which enriches the family of P system. Its chain structure makes it essentially different with other P system; the design of membrane structure of SNPC system is simpler; the SNPC system with skin further strengthen the communication of the membrane in the chain, greatly improving the operational efficiency of the whole system. In this paper, exampled as the SNPC membrane system to achieve basic logic operations, demonstrates the SNPC system computing power and efficiency. For most of the computational problems are based on basic arithmetic and Boolean computation, the basic conclusions of this paper can be used in more complex research areas, such as the construction of a computer chip, or solving some mathematical problems. Membrane computing is considered to be the most promising in solving NP problems, of course, SNPC system also can used to solve NP problems. Literature [8] proposed solving TSP problem by membrane computing, using the algorithm MCTSP, and on this basis, we can use the SNPC system to find a more efficient algorithm for solving TSP. All of these are the future direction and points of the study. Obviously, due to the current of the analog implementation of the membrane system and in reality the corresponding technical support of realizing are too little, calculation based on membrane computing models and methods are more difficult to verify, which makes to solving the problem by membrane computing relatively vague. These have also become challenges and efforts direction for the study of SNPC system.

References

1. Paun G (2002) Membrane computing. An introduction. Springer, Berlin
2. Zhang J, Liu X (2011) Optimization model based on discrete Morse theory. Syst Eng-Theor Pract 31
3. Xing J, Guo P, Zhu Q, Wang C (2009) Research of logic operation in membrane system. Comput Knowl Technol 5(13), 3516–3517, 3526
4. Ionescu M, Păun G, Yokomori T (2006) Spiking neural P systems. Fundam Inform 71(2–3) :279–308
5. Leporati A, Zandron C, Ferretti C, Mauri G (2007) Solving numerical NP-complete problems with spiking neural P systems. Lect Notes Comput Sci 4860:336–352
6. Zhang X, Zeng X, Pan L, Luo B (2009) A spiking neural P system for performing multiplication of two arbitrary natural numbers. Chin J Comput 32(12)
7. Dragos S (2010) P systems with chained rules. Twelfth international conference on membrane computing, pp 447–458
8. Hai-zhu Chen (2011) Application research on membrane computing [D]. Chongqing University, Chongqing

Chapter 3
A Mathematical Model of the Knee Joint for Estimation of Forces and Torques During Standing-up

Zhi-qiang Wang, Yu-kun Ren and Hong-yuan Jiang

Abstract In this paper, the coordinate systems of segments of human were built up to describe the standing-up motion. Based on the coordinates, a mathematical model of knee joint was developed to estimate the forces and torques and contact forces between tibia and femur, muscle forces produced by five significant muscle groups and ligament forces involved into four ligaments of human lower extremity were taking into account. The results showed that the model is efficient to estimate the knee joint force and torques.

Keywords Knee joint modeling · Standing-up motion · Joint force

3.1 Introduction

The biomechanical behavior and estimation of forces of human knee during sitting-to-standing movement play a vital role for designing rehabilitation and assistive training machines. The knee joint is one of the most important and complex joint for human to raise up from sitting position [1, 2].

To avoid overloaded, deformity and unnecessary injury of knee joint of physical impaired persons during standing-up motion and rehabilitation training, it is useful to analyze the forces and torques principle of knee joint elements.

There are several knee joint elements to take into account, such as muscle forces, ligament tension and contact force between femur and tibia [3–5]. The aim of this paper was to develop a mathematical model of the knee joint in the sagittal plane during human quasistatic task of standing up. So the mathematical modeling of knee joint was able to evaluate the property of sit-to-standing (STS) process.

Z. Wang · Y. Ren · H. Jiang (✉)
School of Mechanical and Electrical Engineering, Harbin Institute of Technology, Harbin 150001, China
e-mail: jhy_hit@sina.com

S. Li et al. (eds.), *Frontier and Future Development of Information Technology in Medicine and Education*, Lecture Notes in Electrical Engineering 269,
DOI: 10.1007/978-94-007-7618-0_3,

3.2 Knee Joint Anatomy

Knee joint is one of the most complex but quite important joints of lower limbs to support and load [6, 7], when human raise from sit position. The main parts of the knee joint include the end of the femur, the top of the tibia, articular cartilage AC, meniscus cartilage, four ligaments, tendons and so on. The four ligaments include anterior cruciate ligament (ACL), the posterior cruciate ligament (PCL), the medial collateral ligament (MCL) and the lateral collateral ligament (LCL). There are several large muscle groups in the lower extremity, which can extend or flex the knee joint, such as the quadriceps, hamstring and gastrocnemius muscles.

Hamstring includes three main parts, biceps femoris, semitendinosus and semimembranosus. In our research, we simplify the model and focus on the patellar tendon, hamstring, gastrocnemius muscles, ACL, PCl, MCL and LCL (Fig. 3.1).

So in this paper it is to develop a mathematical model to calculate the forces and torques on the knee joint during standing-up motion in sagittal plane by taking into account of main muscles, ligaments and bone-on-bone contact force.

3.3 Coordinate System of Knee Joint

The origin of the coordinate system was located at the ankle joint during the standing-up motion, due to the movement of ankle joint approximately stable. There are three segments of human body model in sit-to-stand transfer, with three degrees of freedom of motion in sagittal plane and including shank, thigh and HAT (head, arms and trunk). According to the sit-to-stand process, the motion of joints and center of mass were described with four coordinates. The fixed coordinate is

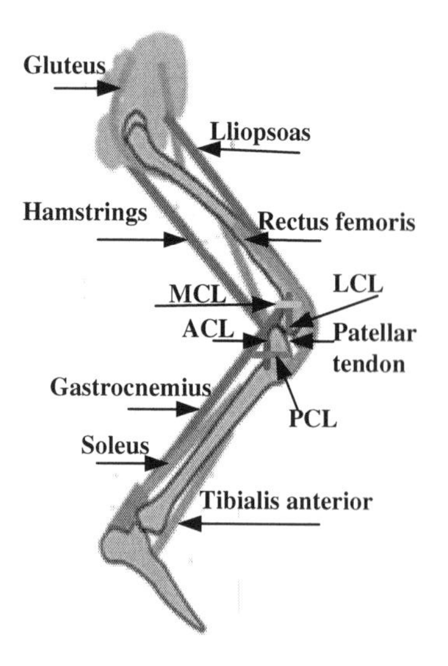

Fig. 3.1 Schematics of muscles and ligaments of lower limbs

connected with ankle joint, and others moving coordinates was fixed with knee joint, centroid of thigh and HAT. Therefore we have the ankle joint coordinate system $\sigma = [O; x, y]$, the knee joint coordinate system $\sigma^{(1)} = [O_1; x_1, y_1]$, the centroid of thigh and HAT coordinate systems $\sigma^{(2)} = [O_2; x_2, y_2]$ and $\sigma^{(3)} = [O_3; x_3, y_3]$. The coordinate systems of lower limbs were shown in Fig. 3.2.

So the motion of moving coordinate systems can be expressed by coordinate vectors and relative rotation angles in the fixed coordinate system. The transformation of the moving coordinates and fixed coordinate is given by the transformation matrix from the coordinate system $\sigma^{(1)}$ to σ was expressed as Eqs. 3.1 and 3.2:

$$\sigma^{(1)} \rightarrow \sigma : \begin{pmatrix} x \\ y \\ 1 \end{pmatrix} = M_{01} \begin{pmatrix} x_1 \\ y_1 \\ 1 \end{pmatrix} \tag{3.1}$$

$$\begin{bmatrix} x \\ y \end{bmatrix} = M_{01} \begin{bmatrix} x_1 \\ y_1 \end{bmatrix} = \begin{pmatrix} c_1 & s_1 \\ -s_1 & c_1 \end{pmatrix} \begin{bmatrix} x_1 \\ y_1 \end{bmatrix} \tag{3.2}$$

So the transform matrix of M_{01} was expressed as:

$$M_{01} = \begin{pmatrix} c_1 & s_1 & l_1 s_1 \\ -s_1 & c_1 & l_1 c_1 \\ 0 & 0 & 1 \end{pmatrix} \tag{3.3}$$

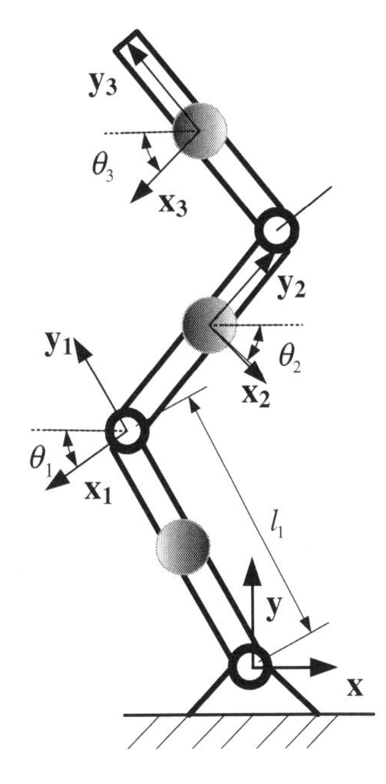

Fig. 3.2 The coordinate system of human body during standing-up motion

The transform matrix of M_{02} was expressed as Eq. 3.4:

$$M_{02} = \begin{pmatrix} c_2 & s_2 & l_1 s_1 + l_h s_2 \\ -s_2 & c_2 & l_1 c_1 + l_h c_2 \\ 0 & 0 & 1 \end{pmatrix} \tag{3.4}$$

The transform matrix of M_{03} was expressed as Eq. 3.5:

$$M_{03} = \begin{pmatrix} c_3 & s_3 & l_1 s_1 + l_2 s_2 + l_t s_3 \\ -s_3 & c_3 & l_1 c_1 + l_2 c_2 + l_t c_3 \\ 0 & 0 & 1 \end{pmatrix} \tag{3.5}$$

The transform matrix of M_{21} was expressed as Eq. 3.6:

$$M_{21} = \begin{pmatrix} c_{1-2} & s_{1-2} & l_1 s_{1-2} \\ -s_{1-2} & c_{1-2} & l_1 c_{1-2} \\ 0 & l_1 + l_h c_{1-2} & l_1^2 + l_1 l_h c_{1-2} + 1 \end{pmatrix} \tag{3.6}$$

Where:

$$c_1 = \cos\theta_1,\ s_1 = \sin\theta_1,\ c_2 = \cos\theta_2,\ s_2 = \sin\theta_2,\ c_3 = \cos\theta_3,\ s_3 = \sin\theta_3$$
$$c_{1-2} = \cos(\theta_1 - \theta_2),\ s_{1-2} = \sin(\theta_1 - \theta_2),\ c_{1-3} = \cos(\theta_1 - \theta_3),\ s_{1-3} = \sin(\theta_1 - \theta_3)$$
$$c_{2-3} = \cos(\theta_2 - \theta_3),\ s_{2-3} = \sin(\theta_2 - \theta_3)$$

The transform matrix of M_{31} was expressed as Eq. 3.7:

$$M_{31} = \begin{pmatrix} c_{1-3} & s_{1-3} & l_1 s_{1-3} \\ -s_{1-3} & c_{1-3} & l_1 c_{1-3} \\ -l_2 s_{1-2} - l_t s_{1-3} & l_1 + l_2 c_{1-2} + l_t c_{1-3} & l_1^2 + l_1 l_2 c_{1-2} + l_1 l_t c_{1-3} + 1 \end{pmatrix} \tag{3.7}$$

The transform matrix of M_{32} was expressed as Eq. 3.8:

$$M_{32} = \begin{pmatrix} c_{2-3} & s_{2-3} & l_1 s_{1-3} + l_h s_{2-3} \\ -s_{2-3} & c_{2-3} & l_1 c_{1-3} + l_h c_{2-3} \\ l_2 s_{1-2} - l_t s_{2-3} & l_2 + l_1 c_{1-3} + l_t c_{2-3} & l_1^2 + l_2 l_h + 1 + l_1 (l_2 + l_h) c_{1-2} + l_1 l_t c_{1-3} + l_t l_h c_{2-3} \end{pmatrix} \tag{3.8}$$

According to the fixed and moving coordinate systems, the centroid of lower limbs' segment and the joints relation were set up by the transform matrix and it is the basis of the next step research for the forces and torques of knee joint during standing-up motion.

3.4 Mathematical Model of Knee Joint During Standing-Up Motion

The motion of sit-to-stand process was the sums of the resultant forces and torques of individual muscle group, ligament and bone-on-bone contact force of the lower extremity. According to the analysis of standing-up motion, the following relationship can be obtained:

$$F_r = \sum_{i=1}^{n} F_{mi} + \sum_{j=1}^{n} F_{lj} + \sum_{k=1}^{n} F_{ck} \tag{3.9}$$

$$M_r = F_r \times r_{Ai} \tag{3.10}$$

F_r was the resultant force at the knee joint, F_{mi} was the force of the ith muscle group, F_{lj} was the force of the jth ligament, F_{ck} was the force of the kth bone-on-bone contact element. M_r was the resultant moment and r_{Ai} was the vector of a moment arm.

Several necessary simplifications will be assumed to make the problem solved reasonably: (1) the tibiofemoral joint was frictionless due to the synovial fluid, (2) the bone-on-bone contact force was applied to the rotation center of knee joint, (3) the patellar tendon was not able to stretch or inextensible.

$$F_{ce} = a{\cdot}f(l)f(v)\cos(\alpha)F_{\max} \tag{3.11}$$

$$F_{\max} = PCSA \cdot \sigma_{\max} \tag{3.12}$$

F_{ce} was the maximum isometric force, a muscle activation; $f_{(v)}$ force–velocity property; $f_{(l)}$ was the force length relation, α was the pennation angle; $F_{\max}$ was the maximum muscle force. Quasi-static conditions during standing-up were assumed, so $f_{(v)}$ is neglected. The value of a muscle activation was set to 1.

Passive force was expressed as Eq. 3.13:

$$F_{pf} = \frac{F_{\max}}{e^{PEsh} - 1}\left(e^{\frac{l_{mus} - l_{muso}}{l_{mus}} \cdot \frac{PEsh}{PExm}} - 1\right) \tag{3.13}$$

l_{muso} was the length of the muscle at optimum fiber length, $PEsh$ and $PExm$, describing the shape of curve, were set to 4 and 0.4 respectively. So the total muscle force of muscle groups were defined as :

$$F_m = F_{ce} + F_{pf} \tag{3.14}$$

Ligamentous elements were simplified by n nonlinear elastic springs with end points connected to the femur and tibia. The direction of the force exerted on the femur and tibia coincides with the direction of the line segment through the insertion point of that spring. The length of spring was equal to the distance of the insertion point and only when its length was larger than initial length L_0. All these

Table 3.1 Lines of action of muscles and ligaments as function of knee joint angle [8, 9]

Function	$\phi_1 = B_0 + B_1\theta + B_2\theta^2 + B_3\theta^3$			
Coefficient	B_0	B_1	B_2	B_3
PT	−74.40	−5.75E−02	−4.75E − 03	3.09E − 05
Bf	275.00	−0.8720	−7.12E − 04	0.00
Sm	260.00	−0.8880	−8.52E − 04	0.00
St	255.00	−0.8160	2.63E − 04	−6.19E − 6
Gn	−90.00	0.00	0.00	0.00
ACL	227.00	−0.4880	0.00	0.00
PCL	−66.00	0.7370	−4.96E − 03	0.00
MCL	259.00	-0.669E−01	0.00	0.00
LCL	71.80	-0.1590	0.00	0.00

elements were assumed to load only when they were in tension. The force of ligaments produced can be expressed as the following equations:

$$F_{lj} = \begin{cases} 0; & \varepsilon_j \leq 0 \\ k_{1j}\left(L_j - L_{0j}\right)^2; & 0 \leq \varepsilon_j \leq 2\varepsilon_1 \\ k_{2j}\left(L_j - (1+\varepsilon_1)L_{0j}\right)^2; & \varepsilon_j \geq 2\varepsilon_1 \end{cases} \quad (3.15)$$

Where k_{1j} and k_{2j} were the stiffness coefficient of the jth spring element for two different regions, L_j and L_{0j} were current and slack lengths. The strain of the jth spring element was specified as 0.03.

Contact force was calculated as Eq. 3.15:

$$F_c = F_{pt} + F \quad (3.16)$$

F_{pt} was the tension in the patella ligament, F was the reaction force and vertical to the line of action of moment arms (Tables 3.1, 3.2).

Table 3.2 Muscle moment arm length as a function knee joint angle [8, 9]

Function	$\phi_2 = A_0 + A_1\theta + A_2\theta^2 + A_3\theta^3 + A_4\theta^4$				
Coefficient	A_0	A_1	A_2	A_3	A_4
Pt	4.71E − 02	4.20E − 04	−8.96E − 06	4.47E − 08	0.00
Bf	1.46E − 02	−9.26E − 05	8.55E − 06	−8.78E − 08	2.38E − 10
Sm	2.84E − 02	−1.61E − 04	6.81E − 06	−8.80E − 08	2.77E − 10
St	-4.11E − 03	5.86E − 04	6.90E − 06	−5.31E − 8	0.00
Gn	1.99E − 02	−3.50E − 04	9.20E − 06	−1.03E − 07	4.07E − 10
ACL	−0.6420	−0.431E − 01	−0.130E − 02	−0.131E − 04	0.475E − 07
PCL	1.840	−0.739E − 01	0.963E − 03	−0.396D − 05	0.00
MCL	0.586-01E	−0.167E − 01	0.130E − 03	0.00	0.00
LCL	0.5580	−0.198E − 01	0.171E − 03	0.00	0.00

PT patellar tendon, *Bf* biceps femoris, *Sm* semimembranosus, *St* semitendinosus, *Gn* gastrocnemius, *ACL* anterior cruciate ligament, *PCL* posterior cruciate ligament, *MCL* medial collateral ligament, *LCL* lateral collateral ligament

3.5 Result and Discussion

According to the parameters and mathematical model mentioned above, the knee joint forces and torques during human sit-to-stand movement were shown as follows.

During human sit-to-stand process, the tibiofemoral bone-on-bone contact force was represented in Fig. 3.3. At the beginning time of standing-up motion, the contact force was climbed up and reached the maximum value approximately 520 N, at the same time human almost standup from sit position. Then the contact force approximately declined to 370 N and fluctuated around it.

The forces of ligaments about ACL, PCL, LCL and MCL during standing-up motion were shown in Fig. 3.4. The peak angle value of ACL was at 70° and LCL 48°, and the maximum force value were approximately 350 and 200 N respectively. Compared with force of ACL and LCL, the MCL and PCL have the smaller force during standing-up process. The MCL and the PCL peak angle value were both at 80°, and the maximum value were approximately both 125 N.

In Fig. 3.5, it was showed that small torques was provided and approximately kept constant torques at the beginning time. However, the torques were greatly increased when human hip joint left seat, and the maximum value of torque was 1.1 Nm/(Kg m). It was turned back to approximately 0 Nm/(Kg m), when human finished the standing-up motion.

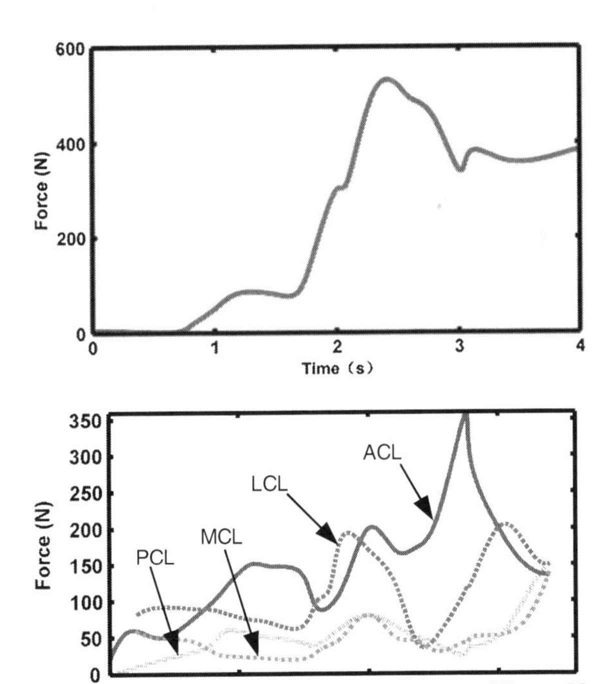

Fig. 3.3 The tibio-femoral bone-on-bone contact force

Fig. 3.4 The force of ligaments and knee angle during standing-up motion

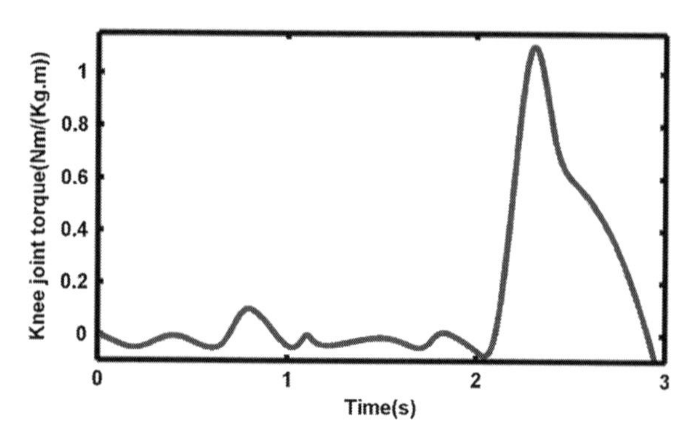

Fig. 3.5 Knee joint torques during standing-up motion

3.6 Conclusion

Compared with others model of knee joint, forces of four ligaments, bone-on-bone contact force, muscle forces and moment arms were considered to develop a comprehensive and multi-factors model in this paper. Knee joint was one of the main forced and loaded joints of human during the standing-up motion, so it is sophisticated to describe the position and orientation by moving coordinate systems relative to fixed coordinate system at ankle joint. In this paper, a mathematical model of knee joint was developed to calculate the forces and torques during standing-up process by taking into account of muscles, ligament and contact force.

References

1. Agrawal SK, Fattah A (2004) Theory and design of an orthotic device for full or partial gravity-balancing of a human leg during motion. J Trans Neural Syst Rehabil Eng 12:157–164
2. Lee H-Y, Kim K, Kim J et al (2011) Requirements of lower-extremity robotic exercise system for severely disabled. In: 8th international conference on ubiquitous robots and ambient intelligence. Songdo ConventiA, Incheon, pp 267–270
3. Ramaniraka NA, Terrier A, Theumann Whitton N et al (2005) Effects of the posterior cruciate ligament reconstruction on the biomechanics of the knee joint: a finite element analysis. J Clin Biomech 20:434–442
4. Thambyah A, Pereira BP, Wyss U (2005) Estimation of bone-on-bone contact forces in the tibiofemoral joint during walking. J Knee 12:383–388
5. Heintz S, Gutierrez-Farewik EM (2007) Static optimization of muscle forces during gait in comparison to EMG-to-force processing approach. J Gait Posture 26:279–288
6. McLean SG, Su A, Van den Bogert AJ (2003) Development and validation of a 3-D model to predict knee joint loading during dynamic movement. J Trans ASME 125:864–872
7. Haut Donahue TL, Hull ML, Rashid MM et al (2002) A finite element model of the human knee joint for the study of tibio-femoral contact. J Biomech Eng 124:273–279
8. Zheng N, Fleisig GS, Escamilla RF et al (1998) An analytical model of the knee for estimation of internal forces during exercise. J Biomech 31:963–967
9. Herzog W, Read LJ (1993) Lines of action and moment arms of the major force-carrying structures crossing the human knee joint. J Anat 182:213–230

Chapter 4
Adaptive Online Learning Environment for Life-Long Learning

Zhao Du, Lantao Hu and Yongqi Liu

Abstract With the rapid development of science and technology, the amount of knowledge is growing exponentially. Therefore, formal learning in educational institutions can no longer meet all needs of people. In order to support life-long learning of people, we propose an adaptive learning environment which is open and learner-centric. In additional to provide engaging learning resources, useful learning services and abundant learning opportunities; it also dynamically tracks and manages the learning needs and learning process of learners to improve their self-management, self-regulation and self-assessment abilities which they will need during their whole lifespan. Furthermore, it helps learners to keep connect with, contribute to, and benefit from social communities of experts and peers with the support of social software tools.

Keywords Online learning · Life-long learning · Collaborative tagging · Recommendation engine

4.1 Introduction

Science and technology are undergoing rapid development in modern knowledge society. They are continuously changing the ways of how we live, learn, work, communicate and collaborate. While the amount of knowledge is growing exponentially, the half-life of knowledge is shrinking. As a result, formal learning in educational institutions cannot meet all developmental needs of people. Because

Z. Du (✉)
Information Technology Center, Tsinghua University, Beijing 100084, China
e-mail: dz@cic.tsinghua.edu.cn

L. Hu · Y. Liu
Department of Computer Science and Technology, Beijing 100084, China

S. Li et al. (eds.), *Frontier and Future Development of Information Technology in Medicine and Education*, Lecture Notes in Electrical Engineering 269,
DOI: 10.1007/978-94-007-7618-0_4,

formal learning outside educational institutions and informal learning are more open, flexible and personalized; they have gained increasing popularity in recent years. They are not only open to all people who wants to learn; but also happens throughout life, at work, play and home [1]. As learners take full responsibility for their own learning outside educational institutions, the effect of learning has strong correlation with the three factors: (1) learners' learning motivation; (2) their self-management, self-regulation and self-assessment abilities; (3) the availability of high-quality learning resources and proper learning facilities.

Online learning is flexible and economic way to support life-long learning. With the widely application of IT in education, online learning has experience rapid development in the past few years. The most striking feature of online learning environments is open. Learning is no longer the process of passive knowledge acquisition for learners, but the process of active knowledge construction during the course of understanding their own experience in specific learning environment [2]. Furthermore, the abilities to connect to the source of information, learn what they need for tomorrow, distinguish between important and unimportant information, and recognize when new information alters the landscape are becoming critical in digital and knowledge economy age [3].

Based on the considerations above, it's significant to provide learners with adaptive online learning environment to support their life-long learning and help them develop the abilities that we mentioned above. Compared with traditional e-learning systems which are close and course-centric or teacher-centric, adaptive online learning environment is open and learner-centric. It's open to all learners of any age, educational background and vocation. Moreover, it aims to assist learners in developing knowledge and skills that they will need during their whole lifespan. Adaptive online learning environment uses data to set learning goals and criteria for learners' success, assesses their learning progress, and provides them with a comprehensive system of personalized developmental supports [4]. It helps learners to become self-regulated learners who can take control of their own learning by providing formative assessment and feedback facilities [5].

4.2 The Evolution of Online Learning Environment

According to the time that online learning environments emerge and the main contributions of them, we can classify them into three categories: resource-centric, course-centric and learner-centric. Resource-centric online learning environment has the longest history. It solves the problem of sharing high quality learning resources to learners conveniently and economically. Course-centric online learning environment has relatively short history. It brings learners and mentors together to create a more realistic course-like online experience to much more learners than traditional courses offered in classrooms. Learner-centric online learning environment is the emerging online learning environment. It's built on the assumption that learners should take full control over their learning outside educational institutions. It's featured by giving learners timely, multi-dimensional, high quality feedbacks to facilitate their self-regulated learning throughout their whole life.

4.2.1 Resource-Centric Online Learning Environment

Resource-centric online learning environment is featured by the aggregation and sharing of huge amount of learning resources. Most of the learning resources are in the form of course materials, and the courses are usually taught by famous professors or faculty members in well-known universities. Course materials usually consist of syllabi, lecture notes, assignments, exams and lecture videos. The contribution of it is that it provides learners with the equal, convenient and economical way of access engaging learning resources. Typical examples of resource-centric online learning environment include MIT's OCW, Stanford Engineering Everywhere and Carnegie Mellon Open Learning Initiative etc. [6].

4.2.2 Course-Centric Online Learning Environment

Course-centric online learning environment focuses on bring learners and mentors together to create a more realistic course-like online experience to a large amount of learners. It usually takes lecture videos of courses as the backbone. It also involves wider online participation of learners and mentors by providing course-centric communication, interaction and collaboration facilities. The key facilities include assessment tools that are embedded in lecture videos, automatic or peer grading tools that can give immediate feedback on grading of coursework, and course communities that can get questions answered. Typical examples of course-centric online learning environment include Coursera, Udacity and edX [7, 8].

4.2.3 Learner-Centric Online Learning Environment

Learner-centric online learning environment focuses on facilitating self-regulated learning. It's built on the assumption that learners should take full control over their learning outside educational institutions. Except for providing engaging learning resources; it allows learners to make decisions on their learning goals, tactics, strategies, routes etc. and helps them to track learning process. Furthermore, it also adds online communication, interaction and collaboration tools to connect learners with experts and peers. Their explicit collaboration such as tagging, evaluation and implicit collaboration such as browsing, searching form collective wisdom on the topic, quality and popularity of learning resources, experts and learners. Typical example of course-centric online learning environment includes NetEase Cloud Classroom.

4.3 Learner-Centric Online Learning

Learner-centric learning puts emphasis on learners' active engagement in learning and their responsibility for the management of learning [8]. Research has shown that effect feedback can lead to better learning gains [9]. Especially, the efforts to improve self-assessment skills of learners and the efforts to improve the quality of feedbacks given to learners are equally important [10]. Based on these researches, our goals are to provide learner-centric online learning environment which can give learners timely, multi-dimensional, high quality feedbacks and to help them to develop their self-management, self-regulation and self-assessment skills.

4.3.1 Learner-Centric Online Learning

Learner-centric online learning includes formal learning and informal learning. Formal learning is organized as a set of personalized learning programs which are made by individual learners and automatically tracked by learning facilities in online learning environment. As shown in Fig. 4.1, there are three types of learning programs in learner-centric online learning: course-based, book-based and topic-based. Every learning program has a corresponding learning program that is automatically generated by online learning environment using learner's behavior data. Informal learning consists of three types of behaviors. The first type concerns browsing, searching, tagging and evaluating learning resources. Learning resources can be provided in forms of online courses, books and documents. The second type concerns browsing, searching, tagging and evaluating, interacting and collaborating with experts and peers. The third type concerns reading and making decisions on the recommendations for learning resources, experts and peers.

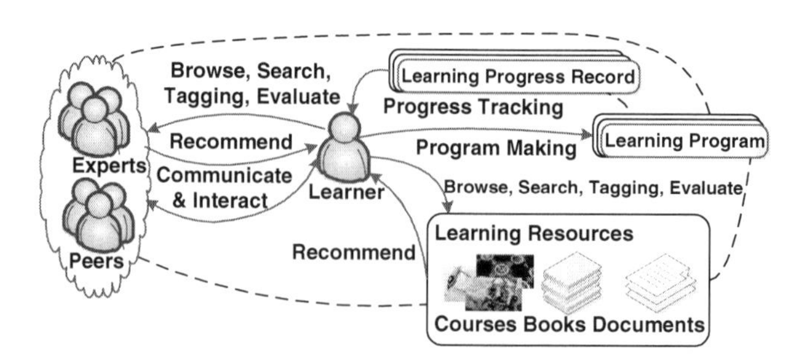

Fig. 4.1 Scenario of learner-centric online learning

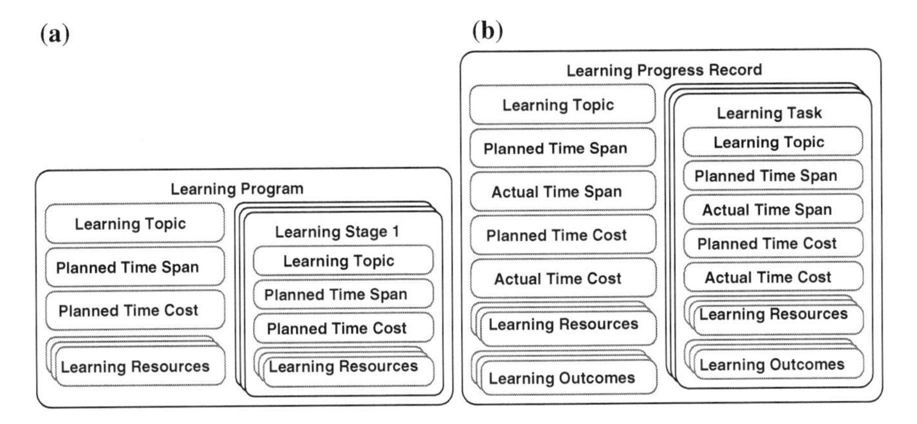

Fig. 4.2 Learning program and learning progress record

4.3.2 Learning Program and Learning Progress Record

As shown in Fig. 4.2(a), a learning program is defined by a learning topic, the planning time span, a set of related learning resources and a few learning tasks. Every learning task has a learning topic, the planning time span, the planned time cost and a set of related learning resources. As shown in Fig. 4.2(b), each learning program has a corresponding learning progress record which adds the actual time span, the actual time cost and the learning outcomes to learning program. The learning progress record can assist learners in getting detailed information about their learning activities. The aggregation of learning programs and learning progress records of a learner constitute his/her learning history; and the aggregation of all learners' learning programs and learning progress records on a specific course, book or topic constitute the learning route and learning curve of them.

4.4 Adaptive Online Learning Environment

Different from traditional e-learning systems such as LMS and CMS which are close and course-centric or teacher-centered, adaptive online learning environments are open and learner-centric. It can not only adapts to different learners' different interest, needs, abilities, level and learning styles; but also can adapts to different interest, needs, abilities, level and learning styles of the same learner in different stage of his/her life.

Adaptive online learning environment has three key features. First, it provides engaging learning resources, useful learning services and abundant learning opportunities which can be accessed everywhere at any time. Second, it dynamically tracks and manages learning needs and learning process of learners to improve their self-management, self-regulation and self-assessment abilities [11].

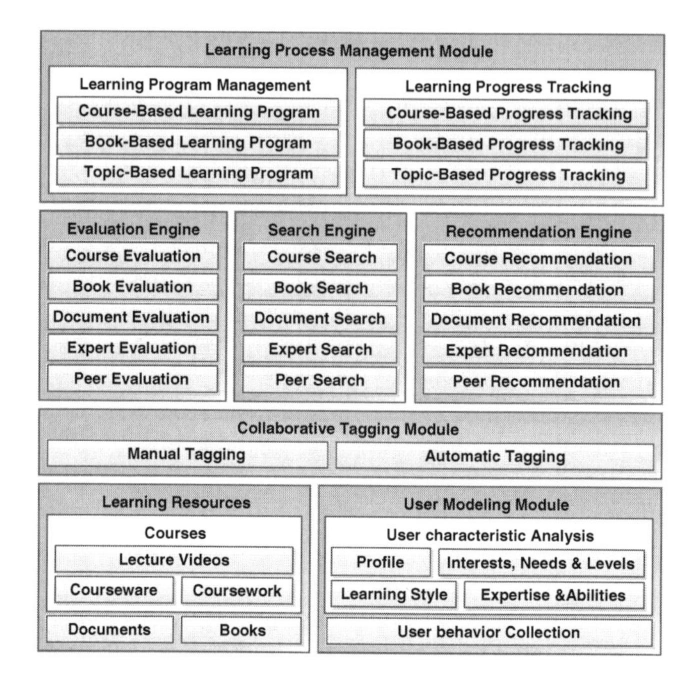

Fig. 4.3 Architecture of adaptive online learning environment

Thirdly, it helps learners to keep connection with, contribute to, and benefit from social communities of experts and peers with the support of social software tools. As shown in Fig. 4.3, adaptive online learning environment has seven components.

4.4.1 Learning Resources

High quality learning resources including courses, books and documents are fundamental components of online learning environment. Learn resources usually include courseware, coursework, lecture videos and value-added information of original learning resources such as tags, comments, evaluation scores, viewing history and learning outcomes of learners etc. The environment can analyze the quality and popularity of learning resources using value-added information with which Learners are expected to make better decisions on selecting proper learning resources.

4.4.2 User Modeling Module

User modeling is the process of exacting users' characteristics through collection and analysis of their profile, tags and behavior etc. It's noteworthy that users in adaptive learning environment can be learners and experts simultaneously. User modeling module is responsible for analyzing users' characteristics that are related to their learning and teaching activities. It provides essential information to offer adaptive learning services to learners. The characteristics include learners' profile data; personal learning styles; current learning interests, needs and levels in interested areas; expertise and abilities with which learners can serve as experts.

4.4.3 Collaborative Tagging Module

Collaborative tagging module allows learners to manually tag learning resources and users. Except for creating tags for courses, books and documents; learners can create tags for experts and peers as well as for themselves. The aggregation of tags is beneficial for learners to get a concise impression of topic, characteristics, quality etc. on learning resources and interests, professional skills, popularity on users. Furthermore, learners' collaborative behavior on tagging can be used by recommendation engine to generate recommendations for learning resources and users.

4.4.4 Evaluation Engine

Evaluation engine processes users' evaluations of courses, books, documents, experts and peers to give up-to-date collective evaluation score and corresponding ranking percentage of them. Adaptive online learning environment adopt a multi-dimensional five-score based evaluation model which is similar to the evaluation model used in many e-commerce systems. For learning resources including courses, books and documents; users can give their evaluations in terms of quality, novelty and difficulty. For experts, learners can give their evaluations in terms of professional capabilities and teaching skills.

4.4.5 Search Engine

Search engine provides search services of courses, books, documents, experts and peers. Search services for learning resources including courses, books, documents and search services for users including experts, peers are independent. The presentation of search results for learning resources should provide tags and evaluation information along with the brief description of learning resources. The presentation of search results for users should emphasize the expertise of experts and the learning interests of peers. The expertise of experts and the learning interests of peers can also described through tags and evaluation information.

4.4.6 Recommendation Engine

Recommendation engine is responsible for giving advises on courses, books, documents, experts and peers to users. It's key to connect users with their potentially interested courses, books, documents, experts and peers proactively. The recommendation is produced using the algorithm of collaborative filtering [12]. Recommendation engine firstly analyze the characteristics courses, books, documents, experts and users. Then it matches the characteristics of recommended objects with the characteristics of users to produce original recommendation list.

4.4.7 Learning Process Management Module

Learning process management module is responsible for the management of learning programs and tracking of learning progress. When making a learning program, a learner should specify a learning topic and several learning tasks. The definition of a learning task includes a learning topic, the planning time span, the planned time cost and a set of related learning resources. The planned time span, planned time cost and related learning resources of a learning program are decided by the planned time span, planned time cost and related learning resources of all learning tasks in the same learning program. There are three types of learning program: course-based, book-based and topic-based. The learning environment will automatically generate a learning progress record for each learning program. Learning progress record includes the actual time span, the actual time cost, the learning outcomes and all information in learning program.

4.5 Conclusion

Online learning is becoming increasingly important to support life-long learning in modern knowledge society. Online learning environments are open and learner-centric. In addition to provide engaging learning resources and create a more realistic course-like online experience, it helps learners develop their self-management, self-regulation and self-assessment skills. Adaptive online learning environment can not only adapts to different learners' different interest, needs, abilities, level and learning styles; but also can adapts to different interest, needs, abilities, level and learning styles of the same learner during his/her whole life-span. The adaptability is achieved through the dynamic modeling of learners, collaborative tagging and evaluation of learning resources and users, proactively made learning programs, automatically generated learning progress records, and personalized recommendation of learning resources and users. Our future work concerns two aspects: the discovery of useful learning programs and effective learning progress feedback strategy, the improvement of evaluation model and recommendation strategies.

Acknowledgments This work is supported by the Beijing Education and Science "Twelfth Five-Year Plan" (No. CJA12134) and the Joint Fund of Ministry of Education and China Mobile (No. MCM20121032).

References

1. Klamma R, Chatti MA, Duval E et al (2007) Social software for life-long learning. Educ Technol Soc 10(3):72–83
2. Driscoll M (2000) Psychology of Learning for Instruction. Allyn & Bacon, Needham Heights, MA
3. Siemens G (2005) Connectivism: a learning theory for the digital age. Int J Instr Technol Distance Learn 2(1):3–10
4. Alliance for Excellent Education (2012) Culture shift: teaching in a learner-centric environment powered by digital learning. http://www.all4ed.org/files/CultureShift.pdf. Accessed 21 Jan 2013
5. Nicola DJ, Dickb DM (2006) Formative assessment and selfregulated learning: a model and seven principles of good feedback practice. Stud High Educ 31(2):199–218
6. Vladoiu M (2011) State-of-the-art in open courseware initiatives worldwide. Inform Educ 10(2):271–294
7. Severance C (2012) Teaching the world: Daphne Koller and Coursera. Computer 45(8):8–9
8. Herman L (2012) Letter from the Editor-in-Chief: the MOOCs are coming. J Eff Teach 12(2):1–3
9. Lea J, Stephenson D, Troy J (2003) Higher education students' attitudes to student centred learning: beyond 'educational bulimia'. Stud High Educ 28(3):321–334
10. Black P, Wiliam D (1998) Assessment and classroom learning. Assess Educ 5(1):7–74
11. Yorke M (2003) Formative assessment in higher education: moves towards theory and the enhancement of pedagogic practice. High Educ 45(4):477–501
12. Adomavicius G, Tuzhilin A (2005) Toward the next generation of recommender systems: a survey of the state-of-the-art and possible extensions. IEEE Trans Knowl Data Eng 17(6):734–749

Chapter 5
A Membrane Bin-Packing Technique for Heart Disease Cluster Analysis

Xiyu Liu, Jie Xue and Laisheng Xiang

Abstract In this paper, we propose a new technique for clustering, which is the combination of membrane computing and Bin-packing technique. A new kind of P system (graph P system) is constructed which is different with the traditional ones. New rules and membrane structure are described. Cluster analysis is transformed by Bin-packing technique. All processes of the algorithm are implemented on this P system, including rules for mutation, swap and the calculation of energy change. Finally we apply the technique in the heart disease data set and obtain some results.

Keywords Cluster analysis · Membrane computing · Bin-packing problem

5.1 Introduction

Membrane systems (P System) are models of computation inspired by the structure and functioning of biological cells [1], which was introduced in 1998 by Păun and since then many results have been obtained [2]. P systems are composed of an hierarchical nesting of membranes that enclose regions in which floating objects exist originally. Each region can have associated evolution rules, symport/antiport rules. From now on, several models have been proposed for solving different problems, such as cell-like P system, tissue-like P system, SN P system, splicing P

X. Liu (✉) · J. Xue · L. Xiang
Shandong Normal University, 250014 Jinan, China
e-mail: sdxyliu@163.com

J. Xue
e-mail: xiaozhuzhu1113@163.com

L. Xiang
e-mail: xLs3366@163.com

S. Li et al. (eds.), *Frontier and Future Development of Information Technology in Medicine and Education*, Lecture Notes in Electrical Engineering 269,
DOI: 10.1007/978-94-007-7618-0_5,

system and so on [3]. P system has been used in various fields, like optimization problems [4] comparison results illustrate that their algorithm is concise and computes fast with high precision [5]; NP problems can be solved in polynomial time. Membrane algorithms are rather new research directions with a well-defined practical interest (Fig. 5.1).

The bin-packing problem (BPP) is a classical discrete mathematics problem and imposes stern difficulties for solving it exactly in a von Neumann architecture based machine [6], since it also belongs to the class NP-Hard in the strong sense.

Clustering is the core problem in data mining, it aims to partition a large number of data into different groups. Cluster analysis is widely used in areas such as market research, pattern recognition, image segmentation, and mesh segmentation [7]. There are several methods are proposed based on different theories, include partitional, hierarchical, density-based, grid-based and model-based clustering algorithms [8]. Since clustering deals with very large databases and high-dimensional data types, it consumes high demands on time and space. However, some existing methods are not suitable for large and high-dimensional databases (Fig. 5.2).

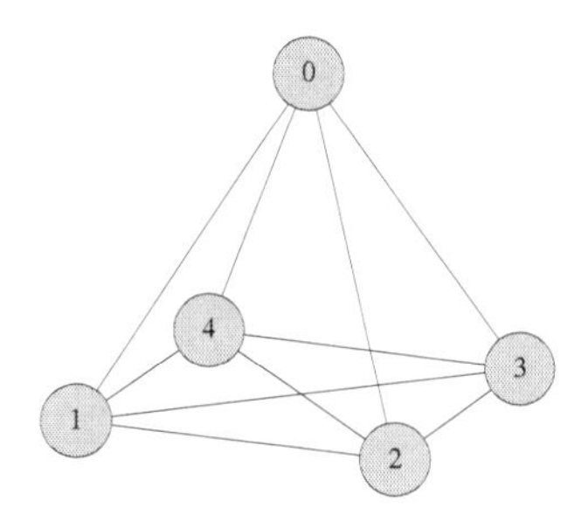

Fig. 5.1 P system with graph structure

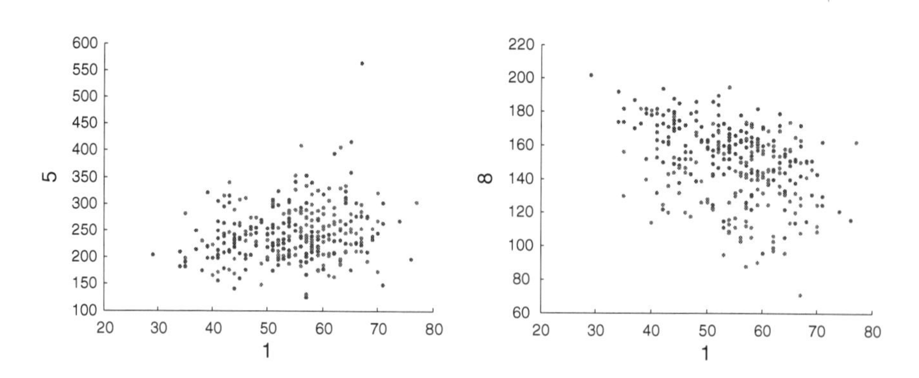

Fig. 5.2 Observation of classifiable attributes

Inspired by the above research, this paper focuses on the joint study of BPP with membrane computing into the analysis of clustering. Our purpose is to propose a new method to solve the clustering problem, which transformed cluster analysis into BPP and carry out in a new graph P system. Up to our knowledge, this is the first paper to extend membrane computing with BPP. Then we use membrane computing in cluster analysis, providing a new approach to data mining. We first propose clustering by BPP. Then we described for the graph P system on. Finally, we present the heart disease analysis (Fig. 5.3).

5.2 Clustering by Bin-Packing Technique

First we present a formulation of the traditional BPP (Fig. 5.4). Given a set of N items $x_1, \ldots, x_N$ with respective weights $w(x_i) = a_i \in (0, c], 1 \leq i \leq N$. The aim is to allocate all items into k bins with equal capacity c where k is predefined [2]. To

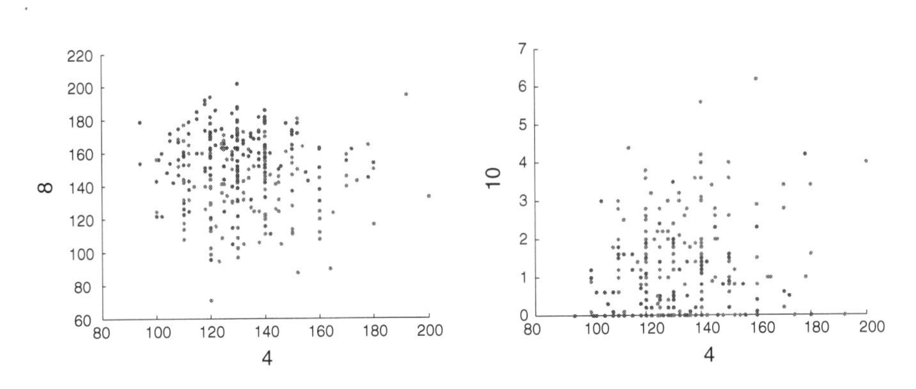

Fig. 5.3 Observation of classifiable attributes

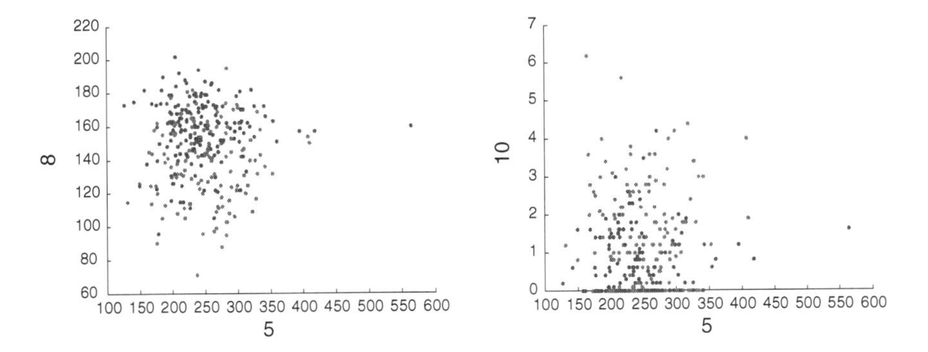

Fig. 5.4 Observation of classifiable attributes

unify the BPP with clustering problem we suppose there is a general data set. Our purpose is to cluster a data set $\Omega = \{x_1, \ldots, x_N\}$ with N points into k clusters where k is to be determined before the process of clustering. The data set is called a spatial data set if $\Omega \subset R^n$, where $x_i = (\xi_{i1}, \ldots, \xi_{in})$ for each $i = 1, \ldots, N$, and R^n be the real Euclidean space of dimension n. A clustering algorithm is to group the data set into k partitions called clusters. If we define an energy as the measurement for the clustering quality, then the problem is to allocate N points into k bins with least energy. In this case there are altogether k^N combinations of allocation and the best solution can be achieved by brute force search (Fig. 5.5).

Now we consider an array $\mathfrak{C}$ of integers

$$\mathfrak{C} = c_1 c_2 \ldots c_N \text{ each } c_i \in \{1, 2, \ldots, k\} \tag{5.1}$$

The i-th bin (cluster) C_i is defined as

$$C_i = \{x_p : c_p = i, p = 1, \ldots, N\} \, for \, i = 1, \ldots, k \tag{5.2}$$

We will identify the allocation $\mathfrak{C}$ with its corresponding partition. In order to guarantee the bins are non-empty, we need to add a restriction that $\#(C_i) > 0$ for valid clusters where $\#(C_i)$ denote the cardinality of the set C_i. Now we define a dissimilarity measure on the data set as $d(x, y)$. In the case where Ω is a spatial data set, the dissimilarity measure can be chosen as the Euclidean distance. Then a dissimilarity matrix D is defined as

$$D = \left[d_{ij} \triangleq d(x_i, x_j) : i, j = 1, \ldots, N\right]_{N \times N} \tag{5.3}$$

To simplify membrane computing, we assume that the dissimilarity measure are nonnegative integers. By this dissimilarity measure we define an energy function to evaluate the quality of clustering

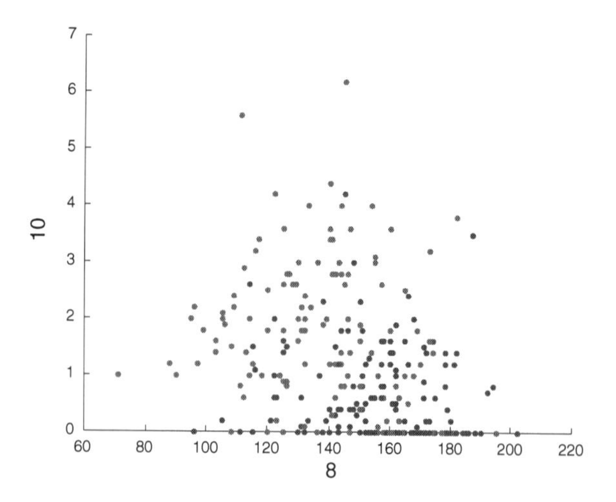

Fig. 5.5 Observation of classifiable attributes

Table 5.1 Clustering algorithm

Steps	Procedures
One	Initiate a random combination $\mathfrak{C}$ of integers in $\{1,\ldots,k\}$ as possible solutions of the clustering problem. Compute the energy $E(\mathfrak{C})$
Two	Perform evolution operations to generate candidate solutions. Compute the cost of energy changes
Three	If the candidate solution is better, then evolve to the new solution. Otherwise discard it and begin new search
Four	Find the best solution with least energy. Store and export the solution

$$E = E(\mathfrak{C}) = \sum_{t=1}^{k} E_t, E_t = \begin{cases} \sum_{i,j \in C_t} d_{ij} & \text{for } C_t \neq \varnothing \\ 0 & \text{for } C_t = \varnothing \end{cases} \tag{5.4}$$

Now we present an algorithm for clustering with the above mentioned technique (Table 5.1).

5.3 Membrane Structure and Computations

In membrane computing, membranes are organized in an architecture. Each membrane is named with associated multisets. We will use $\sigma_1, \ldots, \sigma_N$ to denote all the membranes. Traditional membrane structure of N membranes is a cell-like architecture which can be expressed with parentheses expressions $[[\ldots[\,]_1\cdots]_{N-1}]_N$ (Fig. 5.6).

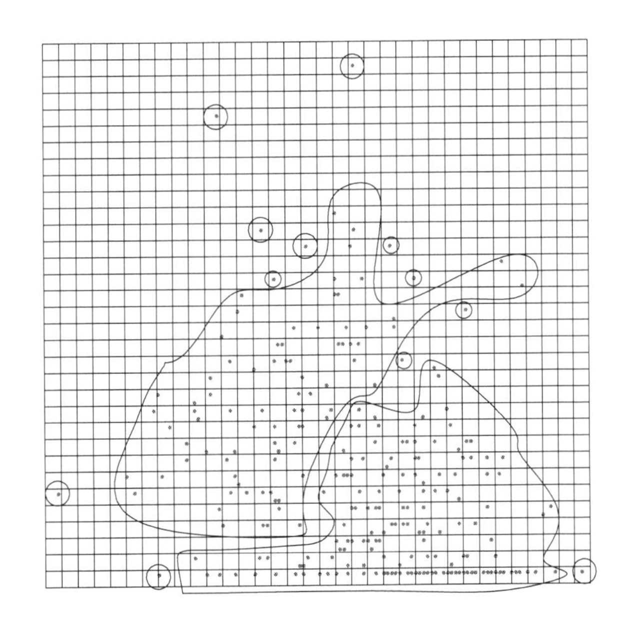

Fig. 5.6 Observation of classifiable attributes

5.3.1 Membrane Structure for Generating Arrays

Now we define a graph-like membrane structure to simulate array generation. Let $G = (V, I)$ be a graph with vertices $V = \{v^0, v^1, \ldots, v^N\}$ and edges $I = \{\sigma^1\}$. If an edge $\sigma = v^1v^2$ joining two vertices, then we call σ the parent of v^1 and v^2 and this relation is written by $v^1, v^2 \prec \sigma$. A vertex or edge is called a membrane. simplex is denoted by its vertices. An edge is the parent of its two vertices. Two vertices are called incident is there is an edge joining them. Two edges are called neighboring if they share a common vertex (Fig. 5.7).

A P system on a graph G, called a graph P system, with antiport and symport rules is a construct

$$\Pi = (N, O, \omega_0, \omega_1, \ldots, \omega_N, R_0, R_1, \ldots, R_N, ch, F(i,j)|_{(i,j)\in ch}, i_0) \tag{5.5}$$

where $N + 1$ is the number of vertex cells labeled with $\sigma_0, \sigma_1, \ldots, \sigma_N$, O is the alphabet, $\omega_0, \ldots, \omega_N$ are initial strings over O of multiset, $R_0, \ldots, R_N$ are symport and antiport rules, $ch \subseteq \{(i,j) : i,j \in \{0, 1, \ldots, N\}\}$ is the set of links, $F(i,j)$ is a finite set of antiport and/or symport rules associated with the link $(i,j) \in$ ch, $i_0 = 0$ is the output cell. The alphabet is as follows

$$O = \{a_1, \ldots, a_k, \alpha, \beta, \alpha_0, \alpha_+, \alpha_-, \alpha_1, \ldots, \alpha_N, d_1, \ldots, d_k, d, E, \Delta, E_1, \ldots, E_k\} \tag{5.6}$$

For our clustering problem, the set of links is $ch = \{(i,j) : i,j = 1, \ldots, N\}$. The output cell has initial configuration $\omega_0 = \lambda$. The initial configuration is shown in (5.8) as follows

$$\omega_i = d^{\varepsilon} d(c_i) E^h(c_i) \alpha^{\kappa_i} \alpha_0 \alpha_1 \ldots \alpha_N \beta^{\lambda_i} a_i^{c_i} \text{ for } i = 1, \ldots, N \tag{5.7}$$

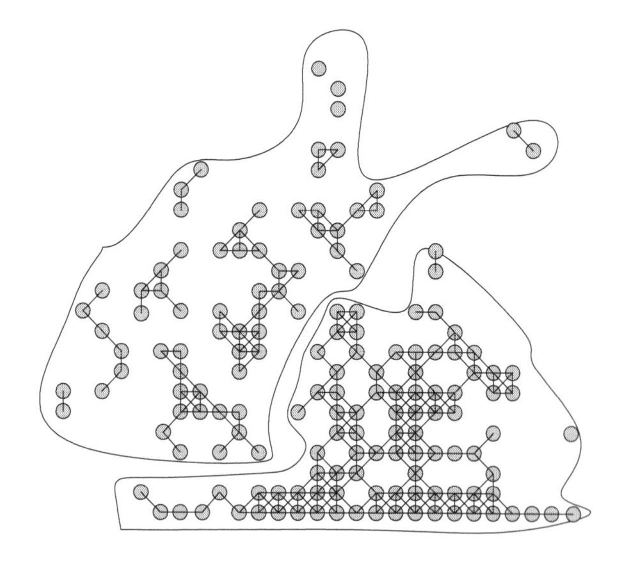

Fig. 5.7 Observation of classifiable attributes

The meaning of symbols in (5.7) is explained below. First the indicator d^{ε} shows if the data point x_i is in a cluster or not, where $\varepsilon = 1$ indicates yes and $\varepsilon = 1$ no. The symbol $d(c_i)$ is the cluster ID where x_i is located. Energy is denoted by $E^h(c_i)$. The symbol c_i is an integer with $c_i \in \{1,\ldots,k\}$, and $\kappa_i = 0, 1, \lambda_i \in Z_2$ where Z_2 is the group with addition module 2. In this configuration the membrane a_i^p encodes a data with integer p while κ_i is an indicator with $\sum_{i=1}^{N} \kappa_i = 1$.

5.3.2 Basic Operations and Rules

Now we define some basic operations needed for our clustering problem. First we define the operation mutation which change the value of a membrane i from p to q, i.e., $\omega_i : a_i^p \rightarrow a_i^q$. In order to do this, we need two adjacent cells $i-1, i+1$. In case when $i = 1$ ($i = N$ resp.) we need only one adjacent cell $i+1$ ($i-1$ resp.). In all cases we use $i-, i+$ to represent adjacent cells, provided they exists. The rule for this operation is as follows where the new integer q is randomly generated.

$$(a_{i-}^r, \alpha a_i^p, a_{i+}^s) \stackrel{up}{\rightarrow} (a_{i-}^r, a_i^q, \alpha a_{i+}^s); \ (a_{i-}^r, \alpha a_i^p, a_{i+}^s) \stackrel{down}{\rightarrow} (\alpha a_{i-}^r, a_i^q, a_{i+}^s) \tag{5.8}$$

The next operation is the swap operation which swaps the value of two adjacent cells. The rule for this operation is as follows.

$$(\beta^{\lambda_-} a_{i-}^r, \beta a_i^p, \beta a_{i+1}^q, \beta^{\lambda_+} a_{i+1+}^s) \rightarrow (\beta^{\lambda_- +1} a_{i-}^r, a_i^q, a_{i+1}^p, \beta^{\lambda_+ +1} a_{i+1+}^s) \tag{5.9}$$

Energy rules $R(\sigma_i, \sigma_j)$ are listed below where $\delta(i,j)$ is the Kronecker symbol.

$$\begin{aligned} R(\sigma_i, \sigma_j) :& \left(dd(p)E^{h_i}(i)\alpha_j, dd(q)E^{h_j}(j)\right) \\ &\rightarrow \left(dd(p)E^{h_i+\delta(i,j)d_{ij}}(i), dd(q)E^{h_j}(j)\right) \end{aligned} \tag{5.10}$$

5.3.3 Configuration and Computation

The main clustering technique here is the agglomerative method. The initial configuration is $\omega_i = d^{\varepsilon} d(c_i) E^0(i) \alpha^{\kappa_i} \beta^{\lambda_i} \alpha_0 \alpha_1 \ldots \alpha_N a_i^{c_i}$ which indicates that energy data is empty. Then the energy rules are applied and $E(i)$ is computed for $i = 1,\ldots,N$ as follows.

$$\begin{cases} R(\sigma_i,\sigma_j) : \left(dd(p)E^{h_i}(i)\alpha_j, dd(q)E^{h_j}(j)\right) \\ \qquad \rightarrow \left(dd(p)\alpha_+E^{h_i}(i)\Delta^{\delta(i,j)d_{ij}}, dd(q)E^{h_j}(j)\right) \\ \qquad j = 1,2,\ldots,N \\ R(\sigma_0,\sigma_i) : \left(E^h, dd(p)\alpha_+E^{h_i}(i)\Delta^{\delta(i,j)d_{ij}}\right) \\ \qquad \rightarrow \left(E^hE^{\delta(i,j)d_{ij}}, dd(p)\alpha_-E^{h_i}(i)\Delta^{\delta(i,j)d_{ij}}\right) \\ R(\sigma_i) : \left(dd(p)\alpha_-E^{h_i}(i)\Delta^{\delta(i,j)d_{ij}}\right) \rightarrow \left(dd(p)E^{h_i}(i)E^{\delta(i,j)d_{ij}}\right) \end{cases} . \tag{5.11}$$

We will now analyze the changing of energy stored in $E^h(c_i)$ when operations are performed. First let us consider mutation $(a^r_{i-}, \alpha a^p_i; a^s_{i+}) \xrightarrow{up} (a^r_{i-}, a^q_i, \alpha a^s_{i+})$. Then the membrane σ_i will evolve as follows

$$\begin{cases} \omega_i = d(p)E^{h_i}(i)\alpha a^p_i \\ d(p)\alpha a^p_i \rightarrow d(q)\alpha_0^N\alpha_1\ldots\alpha_N a^q_i \\ E^{h_i}(i) \rightarrow E^{h'_i}(i) = \lambda \end{cases} . \tag{5.12}$$

Then we apply rules between $R(\sigma_i,\sigma_j)$ and we get

$$\begin{cases} R(\sigma_i,\sigma_j) : \\ \left(dd(q)E^{h_i}(i)\alpha_0\alpha_j, dd(q)E^{h_j}(j)\right) \rightarrow \\ \left(dd(q)E^{h_i}(i)\Delta^{d_{ij}}\alpha_0\alpha_+, dd(q)E^{h_j}(j)\right) \\ \left(dd(q)E^{h_i}(i)\alpha_0\alpha_j, dd(r)E^{h_j}(j)\right) \rightarrow \\ \left(dd(q)E^{h_i}(i)\alpha_0, dd(r)E^{h_j}(j)\right), \qquad r \neq \\ R(\sigma_0,\sigma_i : \\ \left(E^h, dd(q)\alpha_+E^{h_i}(i)\Delta^{d_{ij}}\right) \rightarrow \\ \left(E^hE^{d_{ij}}, dd(q)\alpha_-E^{h_i}(i)\Delta^{d_{ij}}\right) \\ R(\sigma_i) : \\ \left(dd(q)\alpha_-E^{h_i}(i)\Delta^{d_{ij}}\right) \rightarrow \left(dd(q)E^{h_i}(i)E^{d_{ij}}\right) \end{cases} \tag{5.13}$$

Next we consider the swap operation $(a^p_i, a^q_j) \rightarrow (a^q_i, a^p_j)$ where $i \neq j, p \neq q$. Then the rules for this operation are listed as follows.

$$\begin{cases} \omega_i = d(p)E^{h_i}(i)\beta a^p_i, \omega_j = d(q)E^{h_j}(j)\beta a^q_j \\ d(p)\beta a^p_i \rightarrow d(q)\alpha_0^N\alpha_1\ldots\alpha_N a^q_i \\ d(q)\beta a^q_j \rightarrow d(p)\alpha_0^N\alpha_1\ldots\alpha_N a^p_j \\ E^{h_i}(i) \rightarrow E^{h'_i}(i) = \lambda, E^{h_j}(j) \rightarrow E^{h'_j}(j) = \lambda \end{cases} . \tag{5.14}$$

And then we still run rules $R(\sigma_i,\sigma_k), R(\sigma_j,\sigma_k), k = 1,\ldots,N$ as shown in (5.13).

After the operation of mutation and swap, the whole energy of data set is changed, next, we will calculate the new energy and compare it with the old one (In the initial configuration, $E = 0$, comparison can be acted after the second operations of data). Then the rules for this operation are listed as follows.

For membrane σ_i with evolution, after all data act rule (5.13) with σ_i, the new energy will be $(\sum_{j\in 1,2,\ldots,N,j\neq i} d_{ij} \neq h_i)$

$$E^{\sum_{j\in 1,2,\ldots,N,j\neq i} d_{ij}} E^{h_i}(i) \rightarrow E^{\sum_{j\in 1,2,\ldots,N,j\neq i} d_{ij}-1} E^{h_i-1}(i) \tag{5.15}$$

Rule (5.15) subtracts the number of E and $E(i)$ by one and it will go on working until one of the below situation occurring. According to our algorithm, there will be two situations about the change of energy after mutation and swap for membrane σ_i:

(1) After evolution operations, the new solution is much better, which means energy reduces. The new solution instead of the old one.

$$E^{\sum_{j\in 1,2,\ldots,N,j\neq i} d_{ij}} E^{h_i}(i) \rightarrow E(i)^{h_i-(\sum_{j\in 1,2,\ldots,N,j\neq i} d_{ij})+1} Eh \tag{5.16}$$

$$E^{h_i-(\sum_{j\in 1,2,\ldots,N,j\neq i} d_{ij})+1} \rightarrow \lambda \tag{5.17}$$

$$hE \rightarrow E^{\sum_{j\in 1,2,\ldots,N,j\neq i} d_{ij}} \tag{5.18}$$

$$E^{\sum_{j\in 1,2,\ldots,N,j\neq i} d_{ij}} \rightarrow E^{h'_i}(i) \tag{5.19}$$

(2) After evolution operations, the new solution is much worse than the old one or equal to it, which means energy adds. It will be discarded.

$$E^{\sum_{j\in 1,2,\ldots,N,j\neq i} d_{ij}} E^{h_i}(i) \rightarrow E^{(\sum_{j\in 1,2,\ldots,N,j\neq i} d_{ij})-h_i+1} E(i)h \tag{5.20}$$

$$E^{(\sum_{j\in 1,2,\ldots,N,j\neq i} d_{ij})-h_i+1} \rightarrow \lambda \tag{5.21}$$

$$hE(i) \rightarrow E^{h_i}(i) \tag{5.22}$$

In this situation rule (5.12) and (5.14) will do their inverse operation, membrane I or membrane i and j will restore to their pre-operation state.

$$\begin{cases} d(q)\alpha_0^N \alpha_1 \ldots \alpha_N a_i^q \rightarrow d(p)\alpha a_i^p \\ \text{or} \\ d(q)\alpha_0^N \alpha_1 \ldots \alpha_N a_i^q \rightarrow d(p)\beta a_i^p \\ d(p)\alpha_0^N \alpha_1 \ldots \alpha_N a_j^p \rightarrow d(q)\beta a_j^q \end{cases} \tag{5.23}$$

Rules above will continue until there exists $E^{h_i}(i)$that it can not be replaced by any other E. Then, we find the best solution. The cluster ID $d(c_i)$ will be sent to the output membrane $i_0 = 0$ by rule (5.24) for every membrane σ_i

$$R(\sigma_0, \sigma_i) : \\ \left(E^h E^{d_{ij}}, dd(q)\alpha_+ E^{h_i}(i)\Delta^{d_{ij}}\right) \to \left(d(q), d\alpha_- E^{h_i}(i)\Delta^{d_{ij}}\right) \tag{5.24}$$

All $d(c_i)$are read out from the output membrane, we know that x_i is located in $d(c_i)$is best. At this point, we get the clustering result.

5.4 A Heart Disease Analysis

This example is taken from the UCI database with data collected from Cleveland Clinic Foundation, Hungarian Institute of Cardiology, V.A. Medical Center, and University Hospital of Zurich. The names of the principal investigator responsible for the data collection are Andras Janosi, M.D., William Steinbrunn, M.D., Matthias Pfisterer, M.D., and Robert Detrano, M.D., Ph.D.

There are 14 attributes with 303 data points which is listed in Table 5.2.

Now we choose two attributes among the 14 and draw figures to indicate possible classification. By direct observation we know that attribute 1 (age) and attributes 5 (serum cholestoral), 8 (maximum heart rate achieved) are more classifiable.

Table 5.2 Complete attribute documentation

ID	Attribute	Values
1.	Age	age in years
2.	Sex	sex (1 = male; 0 = female)
3.	cp	chest pain type – Value 1: Typical angina – Value 2: Atypical angina – Value 3: Non-anginal pain – Value 4: Asymptomatic
4.	trestbps	resting blood pressure (in mm Hg on admission to the hospital)
5.	chol	serum cholestoral in mg/dl
6.	fbs	(fasting blood sugar > 120 mg/dl) (1 = true; 0 = false)
7.	restecg	resting electrocardiographic results – Value 0: normal – Value 1: having ST-T wave abnormality – Value 2: showing probable or definite left ventricular hypertrophy
8.	thalach	maximum heart rate achieved
9.	exang	exercise induced angina (1 = yes; 0 = no)
10.	oldpeak	= ST depression induced by exercise relative to rest
11.	slope	the slope of the peak exercise ST segment – Value 1: upsloping – Value 2: flat – Value 3: downsloping
12.	ca	number of major vessels (0–3) colored by flourosopy
13.	thal	3 = normal; 6 = fixed defect; 7 = reversable defect
14.	num	diagnosis of heart disease (angiographic disease status) – Value 0: < 50 % diameter narrowing – Value 1: > 50 % diameter narrowing

And attribute 4 (resting blood pressure) is more classifiable with respect to 8 (maximum heart rate achieved), attributes 10 (ST depression induced by exercise relative to rest).

And attribute 5 (serum cholestoral) is more classifiable with respect to 8 (maximum heart rate achieved), attributes 10 (ST depression induced by exercise relative to rest).

Finally attribute 8 (maximum heart rate achieved) is more classifiable with respect to attributes 10 (ST depression induced by exercise relative to rest).

5.5 Results and Discussion

In this paper we use membrane Bin-packing technique to diagnoses of heart disease. Our method clustered data set into two groups, which do a much precise analysis of the disease [num: diagnosis of heart disease (angiographic disease status) value 0: $< 50\ \%$, value 1: $> 50\ \%$]. It also shows the validity of our new algorithm. By membrane Bin-packing technique we can implement the process of clustering significantly, which is especially useful for large database since membrane computing has large parallel ability. Up to authors' knowledge, this is the first paper to extend membrane computing with Bin-packing problems. It provides an alternative solution for this traditional knowledge engineering. We also need to say that in this research, there are many problems waiting to be solved.

Acknowledgments Research is supported by the Natural Science Foundation of China (No.61170038), the Natural Science Foundation of Shandong Province (No.ZR2011FM001), the Shandong Soft Science Major Project (No.2010RKMA2005).

References

1. Păun G (2000) Computing with membranes. J Comput Syst Sci 61(1):108–143. (First circulated as TUCS Research Report No.28, 1998)
2. Cavaliere M, Sedwards S (2008) Decision problems in membrane systems with peripheral proteins, transport and evolution. Theor Comput Sci 404:40–51
3. Păun G, Rozenberg G, Salomaa A (2010) Membr Comput. Oxford University Press, NewYork
4. Huang L, Wang N (2006) An optimization algorithm inspired by membrane computing. Lect Notes Comput Sci 4222:49–52
5. Yang S, Wang N (2012) A novel P system based optimization algorithm for parameter estimation of proton exchange membrane fuel cell model. Int J Hydrogen Energy 37:8465–8476
6. Alonso Sanches CA, Soma NY (2009) A polynomial-time DNA computing solution for the Bin-Packing Problem. Appl Math Comput 215:2055–2062
7. Inform Sci (2009) A new point symmetry based fuzzy genetic clustering technique for automatic evolution of clusters. Inform Sci 179:3230–3246
8. Jiawei H, Kamber M (2006) Data mining concepts and techniques, 2nd edn. Elsevier, Singapore

Chapter 6
Teaching Chinese as a Foreign Language Based on Tone Labeling in the Corpus and Multi-Model Corpus

Zhu Lin

Abstract The paper analyses the different systems of corpus labeling, such as TODI, TOBI, and IVIE, which are three kinds of speech labeling system, and the paper puts forward a suitable labeling system of multi-modal corpus for teaching Chinese as a foreign language. The corpus includes eight levels of character description and labeling of speech tagging system. The system of labeling is applied to the improvement of the labeling method of TIMIT, which has the layer of phonetic transcription, the layer of phoneme layer, the layer of intermittent index, the lay of stress, the layer of target, the layer of phonology, and the layer of the behavior (includes the layer of posture and the layer of movement, and the layer of miscellanea. Finally, we label on the experimental corpus, and it can obtain better results in the process of teaching Chinese phonetic than before.

Keywords Corpus · Labeling · Teaching · Chinese as a foreign language

6.1 Introduction

Currently, there are contradictions between the needs of the limited resources of teachers and personalized service, between the majority of students with limited learning time and a large number of learning content of Chinese language. There is the uneven distribution of the practitioners in the domain of teaching Chinese as a foreign language. There are many teachers from foreign languages, or Chinese professionals in this domain. In order to resolve these conflicts, the building of Chinese language teaching corpus is the core of the Chinese as a foreign language education.

Z. Lin (✉)
The School of International Communication, Beijing International Studies University, 100024 Beijing, China
e-mail: zhulinnini@126.com

S. Li et al. (eds.), *Frontier and Future Development of Information Technology in Medicine and Education*, Lecture Notes in Electrical Engineering 269,
DOI: 10.1007/978-94-007-7618-0_6, © Springer Science+Business Media Dordrecht 2014

The corpus sparkles a revolution in all the areas of linguistics, which is the objective evaluation of the field of linguistics. Corpus studies and language teaching based on corpus are becoming a central topic of linguistics, and language teaching. With the creation of large-scale spoken corpus, especially the establishment of a large speech database for spoken language, the research bids farewell the era of the "field research", and puts into a "digital" era. The new teaching method based on corpus, the use of the new tool (computer, etc.) as well as a variety of new software makes for large-scale speech corpus collection and labeling becomes possible. In addition, the study of the voice labeling system also becomes increasingly important. Therefore, labeling is a core of the corpus construction by characteristics of marked more detailed, and the more support provided by the corpus of language study, and language teaching.

6.2 Analyzing the Different Types of Corpus' Labeling

TODI (Tone Description Index) is the earliest voice labeling system for describing phonetics, and it includes two levels: the layer of word and the layer of intonation, but it still lacks the description for the acoustics on the voice.

TOBI (Tone Break Index) is the first phonetics labeling system for describing rhythm, which is evolved from the TODI. The labeling system was the standard labeling system of English rhythm in 1992. Then, many countries established their system of their rhythm labeling based on TOBI, such as S-TOBI (the Swedish labeling system of rhythm), Japanese J-TOBI, and Korean K-TOBI (Beckman, 1996). The Mandarin phonetic marked C-TOBI 1.0 is established by the Chinese Academy of Social Science. The C-TOBI, the labeling system of rhythm for Chinese, has five levels of labeling: (1) the layer of Chinese characters, (2) the layer of phonetic transcription, (3) the layer of intermittent index, (4) the layer of stress index, (5) the layer of miscellaneous. The layer of intermittent index is to mark the rhythm of Chinese, and it can indicate connection between syllables, which is perceived, and connections between syllables and silent segment; the layer of stress is used to mark each stress prosodic units; the layer of miscellaneous is used to label various vice linguistic and non-linguistic phenomena. Corpus marked example is shown below:

Level Description: (1)the layer of Chinese characters to write; (2) the layer of phonetic transcription; (3) the layer of the phonemes; (4) the layer of intermittent index; (5) the layer of stress index.

But TOBI also has some shortcomings, such as: the opacity on the characterization of some English intonation. For example, in the tone of H*...LL% and the L*...HH%, TOBI is difficult to find the perception of pitch cues due to the existence of the phrase stress; TOBI is difficult to accurately describe phonetics variants due to local variants.

IVIE (Intonational Variation in English) is the system of labeling based on TOBI, which is established by Cambridge University to modify the defect of TOBI mentioned above. The system of labeling can describe variants of English intonation due to local differences. The IVIE compares directly different English rhythm marked under a labeling layer. The different rhythm dues to different accent and the different pronunciation can be realized. IVIE has three levels, the rhythm structure, the acoustic–phonetic structure and phonological structure, as follow:

The layer 1 is for word, and the layer 2 is for prominence, and the layer 3 is for Phonetics trend, and the layer 4 is the phonological layer, and the layer 5 is for Miscellaneous layer.

TIMIT is the corpus based on Gaussian Mixture Model (GMM), which is a speech corpus recorded pronunciation of 630 people. To analyze phonetics on American English word, the phoneme variant is the main purpose of the corpus. Because of one person labeling, the consistency of the corpus is high, so the corpus can reflect greatly on all kinds of phoneme variants, and it is suitable for teaching language. Although it is marked better on Acoustics, phonetics, the marked level is short, and the content of label is insufficient. The example of the Corpus is shown below.

The description: the level 1 is for the phonemes, and the level 2 is for the layer of IPA (international phonetic alphabet) corresponded (Fig. 6.1).

From the labeling of TODI, TOBI, IVOE and TIMIT, it is easily to see TOBI from TODI by improving the description of the acoustics on the phonetics. Compararing IVIE and TOBI, the former is preferable by the layer of prominence and the layer of phonetics trend, but it lacks the layer of intermittently indicating, and the layer of stress description. Description of the phrase in the middle, IVIE can't describe carefully on dividing phoneme, so it can't descript the middle of phrase due to the lack of description of the level of the middle phrase.

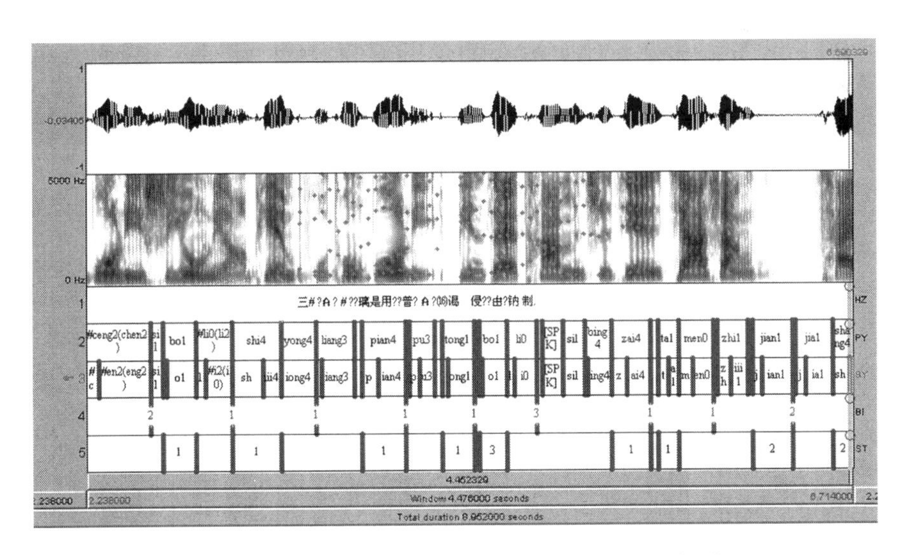

Fig. 6.1 Example of the corpus of TOBI (this figure by the CASS provided)

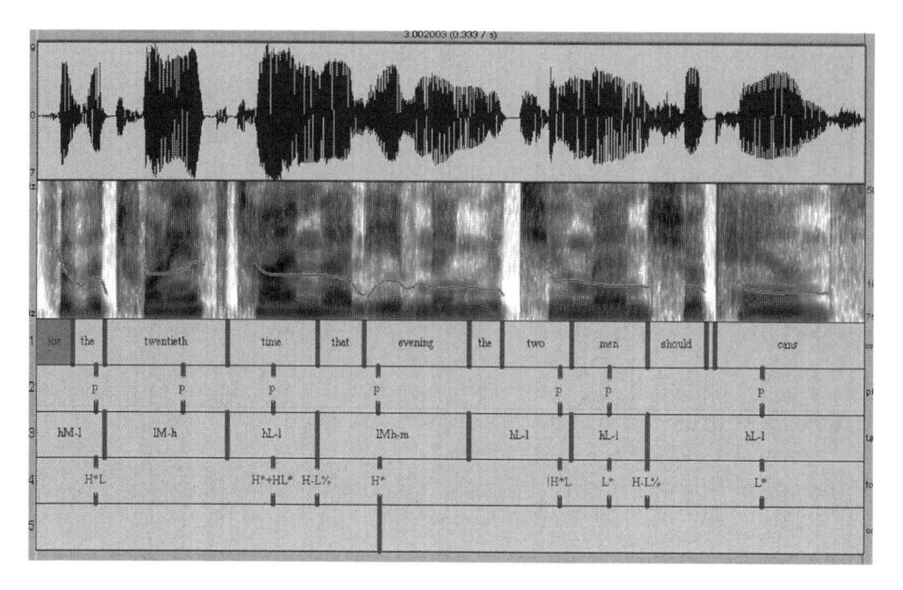

Fig. 6.2 Example of the corpus of IVIE (this figure by the CASS provided)

When labeling, we need to compare between the similarities and differences of the phoneme, especially in teaching language, because the role of this level is extremely obvious in teaching (Fig. 6.2).

6.3 The New Method of Labeling for Teaching Chinese as a Foreign Language

In contrast, the databases form the above, the new method of labeling for Teaching Chinese as a Foreign Language can be combine the labeling of TIMIT, plus the layer of phoneme, the layer of intermittent index, and the layer of prominence like TOBI's labeling method, as follows:

Level Description: the 1st layer is of characters to write; the layer 2 is of the layer of phoneme transcription; the layer 3 is of intermittent index; the 4th layer is of the prominence layer; the 5th layer is of Phonetics trend; the 6th layer is of phonology; the 7th layer is of miscellaneous layer. The labeling is set to accurately describe the voice in teaching Chinese as a foreign language (Fig. 6.3).

In recent years, the construction and development of multi-modal corpus brought a new research for teaching Chinese as a foreign language. The multi-modal corpus is established based on the British linguist Firth (JR Firth) "Discourse Theory" (Utterance Theory). The theory of utterance not only refers to discourse, but also refers to topic-related actions, behavior, occasion, which means an environment for discourse. Building corpus for language must include the real

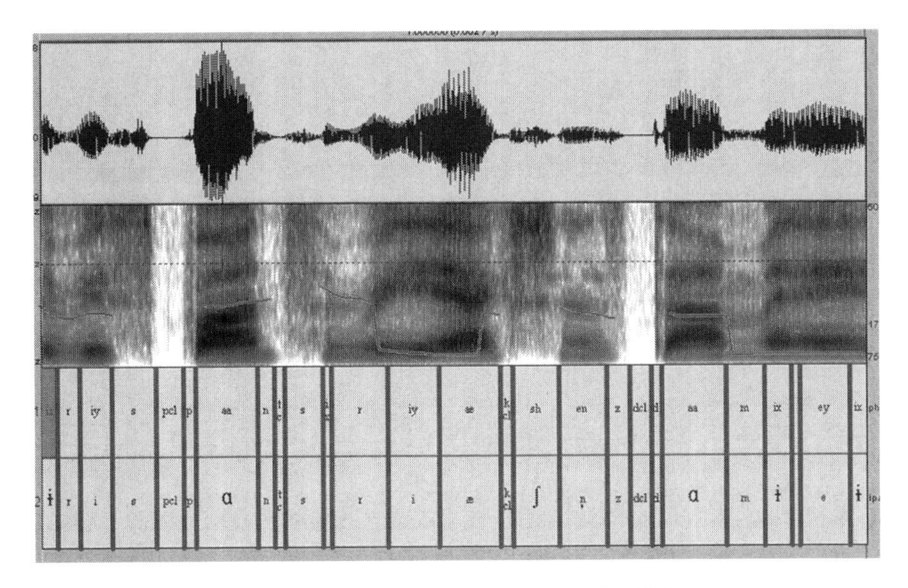

Fig. 6.3 An example of the labeling system from the corpus of TIMIT

context. The corpus above does not consider the factors of contextual, because there are not enough hardware and technology development for coming true (Fig. 6.4).

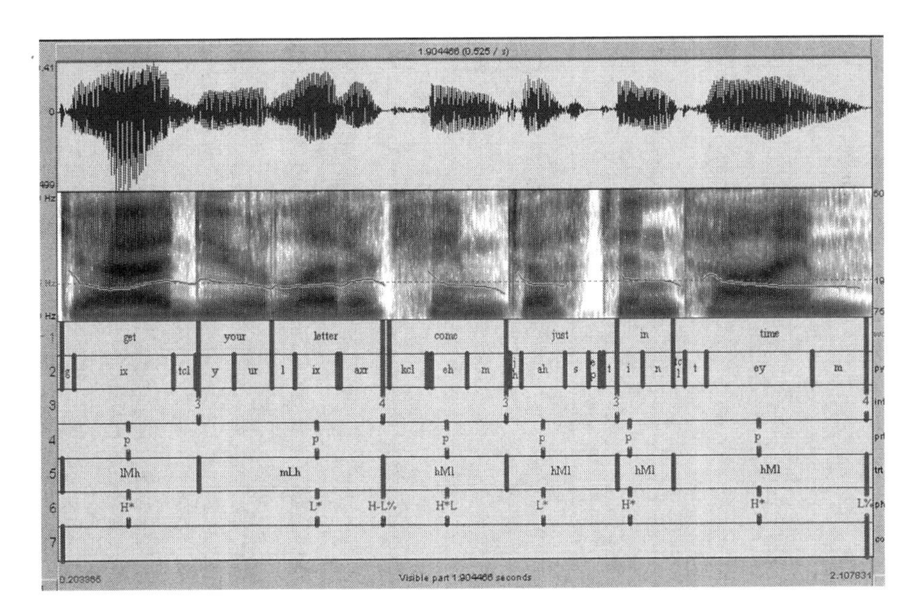

Fig. 6.4 An example of the new labeling system of corpus for teaching Chinese as a foreign language

With the development of technology, current computer can achieve the storage and automated processing of the speech events. Various verbal recording tools (digital cameras, etc.) can be convenient and real-time tracking and also obtain the required corpus. So, the limitation of the database of the text corpus and the voice corpus has become increasingly prominent. Tomorrow the corpus has entered into the era of multi-media corpus, which records audio and visual data in a scene. The Corpus marked example is shown below:

From the Fig. 6.5, it shows that the multi-modal corpus labeling includes a description of the image, sound, movement, the layer of sonic, the layer of acoustic, the layer of word, the layer of miscellaneous, and the layer of visual depictions, which was divided into two sub-levels: the posture layer and the movement layer.

The labeling of Multi-modal corpus provides us with a new labeling which is helpful for teaching language, such as Chinese. It is better to resolve the relationship between sound and entities, or sound and movement. However, I think its description of phonetics and phonological is not enough, so the author should plus the following layers: the phoneme layer, the intermittent index layer, the accent layer, the target layer, and the phonology layer. We can get more accurate description of the utterance by the labeling on corpus, with a wider range using a wider range, greater.

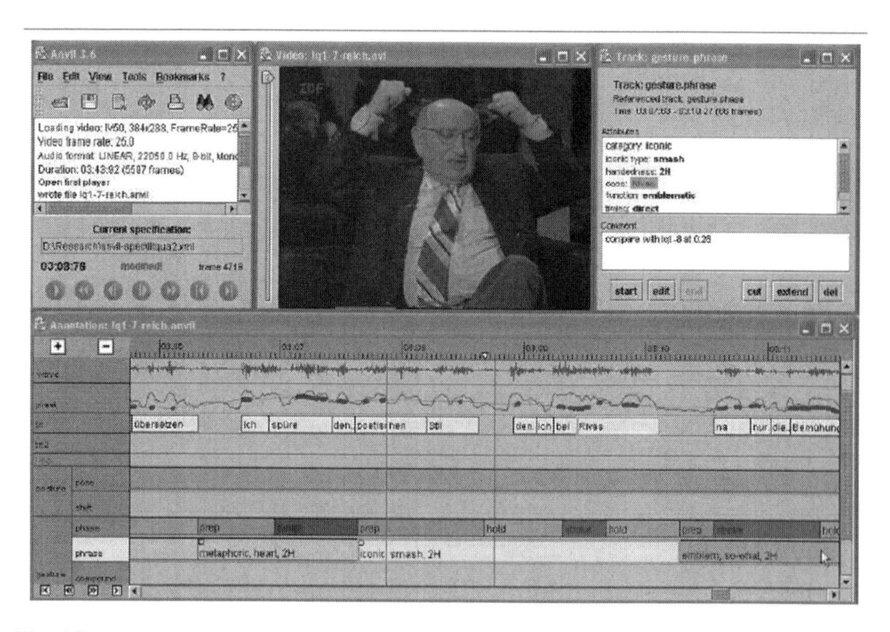

Fig. 6.5

6.4 The Construction of Corpora in Language Teaching of Chinese as a Foreign Language

Existing Chinese learning resources can be divided into three types: (a) the resources of Chinese learning tools, such as dictionaries, terminology translation, automatic translation tools; (b) the systematic, and formal Chinese learning materials, such as network courses; (c) informal additional Chinese learning materials, such as news class, science and technology, culture, class books.

From the summary of the above, the corpus used for the teaching of Chinese as a foreign language needs the following points:

The first point: The function of teaching Chinese phonetics as a foreign language has the following features:

(a) The function of list, such as the Course management, the management of progress in learning, learning styles;
(b) Student speech analysis: (1) the analysis of score achievement (total score, pronunciation, intonation, fluency, volume): displays the scores and the total scores of the student's pronunciation, pronunciation scores, scores of intonation, fluency scores and the volume fraction; (2) the analysis of the Chinese learner's pronunciation: to draw pronunciation squiggles and marked pronunciation problems, the Top Score from Summary pronunciation analysis, 3D animated explanations for problems standard; (3) the analysis of the Chinese learner's tone: to draw tone curve marked tone squiggles, and to analyze the summary of tonal; (4) the analysis of the Chinese learner's rhythm: to draw rhythm curve, waveform curve labeled rhythm to get the Top Score; (5) the analysis of the Chinese learner's sound volume: to draw the volume waveform curve labeled volume, the summary volume analysis of the results of the Top Score.

The Fig. 6.6 shows a new open educational environment, which is a student-centered, teachers-guided model. The teacher's role is the guidance and a facilitator for the students to learn. The way of students' learning can get rid of the

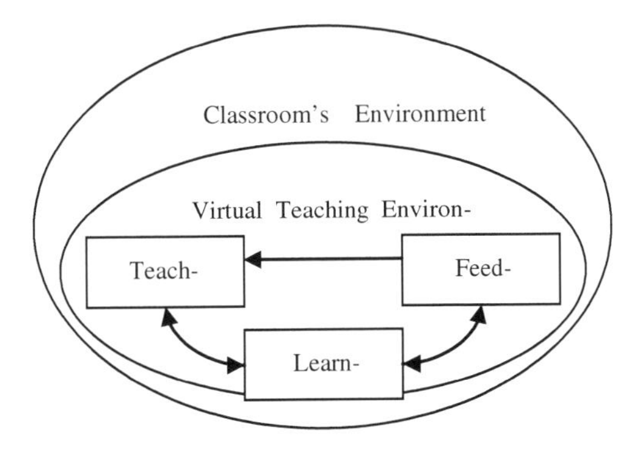

Fig. 6.6 A learning environment

Table 6.1 Performence of spoken language

Difficulty level	Frequency of self evaluating	Total points		Average score on different points			
		Average score	Pass rate	Pronunciation	Intonation	Rhythm	Volum
Junior							
Middle rank							
Senior							
Total							

Table 6.2 The accuracy of pronunciation

Vowel			Consonant		
Phonetic symbol	Standard value	Error rate	Phonetic symbol	Standard value	Error rate

traditional teaching mode from a diverse learning environment. In the learning process, students can break through the limitations of traditional education space and time. With the increase of information, the students' horizons are expanding, and the way of students' learning, the way of thinking gradually are changing, and the status of the students is change to be an active learner from a passive role. Students can learn according to their own dialogue with the teachers in virtual environment, and the students also learn from the real-time tutoring system. The feedback of language learners can be collect, collates, and statistic to teachers by the System Center timely. Teachers and students both can meet their own needs of teaching and learning from diverse resources (Tables 6.1, 6.2).

Table 6.3 Intonation

Item	Standard value	Score
Error freauency of tone of the whole sentence	<20 %	
Average score of the end of sentence intonatotion tone	>75 %	
Fluctuant of intonation	>0.37	

Table 6.4 Rhythm

Item	Standard value	Score
Spoken speed (syllable/a second)	>0.38	
The frequency of unnecessary pause(times a sentence)	<10 %	

6.5 Conclusion

In summary, the research of Corpus is about to enter into a new period, while the labeling will change with the generation of the multi-modal corpus. The multi-modal corpus for teaching Chinese should have eight levels: (1) t the layer of phonetic transcription; (2) the layer of phoneme; (3) the layer of intermittent index; (4) the lay of stress; (5) the layer of target; (6) the layer of phonology; (7) the layer of the behavior (includes the layer of posture and the layer of movement); (8) and the layer of miscellanea. The corpus for teaching Chinese phonetics as a foreign language will improve the classroom teaching efficiency and teaching quality, and help Chinese learners' self-estimation and self-adaption for learning, so it can improve the learner's autonomous learning ability. It supports the Chinese teachers fast, accurate access to phonological teaching resources as well as individual learners and the learning group learning data for the individual guidance and planning adjustment and Tables 6.3, 6.4

Acknowledgments The research has been financially supported by the project of education reform from Beijing International Studies University, which is called "Research on the Mode of Teaching Chinese as a Foreign Language in the Sight of the Cross-Cultural Education Case Studies", and the number of the project is 2013jg1230.

References

1. Beckman M, Elam GA (1997) Guidelines for TOBI labeling (version 3). Linguistics Department, Ohio State University
2. Grabe E, Post B, Nolan F (2000) Modelling intonational variation in english: the IViE system. In: Proceedings of Prosody, Krakow
3. Ladd DR (1996) Intonational phonology[M]. CUP, Cambridge
4. Grabe E, Nolan F, Farrar K (1998) IViE—a comparative transcription system for intonational variation in English. In: Proceedings of the ICSLP, sydney
5. (1998) Evaluation of transcription and annotation tools for a multi-modal[R]. In: Proceedings of the 5th conference on spoken language processing (ICSLP), Sydney. http://www.mpi.nl/tools/elan.html
6. Zhu L (2008) Building a intelligent corpus on teaching middle school based on network environment. China Educ Info 7–9
7. Zhu L (2007) A informational personality foreign language learning platform. Educ Technol Inform
8. Zhu L (2008) Research on personalized teaching model for individual User in ISI: a web based learning systems platforms. In: Paper presented at the international conference on information technology education
9. Jia Y, Aijun-li (2005) Introduce of IViE: a labeling system of corpus. The reacher on phonetics on CASS

7.1 Introduction

There is increasing evidence that Tai Chi or Qigong in Traditional Medicine plays a key role in fighting with diseases and maintain human health [1, 2]. Due to its non-invasive, side effect-free, easy-learning characteristic, more and more people are willing to exercise it. Moreover, in medical society, researchers and educators pay growing attention to playing its role in medicine and education worldwide.

Recently, several surveys reveals that the overall condition of undergraduates' physical and psychological quality is not optimistic, including obvious weaknesses of physical condition and psychological quality, such as endurance and soft quality showing a declining trend, vital capacity cutting down, the rate of obese children and overweight children increasing significantly, and the rate of myopia remaining a high level. Apart from these, anti-setback ability, will power, sense of competition, crisis consciousness, and spirit of cooperation has been worse. While there are significant advances about the traditional health maintenance sports than the west competitive sports in the aspects of physical and psychological health and integrated harmonious development. The effective combination of traditional health maintenance sports and school sports, with the aid of promotion methods of Broadcast Gymnastic Exercise, could integrate the national traditional health maintenance sports into school sports education, which is not only able to promote major undergraduates to inherit traditional culture, but also add more vitality into the development of school sports. In this way, it is able to promote the reform of physical education to develop undergraduates' physical and mental quality, improve the health level and increase the cultural accomplishment.

Broadcast Gymnastic Exercise has been the most widely popularized activity in school, which has been playing a significant role on promoting undergraduates' health and improving the learning efficiency [3]. However, research reveals that the evolution of Broadcast Gymnastic Exercise has experienced a series of important stages. As a representative of the public Broadcast Gymnastic Exercise, "8th Broadcast Gymnastic Exercise" has improved the physical quality, but it is still focusing on the fitness, health maintenance and promoting health, which is not able to reach the purpose of promoting the harmonious development of physical and psychological needs in contemporary undergraduates. Moreover, it dose little association with Tai Chi or Qigong and is hard to inherit the quintessence of Traditional Chinese Medicine. Therefore, it is of significance to create a new kind of Setting-up Exercise fused with the traditional health maintenance sports and Tai Chi or Qigong, which is suitable for the harmonious development of the body and mind. "Chinese Traditional Setting-up Exercise" was elaborately created by professors in sport education department of Beijing University of Chinese Medicine, with following main features: simple actions, clear rhythm, profound connotation, and easy and practical. Each section could pointedly regulate the corresponding internal organ's function so as to relieve fatigue and maintain health.

On the basis of physiologic and medicinal principles, Chinese Traditional Setting-up Exercise belongs to the meridian movement, and its slow gentle movement is able to stabilize and control blood sugar level effectively. However, the scientific evidence of its effectiveness is rarely investigated. Furthermore, its comparison with 8th Broadcast Gymnastic Exercise based on scientific data plays a vital role in popularizing it. When analyzing the collected data sets, information technology, including statistical methods, is a key bridge to communicate the two exercises.

Formally, traditional statistical methods, such as Two-independent samples t test, Pearson Correlation, Linear Regression methods, implemented via information technology by various kinds of programming languages are successfully applied in medical domain to do comparison or compute association. However, due to the complex, multi-dimensional and nonlinear characteristics of exercise data, advanced statistical methods, such as Principal component analysis [4], Random forest [5], should be applied to compare health protection effect of two exercises.

In this paper, we included a group of 200 of undergraduates and randomly separate into two groups. One is of 8th Broadcast Gymnastic Exercise. The other is doing Chinese Traditional Setting-up Exercise. Heart rate (HR), Blood glucose (BG) and Vital capacity (VC) were physically or chemically assayed to compare the effects of two exercises. T test, Pearson Correlation, Principal component analysis, Hierarchical cluster analysis and Random Forest were synthetically applied to analyze the data and evaluate the health protection advantage of Chinese Traditional Setting-up Exercise over 8th Broadcast Gymnastic Exercise.

The paper is organized as following. Section 7.2 is devoted to describing materials and methods used to collect healthy volunteers, assay biological indexes and analyze the associated data. Section 7.3 presents the analyzed results. Conclusion and Discussion were given in Sect. 7.4.

7.2 Material and Method

7.2.1 General Information of Health Undergraduate Volunteer

200 undergraduates, who met the inclusion criteria, had been randomly enrolled from the sophomores in Beijing University of Chinese Medicine from May 2009 to July 2009. They were randomly separated into two groups: case group (Chinese Traditional Setting-up Exercise Group) "and control group (8th Broadcast Gymnastic Exercise Group)" by mean of randomized digital table method. Among the 100 volunteers in the case group, there were 45 males and 55 females, the oldest was 24-year old, the youngest was 16-year old, the mean age was 20.2, the highest was 1.89 m, the lowest was 1.52 m, the mean height was 1.73 m, and the heaviest was 98 kg, the lightest was 44 kg, the mean weight was 61.3 kg; Among the other 100 volunteers in the control group, there were 46 males and 54 females, the oldest

Table 7.1 Basic information of two groups

Group	N	Male/female	Average age (year)	Height (m)	Weight (Kg)
Setting-up exercise	100	45/55	20.2	1.73	61.3
Broadcast gymnastic exercise	100	46/54	20.3	1.72	60.7

was 24-year old, the youngest was 17-year old, the mean age was 20.3, the highest was 1.90 m, the lowest was 1.51 m, the mean height was 1.72 m, and the heaviest was 96 kg, the lightest was 41 kg, the mean weight was 60.7 kg; detailed data was shown in the following Table 7.1. There is no significant difference found between two groups, which indicate that they have homogenous baseline and are comparable.

There was no statistical difference between comparisons of baseline data in two groups ($P > 0.05$) with comparable significance.

7.2.2 Inclusion and Exclusion Criteria

A volunteer meet the following four conditions can be include in the stud:

(1) Sophomore Chinese undergraduates in Beijing University of Chinese Medicine.
(2) Healthy without diabetes, high blood pressure or other serious diseases.
(3) Enough spare time and fond of fitness.
(4) Willing to participate in this research and able to strictly abide by the implementation of the project requirements.

Moreover, there are also three exclusion criteria:

(1) Receiving other relevant treatments, which may affect the effects in this research?
(2) Engagement in other activities or sports may affect this research.
(3) A volunteer is with any irregular habits.

7.2.3 Grouping Method and Practicing Methods

After filling in the basic information, 200 undergraduates were randomly divided into "test group (100 cases)" and "control group (100 cases)" strictly by randomized digital table method, and the test group practiced the Chinese Traditional Setting-up Exercise and the control group practiced the 8th Broadcast Gymnastic Exercise.

(1) Practice period: 1 month (May 26, 2009–June 24, 2009).
(2) Practice time: "Chinese Traditional Setting-up Exercise" and "8th Broadcast Gymnastic Exercise" were practiced three times per week, and each practicing time was 20 min.
(3) Practice site: West playground in Beijing University of Chinese Medicine.
(4) Assay time: The blood glucose value was measured two times respectively before and after the practice.
(5) Processing scheme for the unforeseen circumstances:
In the process of practice, if there were any adverse reactions such as syncope, following methods would be implemented: laying the body, loosening the belt, drinking warm water.
And if these methods were not valid, emergent treatments would be implemented in Chinese and Western medicines. Although these unforeseen circumstances were rare, attention must be paid to.

7.2.4 Assay of Blood Glucose, Heart Rate and Vital Capacity

200 subjects were respectively trained with "Chinese Traditional Setting-up Exercise" and "8th Broadcast Gymnastic Exercise" by special training personnel. During this research, 200 subjects got up at 6 o'clock in the morning every day, receiving the test of blood glucose value by professional personnel, and two groups practiced "Chinese Traditional Setting-up Exercise" or "8th Broadcast Gymnastic Exercise" respectively. 200 subjects would receive the test of blood glucose value by professional personnel at 8 o'clock after movements, and they were not allowed to eat anything until the second test of blood glucose.

Heart rate was measured by using Electronic sphygmomanometer (Omron HEM7101). Vital Capacity was measured by mean of FVC test instrument (EP-FC, Beijing Taimeiquan Inc.)

7.2.5 Systematical Analysis Methods

The index was firstly scaled. T test was employed to compare the variation of index between two groups. Two-independent samples t test was used to detect significant changes between case and control. Pair-sample t test was used to compare significant change of an index before and after an exercise. $P < 0.05$ was considered as significance. Correlation matrix was computed between each pair of the three indexes. Principal component analysis was then employed to separate two groups after exercise and to investigate the importance of indexes. Hierarchical cluster analysis was performed not only on 200 samples, but also on three indexes. Heat map technique was used to intuitionally visualize the cluster results [6]. Random forest classification combined with feature selection was performed to study the interaction between three indexes.

Table 7.2 Comparison of blood glucose change before and after movement in two groups (x ± s)

Biological index	Traditional setting-up exercise group		8th radio gymnastic exercise group	
	Before	After	Before	After
Blood glucose	5.19 ± 1.27	5.00 ± 0.79**	5.14 ± 1.12	5.10 ± 2.26*
Heart rate	2.16 ± 0.97	1.31 ± 0.54**	2.24 ± 1.02	1.66 ± 0.87*
Vital capacity	1.36 ± 0.86	0.40 ± 0.36**	0.90 ± 0.52	0.37 ± 0.32*

Note Comparison within the for group **P < 0.01,*P < 0.05. There were significant statistical differences before and after movement in two groups, and both Chinese Traditional Setting-up Exercise Group and 8th Broadcast Gymnastic Exercise Group could reduce the blood glucose in the view of mean value and clinical literatures to control the stability of the blood glucose

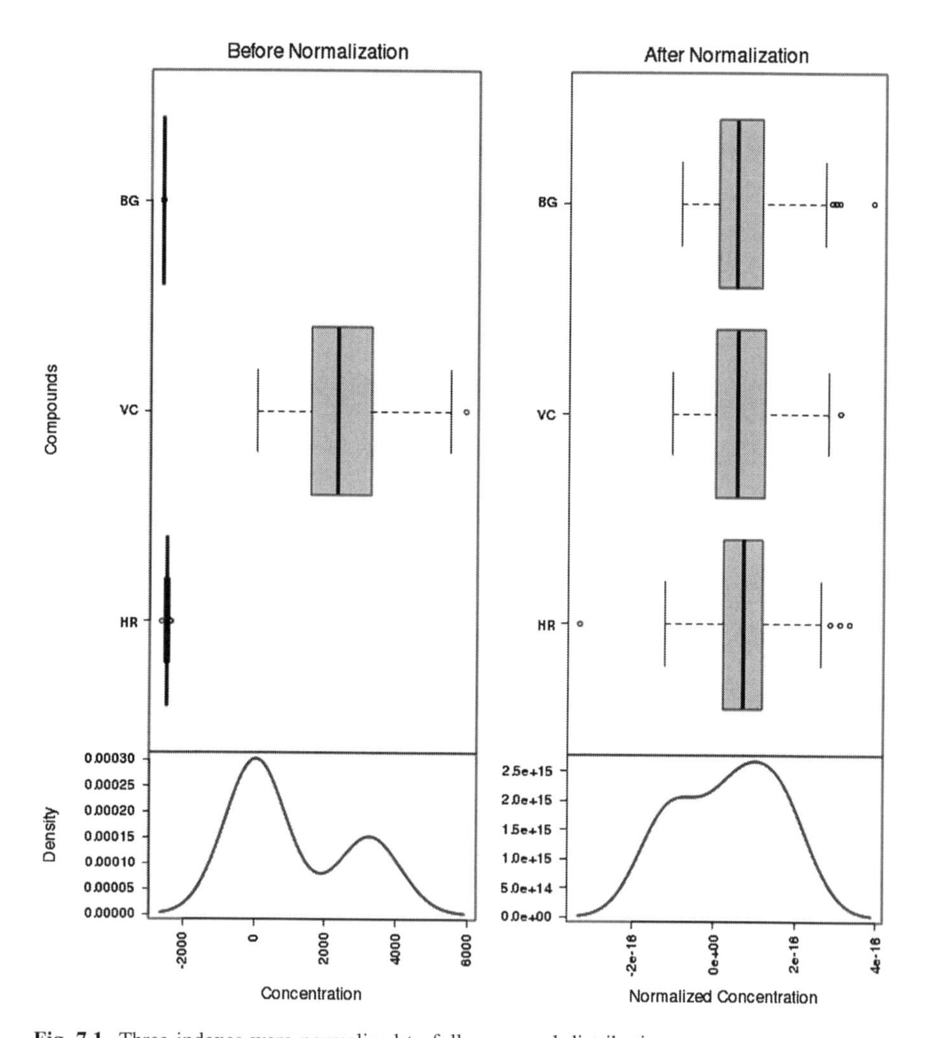

Fig. 7.1 Three indexes were normalized to follow normal distribution

7.3 Results

3.1 Statistical Analysis of Blood Glucose Change before and after Movement in Chinese Traditional Setting-up Exercise Group and 8th Broadcast Gymnastic Exercise Group

As shown in Table 7.2, it was found that three biological indexes have a homogeneous baseline, that is to say, before the two exercises; the mean of each index is with no significant difference. After the exercise, both two groups can significantly improve physical quality of undergraduate students. But the case group performed better than control group. However, the importance and interaction between three indexes were not discovered and needed to be further investigated.

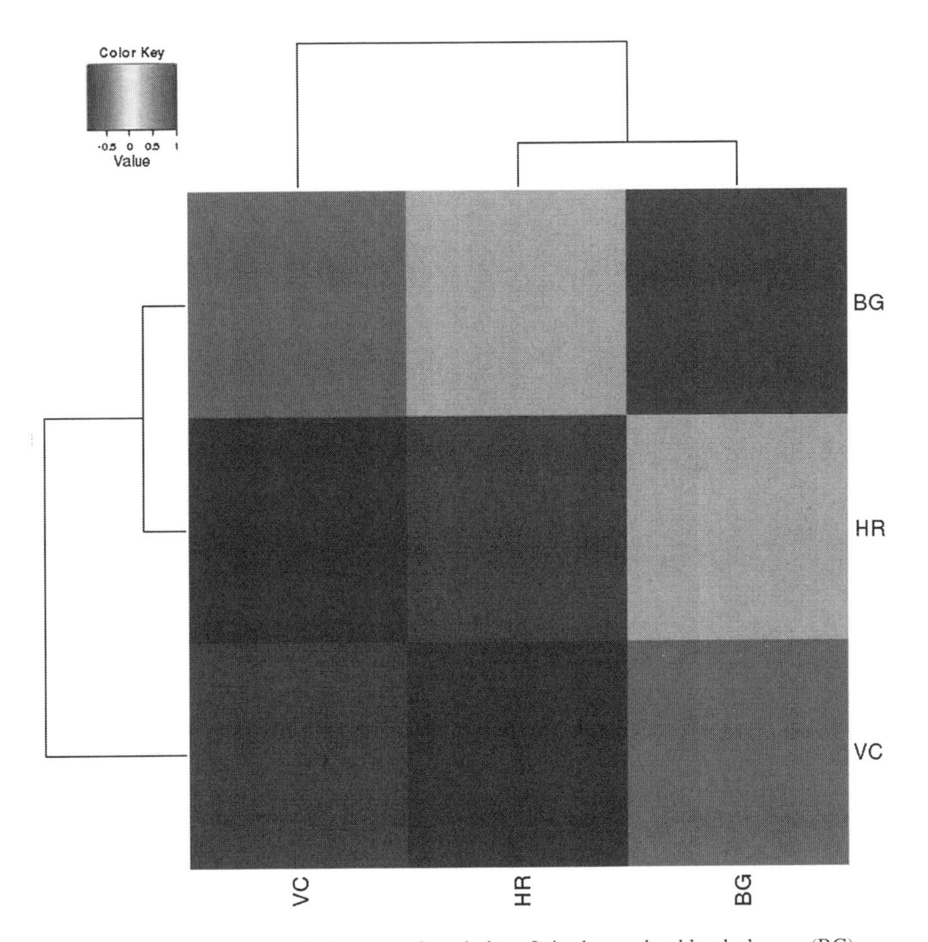

Fig. 7.2 The correlation matrix between three indexesIt is shown that blood glucose (BG) was significantly associated with heart rate (HR). While vital capacity were unrelated with the two indexes

7.3.1 Systematical Analysis Results

Before advanced data analysis, the three indexes should be normalized to a same range scale. As depicted in Fig. 7.1, after normalization, the three indexes were valuing in the same range. And the normalized concentration follows a normal

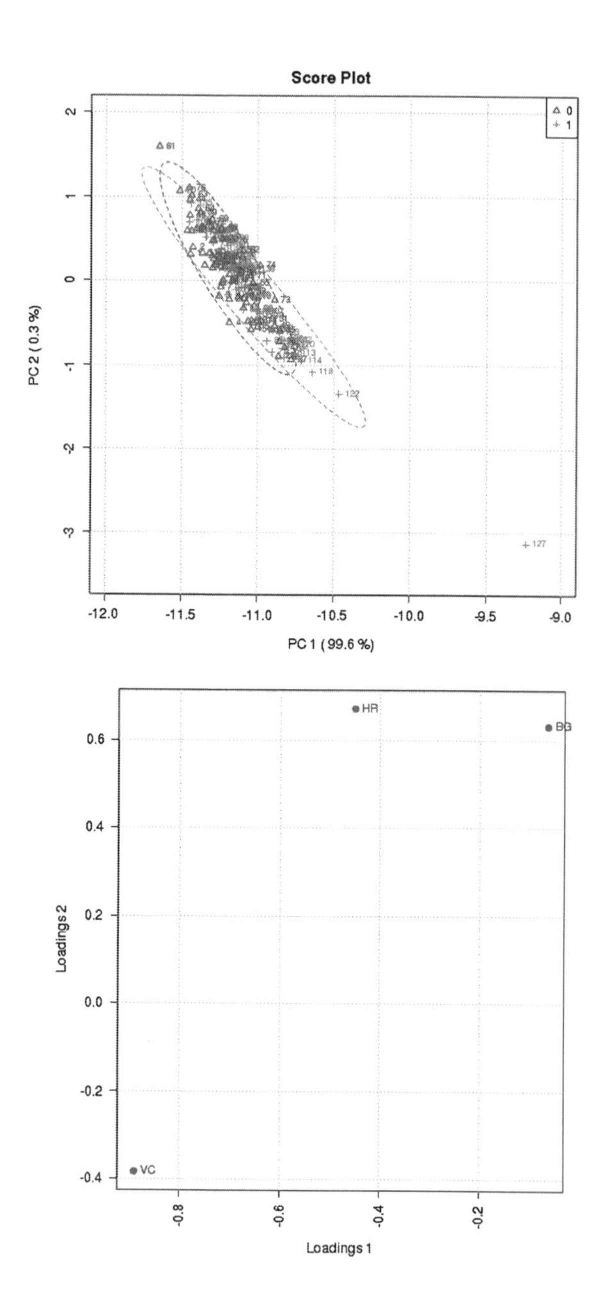

Fig. 7.3 Principal component analysis (PCA) two-dimension score plot indicate that there is a tendency to separate two groups. The loading scoring plot shows that BG is most important

distribution. Therefore, Pearson correlation was used to describe association between each index pair. It was found that BG and HR were associated with each other. But they have a negative association with VC (Fig. 7.2). The three indexes were combined in batch to separate case and control group in an unsupervised way by mean of PCA. It can be discovered that case group were slightly different with control group. The first component occupies a ratio of 96 % in total variance, which meant that it can replace the three indexes. As given in Fig. 7.3, the case group mostly in the right quadrant. The loading plots of PCA showed that BG and HR played a more important role in separating two groups than VC. Moreover, as illustrated in Fig. 7.4, the Hierarchical cluster analysis combined with Heat map depicted that the two groups can be approximately separated (The same color is approximately cluster together).

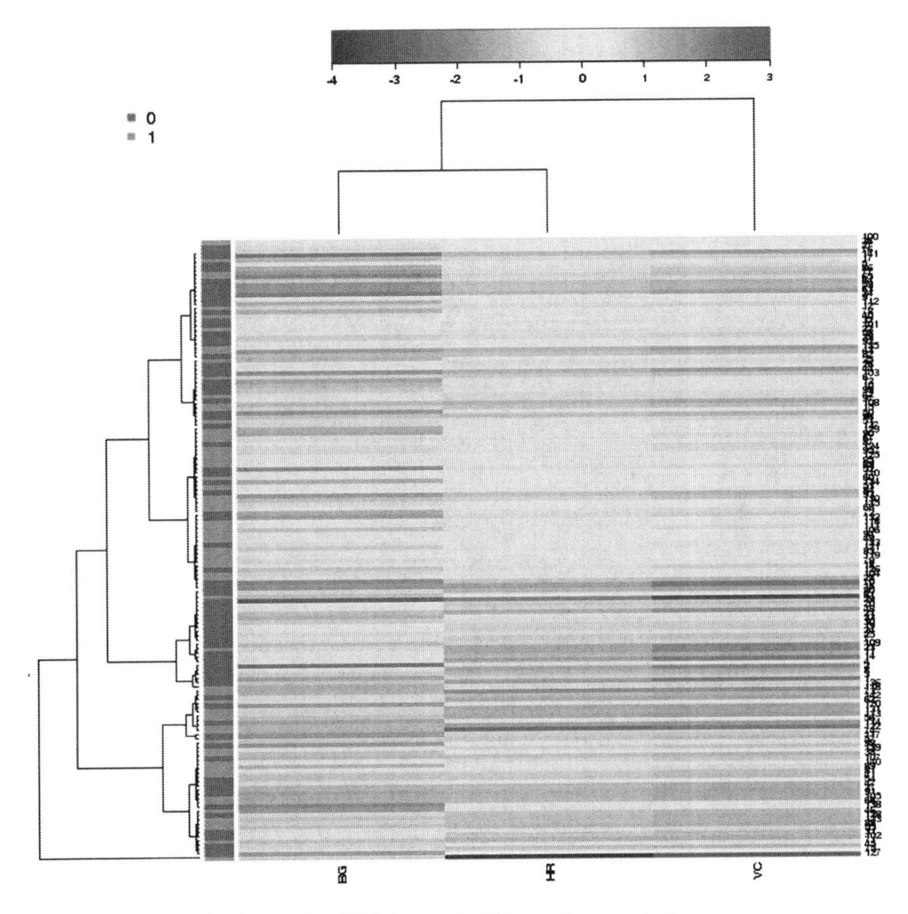

Fig. 7.4 Heat map indicates that CTSE group is different from control group

7.4 Conclusion

In summary, both “Chinese Traditional Setting-up Exercise” and “8th Broadcast Gymnastic Exercise” are able to maintain health care of undergraduate students. But the former performed better than the latter. By mean of systematically data analysis of the two groups, it is found that BG is associated with HR. They combine with VC to separate two groups with an accuracy of nearly 80 %. It is concluded that “Chinese Traditional Setting-up Exercise” can replace "8th Broadcast Gymnastic Exercise” in daily exercise of students.

7.5 Discussion

The traditional health maintenance sports were affected by the chinese traditional culture of Confucianism, Buddhism, Dao, Medicine, and Martial art for thousand years, and gradually formed a profound sports health maintenance system, praising highly the holistic view of body and spirit, and the health care view of Qi-Blood harmony, which had been focusing on the appropriate physical activity, and were suitable for different age groups and different physique. Western sports focus on the body movement, emphasize intaking the energy from outside, and pay attention to the physical form, especially the surface skin and thews, which practice the physical form not the spirit, so it couldn’t establish the real comprehensive health care ideological system.

According to modern medical researches that sports are not only able to improve insulin function and reduce the blood sugar, but also to reduce low-density lipoprotein cholesterol (ldl-c) and improve high-density lipoprotein cholesterol (hdl-c). At the same time, sports have the ability of enhancing the cardiopulmonary function, promoting peripheral circulation, and preventing osteoporosis. Acute sports, such as 100 m race, weight lifting, playing basketball, etc., are able to promote the utilization of glucose in muscle and organs so as to reduce the content of glucose in the blood; however, the blood glucose level lost control without the sports. For undergraduates, it is significant to promote the utilization of sugar in muscles and organs by practicing the Setting-up Exercise daily. Simultaneously, it could reduce the insulin level in blood to control the glucose directly or indirectly and improve insulin resistance. Apart from these, proper movement is better for reducing weight and improving insulin sensitivity to reduce blood sugar, which is particularly obvious for obese undergraduates.

The blood glucose value will rise during the movement or immediately after it, which is responsible for the energy supply and speed up of metabolism. However, if the blood glucose was measured half an hour after the movement, it showed that blood glucose fell down, for the former movement had consumed energy, which is the above issue “Improvement of Insulin Sensitivity”. In fact, this is the corresponding benefit from the long-term exercise, such as the relationship between running and heartbeat, when you are running, the heartbeat will speed up, but if you insist a long-term running, the usual heartbeat will slow down.

The systematical statistical methods were firstly presented here to analyze the data. From single variable (t test), two variables (Correlation methods) to multi-variables (PCA, cluster and classification), we synthesize the data analysis results to uncover the role of an index in separating two groups and the interaction among them. In further work, the sample size and the number of indexes should be enlarged to reach a higher accuracy.

References

1. Wang C, Schmid CH, Rones R, Kalish R, Yinh J, Goldenberg DL, Lee Y, McAlindon T (2010 August 19) A randomized trial of tai chi for fibromyalgia. N Engl J Med 363(8):743–754
2. Leunga RWM, Alisonb JA, McKeoughb ZJ, Petersc MJ (2011) A study design to investigate the effect of short-form Sun-style Tai Chi in improving functional exercise capacity, physical performance, balance and health related quality of life in people with Chronic Obstructive Pulmonary Disease (COPD). Contemp Clin Trials 32(2):267–272
3. Zhao C (2012) The Effects of 8th broadcast gymnastics exercise on heart rate variability and cardiopulmonary function in female undergraduates. Master thesis, Shandong Normal University
4. Gao B, Lu Y, Sheng Y, Chen P, Yu LL (2013) Differentiating organic and conventional sage by chromatographic and mass spectrometry flow-injection fingerprints combined with Principal component analysis. J Agric Food Chem [Epub ahead of print]
5. Yu H, Chen J, Xu X, Li Y, Zhao H et al (2012) A systematic prediction of multiple drug-target interactions from Chemical, Genomic, and Pharmacological data. PLoS One 7(5):e37608. doi:10.1371/journal.pone.0037608
6. Xia J, Mandal R, Sinelnikov I, Broadhurst D, and Wishart DS (2012) Metaboanalyst 2.0—a comprehensive server for metabolomic data analysis. Nucl Acids Res (first published online 2 May 2012)

Chapter 8
Sample-Independent Expression Stability Analysis of Human Housekeeping Genes Using the GeNORM Algorithm

Li Li, Xiaofang Mao, Qiang Gao and Yicheng Cao

Abstract The quantification of mRNAs has been used with great success in many medical research techniques. All of them can use housekeeping genes as internal standards. While most of the commonly used housekeeping genes may have varied expression stability in different human tissue samples or experimental conditions. In this study, 566 housekeeping genes were investigated by conducting a statistical analysis on a large human genome microarray database. The sample-independent expression stability value of every gene was calculated and ranked by using the GeNORM algorithm. Furthermore, microarray expression data of another mammalian model were used to evaluate the variation coefficient of the candidate genes expressed in the mouse models. Most of the candidate housekeeping genes exhibited similar expression stabilities in the two models. This analysis presents the sample-independent expression stability of a set of housekeeping genes.

Keywords Normalization · Housekeeping genes · Internal control · Human genome microarray

---

L. Li · X. Mao · Q. Gao · Y. Cao (✉)
Department of Bioscience and Bioengineering, South China University of Technology, Guangzhou, China
e-mail: yccao@scut.edu.cn

L. Li
e-mail: ottolear@gmail.com

X. Mao
e-mail: xiaofanmao@126.com

Q. Gao
e-mail: gaoqiang201@yahoo.com.cn

S. Li et al. (eds.), *Frontier and Future Development of Information Technology in Medicine and Education*, Lecture Notes in Electrical Engineering 269,
DOI: 10.1007/978-94-007-7618-0_8,

8.1 Introduction

RNA expression analysis is playing an important role in many field of medical research. Microarrays, real-time reverse-transcription polymerase chain reaction, Northern blots, and RNase protection assays are the most commonly used quantitative analysis methods for RNA expression. To correct for sample-to-sample variation, normalization of the expression data is required in all these methods [1]. The conventional way to perform normalization is to select a reference gene whose expression is believed to remain stable across all experimental conditions. The 18s or 28s rRNA molecules are widely considered as the representatives for mRNA integrity because of their capability to remain intact in experiment samples with degraded mRNAs. However, several problems exist with using rRNAs as control genes. First, rRNAs have a different polymerase transcription system from mRNAs. Many changes in the polymerase activity do not affect both types of RNA expressions [2]. rRNA transcription is also reportedly affected by many experimental conditions and biological factors [3, 4], and the effect of partial RNA degradation in 18s rRNA expression levels is smaller than in mRNA expression [5].

Housekeeping genes are also widely used as internal standards in quantitative analysis because their synthesis occurs in all nucleated cell types. Housekeeping genes are necessary for cell survival and are usually essential for cell function maintenance [6, 7]. Compared with rRNAs, housekeeping genes are constitutively expressed at similar levels in all cell types and tissues, and share the same transcribed system with other common mRNAs [8]. However, numerous reports have indicated that the expression of these housekeeping genes varies across tissues and cell types, particularly in routine laboratory applications [9, 10]. Thus, selecting the appropriate control genes for specific tissue samples is vital to a gene expression analysis. Different housekeeping genes have been considered as the only proper reference genes for some specific tissues or experimental conditions, and two or more internal control genes are usually employed in numerous experimental analyses [11, 12]. Speleman et al. [13] developed the GeNORM program, which uses geometric means to calculate the correct normalizing factor from existing housekeeping genes. This algorithm has been widely used as one of the best tools for determining the most stably expressed genes for RNA expression analysis.

After appropriate modifications, the GeNORM algorithm was adopted to evaluate the expression variability of 566 housekeeping genes under various experimental conditions [14]. This work investigated a large set of expression data from 13,629 published human genome gene arrays, which included 18 homo genome microarray platforms, 217 disease types, 475 tissues or cell types, and 430 experimental conditions. The comparison result, sorted by expression stability value, was listed. Furthermore, four sets of mouse genome microarray expression data Gene Expression Omnibus (GEO) dataset accession numbers: GDS3864, GDS3622, GDS2882, GDS2917) were used to evaluate the Coefficient of Variation (CV) of the candidate genes expressed in the mouse models [15]. Most of the housekeeping genes with lower variations in expression level in the human microarray data also exhibited higher expressed stabilities in the mouse microarray data.

8.2 Materials and Methods

8.2.1 Microarray Samples

The microarray samples included the following 18 human genome microarray platforms: Affymetrix Human Genome U95A, U95B, U95C, U95D, U95E, U133A, U133B, U133 Plus 2.0, and U95A V2 arrays; two Affymetrix Human Genome U133A 2.0 arrays, two ABI Human Genome V1, and two V2 arrays; Agilent Human Genome G4112A and G4112F arrays; and General Electric Human Genome array. A total of 16,398 microarray expression data were downloaded from the GEO database of the National Centre for Biotechnology Information. This set of samples comprises the gene expression data of various disease types or stages (e.g., breast cancer, acute myeloid leukemia, hepatoma, hereditary gingival fibromatosis, and others), different tissue samples (e.g., MCF7 breast cancer cell line, skeletal muscle, hepatoma cell line, LM2 breast cancer cell line, among others), and varying experimental conditions (e.g., cigarette smoking, interleukin-20 subfamily cytokine treatment, lung transplant, β-catenin depleted cells, Anaplasma phagocytophilum infection, and others). Probe sets available on all platforms were converted to official gene symbols and average expression values for multiple probe sets targeting the same gene.

8.2.2 Statistical Data Analysis

The GeNORM algorithm defines the internal control gene-stability measurement V as the average paired variation of a particular gene with all the other candidate genes. The genes with the lowest V-values exhibit the most stable expressions. The entire calculation process of the V-value is expressed as the following three functions.

$$\mu_{jk} = \frac{1}{N}\sum_{i=1}^{N}\left(\frac{X_{ij}}{X_{ik}}\right) \tag{8.1}$$

$$\sigma_{jk} = \sqrt{\frac{1}{N}\sum_{i=1}^{N}\left(X_{ij} - \mu_{jk}\right)^2} \tag{8.2}$$

$$V_k = \frac{1}{M}\sum_{j=1}^{M}\sigma_{jk} \tag{8.3}$$

For any given housekeeping gene K, where X_{ik} stands for the expression value of gene k in sample i, X_{ij} represents the same value of another candidate gene j in sample i, N equals the number of microarray samples: 16,398, and M equals the number of candidate genes: 566, then σ_{jk} refers to the standard deviation of the X_j to X_k ratio in every sample, and V_k can be interpreted as the arithmetic mean of j_k of 566 housekeeping genes to gene k. These functions were implemented by using a Perl script [16]. Then, the expression stability values of all the candidate housekeeping genes were obtained. Along with five commonly used reference genes (Beta-2-microglobulin, B2 M; Glyceraldehyde-3-phosphate dehydrogenase, GAPD; tubulin beta 2A, TUBB; Lactate dehydrogenase A, LDHA; Actin beta, ACTB), the top ten genes with the lowest V-values are listed in Table 8.1.

8.2.3 Comparison Analysis

The CV is a useful statistical tool for comparing the scatter of variables measured in different units [17]. This study used CV to investigate the top 100 sample-independent stable expression housekeeping genes obtained from the human microarray data analysis. Four largest mouse microarray datasets of the Affymetrix Mouse Genome 430 2.0 array, which included 347 microarray samples, were downloaded from the GEO [18]. Considering that the probes of the mouse array platform do not include the entire candidate housekeeping genes, four genes were excluded, and the CVs of the remaining genes expressed in all the mouse samples were calculated and ranked. In addition, the distribution of the expression levels of the top ten sample-independent expression stability housekeeping genes expressed in the mouse models was also plotted, as shown in Fig. 8.1.

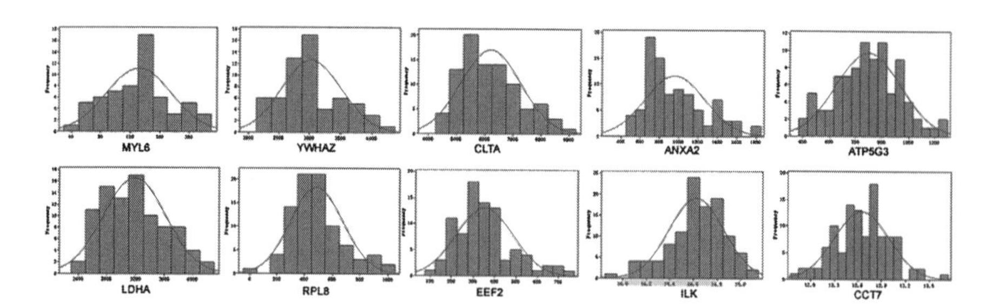

Fig. 8.1 The distribution of the expression levels of *top* ten sample-independent expression stability housekeeping genes expressed in mouse model

8.3 Results and Discussion

Based on the principle that the expression ratio of two ideal reference genes is constant in all samples, independent of the experimental conditions, this study used the GeNORM algorithm to investigate the sample-independent expression stability of 566 housekeeping genes. The paired expression ratio of the given housekeeping genes to any other gene in each of the 16,398 samples was calculated. By comparing the mean values of the standard deviation of these expression ratios, a list of the common housekeeping genes sorted by sample-independent expression stability was obtained. It is available online at http://hpabws.s87.cnaaa1.com/cert/sies.htm. The stability values and other information of the top ten housekeeping genes on the list and five commonly used reference genes are shown in Table 8.1. The result indicates that the commonly used reference genes did not show more significant expression stability than other housekeeping genes. The box plot (Fig. 8.2) presents the standard deviation values of the ten genes. All the ten genes displayed smaller dispersion and lower quantity of outliers, and the distribution areas of each gene presented a gradually increasing trend in the box view.

Table 8.1 Top ten sample-independent expression stability housekeeping genes and five commonly used reference genes

Gene symbol	Accession number	Gene name	Expression stability
MYL6	NM_021019	Myosin, light polypeptide 6, alkali, smooth muscle and non-muscle	0.2143
YWHAZ	NM_003406	Tyrosine 3-monooxygenase/ tryptophan 5-monooxygenase activation protein, zeta polypeptide	0.941
CLTA	NM_001833	Clathrin, light polypeptide	1.016
ANXA2	NM_004039	Annexin A2	1.1297
ATP5G3	NM_001689	ATP synthase, H + transporting, mitochondrial F0 complex, subunit c(subunit 9) isoform 3	1.4017
LDHA*	NM_005566	Lactate dehydrogenase A	1.5274
RPL8	NM_000973	Ribosomal protein L8	1.765
EEF2	NM_001961	Eukaryotic translation elongation factor 2	1.8117
ILK	NM_004517	Integrin-linked kinase	2.313
CCT7	NM_006429	Chaperonin containing TCP1, subunit 7	2.3183
GAPD*	NM_002046	Glyceraldehyde-3-phosphate dehydrogenase	5.5144
B2 M*	NM_004048	Beta-2-microglobulin	6.8382
ACTB*	NM_001101	Actin, beta	31.7909
TUBB*	NM_001069	Tubulin, beta	57.7769

* Five commonly used reference genes

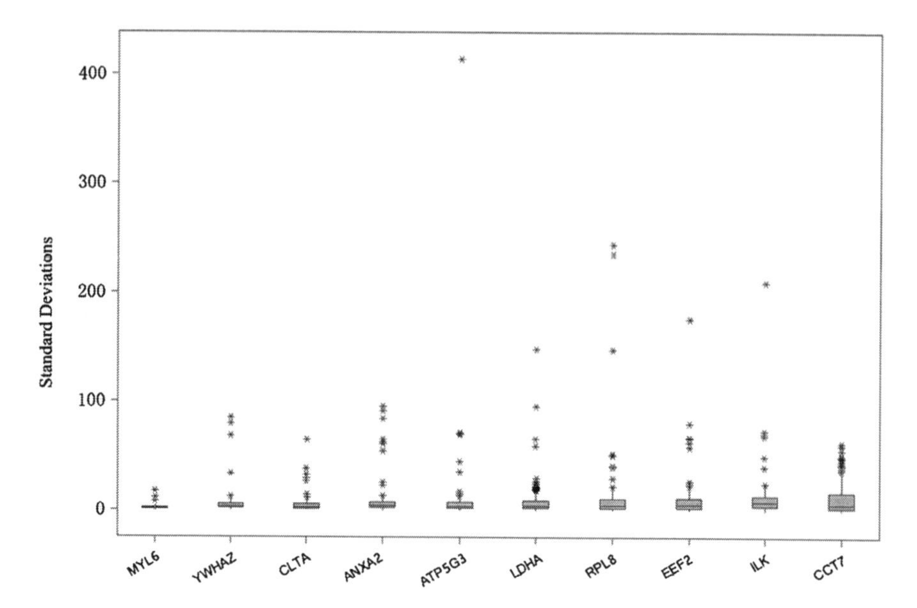

Fig. 8.2 Box plot of standard deviations of *top* ten sample-independent expression stability housekeeping genes

Another mammalian model system (Affymetrix Mouse Genome 430 2.0 Gene Chip) from the GEO databases was adopted, and the CV of the top 100 sample-independent stable expression genes screened was calculated by using the GeNORM algorithm to validate the statistical data analysis method employed in this work. In Fig. 8.3, scatter plot A shows the expression stability values of the top 100 genes expressed in the human model, and the CV of these genes expressed in all the mouse samples are presented in plot B. The baselines of the two scatter plots indicated a similar linear regularity to each other. The results illustrated that the GeNORM algorithm is a feasible method for comparing the expression stabilities of housekeeping genes across various samples and experimental conditions.

The selection of the proper housekeeping genes as internal controls is vital to gene expression analysis. For this reason, 566 housekeeping genes were investigated by conducting a statistical analysis on a large human microarray database, and a comparison of the sample-independent expression stabilities of all the candidate genes was carried out. The top 100 genes with the lowest expression stability values were selected for validation, and the CV values of these genes expressed in four sets of mouse genome microarray data were calculated and plotted. The results indicated that the expression levels of the housekeeping genes expressed in the mouse models have a variation rule similar to those expressed in the human model. Based on the GeNORM algorithm, this paper presents a list of common housekeeping genes, ranked by sample-independent expression stability,

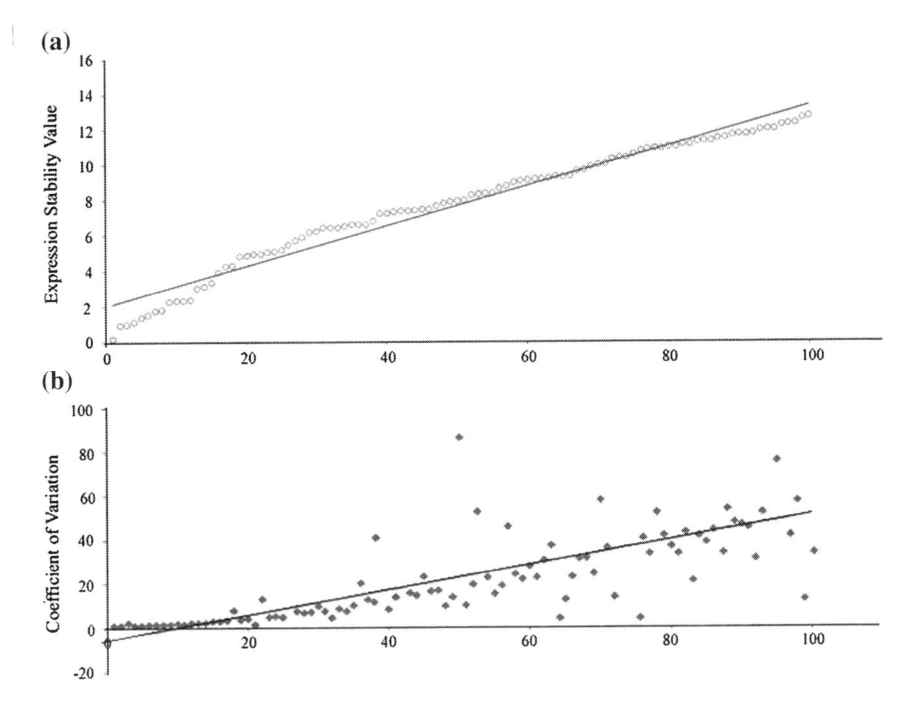

Fig. 8.3 *Top* 100 sample-independent stable expression housekeeping genes. **a** the expression stability value of genes expressed in human microarray data; **b** the coefficient of variation value of genes expressed in mouse microarray data. (X-axis): the gene order in the list obtained by stable expression comparison

and provides a reference tool for selecting the appropriate control gene in human RNA expression experiments.

Acknowledgments This research was supported by the Sciences and Technologies Projects of Science and Information Technology Bureau of GuangZhou. China (Grant No. 2005Z12E4023).

References

1. Suzuki T, Higgins PJ, Crawford DR (2000) Control selection for RNA quantitation. Biotechniques 29:6
2. de Kok JB, Roelofs RW, Giesendorf BA, Pennings JL, Waas ET, Feuth T, Swinkels DW, Span PN (2004) Normalization of gene expression measurements in tumor tissues: comparison of 13 endogenous control genes. Lab Invest 85:154–159
3. Gokal PK, Cavanaugh AH, Thompson EA (1986) The effects of cycloheximide upon transcription of rRNA, 5s RNA, and tRNA genes. J Biol Chem 261:2536–2541
4. Ayrault O, Andrique L, Fauvin D, Eymin B, Gazzeri S, Seite P (2006) Human tumor suppressor p14ARF negatively regulates rRNA transcription and inhibits UBF1 transcription factor phosphorylation. Oncogene 25:7577–7586

5. Brunner A, Yakovlev I, Strauss S (2004) Validating internal controls for quantitative plant gene expression studies. BMC Plant Biol 4:14
6. De Ferrari L, Aitken S (2006) Mining housekeeping genes with a Naive Bayes classifier. BMC Genomics 7:277
7. Nico J, Michel J, Tim P, Annette B (2004) Housekeeping Genes as Internal Standards in Cancer Research. Molecular Diagnosis 8:107–113
8. Thellin O, Zorzi W, Lakaye B, De Borman B, Coumans B, Hennen G, Grisar T, Igout A, Heinen E (1999) Housekeeping genes as internal standards: use and limits. J Biotechnol 75:291–295
9. Lee PD, Sladek R, Greenwood CMT, Hudson TJ (2002) Control genes and variability: absence of ubiquitous reference transcripts in diverse mammalian expression studies. Genome Res 12:292–297
10. Rubie C, Kempf K, Hans J, Su T, Tilton B, Georg T, Brittner B, Ludwig B, Schilling M (2005) Housekeeping gene variability in normal and cancerous colorectal, pancreatic, esophageal, gastric and hepatic tissues. Mol Cell Probes 19:101–109
11. Radonić A, Thulke S, Mackay IM, Landt O, Siegert W, Nitsche A (2004) Guideline to reference gene selection for quantitative real-time PCR. Biochem Biophys Res Commun 313:856–862
12. Banda M, Bommineni A, Thomas RA, Luckinbill LS, Tucker JD (2008) Evaluation and validation of housekeeping genes in response to ionizing radiation and chemical exposure for normalizing RNA expression in real-time PCR. Mutat Res 649:126–134
13. Vandesompele J, De Preter K, Pattyn F et al (2002) Accurate normalization of real-time quantitative RT-PCR data by geometric averaging of multiple internal control genes, Genome Biol 3:research0034.0031–research0034.0011
14. Eisenberg E, Levanon EY (2003) Human housekeeping genes are compact. Trends Genet 19:362–365
15. Barrett T, Troup DB, Wilhite SE, Ledoux P, Rudnev D, Evangelista C, Kim IF, Soboleva A, Tomashevsky M, Edgar R (2007) NCBI GEO: mining tens of millions of expression profiles–database and tools update. Nucleic Acids Res 35:760–765
16. Wall TCL, Orwant J (2000) Programming perl. 3rd edn. O'Reilly Media, Cambridge
17. Reed GF, Lynn F, Meade BD (2002) Use of coefficient of variation in assessing variability of quantitative assays. Clin Diagn Lab Immunol 9:1235–1239
18. Edgar R, Domrachev M, Lash AE (2002) Gene expression omnibus: NCBI gene expression and hybridization array data repository. Nucleic Acids Res 30:207–210

Chapter 9
Development of a One-Step Immunochromatographic Strip Test for Rapid Detection of Antibodies Against Classic Swine Fever

Huiying Ren, Shun Zhou, Jianxin Wen, Xinmei Zhan, Wenhua Liu and Shangin Cui

Abstract An immunochromatographic strip (GICA strip) was developed for the simple and rapid detection of antibodies against classical swine fever virus (CSFV). In the GICA strip, the expressed protein of E2 was labeled with colloidal gold and was used as the detector, and the staphylococcal protein A (SPA) and swine antibody against CSFV blotted on the nitrocellulose membrane were used for the test and control lines, respectively. Conjugation of E2 protein with colloidal gold was optimal at 5.25 μg of protein per mL of colloidal gold. The optimum concentration of the E2 protein applied at the test line was 1.5 mg/mL. The GICA strip was specific for antibodies against CSFV, produced negative results with sera from noninfected pigs or other animals, and was as sensitive or nearly as sensitive as ELISA and HI. According to the comparison of GICA strips with IDEXX ELISA kits, the coincidence rate was 93.26 %. The strips produced results within 5–15 min and can be stored at 4 °C for 3 years or 37 °C 1 year. The strip can be useful for both country veterinarians and field epidemiologists.

Keywords Antibody · Classical swine fever · Rapid test · Strip

---

H. Ren (✉) · S. Zhou · J. Wen · X. Zhan · W. Liu
Qingdao Agricultural University, 266109 Qingdao, China
e-mail: renren0228@sina.com

S. Cui
State Key Laboratory of Veterinary Biotechnology, Division of Swine Infectious Diseases, Harbin Veterinary Research Institute of Chinese Academy of Agricultural Sciences, Harbin, China
e-mail: cuishangjin@126.com

S. Li et al. (eds.), *Frontier and Future Development of Information Technology in Medicine and Education*, Lecture Notes in Electrical Engineering 269,
DOI: 10.1007/978-94-007-7618-0_9,

9.1 Introduction

The classical swine fever (CSF) caused by classical swine fever virus (CSFV), is a highly contagious viral infection of domestic pigs and wild boars, and also one of the most devastating porcine diseases worldwide (Moennig et al. 2003). The disease is endemic in Asia and common in many Central and South American countries as well as in Eastern Europe [5]. Though many countries (e.g., European Union member states) pursue a non-vaccination eradication policy, massive vaccination with attenuated vaccines, such as hog cholera lapinized vaccine (HCLV) (also known as C-strain), has been a major control strategy in China and many other developing countries [4]. In spite of these massive vaccinations, CSF outbreaks still occur in China, and remain as the main disease of swine in China. In recent years, non-typical or chronic CSF caused immunization failures have been frequently reported, mainly due to maternal antibody interference and immunotolerance caused by improper immunization [6].

Traditional methods for the diagnosis of CSFV infection and detection of antibodies to CSFV include indirect hemagglutination (HA) test, fluorescent antibody test, reverse transcription polymerase chain reaction(RT-PCR), enzyme linked immunosorbent assay (ELISA) and hemagglutination inhibition (HI) assay. Although these techniques are highly sensitive and specific for CSFV detection, they are all time-consuming. A practical and rapid method to detect antibodies against CSFV is therefore needed. The colloid gold immunochromatographic strip assay (GICA) is a new immunochromatographic technique in which a cellulose membrane is used as the carrier and a colloidal gold-labeled antigen or antibody is used as the tracer. This technology has several advantages over traditional immunoassays, such as simple procedure, rapid operation, immediate results, low cost, and no requirements for skilled technicians or expensive equipments. These characteristics make the colloidal gold strip test suitable for on-site detection of antibodies or antigens (Peng et al. 2007). In our previous works, we have described colloidal gold strip tests for porcine reproductive and respiratory syndrome virus (PRRSV) [3, 8] and Avian Influenza Virus (AIV) [1, 3]. This paper describes the development, optimization, and evaluation of a novel immunochromatographic strip for the rapid detection of antibodies against CSFV.

9.2 Materials and Methods

9.2.1 Materials

CSFV, porcine epidemic diarrhea virus (PEDV), transmissible gastroenteritis virus (TGEV), porcine rota virus (PRoV), pseudorabies virus (PRV), porcine parvovirus (PPV), PRRSV, and sera with antibodies against them were Provided by Shandong academy of agricultural science. A total of 885 sera samples including 820 swine sera and 15 sera samples from other animals (chicken, duck, goose, and goat) were collected from 36 farms in Shandong province.

Chlorauric acid was purchased from the First Biochemical Reagent Factory of Shanghai(Shanghai China). Nitrocellulose membrane was purchased from Gene Company Limited of Shanghai. CSF ELISA kits were provided by the HVRI, and IH kits were provided by the Lanzhou Veterinary Research Institute(Lanzhou China).

9.2.2 Preparation of Recombinant CSFV E2 Protein

The CSFV E2 fragment was amplified by PCR from the recombinant pMD18T-E2 plasmid. The primers were:

Pf: 5′ tcgaattcatgcgtctagcctgca 3′

Pr:5′ tggtgagtgagtaaagcccccttat3′. The amplified DNA fragment was digested and then ligated into the pET-32a vector (Novagen, Darmstadt, Germany). The ligated plasmid was transformed to *Escherichia coli* BL21 competent cells. The positive clone was grown in LB broth supplemented with 100 g/mL ampicillin and 1 mM isopropyl-d-thiogalactopyranoside (IPTG). After 5 h of induction at 37 °C, cells were harvested by centrifugation and resuspended in 20 mL of lysis buffer (10 mM Tris–HCl, 0.15 M NaCl, 10 mM EDTA, 0.5 mM PMSF, 2 mM DTT, 10 % glycerol, and 400 g/mL of lysozyme pH 8.0).

The cells were sonicated and centrifuged for 20 min at 12000×*g* (SS-34 rotator). The inclusion bodies were collected, purified, denatured, and refolded. The refolded E2 protein was adjusted to 1 mg/mL, and aliquots were stored at -70 °C.

9.2.3 Preparation of Antibodies Against CSFV

Four healthy pigs were intra-subcutaneously injected with Hog cholera lapinized virus (HCLV) obtained from HVRI. Pigs were subsequently booster injected two more times with the vaccine at 2-week intervals. Two weeks after the last injection, sera were collected, and blood samples with high titers of antibodies against CSFV were collected from the immunized pigs. The pig IgG against CSFV was isolated from the immunized sera by sequential precipitation with 50, 40, and 33 % saturated ammonium sulphate (w/v, SAS). After dialysis in 0.01 M PBS (pH 7.2), the titer of the IgG against CSFV was determined to be 1:12800 with a c-ELISA Kit (IDEXX, USA). The purified IgG against CSFV was then stored at -20 °C in 1 mL aliquots.

9.2.4 Preparation of the Colloidal Gold-Labeled Antigen

Colloidal gold was prepared by trisodium citrate reaction. All glassware used in the following procedures was cleaned in a bath of $K_2Cr_2O_7$–H_2SO_4, rinsed thoroughly in double-distilled water, and dried in the air. After 1 mL of a 1 % $HAuCl_4$ solution was added to 99 mL of deionized water and heated to boiling, 2 mL of 1 % trisodium citrate was immediately added to the mixture and was heated for 5–7 min until the mixture turned red. After the mixture was passed through a 0.45-μm micropore filter, the colloidal Au in the filtrate was examined with transmission electron microscopy [7].

Aliquots (1 ml) of colloidal gold and 100 μl of CSFV E2 protein (32.32 μg of protein per ml) were diluted with 0.005 M NaCl in a twofold dilution series with 11 dilutions; each dilution was added to a clear, 10-ml tube. A 12th tube without protein was the control. The concentration of E2 protein in each tube was conform with a spectrophotometer. After 10 min, 100 μL of 10 % NaCl solution was added to each tube, and the contents were stirred. The color of the tubes was observed after incubation at 4 °C for 2 h. The optimal dilution was the maximum dilution of protein that can be visualized by colloidal gold. In practice, to improve the performance of the assay, the protein quantity we used for labeling was 30 % higher than the optimal dilution.

Colloidal gold (100 mL) was prepared and adjusted to pH 9.0 with 0.2 M K_2CO_3. Then, the optimal ratio of CSFV E2 protein (5.25 μg of protein per mL of colloidal gold, see Results) was added to the colloidal gold with moderate stirring for 15 min. Tris –HCl (1 mL, 10 % BSA, 20 mM, pH 7.2) was added to the mixture with moderate stirring for 20 min. After 0.4 mL of 5 % PEG 20000 was added, the mixture was stirred for 15 min and then kept at 4 °C overnight. The colloidal gold -conjugated E2 was centrifuged at 3000 rpm at 4 °C for 30 min, and the supernatant was centrifuged at 12000 rpm for 40 min at 4 °C. The pellet was resuspended in 20 mM Tris –HCl with 1 % BSA (pH 7.2), and the suspension was again centrifuged at 12000 rpm for 40 min at 4 °C. Finally, the supernatant was passed through a 40-μm micropore filter and was stored at 4 °C.

9.2.5 Immobilization of Capture Reagents

Staphylococcal protein A (SPA) (Sigma, Louis, MO, USA) at 0.5 mg/mL and swine antibodies against CSFV at 1 mg/mL (prepared as described above) were dispensed by the Quanti 3000 Biojets attached to a XYZ Biostrip Dispenser (Bio-Dot, Irvine, CA, USA) onto a HiFlow Plus Cellulose Ester Membrane (300 mm × 25 mm, Millipore, Bedford, MA, USA) as the test and control lines, respectively. The test and control lines were situated 0.5 cm apart at the center of the membrane. The membrane has a nominal capillary flow time of 180 s/4 cm and a nominal membrane thickness of 135 μm. These reagents were applied in form of dots at 50 dots/mL/cm on the membrane. After drying for 1 h at 40 °C, the membrane was sealed and stored under dry condition at room temperature.

9.2.6 Preparation and Assembly of the GICA Strip

The strip was assembled as described previously for other viruses [1, 3]; (Zhou et al. 2008) and as shown in Fig. 9.1. Briefly, the sample and absorbent pads were made from nonwoven, 100 % pure cellulose of C048 membrane (Millipore, Bedford, MA, USA). The sample pad was cut into to 15 mm × 300 mm strips, saturated in a buffer (pH 8.0) containing 20 mM sodium borate, 2.0 % (w/v) sucrose, 2.0 % (w/v) BSA, and 0.1 % (w/v) NaN_3, air dried, and stored as

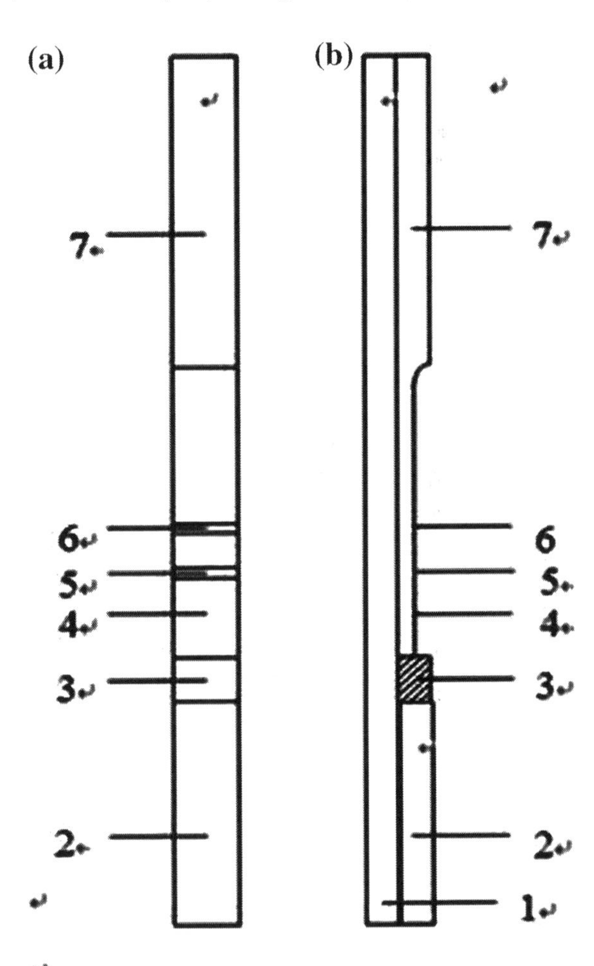

Fig. 9.1 Schematic diagram of gold immumochromatographic strips **a** *top view*; **b** *side view*. *1* Backing plate; *2* Sample pad; *3* Conjugate pad; *4* Nitrocellulose blotting membranes; *5* Test line; *6* Control line; *7* Absorbent pad

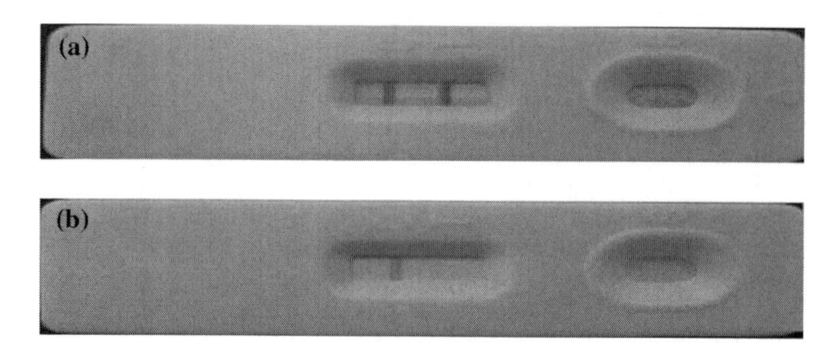

Fig. 9.2 Products of immunocolloidal gold strip. **a** Positive result; **b** negative result

described above. The absorbent pad was cut into 20 mm × 300 mm strips. Then the sample pad, conjugate pad, blotted membrane, and absorbent pad were assembled on the plastic backing support board sequentially with a 1–2-mm overlap to make master cards which were then cut into 4.1-mm-wide strips using a CM-4000 Cutter (Bio-Dot, Irvine, CA, USA). Each assembly was housed in a plastic case that was then sealed in a plastic bag in the presence of desiccant gel and stored at 4 °C.

The sample pad was coated with CSFV E2 protein conjugated by colloidal gold, and SPA and swine antibody against CSFV were blotted on the nitrocellulose membrane for the test (C) and control (T) lines, respectively. When a serum sample containing CSFV antibody is added to the sample pad, the serum moves by capillary action across the conjugated pad where the SPA and CSFV antibody links with the gold-labeled antigen. The complex of the gold-labeled antigen–antibody continues to move through the nitrocellulose membrane and will form two visible lines, one at T and one at C. If a serum sample without CSFV antibody is added to the sample pad, only one line will appear at C, but not at T (Fig. 9.2).

When a serum sample containing CSFV antibody is added to the sample pad, the serum moves by capillary action across the conjugated pad where the SPA and CSFV antibody links with the gold-labeled antigen. The complex of the gold-labeled antigen–antibody continues to move through the nitrocellulose membrane and will produce two lines, one at T and one at C, as shown in A. When a serum sample that does not contain CSFV antibody is added to the sample pad, the serum moves by capillary action across the conjugated pad where the CSFV antibody links with the gold-labeled antigen. The complex of the gold-labeled antigen–antibody continues to move through the nitrocellulose membrane and will produce one line only, at C, as shown in B.

9.2.7 Specificity and Sensitivity of the GICA Strip

The specificity of the GICA strip for CSFV antibody was determined by applying sera samples from swine infected with the following viruses: PEDV, TGEV,

PRoV, PRV, PPV, and PRRSV. Serum from swine infected with CSFV was used as a positive control.

To determine the sensitivity of the assay, 1 ml serum from swine infected with CSFV was diluted with PBS to make two fold dilution series. The samples were added to the GICA strip to determine the minimum concentration that can be detected with the new assay. For comparison, the same samples were also subjected to c-ELISA and HI detection.

9.2.8 Field Tests of GICA Strips

A total of 885 field serum samples were checked for the presence of CSFV with GICA strips as well as ELISA and HI for comparison.

9.2.9 GICA Strip Compares with IDEXX ELISA Kit

In clinical trials, ELISA kit (IDEXX USA) is used as control to examine the coincidence rate of GICA strip. The ELISA kit is operated according to the instructions.

9.2.10 Storage Life of the GICA Strips

GICA strips were placed in desiccated plastic bags with desiccant (silica gel). The bags were sealed and stored at 4 and 37 °C. The storage life of the GICA strips was determined by testing five strips stored at each temperature every month for consecutive 36 months with a CSFV antibody-positive serum and a negative serum.

9.3 Results

9.3.1 Quality of Colloidal Gold

The colloidal gold particles were well dispersed and had a regular shape when examined with the electron microscope (Fig. 9.3). The particle diameter was about 18–20 nm, which was consistent with the requirements of the assay.

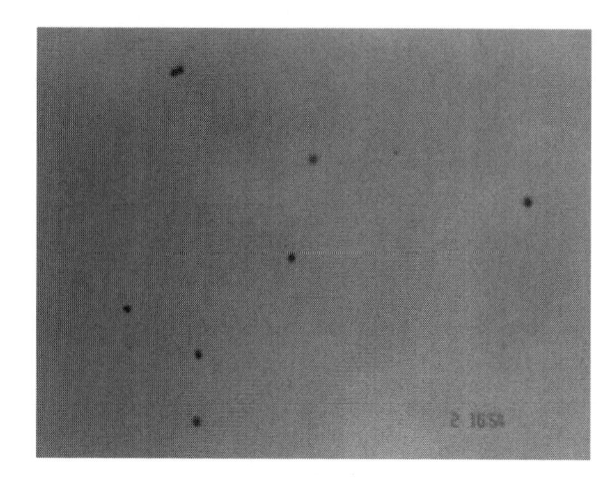

Fig. 9.3 Electron micrographs of colloidal gold particles (20 nm diameter) before conjugation with the CSFV E2 protein

9.3.2 Optimal Concentration of Protein for Colloidal Gold Conjugation

The results shown in Fig. 9.4 indicated that 4.04 μg of protein per ml is the optimal protein concentration for colloidal gold conjugation. For safety, we used 5.25 μg/ml in the GICA strips to ensure the conjugation.

The first tube on the left contains x ug of protein per ml. Each tube to the right represents an x fold dilution, except the last tube on the right, which contains no protein. The lowest concentration of protein that produced a color was x mg/ml (fourth tube from the left).

9.3.3 Optimal Concentration of E2 Protein for the Test Line

The results based on the intensity of the test line showed that 1.5 mg/mL was the optimal concentration for the E2 protein coated on the test line.

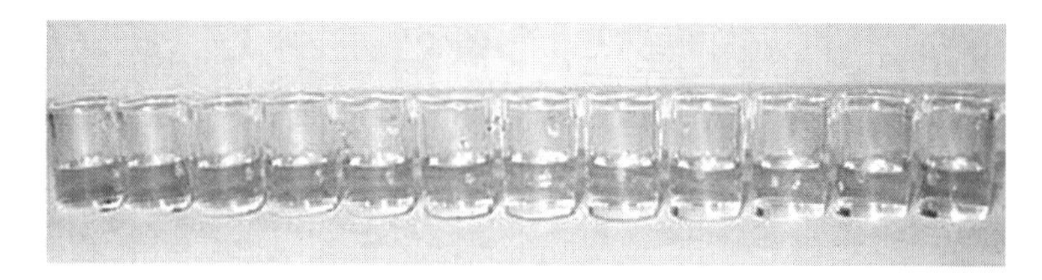

Fig. 9.4 Optimal E2 protein concentration for colloidal gold conjugation

Table 9.1 Detection of antibody to CSFV in a serially diluted serum sample with the GICA strip and with c-ELISA

Method	Dilution of serum							
	1:20	1:40	1:80	1:160	1:320	1:640	1:1280	1:2560
GICA	+++[a]	+++	+++	+++	+++	++	–	–
c-ELISA	–	–	–	–	–	–	+	+++
HI	2^9	2^8	2^7	2^6	2^5	2^4	2^3	2^2

[a] The quantity of antibody detected was assumed to be correlated with the intensity of the color produced. – = no color produced; +, ++, and +++ = light, intermediate, and dark color produced

9.3.4 Specificity of the GICA Strips

Positive results were obtained only with the purified and unpurified sera containing antibodies against CSFV, but not with those against PCV, PEDV, TGEV, PRoV, PRV, or PPV, suggesting that the GICA strips are specific for CSFV.

9.3.5 Sensitivity of the GICA Strip

The results in Table 9.1 showed that GICA strip was able to detect CSFV antibody at a highest dilution of 1:640 (equivalent to 2^4 HA)

9.3.6 Field Tests of GICA Strips

Results from GICA, ELISA, and HI tests were identical for 98.9–100 % of the 885 sera samples from the field (Table 9.2). Among the 825 pig sera samples, the numbers of positive detection of CSFV antibody were 738, 737, and 730 for GICA, ELISA, and HI, respectively. Results were negative for all three assays for all 60 sera from chicken, duck, goose, and goat (Table 9.2).

9.3.7 Comparison of GICA Strips with IDEXX ELISA Kits

In clinical trials, GICA strip and ELISA kit were respectively used to examine the positive and negative rate of 519 samples. The coincidence rate was 93.26 % (484/519) (Table 9.3).

Table 9.2 Detection of antibody to CSFV in clinical samples by GICA, ELISA, and HI

Source of sample[a]	Number of samples	Number of positive or negative samples by method[b]		
		GICA	ELISA	HI
Farm 1	103	92 (+++)	92 (−)	92 (+++)
Farm 2	87	77 (+++)	77 (−)	77 (+++)
Farm 3	114	110 (+++)	110 (−)	106 (+++)
Farm 4	172	161 (+++)	160 (−)	161 (+++)
Farm 5	97	67 (+++)	67 (−)	67 (+++)
Farm 6	124	110 (+++)	110 (−)	108 (+++)
Farm 7	128	121 (+++)	121 (−)	119 (+++)
Chicken sera	15	15 (−)	15 (+++)	15 (−)
Duck sera	15	15 (−)	15 (+++)	15 (−)
Goose sera	15	15 (−)	15 (+++)	15 (−)
Goat sera	15	15 (−)	15 (+++)	15 (−)
Total	885	738	737	730

[a] Except as indicated, all samples are from swine
[b] "+++" = positive; "−" = negative

Table 9.3 Comparison of GICA strips with ELISA

Method		ELISA (IDEXX, USA)		Total
	Results	Positive (+++)	Negative (–)	
GICA	Positive (+++)	260	21	281
	Negative (–)	14	224	238
Total		274	245	519

9.3.8 Storage Life

The GICA strips correctly identified all positive and negative samples after 36 months of storage at 4 °C and after 12 months of storage at 37 °C. The results showed that the strips sealed with desiccant in a plastic bag could be stored for at least 36 months at 4 °C with no significant loss of sensitivity.

9.4 Discussion

We have developed a GICA strip that allows for rapid and inexpensive detection of the antibodies against the CSFV. The GICA strips are sensitive, specific, and reliable. In addition, use of this strip does not require specialized equipment or trained technicians. This GICA strip should overcome the limitations of the routinely used ELISA and IH, which are quite cost- and time-consuming. These strips may find immediate applications in the following sectors as described below.

9.4.1 Monitoring CSFV Antibody Levels in Sows that are Giving Birth

First, if only one line (C, the quality control line) appears on the strips, it indicates that CSFV antibody titers in sows are lower than the minimum level required for protection against virulent attacks. In this case, both sows and the suckling pigs should be vaccinated against CSFV to prevent potential CSFV infection. If two lines appear on the test strips, it indicates a high CSFV antibody titer in the sow and thus immunization of the suckling pigs may not be necessary because the sows can provide CSFV antibody to piglets by vertical transmission.

9.4.2 Detecting Whether the CSFV Immunization is Needed When Buying Pigs

When pigs are being purchased, the herd can be sampled with the CSFV GICA strip. The results will indicate whether CSFV immunization is required.

9.4.3 Monitoring Antibody Levels in CSFV Outbreaks

When CSFV breaks out, the conventional management of the disease involves comprehensive isolation, disinfection, and emergency vaccination. All these actions will significantly affect the antibody titers of the herd, especially that of the breeding herd. Therefore, it is very important to determine the CSFV antibody levels of the herd and establish reasonable immunization program accordingly.

9.4.4 Detection of the CSFV Antigen

At present, the most common method for CSFV detection in China is through the determination of the presence of the antibody against CSFV. This method is useful to the cause of death, however, it cannot detect the presence of CSFV at early stage. Use of the GICA may help to detect the CSFV and its antibodies at early stages, making it possible to avoid major losses by treating the pigs before it is too late.

9.4.5 Determination of Vaccine Quality

Specialized households or large pig farms must buy large quantities of CSFV vaccines from pharmaceutical companies or veterinary stations. In this case, we suggest that the buyer should test the quality of the vaccines using the GICA strip as described below. For each batch of CSFV vaccine, different doses (one, two, three, four, five doses) of CSFV vaccines are injected into pigs of different ages (the suckling pigs, piglets, and breeding pigs). The blood of the immunized animals is sampled 10–15 d after immunization, and CSFV antibody titers are tested with CSFV GICA strips. If all the sera of all the pigs produce positive results on the strip, the pigs have sufficient CSFV antibody against virulent attacks, then the vaccine is suitable. If the CSFV GICA strip produces negative results, the pigs lack sufficient antibody protection against virulent attacks, and the manager should determine whether there is a problem with the vaccine itself, with interference by an immunosuppressed virus (such as PCV2), or some other problem. The manager would then test other batches vaccine to determine whether a batch failure or immunosuppressive virus vaccine interference was the problem.

Acknowledgments The study was supported by grants from the Program of R&D (No. 2011GB2C600011).

References

1. Shangjin C, Chen C, Tong G (2008) A simple and rapid immunochromatographic strip test for monitoring antibodies to H5 subtype avian influenza virus. J Virol Methods 152:102–105
2. Shangjin C, Tong G (2008) A chromatographic strip test for rapid detection of one lineage of the H5 subtype of highly pathogenic avian influenza. J Vet Diagn Invest 20(5):567–571
3. C Shangjin, S Zhou, C Chen, T Qi, C Zhang, J Oh (2008) A simple and rapid immunochromatographic strip test for detecting antibody to porcine reproductive and respiratory syndrome virus. J Virol Meth 152:38–42
4. Xiao-Nan D, Ke W, Zu-Qiang L, Ying-Hua C (2002) Candidate peptide vaccine induced protection against classical swine fever virus. Vaccine 21:167–173
5. Greiser-Wilke I, Blome S, Moennig V (2007) Diagnostic methods for detection of classical swine fever virus—status quo and new developments. Vaccine 25:5524–5530
6. L Yan, Z Jian-Jun, L Na, S Zixue, C Dan, Z Qing-Hu, T Changchun, T Guang-Zhi and Q Hua-Ji (2007) A multiplex nested RT-PCR for the detection and differentiation of wild-type viruses from C-strain vaccine of classical swine fever virus. J Virol Meth 143(1):16–22
7. Thullier P, Guglielmo V, Rajerison M (2003) Short report : serodiagnosis of plague in humans and rats using a rapid test. Am J Trop Med Hyg 69(4):450–451
8. Z Sheng-hua, C Shang-jin, C Chang-mu, Z Chaofan, L Jun, Z Shun, O Jin-Sik (2009) Development and validation of an immunogold chromatographic test for on-farm detection of PRRSV. J Virol Meth 160:178–184

Chapter 10
Cramer-Von Mises Statistics for Testing the Equality of Two Distributions

Qun Huang and Ping Jing

Abstract In the study, two projected integrated empirical processes for testing the equality of two multivariate distributions are introduced. The bootstrap is used for determining the approximate critical values. The result shows that the test statistics and their bootstrap version have the same limit if the null hypothesis is true. A number-theoretic method is applied to the simulation of efficient computation of the bootstrap critical values.

Keywords Bootstrap · Integrated empirical distribution function · Integrated empirical process · Number-theoretic methods · Projection pursuit

10.1 Introduction

In the field of statistical inference, equality of two distributions testing has been drawing great attention. Præstgaard [10] carried out a study about bootstrap Kolmogorov-Smirnov tests for the equality of two distributions. Jing and Dai [8] discussed PP bootstrap Kolmogorov-Smirnov tests for the equality of two multivariate distributions with projection pursuit technique employed. In this paper the bootstrap to another type of statistics was applied to test the equality of two multivariate distributions. Let $X1, \ldots, Xm$ and $Y1, \ldots, Yn$ be independent scalar random variables, where $X1, \ldots, Xm$ are i.i.d. with continuous distribution function F, and $Y1, \ldots, Yn$ are i.i.d. with continuous distribution function G. In [5], the

Q. Huang (✉)
Beijing City University, Beijing 100083, China
e-mail: huangqun72@163.com

P. Jing
China University of Mining and Technology, Beijing 100083, China
e-mail: jping@cumtb.edu.cn

S. Li et al. (eds.), *Frontier and Future Development of Information Technology in Medicine and Education*, Lecture Notes in Electrical Engineering 269,
DOI: 10.1007/978-94-007-7618-0_10, © Springer Science+Business Media Dordrecht 2014

following integrated empirical process was given consideration to test the hypothesis H_0:$F = G$, recently.

$$\overline{\beta}_{mn}(t) = \sqrt{\frac{mn}{m+n}}(\overline{F}_m(t) - \overline{G}_n(t)), \quad -\infty < t < +\infty \tag{10.1}$$

where

$$\overline{F}_m(t) = \int_{-\infty}^{t} F_m(x)dF_m(x), \quad G_n(t) = \int_{-\infty}^{t} G_n(y)dG_n(y)$$

are the so-called *integrated empirical distribution functions*. Here

$$F_m(x) = m^{-1}\sum_{j=1}^{m} I(X_j \leq x) \text{ and } G_n(y) = n^{-1}\sum_{j=1}^{n} I(Y_j \leq y)$$

are the empirical distribution functions of the X-sample and Y-sample, respectively. Based on (10.1), the same authors defined the integrated Kolmogorov-Smirnov (K-S) statistic

$$\overline{D}_{mn} = \sup_{t \in R} \left| \overline{\beta}_{mn}(t) \right| \tag{10.2}$$

as their test statistic for testing the equality of two univariate distributions.

The researcher of the study holds that testing the equality of two multivariate distributions using a bootstrap statistic based on (10.3) should be considered.

To describe the test statistics more precisely, **X**1, ..., **X**m should be p-dimensional i.i.d. observations having underlying distribution P on a probability space (S, ϕ) with **Y**1, ..., **Y**n being independent samples from a distribution Q on the same probability space. It is aimed to test the hypothesis that P equals Q.

Based on the aforementioned integrated K-S statistic (10.2), the known approach adopted is to define the following extended integrated K-S statistic

$$\sup_{t \in R^p} \sqrt{\frac{mn}{m+n}} \left| \overline{F}_m(t) - \overline{G}_n(t) \right|, \tag{10.3}$$

where $\overline{F}_m(t)$ and $\overline{G}_n(t)$ are extensions of $\overline{F}_m(t)$ and $\overline{G}_n(t)$ defined respectively by

$$\overline{F}_m(t) = \int_{-\infty}^{t} F_m(x)dF_m(x), \quad G_n(t) = \int_{-\infty}^{t} G_n(y)dG_n(y)$$

the integrations being understood as multiple integrals based on the multivariate empirical distributions

$$F_m(x) = m^{-1}\sum_{j=1}^{m} I(X_j \leq x) \quad \text{and} \quad G_n(y) = n^{-1}\sum_{j=1}^{n} I(Y_j \leq y)$$

However, it is problematic with statistics of type (10.3) when the dimension p is large. For large p, if the sample size is not large enough, the sparseness of the sample points in a high-dimensional space will usually be encountered [7]. This problem can be solved with the projection pursuit technique, which is well known to be a useful tool for overcoming such problem. In the study two tests based on the integrated empirical processes using the projection pursuit technique were carried out.

Moreover, in order to determine the critical values, the properties of the sampling or at least the limiting distribution of the underlying test statistics should be known. Nevertheless, exact expressions for neither the sampling distribution nor the limiting distribution of our test statistics are analytically tractable. With this considered, the bootstrap [2] was used to estimate the quantities of the null distributions. However, since our bootstrap test statistic is the supremum over the unit vectors on an appropriate high-dimensional unit sphere, exact computation of the statistic is impossible or it is time-consuming. Accordingly, an efficient number-theoretic method adopted by Fang and Wang [3] is adopted to approximate this statistic.

In the paper, Sect. 10.2 introduces both the test statistic and its bootstrap version based on the integrated empirical processes, and the asymptotic null distributions are same for both the original statistic and its bootstrap copy. In Sect. 10.3, results of some simulation experiments are discussed.

10.2 Main Results

10.2.1 Cramer-Von Mises Statistics of Projected Integrated Empirical Distribution

Let S^{p-1} is a unit sphere in R^p, i.e. $S^{p-1} = \{s : \|s\| = 1, s \in R^p\}$, where $\|\cdot\|$ is the Euclidean norm. Let $\mathbf{a}$ be an arbitrary directional vector belonging to S^{p-1}. Let

$$F_{ma}(t) = m^{-1}\sum_{i=1}^{m} I(a^t X_i \le t), \quad G_{na}(t) = n^{-1}\sum_{j=1}^{n} I(a^t Y_j \le t)$$

be the projected empirical distributions determined by $a^t\mathbf{X}_1, \ldots, a^t\mathbf{X}_\mathbf{m}$ and $a^t\mathbf{Y}_1, \ldots, a^t\mathbf{Y}_\mathbf{n}$. Now we define the projected integrated empirical distribution functions as follows denote by

$$\overline{F}_{ma}(t) = \int_{-\infty}^{t} F_{ma}(x)dF_{ma}(x), \quad \overline{G}_{na}(t) = \int_{-\infty}^{t} G_{na}(y)dG_{na}(y)$$

$$\overline{K}_{mna}(t) = \sqrt{\frac{mn}{m+n}}\left(\overline{F}_{ma}(t) - \overline{G}_{na}(t)\right). \tag{10.4}$$

Now we extend (10.2) to define the following projection pursuit integrated Cramer-Von Mises statistic is given by

$$ICVS_{mn} = \sup_{a,t} \int_{R^1} \left(\overline{K}_{mn}(a,t)\right)^2 d\overline{H}_{Na}(t), \; -\infty < t < +\infty \tag{10.5}$$

and projection pursuit integrated C-V-A statistic is

$$ICVA_{mn} = \sup_{a,t} \int_{R^1} \overline{K}_{mn}(a,t)\, d\overline{H}_{Na}(t), \; -\infty < t < +\infty \tag{10.6}$$

where $\overline{H}_{Na}(t) = \frac{m}{m+n}\overline{F}_{ma}(t) + \frac{n}{m+n}\overline{G}_{na}(t)$.

To use the statistic (10.5), (10.6) we first note that testing $P = Q$ is equivalent to the following

$$H_0^a : F_a(\cdot) = G_a(\cdot), \quad \forall a \in S^{p-1} \tag{10.7}$$

where $F_a(\cdot)$ and $G_a(\cdot)$ denote the distribution functions of P and Q in direction a respectively.

To state the main theorem we establish some notations first. For any **a,** let $W_P(\cdot,a,t)$ and $W_Q(\cdot,a,t)$ be independent zero-mean Gaussian processes with continuous sample paths. And for **a,b** $\in S^{p-1}$, with covariance

$$\begin{aligned} Cov(W_P(\cdot,a,t), W_P(\cdot,b,s)) = & \int I(a^tX \le t) I(b^tX \le s) dP \\ & - \int I(a^tX \le t) dP \int I(b^tX \le s) dP \end{aligned}$$

$$\begin{aligned} Cov(W_Q(\cdot,a,t), W_Q(\cdot,b,s)) = & \int I(a^tY \le t) I(b^tY \le s) dQ \\ & - \int I(a^tY \le t) dQ \int I(b^tY \le s) dQ \end{aligned}$$

Now we consider the limiting case when $\frac{m}{m+n} \to \lambda \in (0,1)$ as $m,n \to \infty$. Let

$$W_H(\cdot,a,t) = \sqrt{1-\lambda}W_P(\cdot,a,t) - \sqrt{\lambda}W_Q(\cdot,a,t), \; H = \lambda P + (1-\lambda)Q$$

Theorem 10.1

Suppose that $F_{\mathbf{a}}(t)$ and $G_{\mathbf{a}}(t)$ are continuous with respect to **a** and t. If the null hypothesis H_0 holds, then

$$ICVS_{mn} = \sup_{a,t} \int_{R^1} F_a^3(t)[W_H(\cdot,a,t)]^2 dH_a(t), \tag{10.8}$$

$$ICVA_{mn} = \sup_{a,t} \int_{R^1} F_a^2(t)[W_H(\cdot,a,t)]^2 dH_a(t), \tag{10.9}$$

where the notation $\Rightarrow$ means the weak convergence. If the null hypothesis is false, then the left-hand side of (10.8), (10.9) tends to infinity with probability one as $m, n \to \infty$.

10.2.2 Bootstrap Tests

As illustrated above, the test statistics were constructed with a description of the asymptotic behavior of the statistic. A hard issue is about the analytic tractability of the sampling and the limiting distribution, leading to the difficulty of obtaining the critical values, which are necessary for conducting the test. To get this solved, the bootstrap is proposed.

Let $N = m + n$ and $(\mathbf{Z}_1, \ldots, \mathbf{Z}_N) = (\mathbf{X}_1, \ldots, \mathbf{X}_m, \mathbf{Y}_1, \ldots, \mathbf{Y}_n)$ be the pooled sample. Denote by $\delta_{Z_j}$the probability measure having mass 1 at $\mathbf{Z}_j$, and $H_N = N^{-1} \sum_{j=1}^{N} \delta_{Z_j}$, we note that $H_N = (m/N)P_m + (n/N)P_n$, where $P_m = m^{-1} \sum_{j=1}^{m} \delta_{X_j}$, and $Q_n = n^{-1} \sum_{j=1}^{n} \delta_{Y_j}$, Let $H_{Na} = N^{-1} \sum_{j=1}^{N} I\left(a^t Z_j^* \leq t\right)$, then we have $H_{Na} = \frac{m}{N} F_{ma}(t) + \frac{n}{N} G_{na}(t)$. Let λ, $F_a(t)$ and $G_a(t)$ be given as in the previous subsection. Let $H_a(t) = \lambda F_a(t) + (1 - \lambda) G_a(t)$.

Now let $\mathbf{Z}_1^*, \ldots, \mathbf{Z}_N^*$ be a resample drawn with replacement from $\mathbf{Z}_1, \ldots, \mathbf{Z}_N$. Let

$$F_{ma}^* = m^{-1} \sum\nolimits_{j=1}^{m} I\left(a^t Z_j^* \leq t\right), \quad G_{na}^* = n^{-1} \sum\nolimits_{j=m+1}^{N} I\left(a^t Z_j^* \leq t\right)$$

be the projected bootstrap empirical distributions. A nonparametric bootstrap version of the integrated empirical distributions can be defined naturally as

$$\overline{F}_{ma}^*(t) = \int_{-\infty}^{t} F_{ma}^*(x) dF_{ma}^*(x), \quad \overline{G}_{na}^*(t) = \int_{-\infty}^{t} G_{na}^*(y) dG_{na}^*(y)$$

Similarly, we can define $\overline{H}_{Na}^*(t) = \int_{-\infty}^{t} H_{Na}^*(x) dH_{Na}^*(x)$, where $H_{Na}^* = N^{-1} \sum_{j=1}^{N} I\left(a^t Z_j^* \leq t\right)$. The bootstrap test statistic now takes from

$$ICVS_{mn}^* = \sup_{a,t} \int_{R^1} \left[\overline{K}_{mna}^*(t)\right]^2 d\overline{H}_{Na}^*(t) \tag{10.10}$$

$$ICVA_{mn}^* = \sup_{a,t} \int_{R^1} \overline{K}_{mna}^*(t) d\overline{H}_{Na}^*(t) \tag{10.11}$$

The following theorem states that the $ICMS_{mn}$, $ICMA_{mn}$ test statistics and their bootstrap version have the same limit if the null hypothesis is true.

Let $H = \lambda P + (1 - \lambda)Q$. Under the same conditions of Theorem 10.1, we have Theorem 10.2

$$ICVS^*_{mn} = \sup_{a,t} \int_{R^1} F^3_a(t)\left[\sqrt{1-\lambda}W_H(\cdot, a, t) - \sqrt{\lambda}W'_H(\cdot, a, t)\right]^2 dH_a(t), \quad (10.12)$$

$$ICVA^*_{mn} = \sup_{a,t} \int_{R^1} F^2_a(t)\left[\sqrt{1-\lambda}W_H(\cdot, a, t) - \sqrt{\lambda}W'_H(\cdot, a, t)\right] dH_a(t), \quad (10.13)$$

where $W_H(\cdot, \boldsymbol{a}, t)$ is a zero mean Gaussian process with covariance function given in $W_P(\cdot, \boldsymbol{a}, t)$ with P replaced by H and $W_H(\cdot, \boldsymbol{a}, t)$ is an independent copy of $W_H(\cdot, \boldsymbol{a}, t)$. If H_0 is true, then the right-hand side of (10.12), (10.13) coincides with the right-hand side of (10.8), (10.9). If H_0 is false, then the bootstrap statistic $ICVS^*_{mn}$, $ICVA^*_{mn}$, still (weakly) converges to a certain Gaussian process.

The bootstrap test statistic in Theorem 10.1 and 10.2 defined as the super num of a quantity over the (p-1)-dimensional sphere. To approximately compute this statistic, one may maximize $\overline{K}^*_{mn}(a, t)$ over a suitably chosen finite number of points $a_1, \ldots, a_l \in S^{p-1}$. More specifically, we define

$$\widehat{ICVS}^*_{mn} = \max_{1 \le t \le l} \int_{R^1} \left[\overline{K}^*_{mna_k}(t)\right]^2 d\overline{H}^*_{N,a_k}(t) \quad (10.14)$$

$$\widehat{ICVA}^*_{mn} = \max_{1 \le t \le l} \int_{R^1} \overline{K}^*_{mna_k}(t) d\overline{H}^*_{N,a_k}(t) \quad (10.15)$$

10.2.3 Number-Theoretic Methods

One possible way is to apply a stochastic approximation of the critical values [1]. In this case $\mathbf{a}_1$, …, $\mathbf{a}_l$ is chosen as i.i.d. random vectors distributed uniformly on S^{p-1}. It is noted that the uniformity of $\mathbf{a}_1$, …, $\mathbf{a}_l$ S^{p-1} is important for this kind of approximation. For such chooses points, it can be shown that the discrepancy measure of uniformity (see [3], Chap. 1), is of order O_p ($l^{-1/2}$). Therefore, to have a reliable approximation of (10.14) and (10.15), especially in case of p being large, a large number of l is required for the Monte Carlo approximation using uniformly distributed variables **a**.

In this paper we shall use a more efficient number-theoretic method (NTM) (Fang and Wang [3], p 49) for choosing $\mathbf{a}_1$, …, $\mathbf{a}_l$. Let $u_1, \ldots, u_{p-1}$ be independent random variables distributed on [0, 1], having density functions given by

$$g_j(u) = \frac{\pi}{B\left(\frac{1}{2}, \frac{p-j}{2}\right)}(\sin \pi u)^{p-j-1}, \quad j = 1, \ldots, p-1$$

then we choose $\mathbf{a} = a_1, \ldots, a_p \in S^{p-1}$ according to the following formula.

$$\begin{aligned} a_1 &= \cos(\pi u_1) \\ a_j &= \cos(\pi u_j)\sin(\pi u_1)\ldots\sin(\pi u_j), \quad j = 1, 2, \ldots p-2 \\ a_{p-1} &= \sin(\pi u_1)\ldots\sin(\pi u_{p-2})\cos(2\pi u_{p-1}) \\ a_p &= \sin(\pi u_1)\ldots\sin(\pi u_{p-2})\sin(2\pi u_{p-1}) \end{aligned}$$

For such chosen **a**, it can be shown that the discrepancy measure of uniformity reduces to $O(l^{-1}(\log l)^{p-1})$ compared to the error $O(l^{-1/2})$ of the naive Monte Carlo method; see [3] for a proof of these results.

10.3 Simulation Studies

Simulations using samples from p-dimensional distributions were conducted to investigate the small behavior of the bootstrap test statistic based on the integrated empirical processes. The $l = 7,13$ directional vectors $\mathbf{a}_1, \ldots, \mathbf{a}_l \in S^{p-1}$ were chosen with the number-theoretic method employed as discussed above. Since the computation is quite intensive, only the results for the cases when $p = 3,4$ were elaborated here.

To generate these directional vectors, we used the algorithm of [3] §1.3 in our Monte Carlo studies. Let $l > p$-1. First we choose a generating vector **h**, an integer vector $\mathbf{h} = (h_1, \ldots, h_{p-1})$ satisfying $1 \le h_j < l$, $h_i \ne h_j$ for $i \ne j$. See [3] (Appendix A) for the choice of the generating vectors. Let $\{x\}$ denote the fractional part of x. denote $c_{kj} = \{(2kh_j - 1)/2l\}$ and $\mathbf{c}_k = (c_{k1}, \ldots, c_{k(p-1)})'$ for $k = 1, \ldots, l$ and $j = 1, \ldots, p$-1. Finally we transform the vectors $\mathbf{c}_1, \ldots, \mathbf{c}_l$ using the algorithm of Fang and Wang [3] §4.3 to obtain $\mathbf{a}_1, \ldots, \mathbf{a}_l \in S^{p-1}$.

We considered several cases, (m, n) = (10, 10), (38, 22), (30, 20). The critical values are obtained by the approximate bootstrap test statistic $\widehat{ICVS}^*_{mn}$, $ICVA^*_{mn}$ of (10.14) and (10.15). For each case, 2,000 replications of the bootstrap samples were independently generated for determining the critical values. And, in each case, the samples were repeatedly drawn 1000 times from the respective populations. Here we report the proportions of the values of the test statistics exceeding the 90, 95 %-th percentiles of the bootstrap statistics.

The simulated results are listed in Tables 10.1, 10.2. The pseudo random numbers were generated from the following distributions: (1) The multivariate normal distribution, $MN(\mu_p, \Sigma_p)$; (2) $\chi^2_p = (\chi^2_1, \chi^2_2, \ldots, \chi^2_p)$: where χ^2_i are independent Chi squared variables with two degrees of freedom. (3) $LN = (LN_1, LN_2, \ldots, LN_p)$: where LN_i are independently distributed having the standard lognormal distribution. (4) The multivariate student's t distribution with 5 degrees of freedom, $MT(5; \mu_p, \Sigma_p)$, defined as $MN(\mu_p, \Sigma_p)$divided by $(\chi^2_5/5)^{1/2}$.

In the Tables 10.1, 10.2 the following seven cases are considered: (1) $MN(\mathbf{I}_p, \mathbf{I}_p)$ versus $MN(\mathbf{O}_p, \mathbf{I}_p)$; (2) χ^2_p versus χ^2_p; (3) LN_p versus LN_p;

Table 10.1 $p = 3$, $l = 7$ simulation

(*m*, *n*) α	Statistic	(10, 10) 0.05	(38, 22) 0.05	(30, 20) 0.05	(10, 10) 0.10	(38, 22) 0.10	(30, 20) 0.10
(1)	$ICVS_{mn}$	56	50	43	109	93	94
	$ICVA_{mn}$	54	49	45	109	81	99
(2)	$ICVS_{mn}$	43	45	57	92	97	91
	$ICVA_{mn}$	46	44	54	86	103	91
(3)	$ICVS_{mn}$	51	49	45	106	100	96
	$ICVA_{mn}$	52	51	49	110	106	48
(4)	$ICVS_{mn}$	49	45	55	94	96	105
	$ICVA_{mn}$	50	46	54	93	101	113
(5)	$ICVS_{mn}$	1,000	98	1,000	1,000	993	1,000
	$ICVA_{mn}$	1,000	984	1,000	1,000	995	1,000
(6)	$ICVS_{mn}$	924	1,000	1,000	971	1,000	1,000
	$ICVA_{mn}$	943	1,000	1,000	973	1,000	1,000
(7)	$ICVS_{mn}$	52	57	65	107	119	113
	$ICVA_{mn}$	56	57	65	97	113	115

Table 10.2 $p = 4$, $l = 13$ *simulation*

(*m*, *n*) α	Statistic	(10, 10) 0.05	(38, 22) 0.05	(30, 20) 0.05	(10, 10) 0.10	(38, 22) 0.10	(30, 20) 0.10
(1)	$ICVS_{mn}$	54	57	43	123	111	100
	$ICVA_{mn}$	50	58	46	122	117	101
(2)	$ICVS_{mn}$	46	47	48	107	106	108
	$ICVA_{mn}$	45	46	45	108	100	111
(3)	$ICVS_{mn}$	53	69	43	116	110	93
	$ICVA_{mn}$	52	71	45	119	116	93
(4)	$ICVS_{mn}$	48	53	47	102	113	104
	$ICVA_{mn}$	48	50	59	106	111	109
(5)	$ICVS_{mn}$	1,000	1,000	1,000	1,000	1,000	1,000
	$ICVA_{mn}$	1,000	1,000	1,000	1,000	1,000	1,000
(6)	$ICVS_{mn}$	997	1,000	1,000	999	1,000	1,000
	$ICVA_{mn}$	998	999	1,000	99	1,000	1,000
(7)	$ICVS_{mn}$	48	67	73	113	127	132
	$ICVA_{mn}$	52	68	70	109	127	125

(4) $MT(5; \mu_p, \Sigma_p)$ versus $MT(5; \mu_p, \Sigma_p)$; (5) $MN(\mathbf{O}_p, \mathbf{I}_p)$ versus χ_p^2; (6) $MN(\mathbf{I}_p, \mathbf{I}_p)$ versus LN_p; (7) $MT(5; \mu_p, \Sigma_p)$ versus $MN(\mathbf{O}_p, \mathbf{I}_p)$. In case (1), (2), (3), (4), we can see the two statistics are very effective, because under H_0 for the nominal level $\alpha = 0.05$ and 0.10, number of reject the null hypotheses are close to 1,000α. In case (7), F has symmetric multivariate t distribution with covariance matrix $5\mathbf{I}_p/p$, while G has the identity covariance matrix. The bootstrap tests are not very sensitive to the difference in scale. The remaining two cases concern differences in locations, and the bootstrap tests correctly reject H_0 in all cases.

References

1. Beran R, Millar PW (1986) Confidence sets for a multivariate distribution. Ann Stat 14:431–443
2. Efron B, Tibshirani R (1993) An introduction to the bootstrap. Chapman and Hall, New York
3. Fang KT, Wang Y (1993) Number-theoretic methods and applications in statistics. Chapman and Hall, New York
4. Gin′e E, Zinn J (1990) Bootstrapping general empirical measures. Ann Probab 18:851–869
5. Henze N, Nikitin YY (2003) Two-sample tests based on the integrated empirical process. Commun Stat Theor Methods 32:1767–1788
6. Hofmann-JØrgensen J (1984) Stochastic processes on polish spaces, Unpublished manuscript
7. Huber P (1985) Projection pursuit(with discussion). Ann Stat 13:435–475
8. Jing Ping, chaoshou Dai (1999) Bootstrap tests for the equality of two and K distributions. Math Appl 4:45–52
9. Pollard D (1984) Convergence of stochastic processes. Springer-Verlag and Science Press, New York
10. Præstgaard JP (1995) Permutation and bootstrap Kolmogorov-Smirnov test for the equality of two distributions. Scand J Stat 22:305–322

Chapter 11
Establishment of Craniomaxillofacial Model Including Temporomandibular Joint by Means of Three-Dimensional Finite Element Method

Zhang Jun, Zhang Wen-juan, Zhao Shu-ya, Li Na, Li Tao and Wang Xu-xia

Abstract *Objective* The aim of this study was to establish a finite element model of the craniomaxilloface with higher biological and mechanical similarities for further biomechanical study on maxillary protraction. *Methods* The head was scanned by the spiral CT to acquire two-dimensional images of the craniomaxilloface. Then the original DICOM data from CT were processed by image processing softwares such as Mimics and Magics12.0 and disposed by remesh tool in Magics12.0. Finally the three-dimensional finite element model of the craniomaxilloface was constructed by the special finite element software MSC.Marc2005. *Results* A three-dimensional finite element model of the craniomaxilloface including the mandible and the temporomandibular joint was precisely established. *Conclusions* A three-dimensional finite element model of the ficraniomaxilloface including the mandible and the temporomandibular joint was precisely established. The model has a high accuracy, which will be a ideal model for further biomechanical study of the craniomaxilloface. Besides, the scientific and precise modeling method was achieved.

Keywords Craniomaxilloface · Three-dimensional finite element model · Maxillary protraction · Reacting force · Temporomandibular joint

---

Z. Jun · Z. Shu-ya · L. Tao · W. Xu-xia (✉)
School of Stomatology, Shandong University, 250012 Jinan, China
e-mail: wxx@sdu.edu.cn

Z. Jun · W. Xu-xia
Shandong Provincial Key Laboratory of Oral Biomedicine, 250012 Jinan, China

Z. Wen-juan
Department of Stomatology, Teaching Hospital of Shandong University of Traditional Chinese Medicine, 250011 Jinan, China

L. Na
Department of Orthodontics, Shandong Provincial Qianfoshan Hospital, 250014 Jinan, China

S. Li et al. (eds.), *Frontier and Future Development of Information Technology in Medicine and Education*, Lecture Notes in Electrical Engineering 269,
DOI: 10.1007/978-94-007-7618-0_11,

11.1 Introduction

The finite element method (FEM) is an advanced computer technique of structural stress analysis developed in engineering mechanics, which approximates a real geometry using a large number of smaller simple elements that are connected by points called nodes. Since it was introduced to stomatology by Thresherm and Farah in 1973, [1, 2] this method had been more widely used for stress analyses of jaw bones and teeth biomechanics to evaluate stresses in every field of stomatology. In recent years, the finite element analysis were applied to all kinds of complicated mechanical problems with the rapid development of computer technology and large analysis softwares, which is now well established as an effective tool for basic research and design analysis in oral orthodontic biomechanics [3]. Element types are decided, and each element is assigned material properties to represent the physical properties of the model. The forces and boundary conditions are defined to simulate applied loads and constraint of the structure. The accuracy of the finite element model is an decisive factor in the accuracy and scientific value of he finite element analysis results to a great degree. So the aim of this study was to establish a precise finite element model of the craniomaxilloface.

The last forty years has witnessed increasing use of FEM in orthodontic biomechanics.Miyasaka et al [4] formed three dimensional finite element model of craniofacial complex composed of 2,918 nodes and 1,776 units by using dry skull as modeling materials, and carving it into 14 layer along the horizontal direction mechanical for the first time in 1986. The modeling method was very complex, time-consuming and inefficient.Mechanical cutting caused loss of bone tissue and damaged specimen. However, it was the first time to establish a relatively reliable mathematical model of craniofacial complex. In 2000, Beek [5] established three dimensional finite element model of TMJ with magnetic track instrument measuring the geometry characteristics of the articular cartilage and joint plate surface. Basciftci et al. [6] modeled three-dimensional finite element models of the mandible and the temporomandibular joint with the mesh consisting of 1572 solid elements with 5432 nodes to evaluate stress and displacements in the mandible from various chincup force vectors on the mandible. Bodo Erdmann [7] constructed three dimension finite element model of the mandible in the adaptive finite element technique by CT which copied the mandibular geometry and separated the cortical bone and cancellous bone. It was accurate and efficient.

FEM in orthodontics is mainly used to study craniofacial morphology and biomechanics. Whether the nasomaxillary complex,mandible or TMJ, orthodontic scholars have established a large number of 3D finite element models for biomechanical study. Nevertheless, craniofacial structure is very complicated, so it is hard to establish a model which is the same as the anatomy of human. Therefore, the established finite element models in orthodontics before were single-structure models. In most cases, a single-structure model may be neither accurate nor comprehensive in biomechanics analysis. There is not yet a whole skull mole including the mandible and the temporomandibular joint. In this study, we combined the nasomaxillary complex, the mandible and TMJ to build a relatively complete skull model for future further study of the skull biomechanics.

11.2 Materials and Methods

A health young man was selected and his head was scanned by CT in order to establish a three-dimensional finite element model.The volunteer took a supine position, keeping still. SOMATOM Balance spiral CT machine supporting DICOM 3.0 standard produced by the Siemens company, was vertical to his face vertical axis and scanned the skull from up to down (scanning layer thickness 1.0 mm, layer spacing 0.5 mm, window width 2000, window level 400). Then 1,245 images of CT were received. The image data were stored in the DICOM format and directly sent into the computer.

11.2.1 Image Preprocessing

CT image is a gray image and gray value reflects its bone mineral density. In the process of 3D reconstruction we just cared about the internal and external sketches in each layer of bones, not the gray between them. A skull part without medullary cavity only had external sketch, while a part with medullary cavity had internal and external sketches. Open Mimics, select the File→Import, series of two-dimensional CT image Files were directly stored in DICOM3.0 and medical digital image communication standard were imported into this software.

Select Profile Line, and select the skull part from the upper left Front View (Front View), in whose medium we draw the buttocks, and then Profile Lines dialog popped. Click Start thresholding, select the default threshold, and go on growing. Front view spread to the whole interface and local region was enlarged.

Then image Segmentation and refining processing were achieved by the Segmentation module. The images were divided into different area characterized by different gray fields with slice tools, then the needed target area boundaries were extracted. After that, the internal and external sketches were very rough and serrated, so the dots in the sketch lines should be simplified in order that the image was more real image. Specific steps were as follows:

- Select Erase in the Edit Masks toolbar, then the joint between skull and vertebral bone would be rubbed off to separate each other.
- Use Draw to paint the edges of the skull, especially its top and bottom, and make its edges smooth. After this layer was finished, the other layers of the view were done in the same way. Then use the same method to handle the right vertical view. Figure 11.1 was a completed skull image.

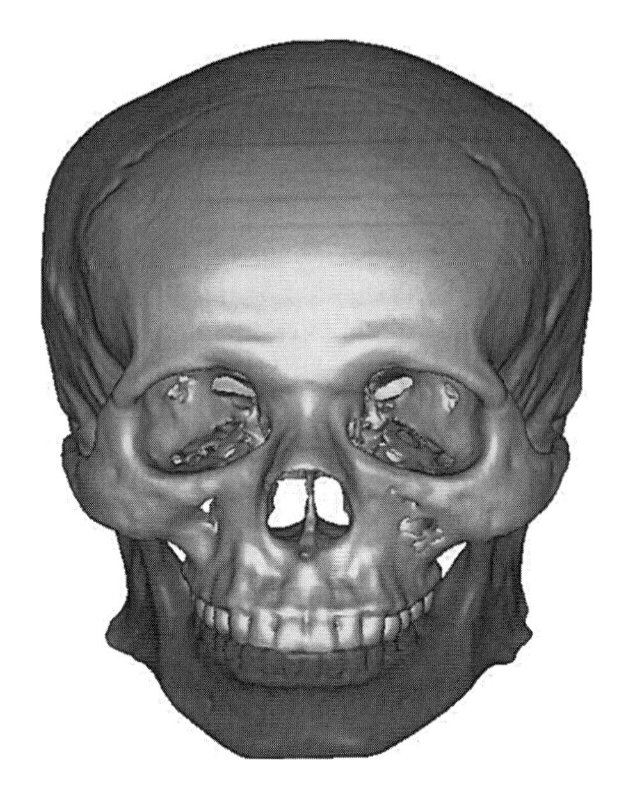

Fig. 11.1 Skull CT image after segmentation and purification (The *yellow* part below is called the maxilla, while *blue* is called the mandible)

Then use 3D skull image generated by Calculate three-dimension toolbar to check the accuracy of the sketch line.According to the above the same steps the maxilla and the mandible were separated, and then 3D model of the mandible was set up.The 3D model was output by Binary STL format for further optimization.

11.2.2 Optimization of Three-Dimension Geometric Model

The 3D Binary STL format data were imported into Magics12.0 (Fig. 11.2). Because of the symmetry of the skull, half of the skull and mandible models were further optimized. Firstly, update information. There would be some useful information after selecting update, such as bad borders, bad sketches, holes, the number of shells, the covered surfaces and the crossing surfaces. Then some optimization were carried out to remove these influences in entity reconstruction. Use the corresponding tools in tool fix pages to correct errors automatically and inspect them repeatedly until shell was one and the other errors were eliminated.

In addition, we could delete something manually and create methods by triangle of the tool fix pages. When the automatic optimization could not eliminate errors

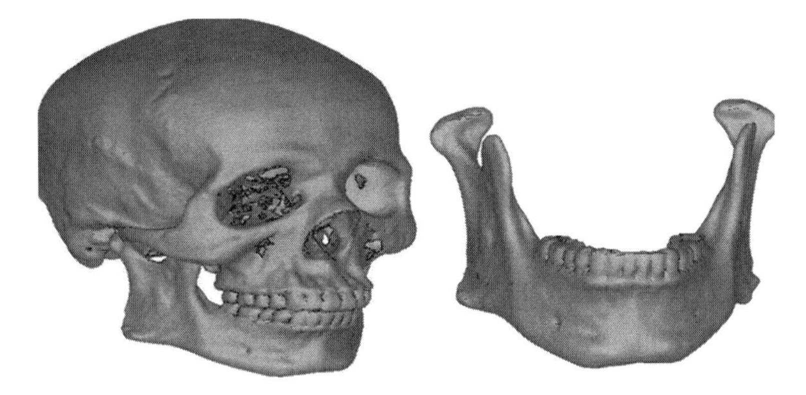

Fig. 11.2 The whole skull model and the mandible before the optimization

any more, it was still necessary to eliminate them manually. Switch display modes of the model which are shade mode and triangle model. There were still some edges in the shade mode, which meant that the triangle surface in the position was not smooth and had sharp edges. These triangle surfaces and the surrounding triangular surfaces were deleted and created to make the model more smooth. Finally the optimized model was achieved, as was shown in Fig. 11.3.

11.2.3 Establishment and Processing of 3D Finite Element Model

11.2.3.1 Generation of Finite Element Surface Mesh and Body Mesh

Select remesh in the magics to divide surface mesh in the mandible model and the whole skull model.

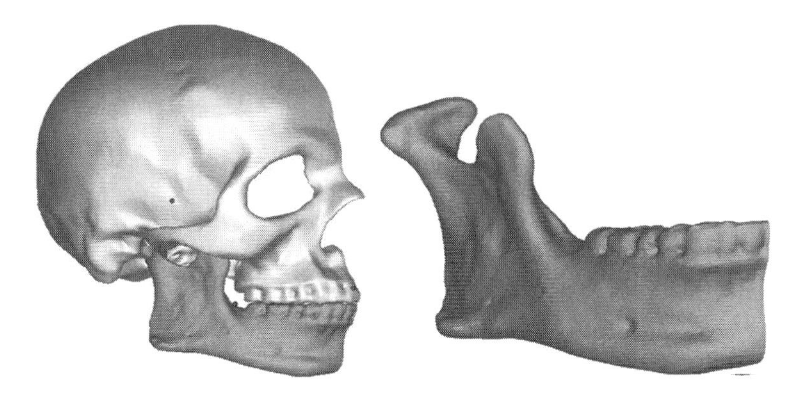

Fig. 11.3 The whole skull model and the mandible after the optimization

Select boolen to subtract the mandible model from the whole skull model after dividing surface mesh to get the maxilla model, which ensured that there were some contact area between the maxilla and the mandible and the grid node was coincident.

The finite element software MSC. Marc2005 was adopted and the geometric model was read from the CAD interface in Mentat. Do the geometry cleaning and repair before dividing mesh automatically because local modification and processing intersection or chamfering may lead to the small geometrical element when geometrically modeling in the CAD system. There were some unnecessary higher density units near these smaller geometrical elements when classifying units automatically was adopted. Besides, there were some defects in the geometric model, such as repeated dots, lines, faces, unclosed surfaces and the unmatched curves. Select geometric repair tools in Mentat, such as: CHECK GEOMETRY, ADD/REMOVE GEOMETRY, CLEAN LOOPS and so on. Clear unnecessary data above and repair the incomplete surface and the unmatched curve to ensure to generate high quality grids.

Select MESH GENERATION > AUTOMESH > SOLID MESH > SOLID TET MESH in Mentat, select all the skull and mandible surface grids and click ok to generate body grids automatically. The model after the formation of the grids was shown in Fig. 11.4.

There were node and unit numbers of the maxilla and mandible in Table 11.1 and the units are all tetrahedron entity units.

The Assumptions of Analysis Condition:

1. Materials of the model and organs were assumed to be continuous, homogeneous and isotropic elastic linear materials. Bone was a kind of anisotropic biological material. Due to too many anisotropic elastic constants, it was simplified as orthogonal anisotropy. Besides, because bone anisotropy is too weak at the same time, so it can be further simplified as isotropy.
2. The material deformation in stress was a small deformation.
3. Influences of masticatory muscle, ligament and gravity were ignored. Suppose in the relax state, the muscle force and gravity of the mandible was in equilibrium in horizontal, vertical, inside and outside directions. So remove influences of muscle,ligament and gravity to the mandible in the paper.

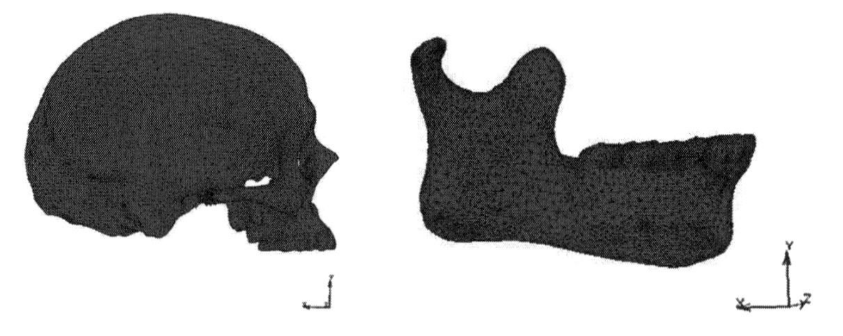

Fig. 11.4 Finite element models of the maxilla and mandible after dividing body grids

Table 11.1 The node number and unit number of three dimensional finite element model

Position	Node number	Unit number
Maxilla	2,0387	7,6892
Mandible	8,353	3,3878

11.2.3.2 The Boundary Conditions and Definition of Material Characteristics

Return to the main menu MAIN, go to the boundary condition submenu BOUNDARY CONDITIONS, and select the type of boundary condition to be the stress boundary condition MECHANICAL and the boundary condition to be a given displacement FIXED DISPLACEMENT. Constraint the displacement of Z direction to be zero and select NODES-ADD, then take all nodes on the symmetry plane of the skull to constraint and confirm. Select FACE FOUNDATION to boundary condition, fill in 1000 in stiffness STIFNESS and choose some mesh surface in the top of the skull to constraint and confirm. Then according to the experiment, something could be applied to the model in the load test (Fig. 11.5).

The material property parameters in the analysis were shown in Table 11.2.

From the main menu into material characteristics definition submenu MATERIAL PROPERTIES, select the type of isotropy ISOTROPIC, define the elastic modulus and poisson's ratio of the maxilla and the mandible according to the parameter in Table 11.2 respectively and assign the MATERIAL PROPERTIES to the corresponding unit.

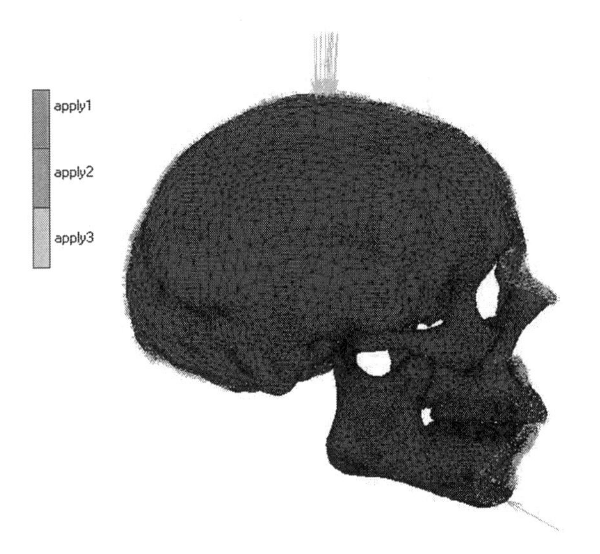

Fig. 11.5 The diagram of boundary condition (The angle between force and occlusal surface was 25 and the force was 3 N)

Table 11.2 Material property parameters

Materials	Elastic modulus(GPa)	Poisson's ratioμ
Maxilla	13.7	0.3
Mandible	13.7	0.3

11.3 Results

The model of human craniomaxilloface containing TMJ was successfully established, which had a high geometric similarity and complete structure. In modeling, the dots in the image contour lines were simplified to make it more real by Mimics. After being optimized by the Magics12.0, the finite element body grids would be generated by MSC. Marc2005. In this model, the maxilla was structured by 20387 nodes and 76892 units, while the mandible was structured by 8353 nodes 33878 units. The shape of the finite element model was very good, and the structure was very similar to the biological entity in geometry. The model materials and organs were assumed to be continuous, homogeneous and isotropic linear elastic and that the materials had a small deformation when stressed. Definite the elastic modulus and poisson's ratio of the mandibular according to the previous researches. Set the boundary constraint condition and the mechanical loading according to the need to mimic the stress and strain of the maxilla and the mandible when people were on the maxillary protraction in the clinical treatment.

11.4 Discussion

The finite element modeling technique is an alternative, indirect mathematical approach. Once the finite element model was established, the stress and strain of the object could be analyzed in different loading conditions, which was more comprehensive, and more accurate than other methods. [8] The method is now well established as a tool for basic research and design analysis in oral biomechanics.

There are about four modeling methods at present. ①Section/slice method. The objects was preprocessed and cut according to certain requirements, and cutting sections were scanned to obtain information for a finite element model. But this method is damage to the object and low accuracy. Therefore this method was less applied. ②3D measurement method. It acquired 3D information by contact or non-contact scanning or holography [9]. Although it can be used to study the object with a complicated morphology and has high accuracy, it need complex softwares and hardwares to support and cannot study interior structure of the object. Hence it is limited. ③Image processing method. The information from CT or MRI are processed by scanning or photography technology and put into the computer.Then they are treated by the related software to establish the model. Compared with the former two methods, this method is no damage to the object, suitable for the living, simple and highly accurate. So it is usually used in the oral biomechanics research.④DICOM data modeling method. It is simpler and more precise and without some subjective factors. This method is used most in finite element modeling of oral biomechanical study, the nature of which is to process images. In this research, we adapted the last one to establish 3D model of the skull.

Class III malocclusion is one of commonly oral clinical disease. As for class III malocclusion caused by maxillary retrusion, one of the best treatments is maxillary protraction. The active force of maxillary protraction is on the maxilla, while reaction force is on the forehead and chin. So the craniofacial skeleton is subjected to complex loading and it would be difficult to assess the mechanical reaction to complex loading in 3D space by using conventional methods, such as strain gauge [10], photoelastic [11] or holographic techniques. FEM would be an effective way to study the biomechanics of craniofacial skeleton in 3D. However, the construction of 3D finite element models of craniofacial complex is quite complicated and still in a confused state. On the early days, some scholars had established finite element models of mandible or TMJ in the section method or CT [12]. Palomar et al. [13] established a finite element model of TMJ by CT and MRI. However, these models are all single-structure. In this research, we established a relatively complete and precise 3D model, of which TMJ and the mandible were included. The model with 20,387 nodes and 76,892 units in the maxilla, and 8,353 nodes and 33,878 units in the mandible helps to go on the further biomechanical study of maxillary protraction. It is more complete than the single-structure model, which will evaluate the stress and strain of the active force and reaction force in the maxillary protraction.

Acknowledgments It was Supported by Shandong Province Natural Science Foundation(Grant No. ZR2011HM036), Science and Technology Development Program of Medicine and Health of Shandong Province(Grant No. 2011QZ023) and Universities and Institutes Indigenous Innovation Program of Jinan(Grant No. 201202032).

References

1. Thresher RW, Saito GE (1973) The stress analysis of human teeth. J Biomech 6(5):443–449
2. Farah JW (1973) Photo-elastic and finite element stress analysis of a restorod axisymmetric first molar. J Biomech 6(5):551—520
3. Fernandez JR, Gallas M, Burguera JM, Viano A (2003) A three-dimensional numerical simulation of mandible fracture reduction with screwed miniplates. J Biomech 36:329–337
4. Miyasaka J, Tanne K, Tsutsumi Set al (1986) Finite element analysis of the biomechanical effects of orthopedic forces on the craniofacial skeleton: construction of a three-dimensional finite element model of the craniofacial skeleton. Osaka Daigaku Shigaka Zasshi 31(2):393–402
5. Beek M, Koolstra JH, van Ruijven LJ, van Eijden TM (2000) Three-dimensional finite element analysis of the human temporomandibular joint disc. J Biomech 33(3):307–316
6. Basciftci FA, Korkmaz HH ,Serdarüsümez et al (2008) Biomechanical evaluation of chincup treatment with various force vectors. Am J Orthod Dentofacial Orthop 134(6):773–781

7. Erdmann B, Kober C, Lang J et al (2001) Efficient and reliable finite element methods for simulation of the human mandible. Berlin, pp 1–15
8. Rick-Williamson LJ, Fotos PG, Coel VK (1995) A three dimensional finite-element stress analysis of an endodontically prepared maxillary central incisor. J Endod 21:362–367
9. Pavlin D, Vukicevic D (1984) Mechanical reactions of facial skeleton to maxillary expansion determined by laser holography. AM J ORTHOD 85:498–507
10. Tanne K, Miyasaka J, Yamagata Y et al (1985) Biomechanical changes in the craniofacial skeleton by the rapid expansion appliance. J Osaka Univ Dent Soc 30:345–356
11. Chaconas SJ, Caputo AA (1982) Observation of orthopedic force distribution produced by maxillary orthodontic appliances. Am J of Orthod 82:492–501
12. Tanaka E, Tanne K, Sakudam A (1994) A three-dimensional finite element model of the mandible including the TMJ and its application to stress analysis in the TMJ during clenching. Med Eng Phys 16:316
13. Perez Del Palomar A, Doblare M (2006) Finite element analysis of the temporomandibular joint during lateral excursions of the mandible. J Biomech 39(12):2153–2163

Chapter 12
The Teaching and Practice for Neutral Network Control Course of Intelligence Science and Technology Specialty

Lingli Yu

Abstract Some main points of teaching and practice innovation for the specialty of intelligence science and technology (IST) specialized course are all described in detail from three aspects of teaching methods, practical teaching and course examination, taking the course of NNC for example, in order to individualized development and strengthen major characteristics. Firstly, teaching methods are innovated for open specialized elective courses, which include interactive syllabi, projects-orient induction combing heuristic with practice and suitable bilingual modes. Secondly, integrating course practice teaching and extended training are proposed to give full play for the leading role of the course and the auxiliary function of the extracurricular activities and projects. The last but not the least, specialized courses examination reform are suggested from three exam essential factors including exam contents, exam methods and grading standards.

Keywords Teaching and practice innovation · Intelligence science and technology (IST) · Neutral network control (NNC) course

12.1 Introduction

After Ministry of Education in China firstly approved the establishment of the undergraduate specialty of 'intelligence science and technology' in Peking University of China in 2004, then this specialty had been sprung up other 13 universities such as Beijing University of Posts and Telecommunications, Nankai University, Capital Normal University, Beijing Science and Technology University and so on [1, 2]. IST is an inter-discipline, which consists of brain science,

L. Yu (✉)
School of Information Science and Engineering, Central South University, Changsha 410083, People's Republic of China
e-mail: llyu@csu.edu.cn

S. Li et al. (eds.), *Frontier and Future Development of Information Technology in Medicine and Education*, Lecture Notes in Electrical Engineering 269,
DOI: 10.1007/978-94-007-7618-0_12,

cognitive science and artificial intelligence for major studying on the intelligence basic theory and implementation technology. The specialty of IST is a multi-interdisciplinary, crossing application field, newly developing, comprehensive and pioneering specialty, which contains strong vitality [2]. In order to survival and development, a new speciality has to form its own unique curriculum system and special courses as soon as possible [3]. Artificial intelligence, intelligent control, robotics and some other core professional courses are the important symbols to distinguish from related disciplines, and IST focus on training the professional basic capabilities of the students. CSU has set up the specialized elective course such as operations research, expert system, neutral network control, web program design, natural language processing, intelligent decision system, intelligent computing, virtual reality and intelligent game, biometric identification etc., for the specialty of IST. It aimed at strengthening practical ability and innovation ability as a fundamental starting point, this paper will describe the innovation from some aspects of teaching method, practical teaching, and course examination one by one, taking the course of neutral network control specialized course for example.

12.2 Some Main Innovation Points of Teaching Methods in the Course of Neutral Network Control

12.2.1 Design of Interactive Syllabi of Specialized Courses

Neural network control is one of the specialized courses of IST. The interactive syllabi could be taken example and introduced and advanced experience could be used, so that interactive syllabi could become the communication medium between students and teachers to improve the situation that the past syllabi exist but not be used or that was payable for leaders' examination, and then turn the static syllabi into the dynamic syllabi.

Interactive syllabi is a kind of advanced teaching management file carried out by western countries which own highly developed advanced education. Early in the neural network control class, every student is to be distributed the syllabi and has a chance to discuss or explain interactively about it in the class so as to make students understand the content of the course and their duty and role in the teaching process. After being revised and approved by both students and teachers, the outline means to reach a teaching and learning agreement between both sides. The teacher and students is looking forward to fulfilling their responsibilities and obligations according to the requirements of this outline in psychological. The core concept is to obtain the ascension of the quality of the teaching in class by use of the 'contract mechanism' of syllabi and to promote the transformation of the teaching centre from teachers to students. In addition to keep the reasonable parts of the traditional syllabi, interactive syllabi have improvements to some other parts, as is shown in Table 12.1.

Table 12.1 The innovation content of interactive syllabi

Inherit the essence	Set the teaching content and progress of specialized course for NNC to make teaching planned
	Make the traditional syllabi as the basic standard for courses teaching to stop randomness of teaching
	The traditional specialized courses syllabi of NNC become an important of teaching evaluation or quality management system
Aspects to improve	The most readers for the former specialized courses syllabi of NNC are leaders and teachers, while the probability of student interaction is limited
	The former syllabi of NNC specialized course lack of clarity of responsibilities and roles for teachers and students in the courses
	The former syllabi of NNC specialized courses lack of detailed design of the content like activities and tasks for students in the courses
	The former syllabi of NNC specialized courses lack of the individualized teaching philosophy and experience that could reflect teachers
	The former syllabi of NNC specialized courses are used as followed or just kept after established so that the syllabi lack of positive dynamic using process
Main points of innovation	The interactive syllabi should focus on students' learning activities, tasks and responsibilities in the courses
	The interactive syllabi could reflect the teaching philosophy and experience of the teachers and definite the role of teachers in the course teaching
	The interactive syllabi come into classroom to make students as main readers and to become the important learning guidebook for students
	The interactive syllabi are distributed to students in the beginning of courses to gain the recognition of students and play its role of contract

12.2.2 Projects-Orient Induction Combing Heuristic with Practice

Project-driven teaching is an education model that the students can complete the relatively small projects under the guidance of teachers actively to acquire knowledge after class. Teaching method of projects-orient induction combing heuristic with practice can enhance cultivation of students' innovation and practical ability, and strengthen students' team cooperation spirit, develop students' independent learning ability, comprehensively assess students' knowledge. The main implementation process is that: take professional planning as the main line, and guide the formation of specialty practice team according to personal preference. Students should not only simply learn the various types of neural network theory knowledge, but also should know the deep reason for every type of network, in addition that they should have targeted when they comprehend the information so as to grasp accurately in the application.

In class, the teacher can map the contents of each paper to corresponding case analysis. For instance, the application of new Google 'unmanned vehicle' are shown in Fig. 12.1. After students have a general understanding of the structure,

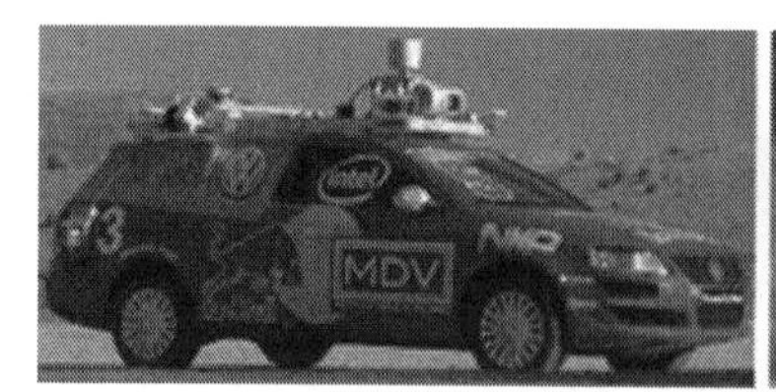

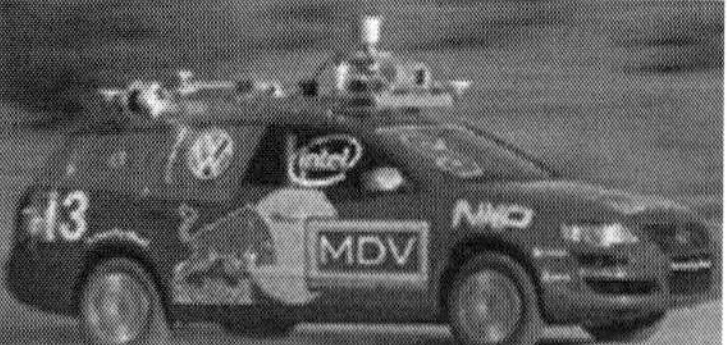

Fig. 12.1 Physical map of unmanned vehicle

control mechanisms and software framework of Google 'unmanned vehicle', it make students to feel that hierarchical control, expert control, fuzzy control, learning control in the intelligent control are no longer the control theory techniques that can not be realized. Of course, the systematic and simple introduction for the development of the most front science and technology can enhance the students' professional courses learning enthusiasm. Certainly, teachers can choose examples related to their own research to induced students stepped into specialization and standardization of specialized courses in a profound but simple way, which is one of the best forms combing heuristic with practice. In fact, the neural network control course can also use similar means to be reformed, but it must note the difference of direct contents system and distinction of architecture between courses. Besides the projects-orient induction in classroom teaching, we can also use the way of big project and interactive discussions to promote teaching.

12.3 Practice Teaching and Extended Training of NNC Course

12.3.1 Teaching Based on Foundation and be Focusing on Comprehensive Design Experiment

The neural network control is designed most for high school students as a specialized elective course, with its experimental courses focusing on the theoretical basis. Students can active thinking through experiment, deepen the understanding, consolidation and improvement of the theoretical knowledge learned in the classroom, and ultimately have the ability to analyze and solve problems. For example: This course experiments design neural networks with the help of Simulink and GUI in Matlab, such as: apply function Gensim() to make BP network generates the network a of Simulink model, as shown in Fig. 12.2. This is one of the classic designs of BP neural network experiments, and the settings for network weights and bias parameters, which require students' classroom theoretical knowledge. At the end of the experiment, the reserve design problems require students to draw the structure of designed BP network in the experimental report.

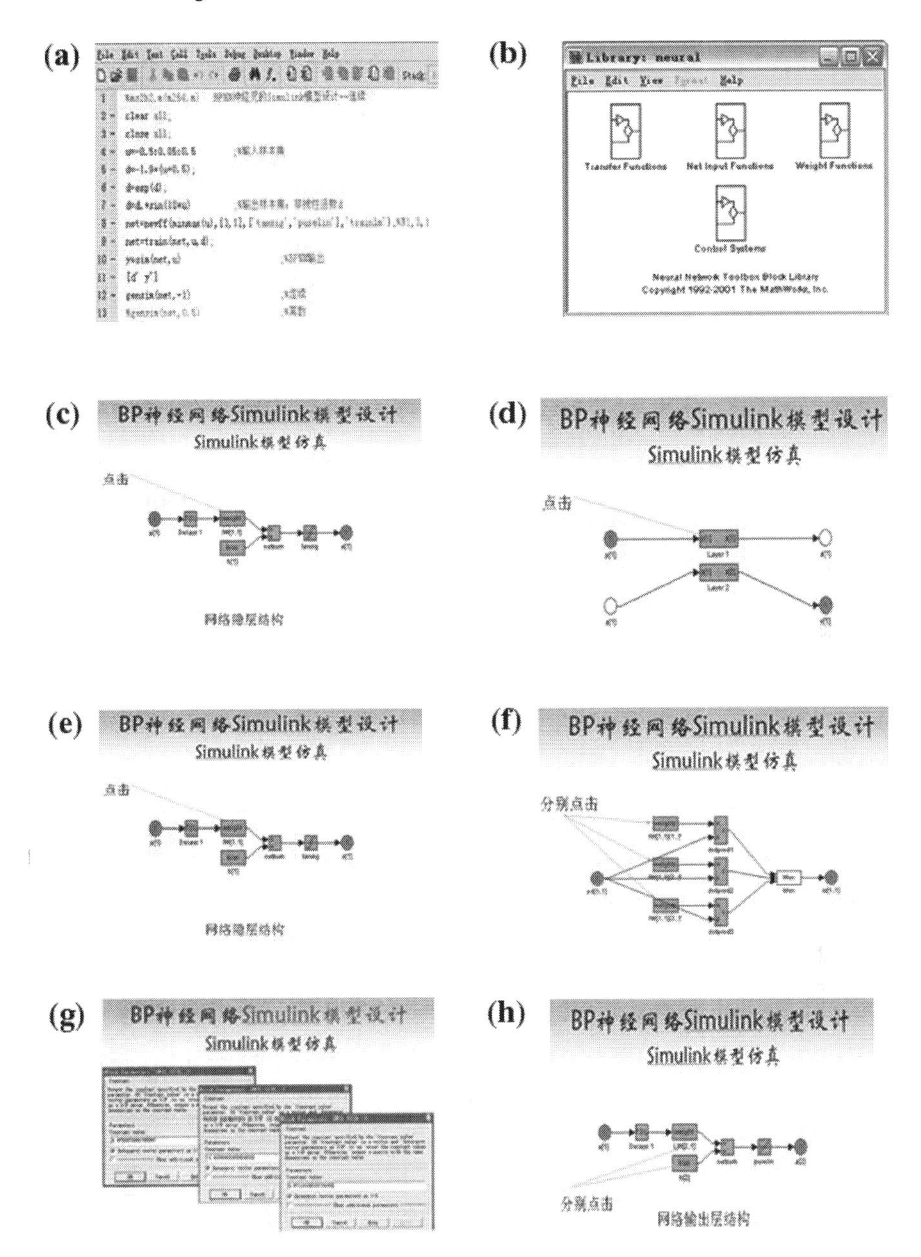

Fig. 12.2 Example of experimental teaching process

Practice teaching system includes the hierarchical experimental teaching and the extending training integrating production practice and scientific research [4, 5]. The hierarchical arrangement mainly reflects the scientific process that the level of experimental teaching from simple to complex, from single to comprehensive, from learning to innovative, and forms the settings manner of 'replication experiment → designed experiment → comprehensive experiments → outward bound → validation experiments → practice innovation'.

12.3.2 Extending Training Integrating Innovation Projects and Competition Driven

At present, innovation and pioneering projects, various academic competitions are continuing without end for undergraduate, students can make comprehensive use of multi-course knowledge to develop hands-on learning, practical and innovative applications, for that it is important for them to improve their manual dexterity and innovation ability. Neural network control of a professional teaching often take advantage of big projects and interactive discussion to guide students in progressive, and design style of project systematic, to lay a solid foundation for the latter part of the extending training.

At same time, our college has offered a number of research laboratories for IST students, such as intelligent robot laboratory, environmental perception laboratory and pattern recognition laboratory, etc., with these laboratories providing experimental environment and hardware support for intelligent control and intelligent automation. Students can choose the research to complete independently or in team, according to advice of the tutor or the direction of interest groups. The establishment of a specialty interest group is to ensure the implementation of the program, so that students can find teammates in the group, or experienced high school students can directly guide primary students. Therefore, the old with the new way of cycle training can improve students' practical abilities group after group in half the work with double results.

Extending training should set up interest groups led by 1–2 teachers, and be in the direction of special courses, such as intelligent game group, intelligent robot team, neutral network algorithm group. Intelligent game groups are designed to enable students to acquire the graphics used in the game, as well as the basic knowledge and principle of artificial intelligence, to master the application of artificial intelligence in the game, to understand and master intelligent game production process and the key technologies, meanwhile to improve students' hands-on programming ability [6, 7]. The intelligent robot team mainly cultivates students' actual capacity of sensor technology, information collection and integration of multi-sensor, and intelligent control and intelligent robotics applications. The neutral network algorithm group cultivate students in using various types of network algorithm for solving the problems of different types and improving the algorithm performance. The three are mutually independent, but closely related. Each group takes their respective closely relating competition as the starting point to further boost vitality and innovation ability of the group. For example, the intelligent robot team can take RoboCup as the main training events, and usually organize the students to participate in small group and simulation group contest of RoboCup. We should form a mutually reinforcing virtuous circle of academic competition and college students innovative experimental projects, to achieve the goal that students can practice the brain (creative thinking), practice hands (manual dexterity), practice mouth (communicate and express), train the mind (mental sublimation).

12.3.3 Suitable Bilingual Teaching Model

As the process of internationalization in institutions of higher learning speed up, the training objectives turn into the complex international talents and prompting the Ministry of Education introduced the bilingual education policy to improve college students' foreign language proficiency and to promote international exchange of expertise. The IST specialized courses are mostly multi-interdisciplinary, newly developing, comprehensive and pioneering. That not only need to borrow foreign language media to learning the advanced foreign technology, but also need to link with international standards to do two-way communicate, and then need to learn from the relevant theory and practice of the abroad, whichever is the essence, for increasing the propellant for strong development of the professional in the country.

After students studied 'Neutral Network Control', we conducted a sample survey, and found that the benefits of bilingual teaching are as the following aspects, as shown in Fig. 12.3. Through professional courses studying, students would enhance their professional knowledge, and expand their understanding of the basic course. Learn to use foreign language skills, and enhance their practical ability and creativity. Enhance their interpersonal skills and team spirit. Foster their confidence and stimulate students' potential to improve their employment competitiveness. Meanwhile, the attitudes towards to english learning are transformation and some other benefits.

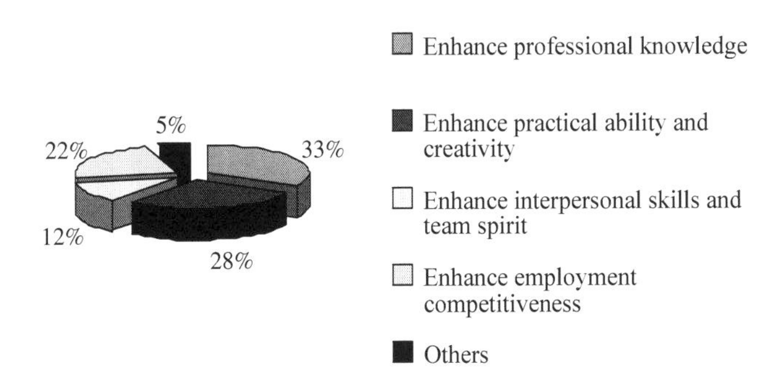

Fig. 12.3 The proportion figure of students' benefit from bilingual education

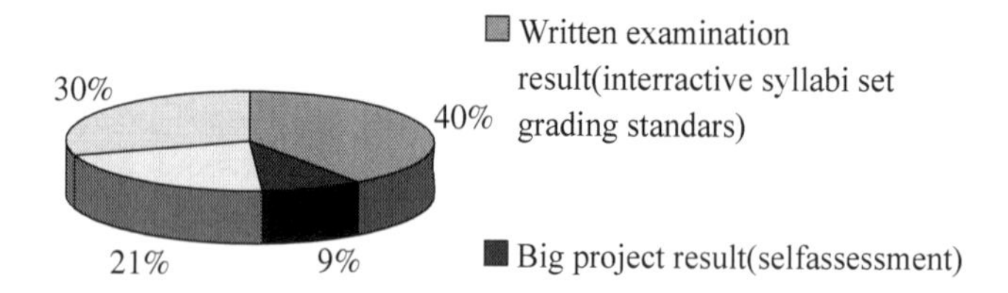

Fig. 12.4 NNC course assessment mechanism

12.4 Open Specialized Elective Courses Examination Reform

As for teaching, examination plays a role of a baton, and exam methods and exam contents directly affect students' learning attitude. Most of the assessments need exam results as an important reference for students. NNC is an optional course for senior students of IST, so the reform form and innovation magnitude can be relatively large. Exam contents, exam methods and grading standards are the three essential factors of examination and the decisive factors to reflect exam significance [8]. The assessment proportion of NNC specialized course is shown in Fig. 12.4, we should focus on cultivating students' practical ability and innovation and enhancing students' ability to work, so that to lay a good foundation for students to engage in engineering practice, engineers, researchers and other roles in the future.

12.5 Conclusion

At present, "neutral network control" specialized course teaching reform is facing the following issues: Firstly, the elective students' number of specialized courses is not many comparing to compulsory limit course. Secondly, it is necessary to clear the features and advantages of intelligence specialty: The intelligence specialized courses are a scientific crosscutting course, with relatively wide setting, includes not only knowledge of the computer, but also knowledge of automation and electronic technology. In this case, specialty orientation should be further clarified.

Although the IST courses reform is facing some difficulties, but if teaching suitable can be implemented deeply, giving full play to the leading role of the class and a supporting role of the second-class, it is sure to be able to improve the situation. Focusing on informal talents training, implementing the cooperation of industry and education, paying attention to effect, to cultivate compound talents with a large knowledge background, wide disciplines vision, high practical ability, strong innovative thinking to meet the country's major strategic talent needs.

Acknowledgments This paper was supported by National Natural Science Foundation of Hunan (13JJ4018, 13JJ4093), the Fundamental Research Funds for the Central Universities (2012QNZT060), and the Science Research Foundation of Education Bureau of Hunan Province (11B070).

References

1. Zhong XY (2009) Set intelligence science and technology as first grade subject of doctoral degree: necessity, feasibility, urgency. Comput Educ 11:5–9
2. Peng Y, Wang WS, HUANG XY (2010) Exploration and practice of construction on intelligence science and technology. Comput Educ 15:133–135
3. Liu HT, Wang GY, HU J (2010) Construction and planning of the course of intelligence science an technology. Comput Educ 19:32–34
4. Chen Y, Wang GY, Yang Q (2010) Reform and development advices for the practical content of intelligence science and technology. Comput Educ 15:119–122
5. Chen WB, Li Q, Peng SH, Li D, SU Z (2010) Construction of the innovation practice system in the intelligent science and technology specialty. Comput Educ 15:114–118
6. Shi ZG, Liu JW, Wang ZL (2009) Discussion on construction of software practical course of intelligence science and technology undergraduate specialty. Comput Educ 11:93–97
7. Jiao LC, Shi GM, Zhong Y (2009) Practice and discussion on construction of intelligence science and technology undergraduate specialty. Comput Educ 11:26–29
8. Xue SZ, Lan JH (2010) Reform for engineering specialized course examination and cultivation for students engineering practice and innovation ability. China High Educ Res 6:80–82

Chapter 13
A New ACM/ICPC-Based Teaching Reform and Exploration of "Design and Analysis of Algorithms"

Yunping Zheng and Mudar Sarem

Abstract The ACM/ICPC (ACM International Collegiate Programming Contest) is famous as the world's largest and highest level of international collegiate programming contest. In this paper, by considering some problems of the traditional teaching mode of the "Design and Analysis of Algorithms" (which is abbreviated as "Algorithms"), we propose a new ACM/ICPC-based teaching reform mode of the "Algorithms". Some principles and characteristics of the exercises based on the ACM/ICPC are presented. And, some merits and features of our reform mode are analyzed. Also, by giving the shortcomings of the ACM online judging system, the corresponding reason and the solving strategy are presented. The ACM/ICPC-based teaching reform mode of the "Algorithms" cultivates the students' interest in participating in the ACM/ICPC, greatly improves the initiative and enthusiasm to learn "Algorithms", and strengthens cultivation of the team spirit and creative ability. Our proposed reform mode improves the teaching quality, which achieves the obvious effect. Also, our mode was highly praised and generally welcomed by students. Therefore, it has some demonstrated functions for teaching reform of the "Algorithms".

Keywords ACM · ICPC · Teaching reform and exploration · Design and analysis of algorithms · Traditional teaching mode

---

Y. Zheng (✉)
School of Computer Science and Engineering, South China University of Technology, 510006 Guangzhou, People's Republic of China
e-mail: zhengyp@scut.edu.cn

M. Sarem
School of Software Engineering, Huazhong University of Science and Technology, 430074 Wuhan, People's Republic of China
e-mail: mudar66@hotmail.com

S. Li et al. (eds.), *Frontier and Future Development of Information Technology in Medicine and Education*, Lecture Notes in Electrical Engineering 269,
DOI: 10.1007/978-94-007-7618-0_13,

13.1 Introduction

13.1.1 Description of "Algorithms" Course

The "Design and Analysis of Algorithms", which is abbreviated as "Algorithms" in this paper, is one of the most important courses for college students majoring in the computer science specialty [1]. An algorithm is nothing more than a set of computational steps that transform a specific input into a desired output. However, to be a computer scientist versus a programmer, you need to know what makes an algorithm efficient, why a particular algorithm is efficient, what kinds of common data structures are involved in various computing problems, how to traverse those data structures efficiently, and a notation for analyzing various algorithms [2, 3]. NP-completeness is the study of problems for which no efficient algorithms have ever been found. These problems are interesting for two reasons. The first is being that even though an efficient algorithm has never been found, there is no proof that one cannot be existed. Second, if an efficient algorithm exists for one of them, then efficient algorithms can be existed for all. Thus, if you can show that the problem is NP-complete, you can work for producing an algorithm that gives a good solution, but it may not be the best possible solution. This kind of knowledge is what distinguishes between a computer scientist and a mere programmer.

13.1.2 Shortcomings of Traditional Teaching Mode for "Algorithms"

The "Algorithms" course is not only a strong theoretical course, but also has strong practical applications. Experimental teaching effects of the "Algorithms" have direct impact to the overall teaching quality. At present, the traditional "algorithms" teaching mode has prevalently the following issues [4–6]:

Firstly, the range of teaching contents is very wide, but with limited credit hours. In fact, in the "Algorithm" curriculum, the course's contents are very rich. The contents include some very classic algorithm design strategies, such as conquer and divide, greedy methods, and dynamic programming methods. Also, they include some advanced algorithm design strategies for solving difficult problems, such as randomized algorithms and approximation algorithms. Therefore, it is very difficult to thoroughly lecture all of the algorithm design strategies in limited credit hours.

Secondly, the students have no interests in a pure theory teaching mode, and generally feel that the "algorithms" course is difficult to learn and hard to use. The real ability of solving practical problems is still very poor after the class. In fact, most teaching methods mainly focus on the theory teaching, and therefore neglect the practice teaching. In the experimental class, there are lacks of the designed and comprehensive experiments. Students often find the answers from the Internet or the books when they are asked to do the exercises. What's more, a small part of the students may directly copy the answers from other students who have finished the exercises. So, these kinds of exercises completely lack of creative thinking ability, lead to failed experiments which just are the process of typing and debugging programs, and finally fail to achieve the teaching objectives. Therefore, the students' innovative ability in the traditional teaching mode of the "Algorithms" course can not be effectively cultured.

Thirdly, for the time being, the vast majority of colleges and universities put the assessment of the "Algorithms" often on results, not on process in general. The final scores are usually composed of two parts. One part is the ordinary score accounting for 30–40 %, which includes quizzes, exercises, reports, attitudes, and participations. The other part is the final written exam score accounting for 60–70 %. Consequently, this situation actually puts too much emphasis on the results, not on the procedure. Therefore, the students' ability to solve practical problems can not be effectively cultured in the traditional teaching mode.

Lastly, the "Algorithms" course, as a basic course in software design, can not culture the teamwork spirit in the traditional teaching mode. During the process of learning the "Algorithms", the relationship between teachers and students is a one-to-many. Some discussions and exchanges among the students can not be effectively formed. The learning experience and the knowledge among the students did not obtain effective dissemination, which leads to low overall efficiency. Since only one computer is shared by three participants during the ACM/ICPC, the contest puts more emphasis on team spirit which is one of the important capabilities that our traditional "Algorithms" teaching mode can not culture.

13.2 Our Analyses of ACM/ICPC-Based Teaching Reform for "Algorithms"

The ACM/ICPC is a multitier, team-based, programming competition operating under the auspices of ACM and headquartered at Baylor University. The contest involves a global network of universities hosting regional competitions that advance teams to the ACM/ICPC World Finals. The contest fosters creativity, teamwork, and innovation in building new software programs, and it enables students to test their ability to perform under pressure. It is the oldest, largest, and most prestigious programming contest in the world. The ACM/ICPC emphasizes not only on the interdisciplinary basis, but also on the comprehensive quality and ability. Compared with other programming competitions, the problems of the ACM/ICPC are much more difficult and put more emphasis on the efficiency of the algorithms. A specific proposition should not only be solved, but also it needs providing a best way to solve the specified proposition. The ACM/ICPC involves extensive knowledge of the computer science, such as the high-level programming languages, discrete mathematics, data structures, artificial intelligence, design and analysis of algorithms, and so on.

Since the ACM/ICPC sets the reasonable race rankings and challenge rules, and provides a complete practice mode to learn and use programming languages and algorithms, so the students who are proficient in programming are proud of their abilities. Therefore, a positive self-learning atmosphere is naturally formed. For the time being, some colleges and universities have applied the ACM mode to the software foundation courses, such as data structure [7], design and analysis of algorithms [8], and high-level programming language C ++ [9], and they have achieved remarkable teaching effects. Before the authors of this paper make a reform about the teaching mode of the "Algorithms", the ACM mode has not been applied to the teaching process of the "Algorithms" in South China University of Technology. By giving the problems of traditional teaching mode of the "Algorithms", it is entirely feasible that we aim to apply the ACM mode to the practical teaching of the "Algorithms" in order to strengthen the theoretical training and practical ability of the students by combining the theoretical knowledge and the practical application.

In this paper, we propose a new ACM/ICPC-based teaching reform mode of the "Algorithms". The proposed reform mode improves the teaching quality, which obtains the obvious effect. Also, the mode is highly praised and generally welcomed by students.

13.3 Our Proposed ACM/ICPC-Based Teaching Reform Mode of "Algorithms"

13.3.1 Our New Online Judging System for Teaching

The ACM online judging system (referred to as the OJ system) is an online real-time submission system which has the functions of program design competition, competition training, course experiments, and so on. During our reform of the "Algorithms", we develop a new OJ system used for teaching the "Algorithms" for the school of computer science and engineering at South China University of Technology. The website of the OJ is http://www.scut.edu.cn/acm/. The new OJ system for teaching can provide a lot of competition exercises or homework for students to contest or practice.

Our general principle for testing problems is as following: By strictly complying with the format of the ACM/ICPC, we provide six exercises per chapter that should be solved by using the design strategy in that chapter on the new OJ system for teaching. The students should complete at least four exercises per chapter.

Moreover, during the process of the ACM/ICPC-based teaching reform mode of the "Algorithms", our compiled exercises or homework have the following features:

Firstly, the ACM/ICPC exercises or homework found in our OJ system directly come from the textbook. The exercises or homework have been adapted or translated from ICPC by ourselves.

Secondly, the key knowledge of each chapter was added into the exercises or homework. Therefore, the students not only mastered the knowledge of each chapter, but also understood the format and style of the ACM/ICPC by submitting their program to the new OJ system.

Finally, the ACM practical teaching can be done through the network independently of time and space constraints. Different from the submitted assignments with document files or papers in the traditional teaching mode, students must write not only a program without compilation or logic errors, but also the input and output formats must comply with the ACM/ICPC format in order to be correctly accepted.

13.3.2 Our Proposed Teaching Reform Measures and Innovation

Our proposed ACM/ICPC-Based teaching reform measures and innovation of the "Algorithms" in this paper are presented as following:

Firstly, in order to enable students to focus on learning process rather than exam results, we increase score proportion of the experimental results and decrease the score proportion of the final exam. For the time being, the vast majority of colleges and universities put the assessment of the "Algorithm" often on results, not on process in general. The final scores usually are composed of two parts. However, in our reform mode, the ordinary score accounts for 60–70 %, which includes quizzes, exercises, reports, attitudes, and participations. The final written exam score only accounts for 30–40 %. In this way, most students will put too much emphasis on the procedure, not on the results. In fact, we think that the actual ability of designing the algorithm and the teamwork should be highlighted in the usual assessment. By paying more attention to the ability of the students during the learning process, the students' active learning will be potentially promoted, and the innovation capability will be effectively cultivated. Therefore, we strongly believe that the teaching effect based on the ACM/ICPC will be very obvious if we reversed the traditional proportion of the final written exam score and the ordinary score. Thus, the students' ability to solve practical problems can be effectively cultured in our ACM/ICPC-based teaching mode.

Secondly, putting the design strategies of each chapter into the exercises makes the students master the knowledge and simultaneously experience programming fun. By strictly complying with the format of the ACM/ICPC, we provide six exercises per chapter that should be solved by using the design strategy in that chapter. The students should complete at least four exercises per chapter. The assignments bare submitted entirely by the OJ system. By enabling students spending more time for programming rather than copying the experimental report, the students' initiative and enthusiasm are effectively improved.

Thirdly, in our ACM/ICPC-Based practical teaching part, we have used the "contests" function that our OJ system provides. Since the contest is carried out with limited hours in the laboratory under the supervision of the teacher, the students nearly have no opportunity to copy the source codes from the Internet or other students. The contest fosters creativity, teamwork, and innovation in building new software programs, and it enables students to test their ability to perform under pressure. The contest is very popular among the students since the contest can reflect their true levels. Therefore, our contest can greatly challenge the students' programming ability, stimulate the competition power, and culture the interest to learn the "Algorithms".

Finally, Our ACM/ICPC-based teaching mode pays more attention to the cultivation of the students' spirit for cooperation, especially the "team spirit". The students are required to communicate, discuss, and cooperate with each other. In our practical teaching, a larger project is usually partitioned into several smaller subtasks which need to be completed by several students together. After the team has finished the project, the students can submit their source codes to our OJ system. By doing this process, the students have not only learned how to deal with larger projects and, more importantly, deeply appreciated the team spirit, and learned to get along with others, but also recognized their personal value in the project.

13.4 Experimental Results and Analyses

During the process of teaching "Algorithm" in 2012, we have done two contests in our computer science and technology classes of South China University of Technology. In these classes, there are 124 students. The number of the problems in each contest is set to three. Also, the time in each contest is limited to 3 h.

The following Table 13.1 presents a contrast of the numbers between the students and the solved problems in the two contests. It can be easily seen that the number of the solved problems is relatively stable in both contests so is the number of the students who can solve the corresponding problems in the two contests. In addition, from the situation of the page place, we know that the students' places in

Table 13.1 Contrast of numbers between students and solved problems

Number of solved problems	Number of students in contest one	Number of students in contest two
3	25	27
2	37	34
1	30	33
0	32	30

both contests are also relatively stable. Therefore, the experimental results in this section show that our contest can really reflect the students' level.

From the table, it can be easily known that

(1) There are 25 and 27 students who solved the whole problems in the contest one and in the contest two, respectively, i.e., accounting for 20.16 and 21.77 %, respectively. In fact, the ordinary scores of these students are also very high.
(2) There are 37 and 34 students who solved the two problems in the contest one and in the contest two, respectively, i.e., accounting for 29.84 and 27.42 %, respectively. That's to say, the ratios of the percents of students who can solve two problems to the percents of students who can solve three problems are about one and half.
(3) There are 30 and 33 students who solved the only one problem in the contest one and in the contest two, respectively, i.e., accounting for 24.19 and 26.61 %, respectively. That's to say, the percents of students who can solve one problem are nearly same to the percents of students who can solve three problems.
(4) There are 32 and 30 students who can not solved any problems in the contest one and in the contest two, respectively, i.e., accounting for 25.81 and 24.19 %, respectively. The reason may be that they can not a design corresponding algorithm for a given problem or that they can not write C ++ programs even if they know the principium of the corresponding algorithm for a given problem. In fact, the ordinary scores of these students are also very low.

Although our ACM/ICPC-based teaching reform has many features and advantages stated above and it is quite popular with students, there is still a problem about the OJ system. The problem lies in that the OJ system can not effectively prevent the copied source codes among students. For the time being, in order to check whether the students' codes are identical or not, what we can do is only to check the database by artificial means. The association of the ordinary score with the exercises done on the OJ system usually inevitably leads to cheating. In order to get a high ordinary score, a small part of the students often directly search for answers from the Internet or some reference books. Even a small part of the students will directly copy other students' source codes and then submit them. Unfortunately, our OJ system can not check whether the students' codes are similar or not.

It is undeniable that most students completed their exercises independently. This part of the students should be given high ordinary score. However, it is fairly unfair to give the cheating students high ordinary scores. Therefore, it is very significant to encourage students to complete the exercises independently in the future. Through the observation of the statistical results from the OJ system, it can be found that some students who did very well in the contest are the students who finished the exercises of each chapter very well, too. Therefore, this part of the students should be given excellent results. However, there were still a small number of students who finished the exercises very poorly in both the contest and the exercises of each chapter. All the students will be very satisfactory with the final results if we consider the situations stated above. What's more, for the sake of fairness, the students hope that teachers can differently treat the final marks of the cheating students and the honest students who finished the exercises independently. Therefore, our solution to the drawback of the OJ system is as following:

Firstly, students must not submit their source codes outside the laboratory. In other words, all students must directly go to the laboratory to submit their source codes under the supervision of the teacher.

Secondly, we are planning to make an improvement on our OJ system by adding a function model which can check and judge the similarities of the source codes submitted by different students. By assigning the repetition rate of the source codes to a certain threshold, the function model will be able to judge the plagiarism among the students.

In fact, the drawback of the OJ system results from the cheating of a small part of the students. Also, most OJ systems do not take the potential cheatings into consideration. If we further make an improvement on our existing OJ system, the drawback will disappear.

13.5 Conclusions and Future Work

The ACM International Collegiate Programming Contest (ICPC) provides college students with opportunities to interact with students from other universities and to sharpen and demonstrate their problem-solving, programming, and teamwork skills. In this paper, by considering some problems of the traditional teaching mode of the "Algorithms", we propose a new ACM/ICPC-based teaching reform mode of the "Algorithms". Some principles and characteristics of the exercises based on the ACM/ICPC are presented. Also, some merits and features of our reform mode are analyzed in details. By giving the shortcoming of the ACM online judging system, the corresponding reasons and the solving strategies are presented. The ACM/ICPC-based teaching reform mode of the "Algorithms" cultivates the students' interest in participating in the ACM/ICPC, greatly improves the initiative and enthusiasm to learn the "Algorithms", and strengthens cultivation of the team spirit and creative ability. Our proposed reform mode improves the teaching quality, which achieves the obvious effect. Also, the mode is highly praised and generally welcomed by the students and therefore, it has some demonstrated functions for teaching reform of the "Algorithms". In the near future, we will design and develop an ACM/ICPC-based examination system used for the final exam of the "Algorithms".

Acknowledgments This work is supported by the Teaching Reform Project of Higher Education of Guangdong Province in 2013, the Major Project of the Teaching Reform of South China University of Technology in 2012 under Grant No. x2jsY1120020, the Research Fund for the

Doctoral Program of Higher Education of China under Grant No. 20120172120036, the Natural Science Foundation of Guangdong Province of China under Grant No. S2011040005815, and the Foundation for Distinguished Young Talents in Higher Education of Guangdong of China under Grant No. LYM11015.

References

1. Cormen TH, Leiserson CE, Rives RL et al. (2010) Introduction to algorithms, 3rd edn. Phi Learning
2. Zheng Y, Zhang J, Sarem M (2012) A new image representation method using nonoverlapping non-symmetry and anti-packing model for medical images. J Comput 7(12):3028–3035
3. Zheng Y, Mudar S (2011) A fast algorithm for computing moments of gray images based on NAM and extended shading approach. Frontiers Comput Sci Chin 5(1):57–65
4. Yu H (2010) Curriculum exploration of algorithm design and analysis in intelligent science and technology specialty. Comput Educ 19:15–18
5. Zheng Y (2012) Teaching mode exploration of design and analysis of algorithms. Study South Chin High Educ Eng 30(2):21–25
6. Li H (2010) Teaching reform and practice of algorithm analysis and design. Chin Electr Power Educ 16:74–75
7. Wu Y, Wang Y, Fu Y et al (2010) Promoting the practice teaching reform of algorithms and data structures relying on the program design competition. Comput Educ 4:53–55
8. Gao S (2008) Curriculum reform in algorithm design and analysis. Comput Educ 14:37–38
9. Zheng Y (2011) A novel method of reform and exploration of C ++ bilingual teaching based on ACM/ICPC. In: Proceedings of 3rd international conference on information, Electron Comput Sci 626–630

Chapter 14
Application Studies of Bayes Discriminant and Cluster in TCM Acupuncture Clinical Data Analysis

Xiangyang Feng, Youqun Shi, Qinfeng Huang, Wenli Cheng, Houqin Su and Jie Liu

Abstract For the acupuncture clinical big samples' data, Bayes discriminant method has been studied and applied to determine comprehensive posterior treatment effects of the same disease samples, and a K-mean cluster algorithm with a tolerance value has been proposed and applied to classify the samples based on a transmutative Euclidean distance function which is proposed in this paper. Differences in terms of acupuncture points and posterior treatment effective gradations between pair of samples are originally introduced into an Euclidean distance function. The analysis methods studied in this paper can service scientific analysis on acupuncture clinical data and provide a newest research way to estimate qualities of TCM acupuncture clinical treatment cases presented in the literatures.

Keywords Traditional chinese medicine · Clinical data · Acupuncture point · Treatment effect · Euclidean distance calculating formula · Estimation · Discriminant and cluster analysis

14.1 Introduction

The acupuncture of Traditional Chinese Medicine (referred as TCM below) is a medicine discipline to research meridians, acupoints, techniques of acupuncture and moxibustion. The meridian theory composed of fourteen meridians, eight extra meridians, fifteen collateral vessels, twelve meridian divergences, twelve meridian

X. Feng (✉) · Y. Shi · W. Cheng · H. Su
College of Computer Science and Technology, Donghua University, Shanghai 200051, People's Republic of China
e-mail: fengxy@dhu.edu.cn

Q. Huang · J. Liu
Shanghai Institute of Acupuncture and Meridian, Shanghai 200030, People's Republic of China

S. Li et al. (eds.), *Frontier and Future Development of Information Technology in Medicine and Education*, Lecture Notes in Electrical Engineering 269,
DOI: 10.1007/978-94-007-7618-0_14,

sinews, twelve cutaneous regions, tertiary collateral vessel, superficial collateral vessel and etc. is formed during the medical treatment practices of acupuncture in the long period, and a set of complete method to treat diseases has been introduced [1]. TCM acupuncture has the rich literature sources; it is an important composing part of Chinese culture legacy and has the precious reference values. Clinical treatment cases of the acupuncture literatures include a large number of treatment examples, but inherent relations and regular patterns among acupuncture points of treatment diseases couldn't be found out in accuracy and science. Therefore, putting the thinking logics of data analysis methods in studying of the clinical treatment data of the acupuncture literatures has a very important meaning.

The work studied and described in this paper was supported by National Basic Research Program of China (973 Program, 2009CB522900).

14.2 Correlation Work

There are a large number of data analysis researches on clinical data in medicinal field inside and outside of China. Cluster methods with multi-dimension data had been used to analyze for albumin and blood platelet of patients outside of China and to obtain the conclusion set of illness data with trouble of chronic hepatitis [2]. There are researches for certain genes to find out relations among their structures and organisms characters, thereby to make an important action for treatment and prevention of hereditary disease [3]. Researches and summarizing of regular patterns for usages of medicinal materials through collecting and reorganizing usage quantities of medicinal materials, observing and treatments and folk prescriptions such as the category of gentle replenishments' science of TCM have provided the reference values for disease treatments in TCM field [4–6], but they are still located at the starting step period compared with western medical field.

Research of the acupuncture clinical data collected by Shanghai Institute of Acupuncture and Meridian can obtain enlightenments. Analysis results of the data can be used to perfect shortages from fortes. The acupuncture clinical treatment cases more than 60,000 have been collected and prepared from 1705 books of journal concerned with TCM or combining TCM with western medicine of 75 kind by the institute, and an information database of the acupuncture clinical treatment cases (referred as DBACTC below) had been established [7].

14.3 Studies of Bayes Discriminant and Cluster Algorithm

14.3.1 Data Selection and Application of Bayes Discriminant Algorithm

14.3.1.1 Data Selection and Expressions

DBACTC is designed and realized following the related standards inside and outside of China and the third normal form (referred as 3NF). Five attributes such as disease symptom code, total number of cases, number of effective cases, acupuncture points and curing ways for each treatment case had been selected as a record attributes of sample. Part records of the samples are shown in Table 14.1.

As shown in Table 14.1, information of acupuncture points and cure ways are expressed by the codes, all the Chinese descriptions of these codes can be retrieved from the corresponding dictionary tables. in DBACTC.

14.3.1.2 Study and Application of Bayes Discriminant Algorithm

A prior treatment effect of clinical treatment cases listed in a literature can be easily obtained through dividing number of effective case by number of all case as shown in Table 14.1. But this kind of prior treatment effect can't objectively reflect an actual treatment effect of the literature. The actual treatment effect should be evaluated in all the collected clinical treatment cases of the same disease symptom in terms of the acupuncture points and cure ways listed in the literature. Therefore, Bayes discriminant is used to determine each actual treatment effect, i.e., each posterior treatment effect. One of its original application aims is objectively to determine the quality of a literature on clinical treatment experiences.

Steps of a Bayes discrisminant algorithm are summarized as the followings:

Step 1 Dividing gradation of prior treatment effect for each record

Suppose n is the total number of record in a samples' set of the same disease symptom, information of *i*th record is abstracted from *i*th literature. M_i and N_i

Table 14.1 Part records of the samples constructed by the five attributes

Name Serial No.	Symptom_Subid	All_ Case	Effective_ Case	Acupuncture_Points	Cureways
1	0028	54	48	CO1,CO4,CO13,CO17,HX1, CO14,CO7,CO18	017, 078
2	0622	45	45	BL10,GV14,GB20,W23,GB4, GB5,GB6,GB8,GB12,EX-HN5,GV20	007, 001
3	0112	240	234	BL12,BL13,EX-B1,CV22,LU10,LU11,ST40,LI11	007

respectively express a value of all case and effective case as shown in Table 14.1. Obviously, $E_i = N_i/M_i$(i = 1,…,n) is a prior treatment effective probability of *i*th record.

Record E = {E_1, E_2,…,E_n}, $E_{\min} = \min_{1 \le i \le n} E_i$ and $E_{\max} = \max_{1 \le i \le n} E_i$, divide [$E_{\min}$, $E_{\max}$] into five value ranges which correspond to five gradations L_1 to L_5 in ascending order.

For example, suppose E_{min} = 60 % and E_{max} = 90 %, a taking value range of L_1 to L_5 can be separately defined as L_1 60 ~ 70 %, L_2 71 ~ 80 %, L_3 81 ~ 83 %, L_4 84 ~ 86 % and L_5 87 ~ 90 %.

Obviously, ith record can be divided into the gradation L_4 if and only if its prior treatment effective value E_i falls in the range [84–86 %].

The prior treatment effective gradations can be separately recorded as $LP_i(E_i) = j$ if and only if the value of E_i falls in the range of the L_j ($\forall E_i \in$ E, j = 1, 2, …, 5).

Step 2 Calculating posterior treatment effective gradations of cure ways and acupuncture points for each record

Suppose ith record has m kind cure ways totally (m ≥ 1), record q[th] (1 ≤ q ≤ m) cure way as C_q.

A posterior effective probability for the cure way C_q of ith record referencing all the prior treatment effective gradation L_j (j = 1, 2, …, 5) of records in the samples' set can be calculated from the following formula:

$$P\left(C_q|_{L_j}\right) = \sum_{1 \le i \le n} LP_i\left(E_i|_{C_q \wedge L_j}\right) \Big/ \sum_{i=1}^{n} LP_i\left(E_i|_{L_j}\right) \quad (j = 1, 2, \ldots, 5,\ 1 \le q \le m) \tag{14.1}$$

Simultaneously, a posterior probability of each prior treatment effective gradation L_j (j = 1, 2, …, 5) referencing all the prior treatment effective gradations can be calculated from the following formula:

$$P(L_j) = \sum_{1 \le i \le n} LP_i\left(E_i|_{L_j}\right) / \sum_{i=1}^{n} LP_i(E_i) \quad (j = 1, 2, \ldots, 5) \tag{14.2}$$

Substitute the value calculated form the formula (14.1) and (14.2) into Bayes formula:

$$P\left(L_j|_{C_q}\right) = \frac{P(L_j)P\left(C_q|_{L_j}\right)}{\sum_{k=1}^{5} P(L_k)P\left(C_q|_{L_k}\right)} \quad (j = 1, 2, \ldots, 5,\ 1 \le q \le m) \tag{14.3}$$

Obviously, a posterior probability of the cure way C_q of ith record under gradation L_j obtained form the formula (14.3) is seemed more objective, fair and overall.

Take $P\left(L_j|_{C_q}\right) = \max_{1 \leq k \leq 5} P\left(L_k|_{C_q}\right)$ $(q = 1, 2, \ldots, m)$ and record a posterior treatment effective gradation of C_q as $LC_q^i\left(L|_{E_i \wedge C_q}\right) = j\,(1 \leq j \leq 5, q = 1, 2, \ldots, m)$.

Suppose ith record has different t ($t \geq 1$) acupuncture points, and separately record as A_r (r = 1, 2, ..., t). Adopting the formula (14.1), (14.2) and (14.3), we can calculate a posterior treatment effective gradation for each acupuncture point A_r and record as $LA_r^i\left(L|_{E_i \wedge A_r}\right) = j(1 \leq j \leq 5,\ r = 1, 2, \ldots, t)$.

Step 3 Take an average value of all the $LC_q^i(L|_{E_i \wedge C_q})$ and $LA_r^i(L|_{E_i \wedge A_r})$ as the posterior treatment effective gradation of ith record

A posterior treatment effective gradation calculating formula of ith record is defined as the following:

$$LNew_i\left(L|_{E_i}\right) = \frac{1}{2}\left(\frac{1}{m}\sum_{q=1}^{m} LC_q^i(L|_{E_i \wedge C_q}) + \frac{1}{t}\sum_{r=1}^{t} LA_r^i(L|_{E_i \wedge A_r})\right) \quad (1 \leq i \leq n) \tag{14.4}$$

An integer will be obtained by rounding when a value of$LNew_i\left(L|_{E_i}\right)$ is a un-integer. Obviously, $LNew_i\left(L|_{E_i}\right)$ is obtained based on all the records in the samples' set, it reflects the treatment effect of the ith literature more objectively and equitably comparing to the prior treatment effect $LP_i(E_i)$.

14.3.2 Study and Application of a K-mean Cluster Algorithm

A K-mean cluster algorithm based on a transmutative Euclidean distance function has been studied in order to classify the records of the same disease symptom, and recognize their treatment effects and ways among the classes.

14.3.2.1 Data Selection

Data which will be applied to a K-mean cluster algorithm can be selected from DBACTC. The posterior treatment effective gradations calculated from the formula (14.4) will be used in a transmutative Euclidean distance function.

Attributes' structure of a samples' set of the same disease symptom is defined in Table 14.2.

Table 14.2 Attributes' structure of a samples' set

Description	Attribute Name	Usage
Codes of disease symptoms	symptom_subid	Unique key to classify different disease symptoms.
Information of acupuncture points	acupuncture_points	Information of acupuncture points for treatment.
Posterior treatment effective gradation	$LNew_i\left(L\vert_{E_i}\right)$	A comprehensive treatment effective gradation of ith record, i.e., ith literature $1 \le i \le n$.

14.3.2.2 A Transmutative Euclidean Distance Function

In DBACTC, a dictionary table about acupuncture point codes and their Chinese terms had been defined and established, in which all the acupuncture point codes are sorted in ascending order. So we can define a binary string to express acupuncture points for any treatment, in which "1" or "0" indicates a point is used or not. At present, about 500 points are used such as 365 meridian points, ear points, scalp points, extra points and etc.

Set A_i^p and A_i^q separately express *i*th acupuncture point of *p*th record and *q*th record for treatment.

A transmutative Euclidean distance function of *p*th record and *q*th record is defined as the following:

$$d(p,q) = \sqrt{\sum_{i=1}^{500} (A_i^p - A_i^q)^2 + \left(LNew_p\left(L|_{E_p}\right) - LNew_q(L|_{E_q})\right)^2} \quad (1 \le p,\, q \le n) \tag{14.5}$$

The former part of function (14.5) can be easily calculated by AND-OR operation, which reflects difference between acupuncture points and between the posterior comprehensive treatment effective gradations of *p*th record and *q*th record.

14.3.2.3 Application of A K-mean Cluster Algorithm with A Tolerance

A symmetrical matrix D_{nxn} of real number can be obtained by using function (14.5) based on pairs of elements in the samples' set. A tolerance value introduced in this paper can classify the elements well.

Set $d_{\min} = \min_{1 \le p,\, q \le n} d(p,q)$, $d_{\max} = \max_{1 \le p,\, q \le n} d(p,q)$, $d_{range} = d_{\max} - d_{\min}$ and the tolerance value $t = \frac{1}{d_{\min} + \frac{1}{5} d_{range}}$ as a boundary value for clustering. $0 < t \le 1$ can be easily proved.

The tolerance value *t* can be adjusted in terms of some special requirement.

For clear description of the clustering algorithm, we define a samples' set as S, S_k ($k \geq 1$) as kth class whose elements belong to S, S_r as a rest samples' set obtained from $S - \overset{k}{\cup} S_k$ in where S_r changes when k changes, e_i as an element of S whose subscript will be determined in terms of its context in S.

A formal K-mean cluster algorithm practiced in this paper is described as the followings:

(1) $k \leftarrow 1$, $S_r = S$, $S_m = \Phi$; //Sm is a miscellaneous class.
(2) $i \leftarrow 1$, $S_k = \{e_{i'} | e_{i'} \in S_r\}$, $S_r = S_r - S_k$; //take an arbitrary element ei' as an element of S_k.
(3) if $\exists e_j \in S_r$ and $i < 2$ and $1/d\{i', j\} \geq t$ then $\{S_k = S_k \cup \{e_j\}$, $S_r = S_r - \{e_j\}$, $i \leftarrow i + 1$, go step 3)$\}$;
(4) if $i < 2$ go step 8); //a class S_k might not be obtained under the tolerance t.
(5) if $S_r \neq \Phi$ then {take $\forall e_j \in S_r$, sort d(i, j) ($e_i \in S_k$, $i = 1, 2, \ldots, |S_k|$) ordered by ascendant, allot e_j to S_k if and only if $1/d(i, j) \geq t$ and a place of the d(i, j) in the sorting should locate in an approximated middle place, $S_k = S_k \cup \{e_j\}$ when it is truth} else go step 7);
(6) $S_r = S_{r-}\{e_j\}$, go step 5);
(7) $S_r = S - \overset{k}{\cup} S_k - S_m$, if $|S_r| > 1$ $\{k = k + 1$, go step 2)$\}$ else go step 9);
(8) $S_r = S_r - S_k$, $S_m = S_m \cup S_k$, if $|S_r| > 1$, go step 2); //changing $e_{i'}$ try to find another class.
(9) if $S_r \neq \Phi$ $S_m = S_m \cup S_r$;//allot the last element of S_r to S_m.
(10) end of this algorithm. //a miscellaneous class S_m might be existed under the tolerance t.

The symbol |S| expresses the total number of element in the set S. Obviously, the reciprocal value of difference for any pair of elements in the miscellaneous class S_m is less than t if $|S_m| > 0$. It can be easily proved that the computing complexity of the algorithm described as the above is $o(n^2)$. Totally k (≥ 1) class can be obtained besides of a miscellaneous class. There is no seed of each class during the clustering procedure, as you see; a sample might be allotted to a class just depending on the 2 conditions. In such a clustering method, similarities among the samples in a class can be well assured with average approximated meanings.

14.4 Experiment Results

14.4.1 Result Analysis of Bayes Discriminant

The result of a typical experiment for eczema cases is used to verify the objectivity of the discriminant analysis. Part of the result of the discriminant analysis on the posterior comprehensive treatment effective gradations on the eczema cases of a skin disease category is listed in Table 14.3.

Table 14.3 Part of the result of the discriminant analysis on eczema of a skin disease category

No.	Subject of Treatment	Acupuncture Points	Posterior Effect	Prior Effect
1	Treatment of Chronic Eczema with Point-through-point Needling plus Pricking- cupping Therapy:A Report of 58 Cases	Dazhui(GV 14) Shenzhu(GV 12) Feishu(BL 13)	5	58/58
2	Treatment of Chronic Eczema with Plum-blossom Needle plus Garlic-partitioned Moxibustion: A Report of 96 Cases	Ashi points	4	88/96
3	Treatment of Eczema due to Varicosity with Fire Needle Therapy: A Report of 31 Cases	Ashi points	5	30/31
4	Clinical Observation on Treating Chronic Eczema by Plum-blossom Needle plus Triamcinolone Acetonide and Neomycin Paste	Ashi points	5	32/33
5	Treatment of Eczema and Neurodermatitis with Auricular Acupuncture plus Induction of Zinc Ion:A Report of 135 Cases (Ear Eletroacupuncture Group)	CO14 ,TF4 ,CO18	2	61/65
6	Treatment of Eczema and Neurodermatitis with Auricular Acupuncture plus Induction of Zinc Ion:A Report of 135 Cases (Ear Acupuncture Group)	CO14 ,TF4 ,CO18	1	34/60

As you see from Table 14.3, No. 2 sample presented the ratio 91.6 % (88/96) as its prior effect for treatment, No. 5 sample 93.8 % (61/65), obviously the prior treatment effect of No. 5 sample is higher than No. 2 sample. But the posterior effective gradation for treatment of No. 2 sample calculated through the Bayes discriminant analysis is 4, No. 5 sample is 2 which is lower than 2 gradations compared with No. 2 sample. This is because that the effective treatment cases of No. 6 sample with similarities of No. 5 sample is partially low obviously; it is the ratio 56.6 % (34/60), and the effective treatment cases presented in No. 3 and 4 sample with similarities of No. 2 sample are partially high. The result listed in Table 14.3 proved the posterior treatment effective gradations are seemed more objective and fair.

14.4.2 Result Analysis of Cluster

Results of Cluster analysis algorithms have some certain reference values; Part of the result of the cluster analysis on the posterior comprehensive treatment effects on leucoderma disease of a skin disease category is listed in Table 14.4.

Samples in the samples' set of leucoderma disease have been classified 5 classes as shown in Table 14.4. 1st class takes primarily the Ashi points, 2nd class the back points, 3rd class the ear points, 4th class the head points and 5th class the four limbs' points of human body for treatment. The similar degree clustered by the algorithm is approximated to the contents presented in the literatures. There are

Table 14.4 the result of the cluster analysis on the samples of leucoderma disease

Class No.	Subject of Treatment	Acupuncture Points	Posterior Effect
1	Clinical Observation on Treating 13 Cases of Vitiligo by Acupuncture plus Electromagnetic Wave	Ashi points	4
	Treatment of Vitiligo with Thread-embedding Therapy plus TDP Radiation: A Report of 7 Cases	Ashi points	5
	Treatment of Vitiligo with Plum-blossom Needle plus Chinese Medicine Administration and External Use: A Report of 25 Cases	Ashi points	5
2	Curative Effect Observation on Treating 83 Cases of Vitiligo with Thread-embedding Therapy	Quchi (LI 11),Yanglingquan (GB 34), Geshu (BL 17),Feishu (BL 13), Weishu (BL 21), Pishu (BL 20), Shenshu (BL 23), Danzhong (CV 17), Guanyuan (CV 4), Waiguan (TE 5), Sanyinjiao (SP 6)	3
	Treatment of Vitiligo with Thread-embedding Therapy: A Report of 30 Cases	Feishu (BL 13), Geshu (BL 17), Pishu (BL 20) Weishu (BL 21), Shenshu (BL 23),Yanglingquan (GB 34), Sanyinjiao (SP 6), Quchi (LI 11), Waiguan (TE 5)	3
3	Treatment of Vitiligo with Auricular Acupuncture: A Report of 18 Cases	CO14 , CO18, AT4, CO15	3
	Clinical Observation on Treating 66 Cases of Vitiligo by Comprehensive Treatment	CO15 ,CO12 ,CO14 ,CO18, Ashi points	4
	Combined Treatment of Acupuncture and Medicine for Vitiligo: A Report of 260 Cases	CO15 ,CO12 ,CO14 ,CO18, Zhongkui (EX-UE 4),Ashi points	4

(continued)

Table 14.4 (continued)

Class No.	Subject of Treatment	Acupuncture Points	Posterior Effect
4	Clinical Observation on Acupuncture plus Vinegar-partitioned Moxibustion for 38 Cases of Vitiligo	Dicang (ST 4), Yintang (GV 29),Hegu (LI 4), Baihui (GV 20), Dazhui (GV 14), Quchi (LI 11), Zusanli (ST 36), Yanglingquan (GB 34), Shangxing (GV 23), Jiache (ST 6), Sanjian (LI 3), Taodao (GV 13), Shousanli(LI 10), Shangjuxu (ST 37), Xuanzhong (GB 39), Sanyinjiao (SP 6)	2
	Treatment of Acupuncture plus Halcinonide Solution for Vitiligo: A Report of 46 Cases	Yintang (GV 29), Dicang (ST 4), Hegu (LI 4), Quchi (LI 11), Yanglingquan (GB 34), Zusanli (ST 36),Xuehai (SP 10), Baihui (GV 20), Dazhui (GV 14), Shangxing (GV 23), Jiache (ST 6), Sanjian (LI 3), Xuanzhong (GB 39), Sanyinjiao (SP 6), Shangjuxu (ST 37), Shousanli(LI 10), Taodao (GV 13)	2
5	Treatment of Vitiligo with Plum-blossom Needling under TDP plus Thread-embedding Therapy: A Report of 58 Cases	Dazhui (GV 14), Zusanli (ST 36), Quchi (LI 11), Fengmen (BL 12), Feishu (BL 13), Ganshu(BL 18), Danshu(BL 19), Shenshu (BL 23), Geshu(BL 17)	4
	Treatment of Vitiligo with Thread-embedding Therapy plus Plum-blossom Needling: A Report of 36 Cases	Feishu (BL 13), Zusanli (ST 36), Quchi (LI 11), Fengmen (BL 12),Waiguan (TE 5), Ganshu(BL 18), Yanglingquan (GB 34), Sanyinjiao (SP 6), Shenshu (BL 23), Ganshu(BL 18), Geshu(BL 17)	4

some certain similarities in each class as shown in Table 14.4. Literatures with some certain similar contents can be classified into a class and be evaluated objectively by using the transmutative Euclidean distance function and the K-mean cluster algorithm with a tolerance studied and proposed in this paper.

14.5 Conclusion

A discriminant analysis method to estimate posterior comprehensive treatment effective gradations for TCM acupuncture clinical treatment cases of the same disease based on Bayes discriminant had been proposed, studied and practiced originally in this paper, in which the transmutative Euclidean distance function is also proposed and introduced for the K-mean cluster algorithm with a tolerance.

Although one of the initial study aims in the project is looking for a method which can be used to estimate qualities of TCM acupuncture clinical treatment cases presented in the literatures automatically. Therefore, the studies in this paper are used to realize the aim. The second aim based on the studies described in this paper is study and realization of an expert system to evaluate or propose TCM acupuncture treatment schemes and to estimate qualities of the literatures automatically. Therefore, a big data of TCM acupuncture clinical treatment cases and some important algorithm studies and applications are very important and meaningful, however,the related reports about the second aim are difficultly to be seen now inside of China.

References

1. Wang J, Yang X, Zhu Q, Li H, Guo Z, Niu X et al (2011) Establishment of acupuncture module in the four diagnoses auxiliary apparatus. World Sci Technol (Modernization of Traditional Chinese Medicine and Materia Medica) 13(2):266–270
2. Hirano S, Tsumoto S (2006) Cluster analysis of time-series medical data based on the trajectory representation and multiscale comparison techniques. In: Sixth IEEE International Conference on Data Mining (ICDM'06), Hong Kong, pp 896–901
3. Yu H, Lu Y (2003) Application of data mining in biomoedical engineering. Foreign Med Sci 2:54–58
4. Fan L, Fu W, Xu N, Liu J, Liang Z, Ou A (2011) Literature measurement data analysis of acupuncture treatment for depression. BMEI IEEE 4:1978–1981
5. Wei Y, Li J, Wang R (2008) The algorithm of rough set-based grid fuzzy clustering and Its application and research in tongue diagnosis of traditional Chinese medicine. In: Fifth International Conference on Fuzzy Systems and Knowledge Discovery, 2008, vol 1. pp 77–81
6. Liu Y, Guo Y, Yongming G, Chen L, Wang C, Wang J, Li.Y (2011) Characteristics extraction and analysis on the electrical signals of spinal dorsal root nerve evoked by acupuncture manipulations. In: 4th International Conference on Biomedical Engineering and Informatics, BMEI 2011, Shanghai, China, 15–17 October 2011
7. Huang Q, Su H (2012) A way of establishing an Information database of TCM acupunctures of Shanghai acupuncture. J Acta Editologica 24(2):66

Chapter 15
Implanting Two Fiducials into the Liver with Single Needle Insertion Under CT Guidance for CyberKnife® SBRT

Li Yu, Xu Hui-jun and Zhang Su-jing

Abstract *Purpose* We implanted four to six fiducial markers before treating liver tumors with CyberKnife® to allow image-guided positioning before treatment and real-time tracking during treatment. In the conventional implanting technique, a needle insertion is required to place each fiducial, i.e., patients would receive four to six needle punctures. To improve efficiency and reduce the time required for the procedure, not to mention the pain and risks of fiducial implantation, we invented a technique whereby two fiducials are implanted with each needle insertion. *Methods and Materials* Liver tumors constitute the most common disease treated at our radiotherapy center. From August 2011 to July 2012, 429 patients with liver tumors underwent fiducial implantation with the technique of one-needle insertion placing two fiducials at a time. Ages varied 19–74 years old. In total, 1252 fiducials were implanted with this technique. For the new technique, an initial CT image of the tumor was used to determine the implanting depth and angle of the first fiducial marker. The first fiducial was placed using an 18-gauge needle, and the needle stylet and set remain stationary for 3–5 min, after which it was slowly pulled 3–5 cm out, and then the second fiducial was released. Another image of the fiducials was acquired to assess the distance between the fiducials, their angle with respect to each other, and their compliance with the requirements of fiducial placement before continuing the procedure. *Results* Among the 1252 fiducials implanted with the technique, 18 (1.44 %) had a distance smaller than 20 mm between each other, 24 (1.92 %) were collinear at 45° vantage point, 17 (1.04 %) migrated to other organs, and the success rate was 95.28 %. With this technique, 626 punctures were required whereas 1252 punctures would have been needed with the conventional technique. Besides, implanting with a 35°–5° angle makes fiducials collinear in the 45° direction. For some patients, for whom the two-fiducial insertion technique required a puncture deeper than 5 cm, the fiducials were inserted one by one. *Conclusion* Dual fiducial insertion doubles the

L. Yu · X. Hui-jun (✉) · Z. Su-jing
Oncology Radiotherapy Center of 302, Military Hospital, 100039 Beijing, China
e-mail: huijunxu2008@sina.com

S. Li et al. (eds.), *Frontier and Future Development of Information Technology in Medicine and Education*, Lecture Notes in Electrical Engineering 269,
DOI: 10.1007/978-94-007-7618-0_15,

implanting efficiency and halves the number of punctures so that the costs and risks are both reduced. The distance between fiducials being smaller than 20 mm and collinear fiducials at the 45° angle direction are the most common complications affecting success rate.

Keywords CT guidance · Fiducial implantation · CyberKnife · SBRT

15.1 Introduction

The CyberKnife® System (Accuray Incorporated, Sunnyvale, CA), which received FDA clearance for treatment in 2001, is used to deliver stereotactic radiosurgery to tumors throughout the body. Combining a linear accelerator, a robotic arm, and an image-guidance system with synchronous respiratory tracking, it allows more angles of incidence and accurate irradiation (the irradiation accuracy to dynamic targets is within 1.5 mm) [1, 2]. As the tumors of soft tissues lack bony structure which can be tracked, fiducial markers are implanted in or beside tumors before CyberKnife stereotactic body radiation therapy (SBRT) so as to be used in the image-guided positioning before treatment and the real-time tracking during treatment delivery [3]. Fiducials can be implanted by several ways, for example, percutaneously under the guidance of ultrasound or CT, or implanted with the guidance of electromagnetic navigation bronchoscopy (ENB). However, these methods can only implant one fiducial per needle insertion [4, 5]. Although fiducial implantation is a minimally invasive surgery, it still exposes patients to pain and medical risks. Conventionally, four to six fiducials are implanted for liver cancer tumors using the same number of punctures. To improve the implanting efficiency and reduce the pain and the risks, we invented a technique of placing two fiducials with one needle insertion based on the conventional 1-fiducial-per-insertion technique. After using the new method for more than a year, we found the success rate as equivalent to the conventional one-fiducial-at-a-time technique. In this article, we describe our experience with this methodology.

15.2 Materials and Methods

15.2.1 Patients

Between August 2011 and July 2012, 429 patients (274 men and 155 women) with hepatocarcinoma were implanted two fiducials with one needle insertion under CT guidance. Average age was 49 years (range, 19–74 years). Altogether, 1,252 fiducials were implanted. Tumor volume ranged from 3.9–978.3 cc. This article is

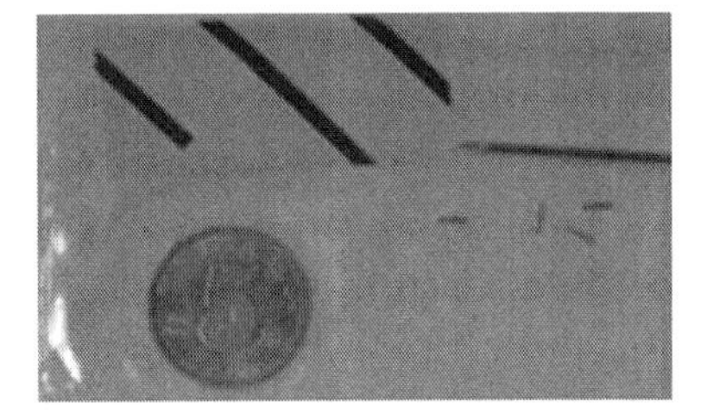

Fig. 15.1 Disinfected and sealed fiducials (4)

concerned only with the evaluation of the fiducials implanted by the two-fiducials-per-puncture technique. However, some patients received fiducials implanted employing both techniques.

15.2.2 Fiducials and Equipment

A fiducial marker, with the dimensions of 0.8 × 5 mm, is a cylinder made of 99.99 % pure gold with whorl on the surface (Fig. 15.1 [6]). We chose an 18-gauge needle with 15-cm length, which was made of a needle stylet, a needle set, and a ring (Fig. 15.2). The necessary equipment in the implantation process included a CT apparatus, puncture guiding device, and position indicator.

15.2.2.1 Fiducial Implantation Parameters

Four to six fiducials were implanted in or near the tumor; the distance between them was smaller than 20 mm; their angle with respect to each other was larger than 15°; the fiducials could not be collinear at a 45° angle view point; and the distance between fiducials and target regions was smaller than 60 mm [7, 8].

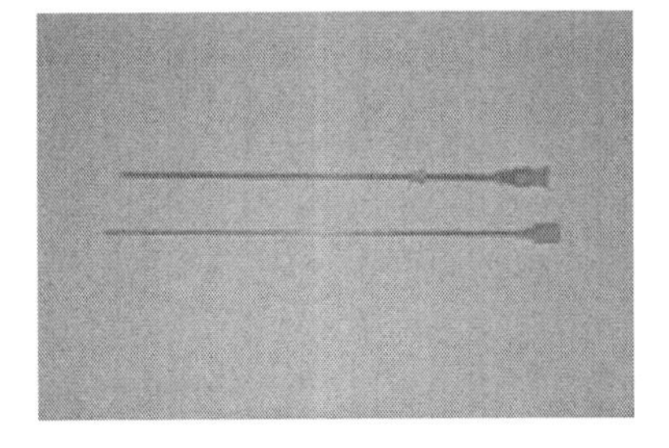

Fig. 15.2 18-gauge puncture needle, consisting of needle stylet, set and ring

15.2.3 Insertion of One Fiducial Per Puncture

Under CT guidance, one fiducial was implanted by a percutaneous puncture. If six fiducials needed to be implanted, the patient would have to bear the pain brought on by six puncture wounds and the associated risk of hemorrhage. This technique is the conventional way of implanting fiducials as it is easy to carry out and has a high success rate.

15.2.4 Evaluation of the Distance Between Fiducials and their Angle with Respect to Each Other

After implanting two fiducials with the two-fiducials-per-puncture technique, an image of the fiducials was acquired and the layer thickness was verified to be smaller than 1.5 mm. Utilizing the measuring tools of "distance" and "angle" on the workstation of CT image apparatus, we measured the distance between each pair of fiducials and their angles with respect to each other on the horizontal plain. What we wanted to accomplish was that the distance between two fiducials was not greater than 20 mm and the markers did not obscure one another when viewed at a 45° angle, before the treatment.

One week after the implantation, during which the fiducials were allowed to settle, the patient would be ready for the treatment using fiducial-assisted respiratory tracking. If two of the fiducials overlapped when viewed at 45°, the distance between the fiducials on one side of the image plane would be too small to be correctly recognized by the computer [9, 10].

15.2.5 Insertion Angle

Unlike the one-fiducial-per-insertion technique, the two-fiducials-per-insertion technique uses coplanar implantation and thus sometimes runs into the problem of fiducials being collinear at 45°. To avoid this situation, we collected data on insertion angles, so that the best available angles could be identified. These angles were grouped into three ranges: 0–35°, 35–55°, and 55–90° (Table 15.1).

Table 15.1 Fiducial insertion angles

Ranges	0–35°	35–55°	55–90°
Fiducial number	382	44	836

15.3 Results

15.3.1 Steps of the Two-Fiducials-Per-Insertion Technique

Disinfect all tools, including the fiducials and puncture needle. The patient lies on the CT couch with hands on either side of the head.

Put the position indicator on the patient's body and acquire images of the liver and position indicator. Use the measuring tools of "distance" and "angle" on the CT workstation to determine the implanting depth of the first fiducial and angle of the two fiducials.

Use the position indicator to choose the coordinates on the left and right of the puncture point, measure the distance between the puncture point and initial point of scanning, and then determine the coordinates in the S/I direction. According to these coordinates, we can pinpoint the puncture point on the patient's skin and mark it (Fig. 15.3a). Open the puncture guiding device and set the direction of the laser in accordance with the puncturing angle which was measured in the CT image (Fig. 15.3b). Move the puncture guiding device so that the laser spot aims at the puncture point, confirm the puncture position and direction, and then start the implantation.

Topically disinfect the implanting position on the patient's skin and apply local anesthesia. Adjust the ring position on the surface of the needle set corresponding to the puncture depth of the first fiducial, as determined in the second step. The puncture needle pierces through the skin and penetrates the liver until the ring reaches the skin. Draw out the needle stylet, put the first fiducial in the needle set, use the stylet to push it into the liver, and finish the implantation of the first fiducial (Fig. 15.3c). Figure 15.4a shows the needle reaching the preset depth, and Fig. 15.4b the image of finishing the first fiducial implantation and backing out the needle a few centimeters.

Slowly back out the needle stylet and set 30–50 mm, and keep them stationary for 3–5 min. Then draw out the stylet, put another fiducial in the set, push it into the liver with the stylet and finish the second fiducial implantation. After the two fiducials have been implanted, we can see them clearly on the same slice of the image (Fig. 15.4c). During the 3–5-min stationary period, we can implant fiducials

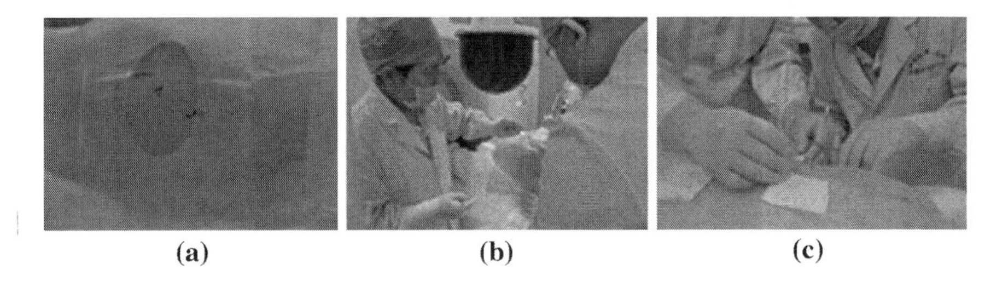

(a) (b) (c)

Fig. 15.3 Fiducial implantation

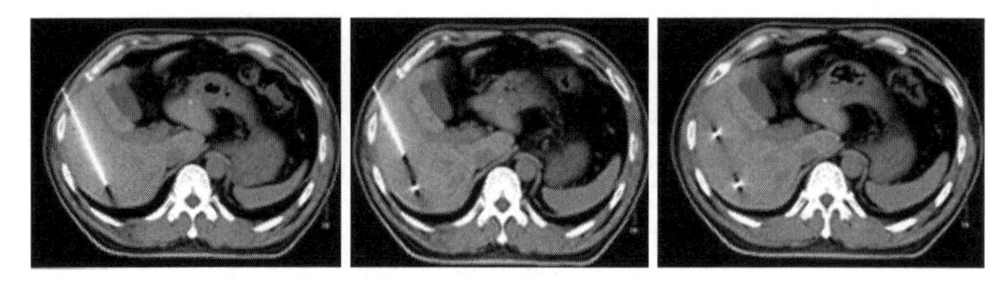

Fig. 15.4 Images taken during the puncturing process

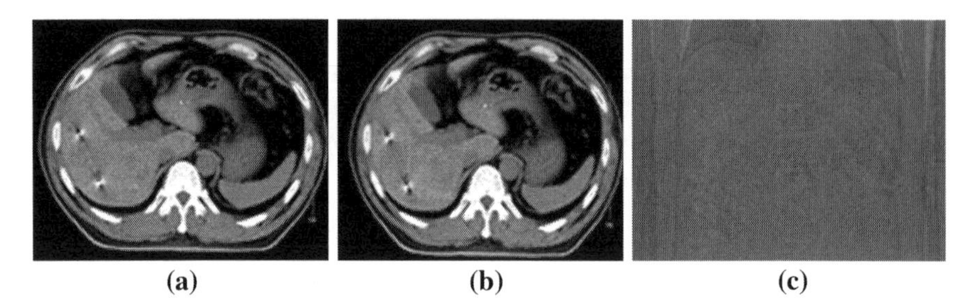

Fig. 15.5 Evaluation of the distance between the fiducials and angle with respect to each other

in other positions so that the entire duration is efficiently utilized. The purpose of the stationary period is to lower the possibility of having a distance smaller than 20 mm between the first and second fiducials. Figure 15.4b shows the aftermath of the procedure, having removed the needle and the airway left by the puncture; Fig. 15.4c is the image of the 3–5-min stationary period and the closed needle passage. The closed passage prevents the second fiducial from sliding down.

Acquire a CT image of the two fiducials after finishing the implantation; measure the distance between them and their angle with respect to each other; and evaluate them in light of the fiducial implantation guidelines. As the two fiducials are positioned in the pathway of one needle, they can easily migrate along this pathway and end up too close to each other. Due to the fact that the two fiducials are implanted in coplanarity, their angle in reference to one another, and the horizontal line, must be measured in order to ascertain that they are not collinear at a 45° angle. Figure 15.5a depicts the measurement of the distance between two fiducials, Fig. 15.5b shows the measurement of the angle of the fiducials with respect to each other, and Fig. 15.5c is a view of all the fiducials.

15.3.2 Results of Fiducial Implantation Using the Two-Fiducials-Per-Insertion Technique

Among the 1252 fiducials implanted by the technique, 18 fiducials (1.44 %) had a distance smaller than 2 cm between them, 24 (1.92 %) were collinear at 45°, and

Table 15.2 Data on fiducials implanted by two-fiducials-per-insertion technique

	Fiducial number
Distance between fiducials <20 mm	18
Collinear on the direction of 45°	24
Migrated fiducials	13

17 (1.36 %) migrated to other organs. The success rate of the implantation was 95.28 % (Table 15.2). With this technique, 626 punctures were required, whereas 1,252 punctures would have been needed had the conventional one-fiducial-per-puncture technique been adopted. Therefore, we can report that the new technique can double the implanting efficiency.

One important factor influencing the success rate of the new technique is collinear fiducials at a 45° angle. According to our data base, 24 of the 1252 fiducials inserted using this technique fell into this category. This problem might lead to a situation in which fiducials cannot be correctly identified during tracking and thus may affect the safety and accuracy of the irradiation. To establish which implanting angles most likely to result in collinearity, we reviewed the records of fiducial implanting angles (Table 15.3). Among the 24 fiducials that ended up collinear at 45°, the point of view of the X-ray cameras, four (16.67 %) were inserted with 0–35° angle; 14 (58.33 %) was in the range 35–55°; and six (25 %) were in the range 55–90°. The risk of collinearity was higher when fiducials were implanted in the range of 35–55°. The problem with collinearity is that the two fiducials appear to have enough distance between each other on one of the orthogonal X-ray images but with a rather small distance on the other image (Fig. 15.6).

When implanting the second fiducial, the needle should be pulled out 30–50 mm. For the purposes of gathering statistics, we divided this range of intended distance between the pair of fiducials into four subcategories: 3–3.5, 3.5–4, 4–4.5, and 4.5–5 cm. The 18 fiducials with a distance smaller than 2 cm in between are shown in Table 15.4. There were four, six, six, and two fiducials in the four ranges, respectively. In other words, the number of fiducials in each category lacked statistical significance.

One week after the implantation, we performed a planning CT for each patient and found that 17 fiducials had migrated (Table 15.5), among which three (17.65 %) had migrated to kidney, four (23.53 %) to spleen, six (35.28 %) to bowel, one (5.89 %) to pelvic cavity, and three (17.65 %) to outside of the body (Fig. 15.7). Fiducials migrating to outside of the body refers to fiducials not being found in a full-body CT scan.

Table 15.3 Number of fiducials collinear on the direction of 45°

Range of implanting angle	0–35°	35–55°	55–90°
Fiducial number	4	14	6

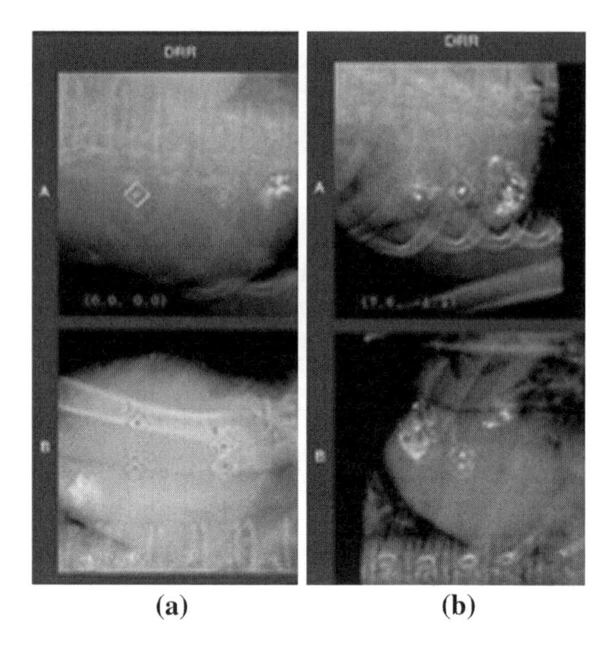

Fig. 15.6 **a** fiducial [1] and fiducial [2] are collinear in the 45° direction; **b** Fiducials have a quite small distance between each other

Table 15.4 The Fiducials having a distance smaller than 2 cm between each other

Moving range (mm)	3–3.5	3.5–4	4–4.5	4.5–5
Fiducial number	4	6	6	2

Table 15.5 Migrating fiducials

Organ	Kidney	Spleen	Bowel	Pelvic cavity	Outside body
Fiducial number	3	4	6	1	3

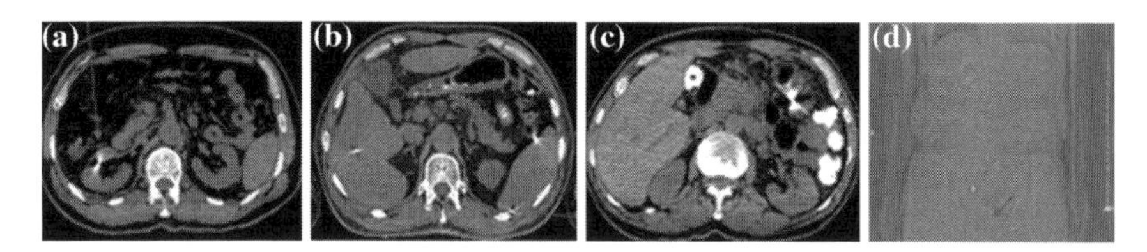

Fig. 15.7 Images of fiducial migration. **a** Fiducials in kidney; **b** In spleen; **c** In bowel; **d** In pelvic cavity

15.4 Discussion

CyberKnife is a frameless image-guided device which delivers stereotactic radiotherapy to tumors throughout the body. It is complemented with an X-ray imaging system which generates two X–ray beams that converge at a 90° angle, and form a 45° angle with the horizontal plane [11]. Furthermore, it uses bony landmarks, such as the skull and spine, in addition to the implanted markers (fiducials) to track tumors [12]. Using the bony landmarks for tracking is non-invasive and painless, but fiducial tracking, even though it's only minimally invasive, still associated with a little pain because of the implantation of the markers. Fiducial implantation is a paracentetic procedure used to place a marker in a specific position in the body through a puncture needle [13, 14]. Conventionally, each needle puncture accomplishes the implantation of only one marker, thus, in a case where four to six fiducials are required for effective tracking, the implantation procedure necessitates as many punctures. In this report, we describe a technique we invented in which two fiducials are placed with every insertion of the needle.

The new technique is not without difficulties. For example, problems of distance between fiducials winding up smaller than 20 mm and fiducials being collinear at the 45° direction did sometimes occur. After some research, we found that, before inserting the second fiducial, backing out the needle for 30–50 mm and keeping it in place for 3–5 min could largely eliminate this problem. At the time of treatment, the patient's position is reset and his or her body may end up in a slightly different position, therefore, it is advisable to avoid puncturing angles of 35–55° in order to circumvent collinearity at 45°.

Because fiducial implantation guidelines require that fiducials have a distance no smaller than 20 mm between each other and, in our technique, the two implanted fiducials actually stay in the pathway of one needle, the puncture needle must be retracted at least 30–50 mm for the benefit of implanting the second fiducial. Therefore, the liver must be thicker than 50 mm at the point of puncture. If the involved part of the liver is thinner than 50 mm, the execution of this technique may be limited. Therefore, some patients received their fiducials using a combination of both techniques. Due to doctors' choice for better implementation, 836 (66.77 %) fiducials were implanted from the angle of 55–90°in total.

Fiducial migration is clearly not unique to the two-fiducial technique and also occurs frequently using other implantation methods because of organ movement, negative pressure in the needle passage, or bloodstream [6, 14]. The statistics of fiducial migration shows that it has no obvious tendency to migrate to kidney, spleen, or the bowel. The migrated fiducials obviously become useless for tracking purposes [15].

On the other hand, the success rate of the two-fiducials-per-insertion technique is almost the same as its conventional counterpart, but the former doubles the implanting efficiency. Placing two fiducials in one needle's pathway with only one puncture cuts in half the number of times the patient is punctured, and greatly reduces the associated pain and other potential complications. Moreover, the puncture needle is disposable and a local anesthetic must be injected before the puncture, so the new technique reduces costs by saving half of the needles and the local anesthetic that would otherwise have been used. Even though fiducial implantation is a minimally invasive surgery, the reduction of puncture times still further brings down medical risks.

15.5 Conclusion

CyberKnife has a rather high accuracy when utilizing fiducials to track tumors. It reduces the amount of margin necessary around target region and thus decreases the dose to normal tissues. Fiducial implantation is a crucial part of the treatment process, and implantation of two fiducials with one needle insertion is safe and of higher efficiency. It doubles the implanting efficiency, and reduces the cost and risks by half through halving the number of punctures. The key factors influencing the success rate were the distance between fiducials and collinearity at 45° angle.

References

1. Kuo JS, Yu C, Petrovich Z, Apuzzo ML (2003) The CyberKnife stereotactic radiosurgery system: description, installation, and an initial evaluation of use and functionality. Neurosurgery 53:1235–1239
2. Chan SD, Main W, Martin DP, Gibbs IC, Heilbrun MP (2003) An analysis of the accuracy of the CyberKnife:a robotic frameless stereotactic radiosurgical system. Neurosurgery 52:140–146
3. Wunderink W, Mendez Romero A, de Kruijf W et al (2008) Reduction of respiratory liver tumor motion by abdominal compression in stereotactic body frame, analyzed by tracking fiducial markers implanted in liver. Int J Radiat Oncol Biol Phys 71:907–915
4. Kim JH, Hong SS, Kim JH et al (2012) Safety and efficacy of ultrasound-guide fiducial marker implantation for CyberKnife radiation therapy. Korean J Radiol 13(3):307–313
5. Anantham D, Feller-Kopman D, Shanmugham LN et al (2007) Electromagnetic navigation bronchoscopy-guided fiducial placement for robotic stereotactic radiosurgery of lung tumors. Chest 132(3):930–935
6. Mallarajapatna GJ, Susheela SP, Kallur KG et al (2011) Image guided internal fiducial placement for stereotactic radiosurgery (CyberKnife). Indian J Radiol Imag 21:3–5
7. Kothary N, Dieterich S, Louie JD et al (2009) Percutaneous implantation of fiducial markers for imaging-guided radiation therapy. AJR 192:1090–1095
8. Berbeco RI, Nishioka S, Shirato H et al (2005) Residual motion of lung tumors in gate radiotherapy with external respiratory surrogates. Phys Med Biol 50:3655–3667
9. Ryu SI, Chang SD, Kim DH et al (2001) Image-guide hypo-fractionated stereotactic radiosurgery to spinal lesions. Neurosurgery 49:838–846
10. Kothary N, Heit JJ, Louie JD et al (2009) Safety and efficacy of percutaneous fiducial marker implantation for image-guide radiation. J Vasc Interv Radiol 20(2):235–239
11. Dieterich Sonja et al (2011) Quality assurance for robotic radiosurgery: report of the AAPM task group 135. Med Phys 38(6):2924–2926

12. Quinn AM (2002) CyberKnife: a robotic radiosurgery system. Clin J Oncol Nurs 6:149–156
13. Lee C (2012) Airway migration of lung fiducial marker after autologous blood-patch injection. Cardiovasc Intervent Radiol 35:711–713
14. Kupelian P, Forbes A, Willoughby T et al (2007) Implantation and stability of metallic fiducials within pulmonary lesions. Int J Radiat Oncol Biol Phys 69:777–785
15. Shirato H, Harada T, Harabayshi T et al (2003) Feasibility of insertion/implantation of 2.0 – mm-diameter gold internal fiducial markers for precise setup and real-time tumor tracking in radiotherapy. Int J Radiat Oncol Biol Phys 56:240–247
16. Sotiropoulou E, Stathochristopoulou I, Stathopoulos K et al (2010) CT-guided fiducial placement for CyberKnife stereotactic radiosurgery: an initial experience. Cardiovasc Intervent Radiol 33:586–589

Chapter 16
On the Statistics and Risks of Fiducial Migration in the CyberKnife Treatment of Liver Cancer Tumors

Li Yu, Hui-jun Xu and Su-jing Zhang

Abstract *Purpose* To gather statistics about the probability of fiducial migration during the process of treating liver tumor with CyberKnife and analyze the risks brought by fiducial migration. *Methods* Between March 2011 and June 2012, 552 patients of liver tumors accepted CyberKnife treatment in the Oncology Radiotherapy Center, among whom the youngest was 21 years old and the oldest was 78. In total, 2378 fiducial markers were implanted in patients, at least 2 fiducials per patient, at most 9 fiducials per patient, and on average, 4.37 fiducials are implanted per patient. We gathered statistics about the fiducial migration before and during the treatment, got the number of cases with fiducial migration and the number of migrated fiducials in these two situations, and studied the risks brought by the migration according to fiducial tracking principle. *Results* 78 of the 552 patients had fiducial migration, with a migration probability of 14.13 %; 93 of the 2378 implanted fiducials migrated, with a migration probability of 3.91 %. Before the treatment, 47 patients had fiducial migration, taking 8.51 % of the total; 58 fiducials migrated, taking 2.44 % of the total; during the treatment, 31 patients (5.62 %) had 35 fiducials (1.47 %) migrated. *Conclusion* The problem of fiducial migration before treatment, which results in the reduction of trackable fiducials, could be resolved by a re-implantation. If fiducials migrate to other organs before treatment, the selection of fiducials used for tracking may be affected, so we need to recognize them carefully. If fiducials migrate during the treatment, the safety and accuracy of treatment may be influenced, and then CT localization shall be implemented when necessary. No matter fiducial migration happens before or during the treatment, we should take measures proactively to avoid influencing the safety and accuracy of radiotherapy.

Keywords CyberKnife · Liver cancer tumors · Fiducials · Migration · Risks

L. Yu · H. Xu (✉) · S. Zhang
Oncology Radiotherapy Center of 302 Military Hospital, VA 100039 Beijing, China
e-mail: huijunxu2008@sina.com

S. Li et al. (eds.), *Frontier and Future Development of Information Technology in Medicine and Education*, Lecture Notes in Electrical Engineering 269,
DOI: 10.1007/978-94-007-7618-0_16,

16.1 Introduction

The CyberKnife® (Accuray Incorporated, Sunnyvale, CA) is used to deliver stereotactic radiosurgery to tumors throughout the body. It has the function of CT guidance before treatment and real-time tracking during the treatment. The 6 MV X-rays emitted by its linear accelerator, which allows robotic manipulation with 6 degrees of freedom and possessed 1920 incident directions (the 4th generation CyberKnife), treat the tumor in a non-isocentric and non-coplanar way so that the dose can be centralized on the tumor while the normal tissues nearby are well protected [1]. The tracking markers of CyberKnife include bony marker (skull and spine), implanted marker (fiducial) and tumor itself (lungs tumor). Its irradiation accuracy to static targets and dynamic targets can be within 0.9 and 1.5 mm, respectively [2]. As soft tissue, the liver has no bony structure which can be tracked, therefore fiducial markers are implanted in or beside tumors so as to track tumors through tracking fiducials [3]. During the treatment, the image registration of fiducials in real-time images and the ones in digital reconstructed radiograph (DRR), which is taken in the stage of designing treatment plans, are implemented, and image-guided localization is also practiced. In the treating process, the images of fiducials are acquired at regular intervals, and the positional deviation is calculated and transferred to the robotic arm to be rectified automatically. Then the movement of fiducials is associated with the movement of patients' body surface so that a respiratory model can be set up [3–5]. During the time of irradiating liver tumors, fiducials are reference objects used for confirming the location and mobility of tumors [6]. The stable relation between fiducials and tumors is crucial for giving safe and accurate irradiation. After fiducials are implanted, they cannot keep stable all the time but may migrate before and during the treatment and thus impact the safety and accuracy of irradiation [7–9]. This paper gathered the statistics of 552 cases of liver cancer tumors along with fiducial migration, and discussed the risks brought by fiducial migration under different conditions.

16.2 Materials and Methods

16.2.1 Case Data

Between March 2011 and June 2012, 552 patients of liver tumors accepted CyberKnife treatment in the Oncology Radiotherapy Center, among whom the youngest was 21 years old and the oldest was 78. In total, 2378 fiducial markers were implanted in patients, at least two fiducials per patient, at most nine fiducials per patient, and on average, 4.37 fiducials are implanted per patient. The data of patients being implanted different number of fiducials, see Table 16.1.

Table 16.1 The number of implanted fiducials

Number of implanted fiducials	2	3	4	5	6	7	8	9
Number of cases	8	29	268	172	45	8	1	1

16.2.2 The Fiducial Size and Implanting Method

A fiducial marker is a cylinder made from 99 % pure gold with whorl on the surface. The size of it is 0.8 × 5 mm. Under the guidance of computed tomography (CT) and puncture device, using an 18-gauge puncture needle to implant fiducials into the patient's liver [8].

16.2.3 Definition of Fiducial Migration

Fiducial migration before treatment: carrying out CT localization one week after fiducials were implanted into the liver, and it can be found that fiducials migrate to other organs or out of the body from the liver [8, 9].

Fiducial migration during treatment: fiducials migrate during the time of accepting CyberKnife irradiation. Fiducial tracking algorithm utilizes rigid error and X-axis pairing tolerance to check whether fiducials migrate or not. For two or more fiducials, the algorithm calculates the distance between every pair of fiducials in the X-ray real-time images, and compares it with the distance between relevant fiducials in DRR which is generated by CT [10, 11]. The difference between these two distances is called rigid error, and the threshold is 0.5–5 mm. The fiducial migration during treatment can be classified as single-fiducial migration and double-fiducials migration.

16.2.4 Influence

Because fiducials are reference objects, the changed tracking targets caused by fiducial migration will affect the safety of treatment. With less than three fiducials, only three shifting deviations can be calculated; with three or more fiducials, six-dimensional deviation can be calculated [11]. The migration may lead to a result that less than three trackable fiducials are left and the irradiation accuracy drops down.

16.3 Method

Count the number of cases with migration and migrated fiducials among the 552 cases, and discuss the risks brought by the migration before and during the treatment process.

16.3.1 Results

We gathered statistics about the 552 cases of liver tumors with fiducial migration, including the migration before and during treatment (Table 16.2). The probability of patients having fiducial migration was 14.13 %. In all implanted fiducials, the probability of migration was 3.91 %.

The risks brought by fiducial migration before and during treatment are different, therefore we collated the data respectively. Among the 78 cases with migration, 47 had migration before the treatment and 31 had it during the treating process, taking 8.51 and 5.62 % of the total cases, respectively (Table 16.3).

Among the 47 cases with migration before treatment, 34 cases had fiducials migrated to other organs and 13 cases migrated out of body, taking 6.7 and 2.36 % of the total (Table 16.4). When puncture needle is pulling out of the body, the negative pressure and blood flow emerging in the needle track and organs movement may cause fiducial migration. When implementing CT localization, some fiducials were found having migrated to bowel (Fig. 16.1a), kidney

Table 16.2 Data of the patients with fiducial migration

	Sum	Number of migration	Probability (%)
Number of cases	552	78	14.13
Number of fiducials	2378	93	3.91

Table 16.3 Data of fiducial migration before and during treatment

	Before treatment		During treatment	
	Case number	Fiducial number	Case number	Fiducial number
Number of migration	47	58	31	35
Probability of migration (%)	8.51	2.44	5.62	1.47

Table 16.4 Data of cases with fiducials migrated to other organs and out of body before treatment

	Other organs		Out of body	
	Case number	Fiducial number	Case number	Fiducial number
Number of migration	37	40	13	18
Probability of migration (%)	6.70	2.44	2.36	0.76

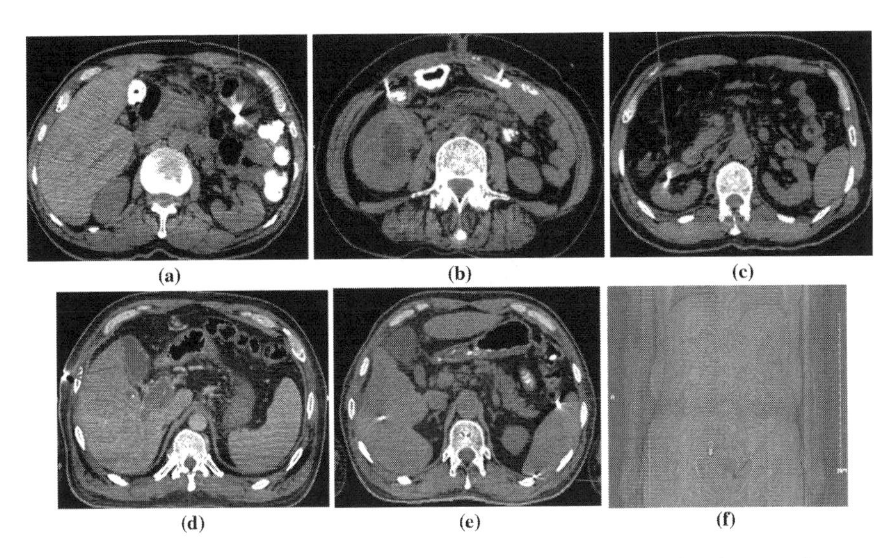

Fig. 16.1 **a** Fiducials migrated to bowel, **b** 2 fiducials migrated to bowel at the same time, **c** to kidney, **d** to thoracic wall, **e** 2 fiducials migrated to spleen at one time, **f** to pelvic cavity

(Fig. 16.1c), thoracic wall (Fig. 16.1d), spleen (Fig. 16.1e) and pelvic cavity (Fig. 16.1f) (Table 16.5). The fiducial migration out of body can be divided into two situations: all-migration and partly-migration. Two cases had their implanted fiducials all migrated out of the body.

From Table 16.4, we can see that 50 cases had migration. The three more cases appeared because one same patient had several kinds of migration: one patient had a fiducial migrated out of body and another migrated to bowel; one patient had a fiducial migrated out of body and another to thoracic wall; and one patient had a fiducial migrated to thoracic wall and another to bowel. Among the 13 cases with fiducials migrated out of body, one patient had three migrated fiducials, three patients had two migrated fiducials per person and eight patients had one migrated fiducial. Among the 18 cases with fiducials migrated to bowel, two patients had two fiducials migrated per person (Fig. 16.1b). One patient had two migrated fiducials among the four cases with fiducials migrated to spleen (Fig. 16.1e).

For the migration during treatment, the fiducial couldn't be utilized as rigid error surpassed threshold, and then CT localization is necessary to re-confirm that

Table 16.5 Different situation of fiducial migration before treatment

Migration organs						
	Bowel	Spleen	Kidney	Thoracic wall	Pelvic cavity	Out of body
Number of migrated cases	18	4	6	8	1	13
Number of migrated fiducials	20	5	6	8	1	18

Table 16.6 Fiducial migration during the treatment

Implanted fiducials	2	3	4	5	6	7	8	9
Number of cases	8	29	268	172	45	8	1	1
Number of cases with fiducial migration	2	7	16	9	1	0	0	0

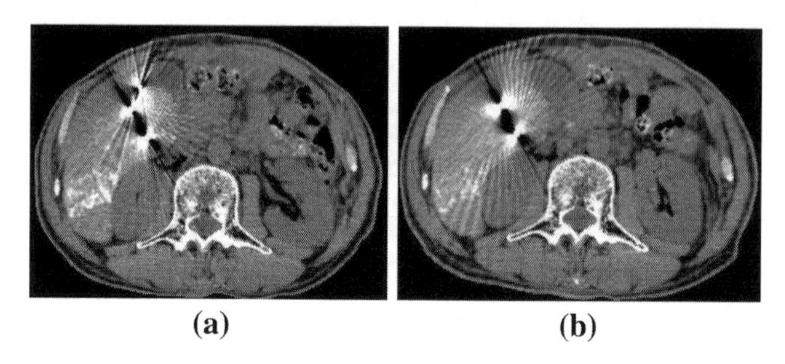

Fig. 16.2 **a** 3 fiducials trackable at the first time of treatment, **b** 1 fiducial migrated and 2 *left* for tracking

it had migrated. When using two fiducials for tracking, one of them migrates but can't be calibrated for the rigid error exceeds the threshold. Besides, the migrated fiducial cannot be confirmed because no reference object is available. When using three fiducials for tracking, the migration of one fiducial leads to a consequence that less than three fiducials are trackable and the rotation error can't be calculated. When four or more fiducials are used for tracking, one of them migrates and the other three are still trackable. CT localization is in need for re-confirming whether the fiducial migrates or not. 31 of the 552 cases had fiducial migration during the treatment (Table 16.6) (Fig. 16.2).

16.4 Discussion

Before the treatment, image-guidance is utilized for positioning and fiducials are calibrated as a group. The fiducial group chosen as the tracking target is what available in real-time tracking during the treating process [12, 11]. The stability of fiducial is crucial as the migration shall directly cause the reduction of trackable fiducials and the change of targets' position [8, 13]. Although fiducial has whorl on the surface, migration still exists [8]. From Table 16.2 we can see that 14.19 % of all the cases and 3.91 % of all the fiducials migrated.

According to Table 16.3, 8.51 % of all the cases and 2.44 % of the fiducials migrated before treatment. Less than 3 trackable fiducials caused the decrease of tracking accuracy; only 1 trackable fiducial influenced the safety of treatment becasue no reference object is available and we cannot realize if migration actually appears. Dealing with the migration before treatment, a re-implantation would make up and will not impact the safety and accuracy of irradiation.

If fiducials migrate to other organs or out of body, patients could have one or more fiducials migrates (Table 16.4), and the migrated ones are untrackable. If the fiducials which migrated out of body can't be displayed on the CT image, it would not impact the fiducial choosing when designing treatment plans. If fiducials which migrated to other organs can be seen on the DRR and real-time image, it requires a second consideration to make the right decision. It can be seen from Table 16.5 that there were more cases with fiducials migrated to bowel, but no obvious tendency.

The major sign of fiducial migration during treatment is that rigid error exceeds threshold (5 mm) [14, 15]. When tracking many fiducials, some of the implanted ones are not utilized doesn't mean that they migrate [15–17]. The fiducial migration during treatment has much more impact on the cases using three or less fiducials for tracking: if one of the two fiducials migrates, we can't realize exactly which one migrates as no reference object exists, but a wrong decision affects the safety and accuracy of treatment; one of the three fiducials migrates will decline the accuracy of treatment. However, taking four or more fiducials for tracking can avoid the influence to treatment brought by a single migrated one.

In conclusion, fiducial migration before treatment causes the decline of available fiducials, but a re-implantation can solve this problem. Once fiducials migrate to other organs before treatment, it requires careful observation because it may impact the fiducial choosing. Fiducial migration during treatment affects the safety and accuracy of treatment and CT re-localization should be taken if needed. All in all, whenever the migration appears, we must adopt useful measures positively so as to assure the safety and accuracy of radiation therapy.

References

1. Kuo JS, Yu C, Petrovich Z, Apuzzo ML (2003) The CyberKnife stereotactic radiosurgery system: description, installation, and an initial evaluation of use and functionality. Neurosurgery 53:1235–1239
2. Quinn AM (2002) CyberKnife: a robotic radiosurgery system. Clin J Oncol Nurs 6:149–156
3. Wunderink W, Romero AM, de Kruijf W et al (2008) Reuduction of respiratory liver tumor motion by abdominal compression in stereotactic body frame, analyzed by tracking fiducial markers implanted in liver. Int J Radiat Oncol Biol Phys 71:907–915
4. Hoogeman M, Prevost JB, Nuyttens J et al (2009) Clinical accuracy of the respiratory tumor tracking system of the Cyberknife: assessment by analysis of log files. Int J Radiat Oncol Biol Phys 74:297–303
5. Ho AK, Fu D, Cotrutz C, Hancock SL, Chang SD, Gibbs IC, Maurer Jr CR (2007) A study of the accuracy of CyberKnife spinal radiosurgery using skeletal structure tracking. Neurosurgery 60, ONS147-156 discussion ONS156
6. Pantelis E, Petrokokkinos L, Antypas C (2009) Image guidance quality assurance of a G4 Cyberknife robotic stereotactic radiosurgery system. JINST 4 P05009

7. Yu C, Main W, Taylor D, Kuduvalli G, Apuzzo ML, Adler JR Jr (2004) An anthropomorphic phantom study of the accuracy of Cyberknife spinal radiosurgery. Neurosurgery 55:1138–1149
8. Sotiropoulou E, Stathochristopoulou I, Stathopoulos K et al (2010) CT-guided fiducial placement for CyberKnife stereotactic radiosurgery: an initial experience. Cardiovasc Intervent Radiol 33:586–589
9. Kupelian P, Forbes A, Willoughby T et al (2007) Implantation and stability of metallic fiducials within pulmonary lesions. Int J Radiat Oncol Biol Phys 69:777–785
10. Mallarajapatna GJ, Susheela SP, Kallur KG et al (2011) Image guided internal fiducial placement for stereotactic radiosurgery (CyberKnife). Indian J Radiol Imaging 21:3–5
11. Antypas C, Pantelis E (2008) Performance evaluation of a CyberKnife® G4 image-guided robotic stereotactic radiosurgery system. Phys Med Biol 53:4697–4718
12. Change SD, Main W, Martin DP, Gibbs IC, Heibrun MP (2003) An analysis of the accuracy of the CyberKnife: a robotic frameless stereotactic radiosurgical system. Neurosurgery 52:140–147
13. Dieterich Sonja et al (2011) Quality assurance for robotic radiosurgery: report of the AAPM task group 135. Med Phys 38(6):2924–2926
14. Shirato H, Harada T, Harabayshi T, Hida K, Endo H, Kitamura K et al (2003) Feasibility of insertion/implantation of 2.0 mm-diameter gold internal fiducial markers for precise setup and real-time tumor tracking in radiotherapy. Int J Radiat Oncol Biol Phys 56:240–247
15. Kim JH, Hong SS, Kim JH et al (2012) Safety and efficacy of ultrasound-guide fiducial marker implantation for CyberKnife radiation therapy. Korean J Radiol 13(3):307–313
16. Kothary N, Dieterich S, Louie JD et al (2009) Percutaneous implantation of fiducial markers for imaging-guided radiation therapy.AJR 192:1090–1095
17. Lee Christopher (2012) Airway migration of lung fiducial marker after autologous blood-patch injection. Cardiovasc Intervent Radiol 35:711–713

Chapter 17
The Comparative Analysis with Finite Element for Cemented Long- and Short-Stem Prosthetic Replacement in Elderly Patients with a Partial Marrow Type I Intertrochanteric Fracture

Wang Shao-lin, Tan Zu-jian and Zhou Ming-quan

Abstract *Objective* This study investigated the stress distribution in a femur after a cemented prosthetic replacement surgery in elderly patients with a partial marrow type I intertrochanteric fracture and compared the differences in stress distribution between a long- and short-stem prosthetic replacement. *Methods* A spiral computed tomography (CT) scan was used on the volunteer's right femur to obtain image data, which were processed with the Mimics software and the modeling software to reconstruct a three-dimensional model of the femur. On this basis, the three-dimensional physical models for a partial marrow type intertrochanteric fracture, long- and short-stem femoral prostheses, and the mantle layer of cement were established. Finally, the three-dimensional finite element models of the long- and short-stem femoral prostheses as a treatment of an intertrochanteric fracture were established using the software for finite element analysis, and the biomechanical analysis was implemented for the models. *Results* The stress distribution in the femur after the cemented long- or short-stem prosthetic replacement did not change significantly; it still gradually increased from the proximal end to the distal end, reaching the peak value at the lower 1/3 of the medial and lateral junction, and then decreased to the end. Although a stress concentration zone formed in the medial and lateral end of the bone cement-prosthetic stem interface in the short-stem prosthesis, which had a lateral peak value of 15.3 MPa, it did not exceed the fatigue strength of the bone cement. Alternatively, a stress concentration zone formed in the distal medial and lateral end of the bone cement-prosthetic stem interface and the medial middle part of the shaft in the long-stem prosthesis, which showed a peak value that was also lower than the fatigue strength of the bone cement. No significant stress concentration zones were found in the femoral calcar reconstructed by bone cement. *Conclusion* The stress

Fund: medical research project of Chongqing Health Bureau, No. 2011-2-371.

W. Shao-lin (✉) · T. Zu-jian · Z. Ming-quan
Department of Orthopedics, Chongqing Zhongshan Hospital, Yuzhong, China

S. Li et al. (eds.), *Frontier and Future Development of Information Technology in Medicine and Education*, Lecture Notes in Electrical Engineering 269,
DOI: 10.1007/978-94-007-7618-0_17, © Springer Science+Business Media Dordrecht 2014

distribution in the femur did not change significantly after cemented long- and short-stem prosthetic replacements were used for elderly patients with a partial marrow type I intertrochanteric fracture. The probability of loosening of the cemented long-stem prosthesis was comparable to that of the short-stem prosthesis, but the latter may be more suitable for treating elderly patients with a partial marrow type I intertrochanteric fracture due to the shorter surgery time, minor trauma, and fewer complications.

Keywords Arthroplasty · Replacement · Hip fracture · Finite element analysis · Fracture classification

With the advent of an aging society in China, the elderly intertrochanteric fracture has become increasingly common. It has been reported that its incidence accounts for 31–51 % of the hip fractures [1]. Its treatments mainly include conservative traction, reduction and internal fixation after incision, and artificial joint replacement. The first two methods have the disadvantages of the patient being bedridden for a long time and many complications, while cemented arthroplasty as a treatment for elderly intertrochanteric fractures has the advantages of minor trauma, shorter time for the patient being bedridden, and a rapid postoperative recovery with fewer complications; therefore, it is increasingly favored by the majority of patients and doctors. Cemented or biological long-stem prostheses has been generally applied in artificial joint replacement for elderly intertrochanteric fractures. We have explored the treatment for partial marrow type I fractures [2] using an ordinary biological stem (short-stem) prosthesis. We encountered the following important issues: whether to use a common stem or a long stem; whether to use a long stem similar to other surgeons for insurance purposes; the disadvantages of abusing a long-stem prosthesis (for example, an increased amount of bone cement will increase the surgical risks, such as the reduced blood pressure due to bone cement or even sudden death); and which case should an ordinary stem versus a long stem be used for. However, little research had been performed on the biomechanical characteristics of a femur after a cemented artificial joint replacement for an elderly intertrochanteric fracture, and no comparative study on the long-stem prosthetic replacement and short-stem prosthetic replacement based on the partial marrow classification [2] has been reported. Therefore, in this study, the femoral biomechanics after a cemented artificial joint replacement for an elderly partial marrow type intertrochanteric fracture was analyzed using the three-dimensional finite element analysis method. In addition, after the prosthetic replacement, biomechanical differences in the femur between the long-stem and short-stem prostheses were observed, with which a theoretical basis for a reasonable choice of the prosthesis can be provided.

17.1 Materials and Methods

17.1.1 General data

A 75-year-old healthy male volunteer, who had a height of 170 cm and weight of 65 kg, was selected as the subject for the modeling. This volunteer was healthy and had no history of hip or femur injuries, with no abnormalities shown in the bilateral hip and femur x-ray examination.

The equipment and software used in this study included: a Somatom Balance Nano 128-slice spiral computed tomography (CT) machine that supported the Dicom 3.0 standards (Philips Company), Internet Core Duo computer, the image processing software Mimics 8.1, the large CAD/CAM/CAE (computer-aided design/computer-aided manufacturing/computer-aided engineering) modeling software Unigraphics (UG), and the finite element analysis software ABAQUS 6.5 and Ansys 11.0.

17.1.2 Model Establishment

17.1.2.1 Establishment of a Three-Dimensional CAD Model for the Human Femur

The spiral CT, which was perpendicular to the longitudinal axis of the volunteer's right femur, was scanned from the proximal end above the femoral head to the distal end of the femoral shaft, with a slice thickness of 1.0 mm, an interlayer spacing of 0.8 mm, a window width of 2000, a window level of 400, and a total of 248 tomographic images over the length of 448 mm. Then, the image data were directly inputted into the computer in the DCM (Digital Imaging and Communications in Medicine) format, and femoral data files in the IGES (Initial Graphics Exchange Specification) format were outputted after the images were preprocessed using the Mimics software. Finally, they were inputted into the CAD/CAM/CAE integrated software UG to establish the physical simulation model.

17.1.2.2 Establishment of a Three-Dimensional CAD Model for a Partial Marrow Type I Intertrochanteric Fracture, Artificial Femoral Stem Prostheses of Different Lengths, and Bone Cement

According to the definition of a partial marrow type intertrochanteric fracture (a cis tuberosity fracture with intact trochanter ring and lesser trochanter base) and the location of the calcar, a femoral osteotomy was used on the greater trochanter tip to the lower edge of the lesser trochanter tip for the model, in which the area above the osteotomy plane included removal of the femoral head, a partial removal bone in the femoral neck, and a defect in the calcar. The prostheses (Zimmer Co., United States) chosen for this study had the following parameters: the short-stem prosthesis had a stem length of 140 mm and a neck length of 39 mm, and the long-stem prosthesis had a stem length of 180 mm and a neck length of 41 mm. The neck shaft angles of the two prostheses were both 135°, and both prosthetic stems were flat cones with a thickness of 13 mm. Similar to the femoral neck of the volunteer, the femoral neck of the prosthesis had an anteversion of 15°. According to the above parameters and using the shaping characteristics of the input variables, the femoral neck and femoral stem of the prosthesis were individually built, and the prosthesis model was established by assembling the various parts through Boolean operations. Then, by taking the greater trochanter tip as the datum and maintaining the top center of prosthesis neck at the same level as that of the greater trochanter tip, the prosthesis and the femur model of intertrochanteric fracture were assembled. Based on clinical experience, to reduce the loosening of the prosthesis, the intramedullary bone cement around the prosthetic stem was set as a 3-mm cylinder, and the bone cement thickness in the extramedullary area, which is the bone defect area of the calcar, was set to be 5 mm. The top plane of the bone cement was consistent with the conventional osteotomy plane in the prosthetic replacement of the femoral neck, and the reamed length was 10 mm longer than the intramedullary stem.

17.1.2.3 Establishment of a Three-Dimensional Finite Element Model

The software ABAQUS 6.5 defines the mesh for each model using the modified quadratic tetrahedral element C3D10 M. In this study, the mesh was automatically divided using a software program, with a unit number of 58648 for the short-stem prosthesis model and 63868 for the long-stem prosthesis model. For the critical parts, such as the contacting surface of the femoral prosthesis and bone cement and the contacting surface of the bone cement and femur, the mesh was refined and the sharp edges were polished to improve the accuracy of the analytical results.

17.1.3 Definitions of the Material Properties

The properties of the modeling material were set in accordance with the relevant material parameters of the finite element analysis in the literature [4], as shown in Tables 17.1 and 17.2.

Table 17.1 The parameters of the various materials

Material	Modulus of elasticity (MPa)	Poisson's ratio
Cobalt-chromium-molybdenum alloy	220000	0.3
Bone cement (PMMA)	2620	0.35
Cancellous bone	2130	0.3

Table 17.2 The performance parameters of cortical bone

Material	Young's modulus of elasticity (MPa)	Shear modulus of elasticity (MPa)	Poisson's ratio
Cortical bone	E1 = E2 = 11500, E3 = 1700	G1 = 3600, G2 = G3 = 3300	υ1 = 0.51, υ1 = υ3 = 0.31

17.1.4 Imposition of Boundary Conditions

It was assumed that the contacting surfaces of prosthesis-bone cement and bone cement in the femur were firmly fixed in the early postoperative period with no relative sliding. Boundary conditions were imposed on the distal plane of the femur, and the degree of freedom was fully constrained. Loading was based on a body weight of 65 kg. The stress distribution among the prosthesis, the bone cement, and the femur was simulated for a landing with one leg during normal walking, regardless of the muscle loading.

17.1.5 Three-Dimensional Finite Element Analysis

The software programs ABAQUS 6.5 and Ansys 11.0 were applied to analyze the stress distribution in the femur, the interface of the bone cement and prosthesis, and the reconstructed calcar after the prosthetic replacement, and a contour graph of the equivalent stress and a stress curve were plotted. The strength of the stress is presented as the peak value and the regional average, which was calculated by 4 stress values at a corresponding point for every 5 mm proximal to the peak.

17.1.6 Statistical Analysis

The strength of the stress is presented as the peak value and the regional average ($\bar{x} \pm s$), and the obtained data were statistically analyzed using the SPSS 13.0 statistical software package (SPSS Inc., USA). The t-test was applied to compare the difference in average values at the corresponding location of the femur and the interface of bone cement-prosthesis between the long-stem and short-stem prosthetic replacement. $P < 0.05$ was considered statistically significant.

17.2 Results

17.2.1 The Stress Distribution of the Femur After a Prosthetic Replacement

A contour graph of equivalent stress for the femoral model is shown in Figs. 17.1–17.4. The stress distribution of the femur gradually increased from the proximal end to the distal end (color turns from blue to red). At the lower 1/3 of the medial and lateral junction in the femoral shaft, the stress was obviously concentrated, which then decreased to the end. The red area of the lateral interface in the stress contour graph was significantly greater than that of the medial interface. The medial and lateral peak stresses were 83.29 and 95.76 MPa, respectively, for the short-stem prosthesis and 82.22 and 94.768 MPa, respectively, for the long-stem prosthesis; the medial and lateral regional averages were 78.36 ± 5.043 MPa and 89.67 ± 6.75 MPa, respectively, for the short-stem

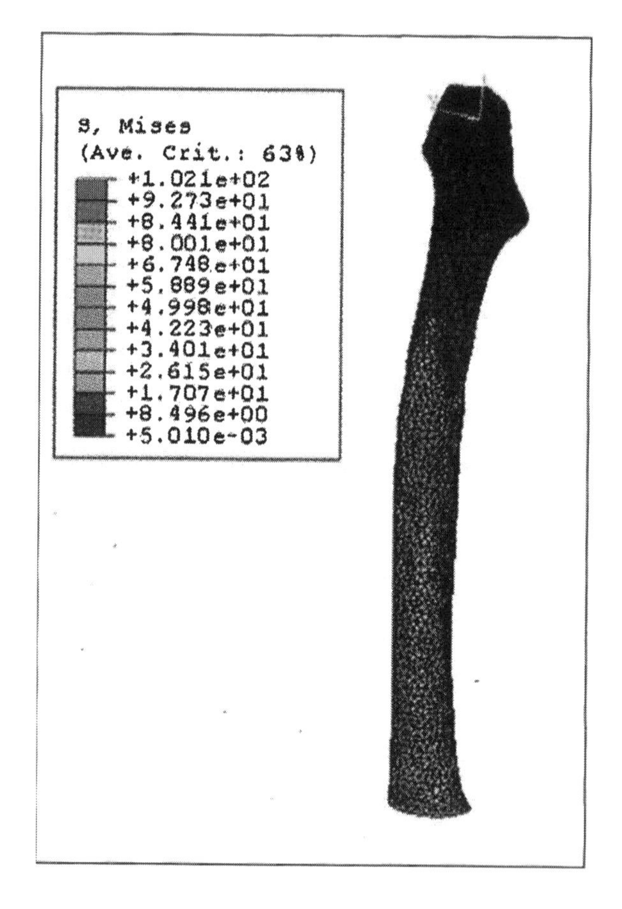

Fig. 17.1 A medial stress contour graph of a femur after a short-stem prosthetic replacement (the stress gradually increased from *blue* to *red*, which is the same for the following figures)

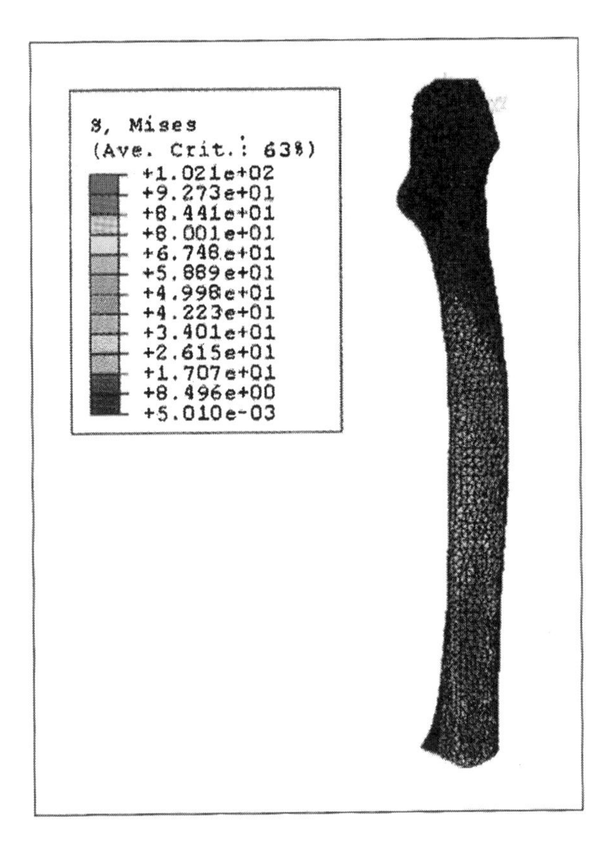

Fig. 17.2 A lateral stress contour graph of a femur after a short-stem prosthetic replacement

prosthesis and 77.23 ± 4.26 MPa and 86.85 ± 7.31 MPa, respectively, for the long-stem prosthesis. Based on the t-test, the medial and lateral regional averages for the long- and short-stem femoral prosthesis replacement were not statistically different (medial $t = 0.398$, $P > 0.05$; lateral $t = 0.678$, $P > 0.05$).

17.2.2 The Stress Distribution in the Interface of the Bone Cement and Prosthetic Stem

Figures 17.5–17.8 show the stress contour graphs for the interface of the bone cement and prosthetic stem corresponding to the long- and short-stem prostheses. The stress of the medial interface of the bone cement corresponding to the short-stem prosthesis slowly increased from the calcar area (separately analyzed) downward to the distal end, and the stress rapidly increased and reached its peak value of 9.7 MPa at approximate 5 mm from the most distal end of the prosthesis. Then, it decreased to the distal end. The regional average of this stress concentration region was 5.68 ± 3.14 MPa. Similarly, the stress of the lateral interface

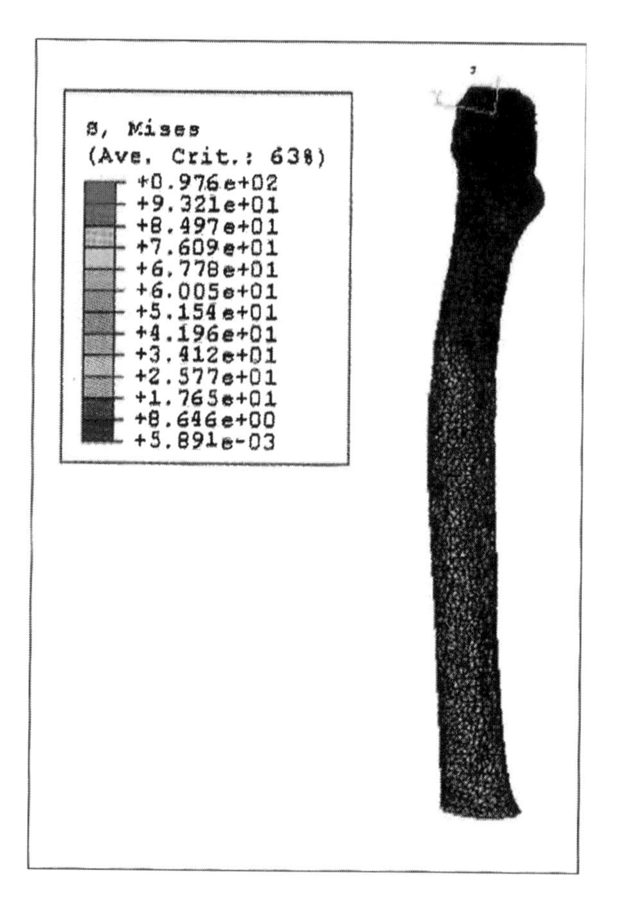

Fig. 17.3 A medial stress contour graph of a femur after a long-stem prosthetic replacement

gradually increased from the proximal end to the distal end, reaching a peak value of 15.3 MPa at the region corresponding to the end of the prosthesis stem, which did not exceed the fatigue strength of the bone cement, and the regional average in the lateral interface was 11.98 ± 4.12 MPa. The stress of the medial interface of the bone cement corresponding to the long-stem prosthesis slowly increased from the calcar region downward, reaching the first peak at the middle of the shaft with a value of 4.97 MPa, and the regional average was 4.45 ± 0.15 MPa. The stress gradually decreased and then increased again to reach the second peak at the distal end, which had a peak value of 2.56 MPa and a regional average of 1.96 ± 0.41 MPa. The difference in the regional average between the long- and short-stem prostheses was not statistically significant ($t = 0.12$, $P > 0.05$). The lateral interfacial stress also gradually increased from the proximal end to the distal end, reaching its peak value at the corresponding region in the end of the prosthesis with a peak value of 14.93 MPa, and the regional average was 12.56 ± 1.48 MPa. Both the peak value and regional average did not exceed the

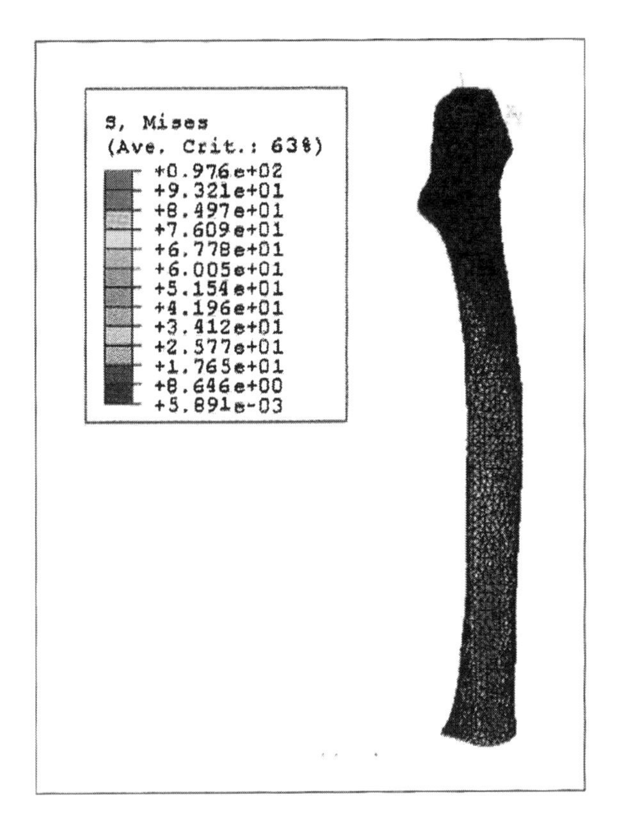

Fig. 17.4 A lateral stress contour graph of a femur after a long-stem prosthetic replacement

fatigue strength range of the bone cement. Compared with the regional average at the corresponding region of the short-stem prosthesis, the difference was not statistically significant ($t = 0.029$, $P > 0.05$).

17.2.3 The Stress Distribution of the Bone Cement in Calcar

Stress contour graphs of the corresponding internal and external mantle layer of cement in the calcar of the long-stem and short-stem prostheses are shown in Figs. 17.9–17.12, in which the top views show the internal stresses while the rear views show the external stresses. Analysis showed that the stress distributions in both the medial and lateral interfaces of the mantle layer of cement were similar, i.e., the posteromedial stresses were relatively high in the transition region of the thick and thin bone cement and the top of the mantle layer, but the stress was not significantly concentrated. The regional peak stress values in the relatively concentrated region of the medial interface were 4.56 MPa for the short-stem prosthesis and 5.89 MPa for the long-stem prosthesis, while the regional peak stress

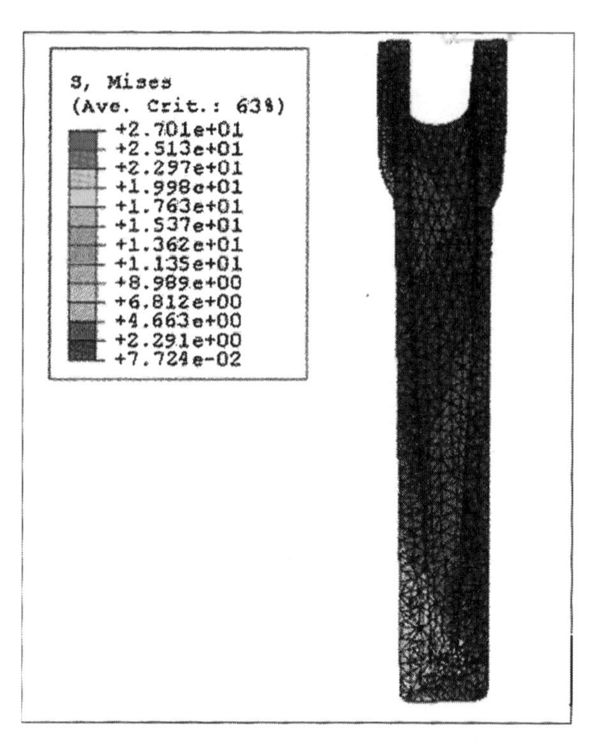

Fig. 17.5 A stress contour graph of the medial cement-short-stem prosthesis interface

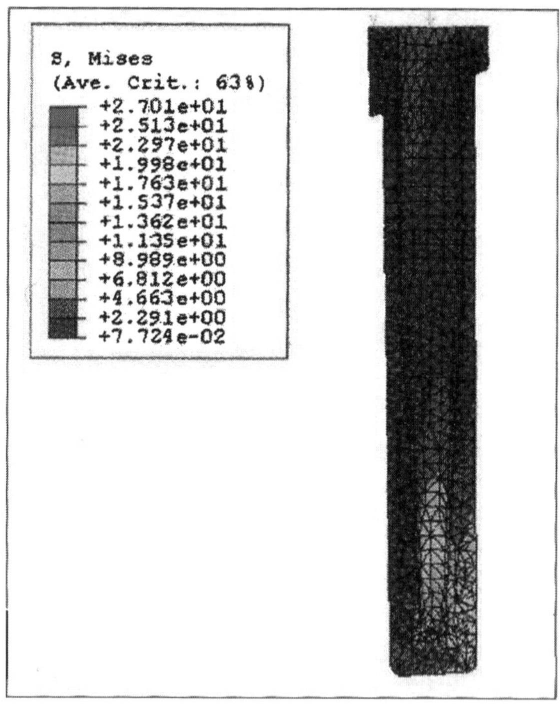

Fig. 17.6 A stress contour graph for the lateral cement-short-stem prosthesis interface

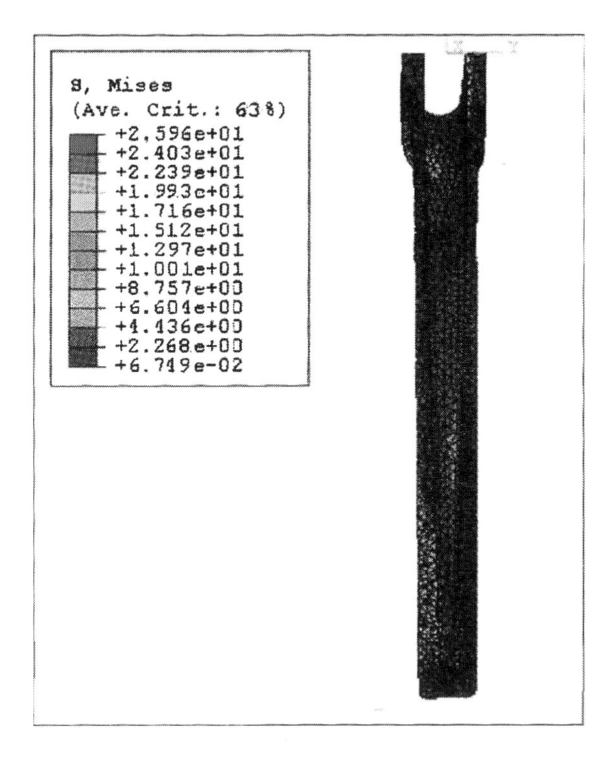

Fig. 17.7 A stress contour graph of the medial cement-short-stem prosthesis interface

values in the relatively concentrated region of the lateral interface were 10.18 MPa for the short-stem prosthesis and 12.87 MPa for the long-stem prosthesis. None of these values exceeded the fatigue strength of the bone cement.

17.3 Discussion

17.3.1 The Origin and Principle of Partial Marrow Classification

Regarding the situation and limitations of the current classification, the AO classification (Arbeitsgemeinschaft für Osteosynthesefragen [Association for the Study of Internal Fixation]; 1981), which has been in use for 30 years, is the latest of the commonly used classifications [5]. In the previous 30 years, bone science has undergone tremendous changes. The current common classification for inter-trochanteric fractures is generally based on the trace of the fracture line (shape) and the degree of the fracture fragmentation (crushing). An integrity assessment for the remaining ring structure of the bone marrow cavity after the fracture is ignored. Therefore, there are inherent limitations in the AO classification. We believe that bone fracture classification is at the eve of a dramatic change.

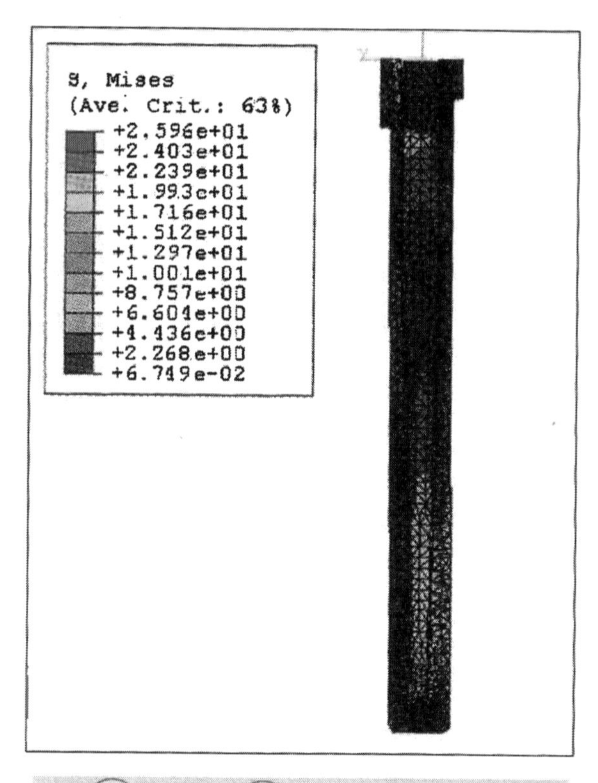

Fig. 17.8 The stress contour graph for the lateral cement-short-stem prosthesis interface

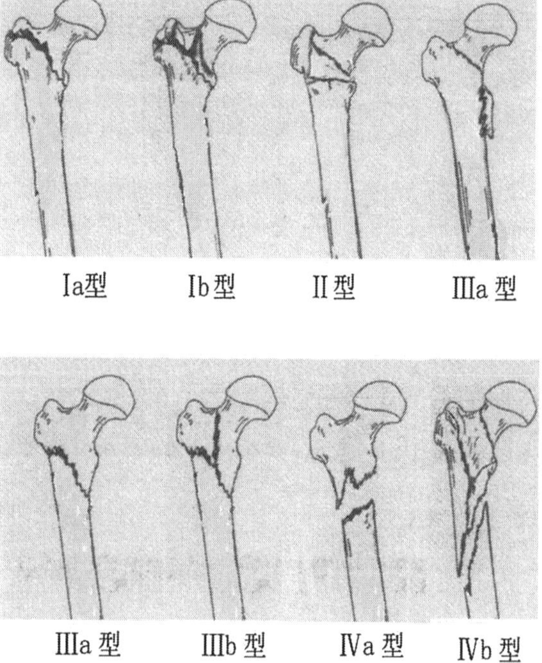

Fig. 17.9 Schema of the partial marrow classification for an intertrochanteric fracture.

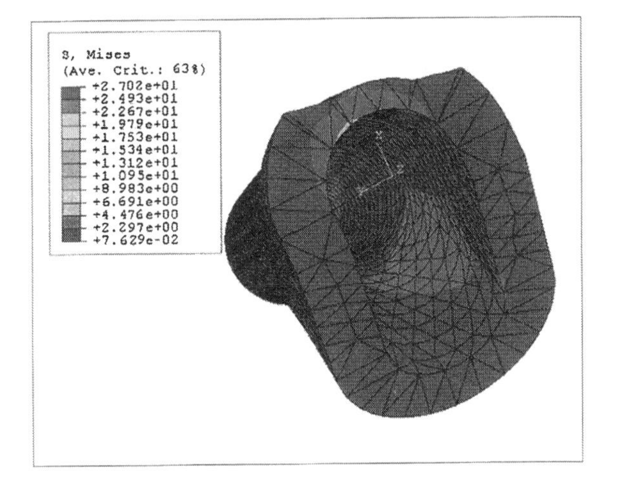

Fig. 17.10 An internal stress contour graph of the bone cement mantle layer in the calcar region of a short-stem prosthesis (top view)

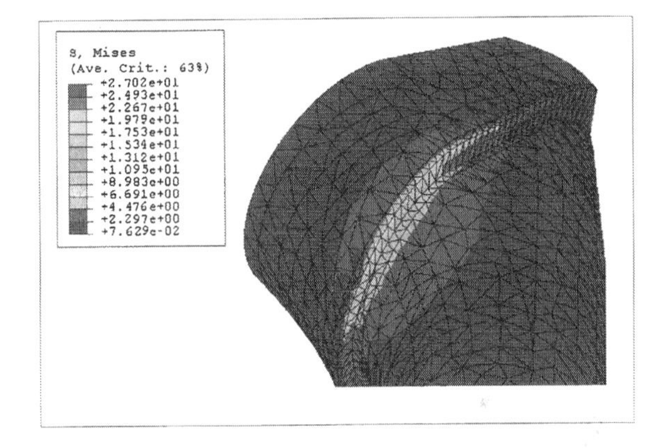

Fig. 17.11 An external stress contour graph of the bone cement mantle layer in the calcar region of a long-stem prosthesis (rear view)

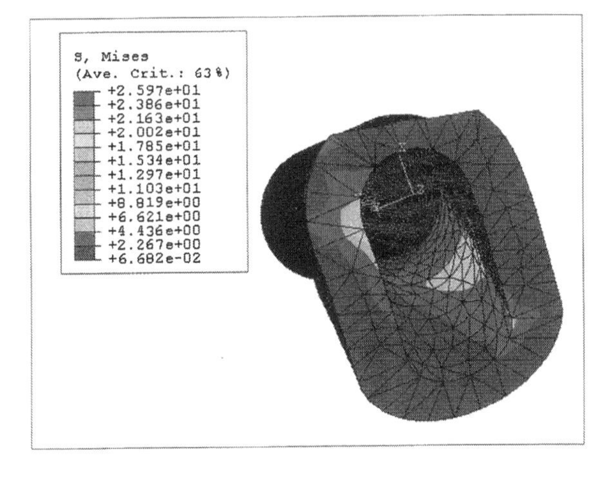

Fig. 17.12 An internal stress contour graph of the bone cement mantle layer in the calcar region of a long-stem prosthesis (top view)

With the wide use of intramedullary fixation systems for fractures, such as the interlocking intramedullary nail, gamma nail, and reconstruction nail [6], e.g., proximal femoral nail antirotation (PFNA) [7], modern bone science currently has an urgent need for a classification method for fractures with an integrity assessment for the remaining ring structure of the bone marrow cavity after the fracture. Meanwhile, the emergence and wide use of a large number of fastening systems inserted in the marrow cavity, such as artificial joints, greatly requires a classification method for fractures with an integrity assessment for the remaining ring structure of the bone marrow cavity after the fracture. These two important reasons promote an inevitable change of the fracture classification. We have named this new fracture classification method a three-dimensional partial marrow classification, which is a three-dimensional digital fracture classification with an integrity assessment for the remaining bone marrow cavity after the fracture as a standard, and a CT reconstruction as a base for the final diagnosis. In primary hospitals without CT reconstruction, the three-dimensional partial marrow type can be classified with only CR anteroposterior and lateral radiographs, which is a simplified classification method of the three-dimensional partial marrow typing. The new classification of intertrochanteric fractures has been tentatively named as partial marrow classification[8], which is a classification method with an emphasis on the integrity assessment of the ring structure of the remaining bone marrow cavity after the fracture. This new classification is our preliminary exploration under the guidance of this new concept. At the same time, the new concepts of an intertrochanteric ring (a ring structure of bone surrounding the inner wall of the marrow cavity of the trochanteric bone), the femoral neck (calcar) ring (a ring structure of bone 1.5 cm from the distal end of the femoral neck or a ring structure of bone formed by both the calcar and the greater trochanter), and the lesser trochanter base (a bony structure constituted by both the lesser trochanter and the adjacent marrow cavity) were proposed as basic terms and concepts for partial marrow classification.

The intertrochanteric fracture is divided into four types based on partial marrow classification (Fig. 17.13):

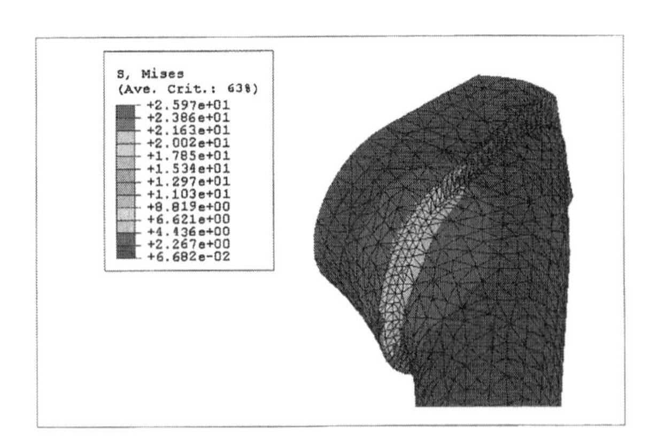

Fig. 17.13 An external stress contour graph of the bone cement mantle layer in the calcar region of a long-stem prosthesis (rear view).

(1) Type I: The trochanter ring and the lesser trochanter base in the femur are both intact. Subtypes: Ia: the intertrochanteric ring, the femoral neck ring, and the lesser trochanter base in the femur are all intact; and Ib: the femoral neck ring is not intact.
(2) Type II: The intertrochanteric ring is not intact, while the lesser trochanter base is intact.
(3) Type III: The lesser trochanter base in the femur is not intact. Subtypes: IIIa: the lesser trochanter base is not intact; and IIIb: the lesser trochanter base together with the tuberosity ring of other parts (not at the lesser trochanter) are not intact.
(4) Type IV: The trans-trochanteric fracture and subtrochanteric fracture (subtrochanter $\leq$ 5 cm). Subtypes: IVa: the trochanter ring is intact; and IVb: the trochanter ring is not intact.
The integrities of the intertrochanteric ring, the femoral neck (calcar) ring, and the lesser trochanter base (more precisely, it should be described as the remaining integrity of the ring structure of the bone marrow cavity after fracture, hereinafter referred to as integrity) have been defined.

The standards for the integrity of the intertrochanteric ring, the femoral neck (calcar) ring, and the lesser trochanter base are as follows:

① For a fracture in the lesser trochanter, the standard of integrity for the lesser trochanter base is the height of the lesser trochanter fracture $\leq$ 1.5 cm.
② The integrity standard of the trochanter ring is the width of the narrowest point of the trochanter ring $\geq$ 0.5 cm.
③ The integrity standard of the femoral neck ring is the narrowest point $\geq$ 0.3 cm.

We had studied the various classifications of intertrochanteric fractures [9], such as the AO classification, Evans classification, Jensen classification, Kyle classification, and Boyd-Griffin classification. Based on an analysis of different surgical procedures and their efficacies, the advantages and disadvantages of commonly used classification methods [10] were investigated, and the partial marrow classification was proposed for clinical application. Additionally, a partial marrow classification for intertrochanteric fractures involving the femoral shaft was proposed [11].

The intertrochanteric fracture is a common disorder with a high incidence in elderly people. The cemented prosthesis is now generally used in arthroplasty for these patients. However, few studies on long-stem biological artificial femoral head replacement [12] or artificial joint replacement with the greater trochanter stem [13] have been reported. With the widespread launch of artificial joint surgery using bone cement, many problems have been exposed, some of which are serious. In addition to the long surgery, major trauma, and difficulty for second refurbishment by using bone cement, a more serious consequence is that bone cement use would lead to bone cement syndrome, including cardiac toxicity, decreased blood pressure to shock, and even sudden death. Therefore, minimizing surgical trauma (e.g., by reducing the reamed length and amount of bone cement, such as by replacing a long-stem bone cement prosthesis with a short-stem prosthesis) has become an important research topic and is also a major issue explored in this study.

17.3.2 The Analysis of Femoral Stress Distribution After Long- and Short-Stem Prosthesis Replacement

After an artificial prosthetic replacement, the mechanical pathway in the femur changed. Unlike the conduction of joint stress under normal physiological conditions, the joint stress is transmitted to the bone cement and then to the femur by the prosthesis. If the implanted prosthesis does not meet the requirements of human biomechanics, it is likely to form stress shielding, causing bone absorption and atrophy, which leads to complications such as a loosening of the prosthesis and femur fracture [14]. Many studies have shown that [15, 16] the stress distribution of a normal human femur is concentrated in the lower 1/3 of the medial and lateral junction in the femoral shaft and at the junction of the middle and lower part of the femoral neck with the top of the lesser trochanter. The stress value of the former is higher than that of the latter. The stress in the femoral shaft is concentrated in the lower 1/3 of the medial and lateral junction mainly because this region is the transitional region for the cross-section of the femoral shaft as it shifts from circular to quadrilateral, with a rapid thinning of the cortical bone in the medial and lateral femoral shaft, thereby significantly increasing the marrow cavity and suddenly changing in cross-section. Based on mechanical principles, the stress concentration is easily formed in this site [17]. The results of this study indicated that after the surgery for a prosthesis replacement for the intertrochanteric fracture, regardless of whether it was a long-stem prosthesis or a short-stem prosthesis, the stress distribution in the remaining part of the femoral shaft did not generally change. The lower 1/3 of the medial and lateral junction in the femoral shaft still showed a significant concentration of stress, and the lateral femoral stress close to the knee was greater than the medial stress, which is consistent with the stress distribution in a normal human femur. This may be related to the fact that a prosthetic replacement does not change the bending moment and the shape of the middle-lower part of the femur.

17.3.3 Stress Distribution of the Bone Cement-Prosthesis Interface

A loosening of the prosthesis is still the leading cause of hip replacement failure. Fragmentation and de-bonding of the bone cement that first occurs in the bone cement-prosthesis interface is considered to be the initiation of the aseptic loosening of the prosthesis [18]. The studies by Jansson and Refior [19], Breusch et al. [20], and Kawate [21] all indicated that the stress value at the interface of the bone cement and the femur is less than that at the interface of the bone cement and prosthesis, and the de-bonding and loosening at the bone cement-femur interface are basically unrelated to the stress of the bone cement. Instead, they are secondarily generated with the osteolysis that is caused by debris in the interface of the bone cement and prosthesis. After a fracture of the bone cement, the potential debris will reach the bone through the fracture path, triggering the immune response to induce osteolysis. Thus, the loosening of the bone and bone cement interface is a secondary harmful biological response initiated by the debris produced in the prosthesis-bone cement interface, while the loosening of the bone cement-prosthesis interface is mainly the result of high stress. Therefore, a stress analysis of the bone cement-prosthesis interface is particularly important.

Finite element analysis, laboratory research, and clinical studies have all shown that after a conventional arthroplasty, the maximum stress in the bone cement layer around the femoral prosthesis is at the lateral distal end of the prosthesis-bone cement interface, which is followed by at the medial proximal end of the bone cement [18, 22, 23]. The results of this study showed that after a cemented long- or short-stem prosthetic replacement surgery, the stress distribution in the bone cement-prosthesis interface was basically the same for both prostheses. The stress distribution in the interface of the bone cement-prosthesis for the long-stem prosthesis was mainly concentrated in the medial and lateral distal end and the middle of the medial interface. The stress distribution in the interface of the bone cement-prosthesis for the short-stem prosthesis was concentrated in the medial and lateral distal end. The difference between the stress averages at the medial distal end of the short-stem prosthesis and the long-stem prosthesis was not statistically significant by a t-test. In addition, the peak value for the distal lateral stress in the bone cement-prosthesis interface of the short-stem prosthesis was 15.3 MPa, which did not exceed the fatigue strength of the bone cement. Fatigue strength is currently considered to be the most important mechanical property of the bone cement [24], and the intensity range of the bone cement fatigue tolerance reported in the literature is 8–17 MPa [25, 26]. Studies have shown that the de-bonding and fracture of the bone cement in the bone cement-prosthesis interface occur mainly because the stress on the bone cement exceeds its fatigue strength [22]. Accordingly, compared with the long-stem prosthesis, the probability of an occurrence of osteolysis and loosening after the short-stem prosthetic replacement did not increase, suggesting that both the long-stem and short-stem prostheses are suitable for the treatment of intertrochanteric fractures in the elderly.

17.3.4 Stress Distribution in the Bone Cement at the Reconstructed Calcar

The finite element analysis revealed that the stress distribution in the femur did not change significantly after a long- or short-stem prosthetic replacement, and the internal and external areas of the calcar reconstructed with bone cement had no obvious zones of stress concentrations. Although the distal medial stress in the interface of the bone cement-prosthesis after the short-stem prosthetic replacement was greater than that for the long-stem prosthesis, the peak value of the lateral stress in the interface of the bone cement-prosthesis of the short-stem prosthesis did not exceed the fatigue strength of the bone cement, and neither did the interfacial stress peak value of the long-stem prosthesis. Accordingly, the probability for a loosening of the short-stem prosthesis is comparable to that of the long-stem prosthesis, indicating that both the long- and short-stem prostheses are suitable for the treatment of intertrochanteric fractures in the elderly.

Above all, the partial marrow type I fracture is characterized as a cis trochanteric fracture with an intact trochanter ring and lesser trochanter base. According to the preliminary clinical practice of the Department of Joint and Orthopedics in our hospital, a cemented short-stem prosthetic replacement is the preferred treatment for this type of fracture, which was initially confirmed in this study. In recent years, a comparative analysis using a three-dimensional finite element to study the cemented long- and short-stem prosthetic replacements as the treatment of femoral intertrochanteric fractures [27] was reported, and it was inferred that the loosening probability for the short-stem prosthesis was relatively higher, with the conclusion that a long-stem prosthesis may be more suitable for the treatment of intertrochanteric fractures. However, based on the new classification for intertrochanteric fractures (partial marrow classification), it is now necessary to perform further in-depth research in this area. One of the fundamental purposes of this research project was to determine the rationality of using a short-stem prosthetic replacement with bone cement for a partial marrow type I fracture through a comparative analysis with a three-dimensional finite element from a biomechanical point of view. If the results of the comparative analysis with the three-dimensional finite element suggest no significant difference in efficacy, including data related to biomechanical stability, between the long- and short-stem prosthetic replacements for the treatment of the partial marrow type I intertrochanteric fractures, their efficacies and biomechanical stabilities can be considered comparable, which means that partial marrow type I fractures can be treated with a cemented short-stem prosthetic replacement instead of a cemented long-stem prosthesis replacement, with several obvious advantages, such as the shorter surgery time, decreased trauma, reduced bleeding, and smaller amount of bone cement (thus reducing the occurrence of bone cement syndrome). This was preliminarily confirmed by the results of this study.

References

1. Haidukewych GJ, Israel TA, Berry DJ (2001) Reverse obliquity fractures of the intertrochanteric region of the femur. J Bone Joint Surg 83(5):643–650
2. Wang S, Tan Z, Zhou M et al (2012) New fracture classification and guidance treatment for femoral intertrochanteric comminuted fracture with locking plate. Chin J Bone Jt Inj 27(2):103–106
3. Ramaniraka NA, Rakotomanana LR, Leyvraz PF (2000) The fixation of the cemented femoral component: effects of stem stiffness, cement thickness and roughness of the cement. bone surface. J Bone Joint Surf 82(2):297–303
4. Kowalczyk P (2001) Design optimization of cementless femoral hip prostheses using finite element analysis. J Biomech Eng 23(5):396–402
5. Liu Y-P, Liu X, Yu H et al (eds) (2002) The diagnostic classification and functional assessment standards for bone and joint injuries and diseases, 1st edn. Tsinghua University Press, Beijing, pp 71–73
6. Zhang W, Zou J, Luo C et al (2004) The comparative study of the treatment to intertrochanteric fractures and subtrochanteric fractures of the elderly patients. Chin J. Orthop (11):649–652
7. Simmernacher RK (2008) The new proximal femoral nail antirotation (PFNA) in daily practice: Results of a multicentre clinical study. Injury 39(8):932–939
8. Wang S, Jiang D, Tan Z et al (2011) New classification of intertrochanteric fracture and its applications in artificial joint replacement. Chin J Bone Jt Inj 26(10):884–886
9. Wnag X, Feng G et al (2007) Classification of intertrochanteric fracture and selection of the internal fixation methods. Chin J Bone Jt Inj 22(10):814–816
10. Chen D, Li X (2009) Classification and treatment progress of intertrochanteric fracture [J]. Asia-Pacific Tradit Med 5(6):148–150
11. Wang S, Tan Z, Zhou M et al (2012) Treating femoral intertrochanteric and subtrochanteric fractures combined with femoral shaft fractures using anatomic locking plate. Chin J Orthop 32(7):626–631
12. Wang X, Dong Q, Zheng Z et al (2007) Long-stem bipolar femoral head prosthetic replacement for elderly patients with femoral intertrochanteric fracture. Chin J Bone Jt Inj 22(9):714–716
13. Luo J, Zhu G, Chen D et al (2006) Hemiarthroplasty treatment for elderly patients with unstable intertrochanteric fracture. Chin Bone Jt Inj 21(1):60–61
14. Li Y, Zhang L, Yang G et al (2007) Progress in the finite element analysis for biomechanics of total hip arthroplasty. Chin J Orthop Trauma 9(3):277–289
15. Liu A, Zhang Y, Wang C et al (2001) Three-dimensional finite element analysis for the biomechanical properties of human femur. J Xi'an Med Univ (Chinese) 22(3):242–244
16. Ma JX, Ma XL, Zhang QG et al (2008) Three-dimensional finite element analysis of femur's biomechanics in normal standing position. J Clin Rehabilitative Tissue Eng Res 12(35):6823–6826
17. Dong Y, Huang T, Li W et al (2002) Image anatomy of femoral marrow cavity in adults and its clinical significance. Chin J Clin Anat 20(1):18–20
18. Estok DM 2nd, Harris WH (2000) A stem design change to reduce peak cement strains at the tip of cemented total hip arthroplasty. J Arthroplasty 15(5):584–589
19. Jansson V, Refior HJ (1993) Mechanical failure of the femoral component in cemented total hip replacement-a finite element evaluation. Arch Orthop Trauma Surg 113(1):23–27
20. Breusch SJ, Lukoschek M. Kreutzer J et al (2001) Dependency of cement mantle thickness on femoral stem design and centralizer. J Arthroplasty 16(5):648–657
21. Kawate K, Ohmura T, Nakajima H et al (2001) Distal cement mantle thickness with a triangular distal centralizer inserted into the stem tip in cemented total hip arthroplasty. J Arthroplasty 16(8):998–1003

22. Ayers D, Mann K (2003) The importance of proximal cement filling of the calcar region: a biomechanical justification. J Arthroplasty 18(7 Suppl 1):103–109
23. Powers CM, Lee IY, Skinner HB et al (1998) Effects of distal cement voids on cement stress in total hip arthroplasty. J Arthroplasty 13(7):793–798
24. Lewis G, Austin GE (1994) Mechanical properties of vacuum-mixed acrylic bone cement. J Appl Biomater 5(4):307–314
25. Lewis G (2003) Fatigue testing and performance of acrylic bone-cement materials: state-of-the-art review. J Biomed Mater Res B Appl Biomater 66(1):457–486
26. Krause W, Mathis RS (1988) Fatigue properties of acrylic bone cements: review of the literature. J Biomed Mater Res 22(A 1 Suppl):37–53
27. Wang S, Liu S, Liu W et al (2010) The finite element analysis of cemented long- and short-stem prosthetic replacement in aged patients with comminuted intertrochanteric fracture. Chin J of Ortho 30(11):1144–1150

Chapter 18
The Exploration of Higher Undergraduate Education Mode Based on University-Enterprise Cooperation

Yunna Wu, Jianping Yuan and Qing Wang

Abstract In recent years, with the rapid development of higher undergraduate education, China has begun to enter the period of education popularization. The undergraduate students have lost the previous pride. The current situation that graduates are difficult to meet the requirements of enterprises has become a growing concern in the current society. More and more people have the requirement of higher undergraduate education reform. It is the inevitable requirement for exploring the reason of the said problem and promoting China's higher undergraduate education healthily to study the current higher undergraduate education mode and the graduates' employability. Based on the research of status quo of undergraduate students and with reference to the current solutions, paper proposes higher undergraduate education mode based on the cooperation of universities and enterprises, which can make modern higher undergraduate education more adapted to the modern society.

Keywords Undergraduate education · Specialist college education · Closed-loop Education · Employability

Y. Wu · J. Yuan (✉) · Q. Wang
School of Economics and Management, NCEPU, Beijing, China
e-mail: 1021431168@qq.com

Y. Wu
e-mail: yys8629823@gmail.com

Q. Wang
e-mail: w20070627@126.com

S. Li et al. (eds.), *Frontier and Future Development of Information Technology in Medicine and Education*, Lecture Notes in Electrical Engineering 269,
DOI: 10.1007/978-94-007-7618-0_18,

18.1 Introduction

Higher education increasingly magnified so that the government and society is increasingly worried about the quality of higher education issues. Society hopes for reform in higher education and enhance the quality of higher education [1]. On January 9, 2005, in the 15th work report meeting of universities directly belonging to Ministry of Education, the minister of education made it clear that emphasis should be earnestly put on the improvement of education quality to deepen teaching reform and advance the quality of higher education [2, 3]. Therefore, how to improve the quality of education to make graduates meet the requirements of the modern enterprises has become an urgent problem for universities. Higher undergraduate education plays an important role in the country's higher education. The higher undergraduate education affect the country's future personnel reserve and is also the source of senior personnel for enterprise, which has a major impact on the future development of the enterprise. However, in the field of higher undergraduate education, graduate employability is not given enough attention as they should. And hardly any university has taken the pace of innovation.

This paper studies the status quo of undergraduate, universities and enterprises and refers to the current solution of higher education in order to seek out a practical higher undergraduate education mode based on university-enterprise cooperation, of which the objective is improve graduate employability. In this mode, cultivating undergraduates is not only the task of universities, but the responsibility of undergraduates, universities, enterprises and even society. The aim of this mode is to make graduate employability improving continuously through the interaction energy between the parties, so that today's higher undergraduate education is more suited to today's social development.

18.2 The Difference Between Personnel Cultivated by Universities and Personnel Needed by Enterprises

In March 2011, the Minister of Human Resources and Social Security Yin Weimin said at a press that the initial employment rate of graduates is between 70 and 75 % in recent years [4]. The Graduate Employment report written by the MyCOS Institute indicated that the employment rate was 88.0 % in the 6 months after graduation. In recent years, there are still more than 10 % of undergraduates who cannot be employed in 6 months after graduation. From the actual situation, even though the employment situation is grim, it does not mean "graduates oversupply". The number of those with higher education in the United States accounts for 35 % of the national population and 23 % in Japan. But now China is only 5 %.Nowadays the existing phenomenon is that graduates cannot find a suitable job and enterprises cannot find the right personnel [5, 6]. There is a structural contradiction between the graduates' professional skills and the needs of society.

The lack of graduate employability contributes to the grim situation of graduate employment, which results in the phenomenon that graduates cannot find a suitable job and enterprises cannot find the right personnel.

18.2.1 The Status Quo of Undergraduates

In China, students rarely think about their own future ideal and future planning before entering universities. Most people bury themselves in learning without thinking about other things that parents and teachers will help them solve. Almost everyone has just a common entrance examination target. However, when entering the University, undergraduates have no the hands-s' guide of teachers and parents so that they lose the forward direction and the goal of the struggle. If undergraduates have no timely adjustment, they will inevitably produce a confused state of mind [7].

Graduates' confusions are mainly university studies confusion and employment confusion. The first and foremost confusion is their university studies. Many students do not understand their own majors and future enterprise requirements and have no idea that what job skills they have to possess at university. As a result, undergraduates lack a sense of employment crisis so that they don't pay attention to learning as they should. In the survey, 56 % of the students consider themselves uninterested in learning, and 25.9 % of the students want to learn, but they think themselves mediocrities, which is very different with their expectations and makes them lost and confused. So some undergraduates become bored with learning and skip class. Then these people develop as internet addiction. The undergraduates who develop as internet addiction will skip further and enter a vicious cycle. There are also some students in class who pay no attention to class and do other things. The second confusion is their employment. This confused sense results from their university studies confusion. The university studies confusion contributes to undergraduates' poor university studies. The students find themselves incapable of the company's work when graduating from university, which makes graduates overwhelmed in the face of employment and employer. There are also some students at university who seriously study but still don't know the functional needs of future enterprises, resulting in learning unfocusedly and low efficiency.

18.2.2 The Status Quo of Graduate Staffs that China's Enterprises Face

In fact, China's enterprises are also faced with the problem that how to select qualified staffs from graduates. Recently, Donghua University conducted a survey of 152 enterprises in Jiangsu, Zhejiang, Shanghai, covering the field of government, education, information, finance, etc., and 11 personnel market, which reflects that fresh graduates lack of employability in several aspects.

(1) Lack of professional skills. Professional skills are the basis of sustainable development and the capital of entering the job market for graduates. It is also considered as a key factor in the employer hiring personnel. Through a rigorous professional training, graduates should be able to master the basic theories and methods of the discipline comprehensively and systematically and apply professional knowledge and skills into the actual work. However, in fact, most of today's graduates' professional skills are weak and they only have a smatter of lots of things. What's more, the undergraduates pay insufficient attention to the training of their professional skills, leading to the lack of the skills, ability to learn and innovation capability.
(2) Lack of practical ability. Practical ability that mainly refer to graduates operating capacity and manipulative ability also includes the abilities of problem-analyzing and problem-solving. The important reason why some enterprises express indifference to graduates is that their lack of practical work experience. Lack of work experience and practical ability become the bottleneck of graduates when seeking jobs. Some graduates put emphasis on theoretical learning and pay little attention to practical training, which makes them have grandiose aims but puny abilities. Thus difficulty of seeking job is inevitable.
(3) Lack of humanities accomplishment. Comprehensive, high-quality humanities accomplishment, a good work ethic, career awareness and professionalism are the basic quality that professional people should have and are also the primary criterion for selecting graduates. However today's undergraduates is poor in knowledge of history and culture. They have confused moral ideal value and purse utilitarian values. Many undergraduates ignore improving their own cultural accomplishment and cannot be addicted to work. Whether graduates possess humanities accomplishment has become an important factor for seeking jobs.

Therefore, universities and enterprises should cooperate actively and work together to create a "university + enterprise" teaching mode which makes students enhance employment crisis at university and focus on their own academic learning. The mode can contribute to the result that graduates solve the employment problem and enterprises find a suitable staffs, achieving a win–win goal.

18.3 Higher Undergraduate Education Mode Based on University-Enterprise Cooperation

18.3.1 The Current China's Education Status Quo Based on the Cooperation of Specialist Colleges and Enterprises

Currently, the school-enterprise cooperation training skilled personnel is only developed for specialist colleges and reflects in the following three forms: (1) order training, enterprises book training plan to specialist colleges on the basis of corporate demand for skilled personnel. Specialist colleges employ engineering and technical personnel of enterprises to involve in the discipline building and modify the teaching program and adjust the curriculum in a timely manner according to the students' future career development needs and industry dynamics. (2) joint schools, on the basis of teaching plans and models, specialist colleges train teachers regularly and strengthen the construction of training facilities and make use of project teaching methods to train senior skilled personnel urgently needed by the market. (3) comprehensive training, specialist colleges train students with turners, fitters, welders, CNC, etc. professional issues at different levels in the school's practice facility, making students possess sustainable development of comprehensive vocational ability. However, these modes are only developed for specialist colleges and vocational institutions. This open-loop mode of higher education itself has its limitations.

As is known, there is essential difference between undergraduate education and specialist college education. Both educations have qualitatively different training objectives. Specialist college education training aims are to train senior personnel with some professional knowledge and skills. The students who graduate from specialist colleges should be adapted to the front-line of production, management, service and apply technology to the rural work. College education makes students equipped with a certain specialized skills and be able to engage in a certain kind of career or a certain type of work. The purpose of knowledge taught by specialist colleges is for use at work. The undergraduate education training aims are to cultivate students to develop a solid understanding of the basic theory of the discipline, specialized knowledge and basic skills, and to have the initial capacity of undertaking scientific research or specialized technical work. The graduates should have a reasonable knowledge structure, master the general method of scientific work, judge and solve practical problems aright and have the ability and habit of lifelong learning. They can be also competent to carry out varied field of works. Undergraduate education teaching knowledge not only emphasizes disciplines depth development but also pay attention to horizontal linkages between disciplines. At the same time, undergraduate education pays attention to cultivating students' scientific thinking skills, creative ability, the spirit of innovation and entrepreneurship.

18.3.2 The Proposal of Higher Undergraduate Education Mode Based on University-Enterprise Cooperation

The fact that undergraduate education is essentially different from college education determines universities cannot copy the mode of specialist college when conducting cooperation with the enterprises. Undergraduate colleges need to find out higher education mode which is in linc with thc characteristics of undergraduate education. This article explores a kind of higher undergraduate education mode based on university-enterprise cooperation which is in line with the original intention of the undergraduate education.

At the beginning of students' enrollment, university, its joint enterprises and fresh undergraduates reach an agreement to ensure that undergraduates can get a internship opportunities on condition that undergraduates complete the first 2 years of their studies and achieve enterprise standard. Then the students begin university studies learning. 2 years later, the students select the relevant corporate internship on the basis of their specialties, achievements and interests and hobbies. The stage when undergraduate is in the internship is counted as the future internship period if undergraduate finally works for the enterprise in the future. In the internship phase, undergraduates understand their specialties and vocational needs of the enterprise, as well as the gap between their abilities and enterprise demand, which can inspire undergraduates' employment crisis and learning morale. Meanwhile, students can also find professional issues in practice in the internship, enhancing students' interest in the in-depth study of the specialty. A year later, the students returned to school for re-education after the end of the business practices. During this time, undergraduates have understood their specialty clearly.

At this point, students have emotional understanding of their professional clearly. At the same time, undergraduates recognize the urgency of learning. Thus undergraduates can start from the gap between their own ability and enterprise demand and the professional issues found in the internship to achieve the target that undergraduates learn knowledge with clear purpose and motivation. This higher undergraduate education mode can inspire students to delve into the knowledge and eliminate the students' sense of employment confusion at university. The students eventually use a high-quality paper to embody the results of their study and research. As shown in Fig. 18.1

The higher undergraduate education mode based on university-enterprise cooperation is a closed-loop model of higher education. It is different from the open-loop college-enterprise cooperation education mode. College students learning is for use at work. But higher undergraduate education mode based on university-enterprise cooperation is better for studying, then studying contributes to work in turn, which is in line with the purpose that universities should cultivate senior personnel who have a more solid understanding of the basic theory of the discipline, specialized knowledge and basic skills, and have the initial capacity of engaging in scientific research or undertaking the specialized technical work.

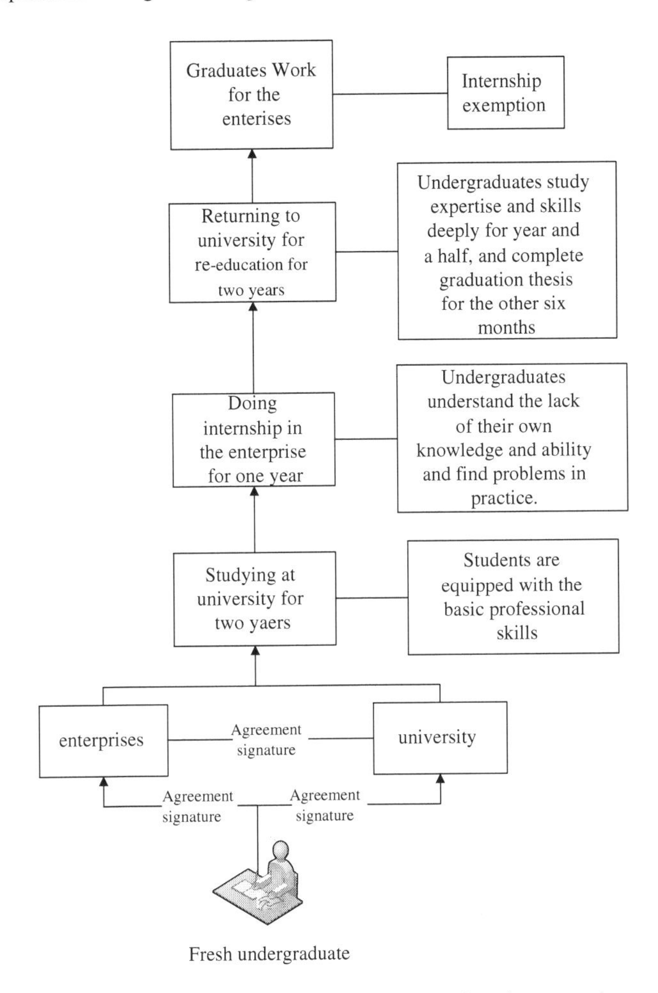

Fig. 18.1 Higher undergraduate education mode based on university-enterprise cooperation

At the same time, this closed-loop model of higher education improve the integrity of higher education, which help undergraduates associate the learning as a whole and improve their professional skills and the ability to solve problems effectively in the loop. This closed-loop model of higher education is in line with the human progressive cognitive philosophical thinking of "theory study–theory practice–theory improvement", on the basis of which, undergraduates learn more systematically and pointedly and the learning is more closely combined with the actual situation. As shown in Fig. 18.2.

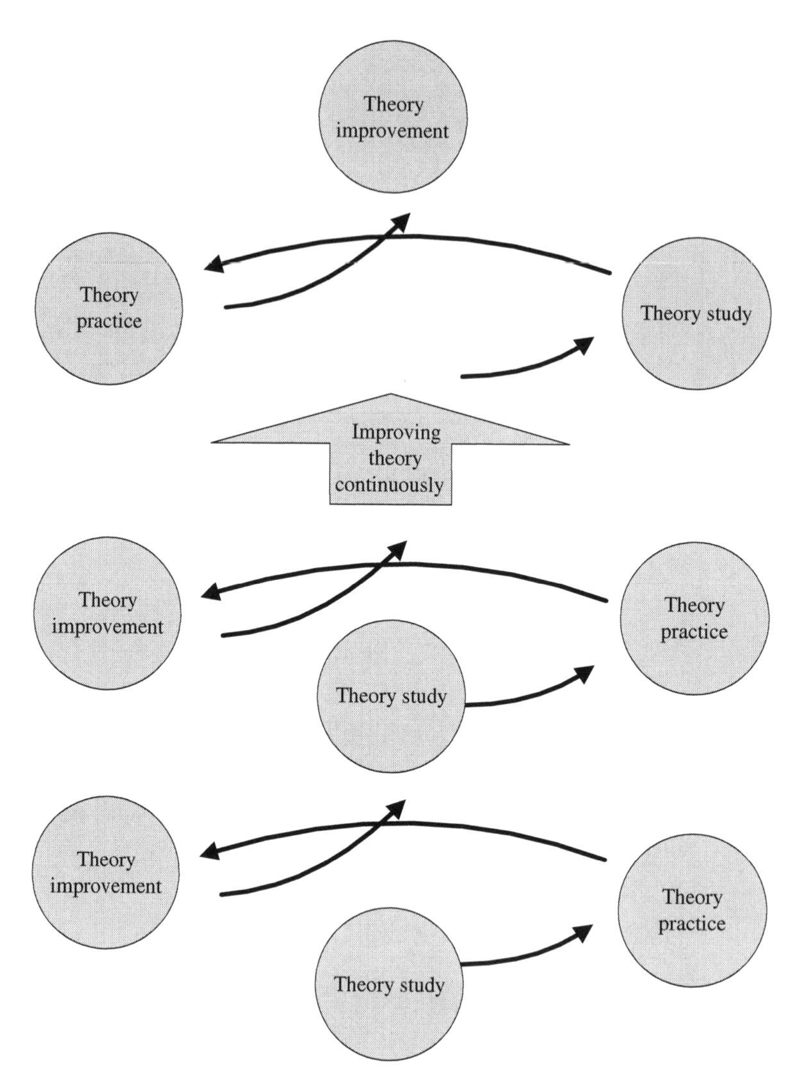

Fig. 18.2 The process of students' learning and cognition in higher undergraduate education mode based on university-enterprise cooperation

18.4 Conclusion

With the development of China's economy, the quality of corporate demand for personnel is improving. Higher undergraduate education reform task becomes urgent. Taking into account the difference between undergraduate education and specialist college education, this paper explores a higher undergraduate education mode based on university-enterprise cooperation on the basis of the characteristics and the nature of undergraduate education. This mode can provide enlightenment for China's university-enterprise cooperation. The higher undergraduate education mode based on university-enterprise cooperation changes the traditional undergraduate education mode that depends only on the university itself. It enables students, universities and enterprises to participate in higher undergraduate education. Each party plays their own role and jointly shoulders the responsibility of training qualified undergraduate, so that Chinese universities foster a growing number of higher education personnel who can adapt themselves to the modern society.

Acknowledgments This paper is sponsored by the special funding of Beijing Municipal Commission of Education for joint projects with North China Electric Power University of 2012 and the authors also would like to acknowledge the supports by Chinese National Nature Science Foundation of China (No.71271085) and Beijing Twelfth Five Year Plan Project of philosophy and social sciences (No.12JGB044).

References

1. Nong R, Meng Z, Hui Z (2006) College cracking university graduates employment predicament ideas. Guangxi Youth Leaders Coll 2006(14)
2. Zhao Z, Chen X (2006) College Students' employability and competitiveness of its upgrade. Heilongjiang High Stud 2006(4)
3. Gu X (2006) Constructing the university vocational guidance system and deepening the reform of vocational guidance. Chin Vocat Tech Edu 2006(4)
4. Huang J (2006) Student career guidance–a special kind of human resource development. Furth Edu Study 2006(2)
5. Jing H, Guisong, Wang et al (2006) The investigation and analysis of college students' career guidance. Hefei Univ Tech J (Social Sciences) 2006(4)
6. Ma S (2005) School-enterprise cooperation and actively explore new modes–practice and thinking of Jinhua college of vocational and technical schools. Qiushi 2006(5)
7. Human resources ministry and social security ministry of highly skilled training joint committee (2008) Promoting school-enterprise cooperation guidebook. China Labor and Social Security Publishing House, Beijing
8. Gu X (2001) College vocational guidance progressive target. Edu Career 2001(12)
9. Zhou J, Xie F (2008) Vocational colleges open cooperative education research and practice. Zhejiang University Press, Hangzhou

Chapter 19
Higher Education Quality Supervision System Research

Yunna Wu, Jinying Zhang, Zhen Wang, Jianping Yuan and Yili Han

Abstract In recent years, with the rapid development of higher education in China, the higher education quality has aroused extensive attention over the whole society. Hence how to supervise higher education quality becomes a difficult theoretical and practical problem that should be solved urgently. Study on Chinese higher education quality supervision system will promote the development of higher education quality. This article puts forward a higher education quality supervision system over college quality control, on the basis of which the multi-party involved supervision domains are formed.

Keywords Education · Quality · Supervision · Whole-process

19.1 Introduction

The government and the society became more and more concerned about the improvement of higher education quality. On January 9, 2005, in the 15th work report meeting of universities directly belonging to Ministry of Education, the

---

Y. Wu · J. Zhang · Z. Wang · J. Yuan (✉) · Y. Han
School of Economics and Management, NCEPU, Beijing, China
e-mail: 1021431168@qq.com

Y. Wu
e-mail: yys8629823@gmail.com

J. Zhang
e-mail: zhangjinying8899@163.com

Z. Wang
e-mail: jianpingsafety@126.com

Y. Han
e-mail: hanyilibj@126.com

S. Li et al. (eds.), *Frontier and Future Development of Information Technology in Medicine and Education*, Lecture Notes in Electrical Engineering 269,
DOI: 10.1007/978-94-007-7618-0_19,

minister of education made it clear that emphasis should be earnestly put on the improvement of education quality to deepen teaching reform and advance the quality of higher education. Therefore, how to improve education quality becomes an urgent problem. However, in the current higher education field, the education quality is not a clear understanding, and there is also no comprehensive quality control system of higher education yet from the angle of management and supervision.

This article puts forward a feasible whole-process control mode through studies on the higher education quality mechanism to coordinate quality control and quality supervision, and establishes higher education quality supervision mechanism in accordance with the situation of our country and objective law of higher education, aiming to use the supervision energy to promote the continuous development of education quality.

19.2 Higher Education Quality Management Regulatory System Framework Design

19.2.1 *The Basis of the Quality Management Supervision*

(1) The regulatory based on Higher education policy and regulations
Our country puts high emphasis on higher education quality supervision. In 2007, the state council, the Ministry of Education and the Ministry of Finance jointly issued the "No. 1 files" and decided to implement "quality project", namely "higher school undergraduate teaching quality and teaching reform project". At the same time, the Ministry of Education issued "opinions of the Ministry of Education on further deepening the reform of the undergraduate teaching course quality", and issued "opinions of the Ministry of Education on improving the quality of higher education", "Beijing long-term education reform and development plan outline" etc., implying the specialty structure adjustment of personnel training mode, curriculum and teaching materials construction, reforming practice teaching and personnel training mode, building high level teacher teams, and establishing the teaching quality supervision and evaluation system. As the main regulator, the Ministry of Education has to meet the basic requirements of supervision according to law and make clear the scope and depth of work, guiding and controlling the reform direction of higher education, and not excessively intervening the autonomic regulation function of colleges and universities.

(2) The whole-process (prior supervision, a matter of supervision and subsequent supervision) and multi-way regulatory principles
Implement supervision needs to respect supervision object characteristics, only the whole- process and multi-way supervision can achieve good results. For higher education quality management, the government needs to

understand and supervise their implementation details. Only the whole-process supervision can achieve this effect, the importance of which is especially outstanding. Switching to the view of colleges and universities, they will face how to cooperate with the government supervision without interfering with their normal management when they perform education work and promote education teaching practice. In addition to the universities trying to outside coordination, the government should work hard in choosing the way of supervision and regulation. The whole process and multi-way supervision principles, on the one hand, require the government to attach great importance to and carry out their own the responsibility of supervision and regulation, on the other hand, also suggest the government should exercise regulatory power flexibly and effectively in a reasonable range.

(3) Closed-loop regulatory principles
Each phrase of government supervision implementation needs to collect the information associated with the then process of education improvement. Only through careful information analysis and comparison can the government learn about the reality about the quality of stage work in colleges and universities, and give reasonable supervision advice. Therefore, the government should be objective about measuring, analyzing and dealing with the monitoring results in order to ensure a smooth transition between this stage of regulatory supervision and the next stage, which can format closed-loop control and implement supervision. Closed-loop supervision can help ingrate the various stages of the supervision process into a whole, on the basis of which the monitoring results can be properly dealt with. Therefore, it is obvious that closed-loop supervision and the whole-process and multi-way supervision supplement each other. The higher education management regulatory system framework design is shown in Fig. 19.1.

19.2.2 The Basic Framework of Quality Supervision System of Higher Education

The basic framework and steps of agent construction higher education quality supervision system is shown in Fig. 19.2.

(1) Regulatory supervision content. Government regulatory supervision content is the development of higher education quality management, including basic elements and management elements. Basic elements refer to human, environment, work, risk, and management fundamentals, etc. And management elements refer to culture, behavior, information, etc. The government should make clear the supervision content and purposes before implementing the supervision.
(2) Supervision implementation. Government monitors colleges and universities management in an appropriate manner. It will collect regulatory information,

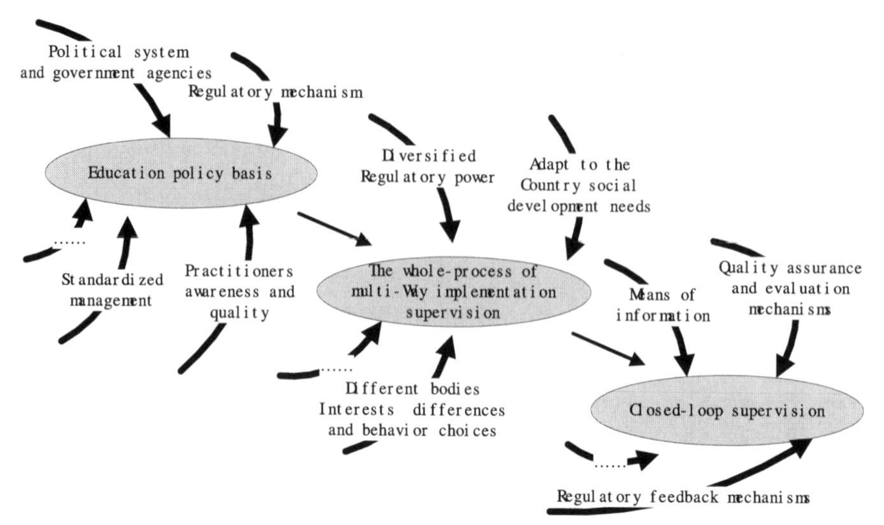

Fig. 19.1 Higher education quality management supervision route and its extension scope

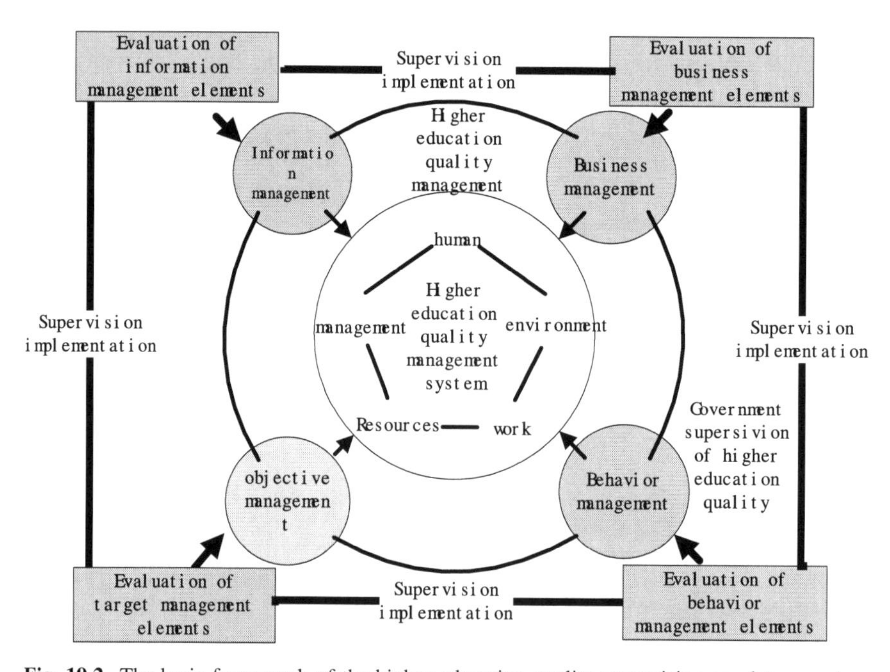

Fig. 19.2 The basic framework of the higher education quality supervision regulatory system

analyze regulatory data and assess monitoring results. The higher education quality management elements are regarded as core elements in the regulatory implementation for the reason that regulatory content is the quality management of higher education.

(3) Regulatory evaluation. Regulatory evaluation is used to aid government supervision. Based on the extracted evaluation indicators, the government grades the elements of higher education quality management and comprehensively evaluates the present situation of higher education quality management. The comprehensive evaluation results are the basis of evaluating and dealing with supervision results.

19.3 The Division of the Higher Education Quality Management Regulatory Constitution

19.3.1 Higher Education Quality Management Supervision Decomposition

Higher education quality is the final result after a series of activities, and is embodied by the knowledge and ability with which students are equipped. With the prerequisite of meeting the demand for resources required by the education activities, higher education quality control is, according to the talent training scheme, to take a series of measures to supervise and control various activities happening in training process, correct the deviation at any time and summarize the experience to ensure the realization of the quality objective. Therefore, higher education quality control system is mainly colleges and universities internal quality control, on the basis of which the whole supervision is established to play the role of internal cause. The latter is the important external guarantee of standardizing teaching activities and comprehensively promoting the education level.

Considering our higher education actual situation and in the guiding ideology of Ministry of Education's "opinions of the Ministry of Education on improving the quality of higher education" and "Beijing long-term education reform and development plan outline", this article develops out quality supervision WBS structure figure which is shown as Fig. 19.3, making higher education quality supervision work perform throughout the full process of universities personnel training and constitute a clear masterstroke which continues adjustment and change. According to the higher education process, quality supervision content includes all elements from admissions, training preparations to participate in their jobs. The supervision score is personnel training.

In order to respond to the call for the Ministry of Education to strengthen the experimental teaching and implement innovation and entrepreneurship education, the practice\business is introduced into the personnel training plan, which is in line with the requirement that Higher Education should be based on the overall development of students and meet the needs of the community; the curriculum arrangement department explicitly indicates that ideological and political course and its lecture professors should be under the supervision so as to meet the demand

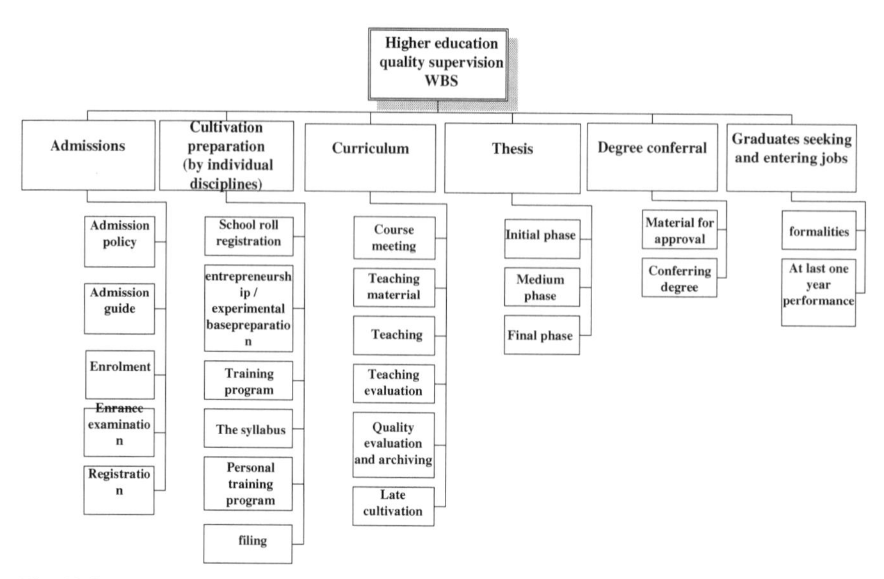

Fig. 19.3 Higher education quality supervision WBS structure figure

for strengthening ideological and political education; teaching share is incorporated into the scope of quality supervision to comprehensively improve the quality of higher education; teaching quality evaluation responds to the Beijing Municipal Education plan and incorporates the comments of the students and teachers; in addition, this article regards the employers' evaluation as the important post evaluation, and the employers' opinions of the evaluation to some extent reflects the social demand for personnel.

19.3.2 Hierarchical Division of Education Quality Supervision

The collaborative supervision system should be founded. The supervision bodies include three levels, namely the government level, the society level and the employer level. ① the government level. The government departments include Ministry of Education, National Development and Reform Commission, Ministry of Finance, the National Audit Office, the State Council Academic Degrees, etc. Led by the Ministry of Education, all the government departments compose the collaborative supervision group. Combining on-the-spot investigate and the feedback information of the society and employers, the supervision group supervises the quality of higher education in the landmark every school year. And the supervision mainly refers to comprehensive evaluation. ② the society level. The society including parents and media carries out the whole process of the higher education quality supervision. The parents and media can offer advice and questions about the apparent or potential quality problems in order to assist higher education quality improvement. ③ the employer level. In addition, the employers who cooperate with universities or are authorized by universities perform post-evaluation when students work for at least a year, according to the student's performance, integration into the work and work ability. The employer's evaluation guides college training plan, improve educational practice and make higher education develop towards the direction to meet the needs of the community.

Each participant of horizontal supervision of the education quality in the time range covers the whole process of personnel training. In the regulatory process, each participant should focus on the implementation of personnel training quality plan and seize the key aspects of the supervision implementation in the regulatory process. The optimization of the various regulatory point targets should be achieved on the basis of implementation of the training program. Parties to participate in training quality horizontal supervision should clear regulatory responsibilities, which can minimize unnecessary regulatory aspects and phenomenon of regulatory overlap. The involved parties should make greater use of the inner and inherent constraints and incentives for training quality to realize the quality-driven higher education personnel training goals.

19.4 The Proposal and Application of Education Quality "Supervision Domain"

Based on the analyzed supervision level and higher education personnel training stage, this article puts forward the concept of "supervision domain", which is used to define the scope of supervision on a certain basis. In the same supervision domain, the supervision work has similar properties.

The supervision source of higher education is divided into three levels. There are different advantages and limitations in each supervision levels, the function of which are different, too. The government should make clear its own role and function. The supervision domain is divided by specific supervision level and supervision factors, as is shown in Table 19.1.

Supervision domain can be understood from two aspects as follows.

First of all, in a certain supervision domain, certain supervision content can be extracted, according to which targeted supervision methods can be drawn. e.g. when supervision domain is divided by higher education personnel training stage, in the recruit stage, for example, time point supervision can be applied as main approach and process supervision can be used as auxiliary supervision means, in which way supervision resources can be saved; in cultivate and course stage, time point supervision is still important. However it is unable to have full grasp of quality only in this way and the efficiency of quality management could be affected if the supervision at time point is too strict. Hence Regulators should take process

Table 19.1 The division of regulatory domain of higher education personnel training based on regulatory resource

	Regulatory authority	Regulatory nature	Regulatory role
Government level	Administrative powers	Direct supervision	Supervise universities to comply with the law and control the quality objectives
Society level	Civil rights	Direct supervision Indirect regulation	Supervise universities to standardize the quality management in accordance with the policies and regulations
Employer level	Civil rights	Indirect supervision Indirect supervision	Supervise universities to make their quality management activities more in line with employers' demands

supervision as main approach, and at the same time reduce supervision strength in order to save supervision resources and avoid interrupting management of colleges and universities.

Similarly, when supervision domain is divided by supervision level, the government level possesses substantial supervision power. However as regulatory resources are limited, supervision at time point should be carried out strictly to establish the authority of government supervision. Process supervision can be regarded as auxiliary means to some extent. On society supervision level, citizens produce supervision effect through various channels on the basis of being informed of the relevant information, so process supervision and time point supervision are equally important in this condition. Enterprise level supervision will generate effect as making tracking evaluation on graduates, which will apply process supervision and time supervision as the main means.

Meanwhile, various regulatory domain divisions don't have completely clear boundaries. There are indistinct boundaries between different domains due to the necessity of interactive cooperation and exchange of information. In the actual implementation of the supervision, regulatory domains are linked as a whole supervision force instead of being independent from each other. The government has to play a role as the leader and guide the other domains consciously in the implementation of the supervision work in order to form the joint supervision force.

Regulatory domain division can help clear the supervision philosophy for government and provide guidance in improving the way of supervision and regulation.

Acknowledgments This paper is sponsored by the special funding of Beijing Municipal Commission of Education for joint projects with North China Electric Power University of 2012. And the authors also would like to acknowledge the supports by Chinese National Nature Science Foundation of China (No.71271085) and Beijing Twelfth Five Year Plan Project of philosophy and social sciences (No.12JGB044).

References

1. WangHuan A (2011) China's higher education system reform lack effective why. J High Educ Res 19404(32):30–36
2. Lei H (2007) China's higher education quality problem in popularization stage education. J Tsinghua Univ Educ Res 9804:107–113
3. Wang SJ, Zhao JF (2009) China's higher education popularization— ten years inventory and reflection. J High Educ Res 17004(30):25–33
4. Wu JP (2011) Theory under the guidance of the scientific concept of development of higher education quality. J Tsinghua Univ Educ res 12002(32):1–33
5. Guo P (2011) Quality assurance system present situation and the countermeasures. J High Educ Res 22012:25
6. Wang Y (2010) Higher education quality guarantee system in government duty. Heilongjiang university, Harbin
7. RuanPing S, Zhao Q (2007) Private higher education in the development of supervision mechanism analysis. J Tsinghua Univ Educ Res 9501:25–51
8. Che L (2008) Subject under the perspective of higher education quality monitoring mechanism research. Xiamen university, Xiamen
9. Yongjun S (2003) Comprehensive evaluation research of engineering project management effect. Xi'an University of Science and Technology, Xi'an
10. Biao L, Hong C (2006) Agent construction unit selection method based on the improved fuzzy optimization model. Hohai Univ J (JCR Sci Ed) 34(2):231–234

Chapter 20
Micro-blog Marketing of University Library Based on 4C Marketing Mix

Feng Qing, Shang Wei and Chen Huilan

Abstract Micro-blog has become a popular marketing tool for many institutions including university library to promote their products and services. This paper analyzes micro-blog marketing of university library in the 4C perspective and proposes several micro-blog marketing strategies for university library.

Keywords Micro-blog marketing · University library · 4C marketing mix

20.1 Introduction

With the environment change brought by the age of technology, organizations have built their relationships with customers through information systems. Recently, micro-blog service providers such as Twitter are hot topics for news and have accumulated a large amount of users. Micro-blog enables users to share news and make friends by mobile phones, email and other client servers. It combines key features of blogging, the practicality of instant messaging and the mobility of Short Message Service texting, and displays particular strengths as a new weapon for customer marketing. The primary aim of this paper is to provide limited insight into micro-blog marketing of university library. After the literature review, the exploration of micro-blog marketing of university library is analyzed following the 4C marketing mix. Based on the analysis, it proposes several strategies of micro-blog marketing for university library.

F. Qing (✉) · S. Wei · C. Huilan
Donghua University Library, No.2999 North Renmin Road, Shanghai, Songjiang District, China
e-mail: fengqing@dhu.edu.cn

S. Li et al. (eds.), *Frontier and Future Development of Information Technology in Medicine and Education*, Lecture Notes in Electrical Engineering 269,
DOI: 10.1007/978-94-007-7618-0_20,

20.2 Literature Review

20.2.1 4C Marketing Mix

The marketer E. Jerome McCarthy stated that "developing a marketing mix must be an integral part of selecting a target market" and all elements must be set at the same time to coordinate with the marketing strategy to make the strategy successful. "The four major ingredients of marketing mix are the four P's, i.e. product, price, place and promotion" [1]. With market competition shifting from product-oriented into customer-oriented, some defects of 4P emerge. Under this condition, Robert F. Lauterborn proposed the 4C marketing mix model [2] in 1993 as a more consumer-oriented model than 4P that attempts to better fit the movement from mass marketing to niche marketing. Consumer wants and needs, cost to satisfy, convenience to buy and communication are the catechism for our times [3]. This model considers a marketing problem from the consumer perspective [4]. The 4C marketing mix model is the combination of four elements: customer, cost, convenience, and communication. All four Cs are important elements of the marketing mix, and each of them is significant and equal. Institutions modify each element in the marketing mix to establish an overall brand image and unique marketing point that makes their products stand out from the competition.

20.2.2 Micro-blog and Micro-blog Marketing

Micro-blog is a new tool for communication in which users can broadcast news in short posts distributed by mobile phones or the web site. Increasingly popular micro-blogs such as twitter offer a short-winded platform for sharing information with patrons by combining the interacting. Beaumont defines that micro-blogging has taken the concept of blogging which is sharing thoughts and opinions, inviting discussion and telling people about your life [5]. While on the contrary to conventional blog's unlimited length, micro-blog only allows posts of up to 140 characters per message which is short, sharp and to the point. The most significant feature of micro-blog, besides the limitation length of the posts, is the unique concept of fans [6]. Once a user considers the posts of another person as particularly relevant or interesting, he can become a "fan" of that person without any restriction. One author's posts are automatically pushed onto the main page of all his fans. In some cases, the receiver of the message might find the news so interesting that they decide to re-post it to their own fans. The initial message can then cascade down from one user's fans network to another's, and on the way transform from a simple bit of information to word-of-mouth [7].

The characteristic of micro-blog make micro-blog marketing being an effective way of marketing. Kaplan point out that micro-blog can generate value for companies along all three stages of the marketing process: pre-purchase, purchase, and post-purchase [7]. In the pre-purchase stage, the micro-blog provides the potential to easily obtain customer feedback for marketing research. In the purchase stage, micro-blogging entails posting advertising and other brand-reinforcing messages to communicate externally with the potential or current customers. In the post-purchase stage, micro-blogging can improve the customer service and complaint management processes by managing the positive feedback and recommendations and handling the negative customer comments as early as possible. Micro-blog marketing has become a choice for many institutions to promote their products, so do the libraries. According to Library Success, NFI and Lindy Brown, more than 700 libraries all over the world are conducting micro-blog marketing such as Yale university library, Yonsei university library, and so on [8]. Sina micro-blog platform is the largest and most popular of the micro-blogging site in China. Up to April 2, 2012, there are 224 libraries using the Sina micro-blog for marketing and 79 of them are university libraries [9].

20.3 University Library's Micro-blog Marketing in the 4C Perspective

20.3.1 Customer

According to Lauterborn's definition, customer means "what the customer want should be sold rather than what you can manufacture". Generally, the demand of university library's customer is the needs for its space and resources. It could be physical or psychological. University library connects the customers and their demands together, and its goal is using the existing resources to meet the various demands of the actual customers and to mine the potential customers and demands. In traditional university library marketing, the marketing object is the actual customer who goes to the library for information, training, consulting and other activities. As for micro-blog marketing, the object is all internet users.

20.3.2 Cost

In the 4C marketing mix, cost means "enterprise should take every effort to decrease the cost of fulfilling the customer's demand". For university library, micro-blog marketing greatly reduces the marketing costs. After registering a micro-blog account, relevant information about library can be posted online and diffused rapidly through its fans' constantly forward. For customers, most of university library services are free of charge, thus the cost is more non-monetary such as the time and effort they take when using the services of the library, the wasted time caused by the unfriendly system or the change of opening hours in holiday. In the micro-blogging marketing, university library can take full advantage of the micro-blog's broadcast and interactive function to save the reader's time and effort as much as possible.

20.3.3 Convenience

Lauterborn defined convenience as "enterprise should take every effort to give convenience to customer for purchasing". Micro-blog is a powerful information dissemination platform and resource repository which can release, browse, retrieve information, reply, and leave comments. University library can take advantage of these functions to push relevant information to its fans initiatively at the first time, and timely get fans' reviews and comments. Micro-blog reduces the difficulty of information accessing, and provides great convenience for both the library and customer.

20.3.4 Communication

Communication means "communication with customer is more important than promotion". Micro-blog with the interactive feature strengthens the interaction between university library and the customers. Different to the traditional one-way marketing pattern, micro-blog marketing provides a face-to-face environment for communication. The environment narrows the distance between each other, makes the customers to be more intimacy, allows library to get first-hand feedback from customers. Effective communication is very important to improve the customers' satisfaction and loyalty.

20.4 University Library's Micro-blog Marketing Strategy

Customer, cost, convenience and communication are important elements of university library's micro-blog marketing, and each of them can directly influent the marketing effect. In this paper, we discuss strategies of university library's micro-blog marketing based on the 4C marketing mix theory.

20.4.1 Customer

20.4.1.1 Building Trust

A certain amount of customers is the most important factor in micro-blog marketing as popularity is the necessary premise to expand marketing. As for customer, trust is a key issue when they are intending to accept the micro-blog service. For this reason, trust building should be an integral part of micro-blog marketing strategy. Trust can be built through strong brand recognition. Using formal account name and logo, such as the full name and landmark of the library, applying for official certification to reflect its authority, and announcing the new form of communication on its website will help university library built trust and attract more attention.

20.4.1.2 Providing Valuable Content

The greatest reason for customers to pay close attention to university library's micro-blog is that they require valuable information. The content that university library posted directly decide its micro-blog's authority and customers' attitude. A survey of micro-blogs hosted by university libraries found that their content mainly involves several kinds: news, resources introduction, push service, reference, education and training, subject service and promotions [9]. The customers are eager for fast, accurate and authoritative information about the library and relative industry. Only university library meets the customers' demands by micro-blogging, it could draw more attention and result in higher social acceptance.

20.4.1.3 Building Customer Community

The core of micro-blog marketing is based on the attributes of the customers' socialization. Micro-blog is ideal for gathering customers with similar interests and tasks into communities. When folks with similar interests gathering at micro-blog to discuss issues, the value they receive in both information and social bonding keeps them returning. If university library builds the customer community, it can present topics and messages customized to the group's interests. By using the label function (# #) of micro-blog, a crowd of customers (such as library peers, scholars and institutions) can be collected because of the same interest in the topic. By using the "fans" function, university library can establish a friendship with these customers to enhance its visibility and promote profession exchanges. Besides, through the vote function, university library not only can publicize information, but also can understand the customers' attitudes and needs.

20.4.1.4 Launching Customer Investigation

In order to lock the target customer community and attract more customers, university library needs to carry out a survey on its current and potential customers, investigating their occupation, gender, age, micro-blogging time and purpose, and other information. Complete survey is important to understand the customers' demands and provide targeted service, therefore enhancing customers' satisfaction, maintaining present customers and expanding the potential customers.

20.4.2 Cost

20.4.2.1 Extracting Message

The micro-blog's limitation of 140 characters per message can be considered as a great bonus for the customers. Instead of reading a large segment of words, the customers only need a few seconds to obtain the important information. The character limitation will greatly save the customers' cost of time, while put forward higher requirements to university library. University library is forced to extract information to be short, sharp, correct and to the point. As supplementary, they can disseminate pictures, audio, video and other forms of information on micro-blog. Besides, they can also provide link to other online resources.

20.4.2.2 Conducting Online Investigation

As well as posting information, university library also can conduct free customer investigations through micro-blog. Using the label, reply and vote functions of the micro-blog, the investigation can be diffused rapidly and widely. It not only reduces the cost of investigation, but also improves the investigation efficiency through the direct communication with respondents.

20.4.2.3 Realizing Open Real-Time Reference

As an important platform of releasing information, the micro-blog offers librarians an effective way to provide reference services. In addition to answering the customers' questions online, librarians also can forward some general questions and answers to more customers. It not only can save the customers' time to ask question and wait for a reply, but also reduce the duplicated work of librarians. Besides, university library can encourage customers to answer questions and forward answers to realize the open real-time reference service.

20.4.3 Convenience

20.4.3.1 Pushing Active Service

Due to the "fan" function of micro-blog, the content posted by university library displays automatically on its "fans" homepage and allows commenting and forwarding. This function will be useful to change the passive services to active services that pushing library resources and service information to customers. Without leaving their workplace or entertainment environment, or accessing to the library website, the customers can receive important information of university library efficiently and accurately at anytime and anywhere. The active services provide great convenience for the customers to access information about university library.

20.4.3.2 Synchronizing with Library's Website

One of the strongest motivators for customers to use micro-blog service is the efficient and timely process. By real-time synchronizing with the library's website, micro-blog can deliver information more timeliness. Customers can be participated in the activities through micro-blog directly, their comments and performance can be on the website at the same time. Participating in the activities of university library can be much easier.

20.4.4 Communication

20.4.4.1 Conducting Interactive Marketing

The biggest difference of Micro-blog marketing to traditional marketing is its interactive feature which makes it become a great platform to carry out customer service. University library needs to take advantage of the interactivity and openness of micro-blog to deliver resources and service information to the customers and reply their comments timely. The customers can also use the "@" function and comment function to transmit personal aspirations to university library. The interaction will help university library narrow the distance with the customers, understand the customers' needs and its own lack, and enhance its affinity and quality of service.

20.4.4.2 Listening to the Customers' Voice

Through collecting the comments and posts released on the micro-blog by the consumers, university library can understand the concerns of the target customers, analyze their behaviour, and gain valuable customer information and demands. It is important to university library to provide services and design marketing plan from the customers' perspective. In addition, university library can also forward the positive comments of the customers, such as their laudation to the library, thereby enhancing its reputation. As for negative voices, university library must be sensitive, as customer dissatisfaction can spread very quickly on the Internet with just a few keystrokes. Communication with the customers, responding their questions and appeasing their discontent in time will be necessary in improving customer satisfaction.

20.5 Conclusion

Micro-blog provides a new platform for exchanging information and helps realize a face-to-face communication with the customers. The low-cost, interactive and rapid-spread features of micro-blog create an excellent marketing opportunity for university library to promote its services and enhance the relationship with customers. This paper analyzes the micro-blog marketing of university library in four aspects: customer, cost, convenience and communication. It reveals that micro-blog can be taken as a formal tool for marketing purpose and play an important role in promoting the influence, service quality and customers' satisfaction of university library. However, the application of micro-blog marketing is also facing many challenges, such as the privacy issues and technical problems, and needs the further study.

Acknowledgments The authors wish to express their sincere gratitude to "the Fundamental Research Funds for the Central Universities" (13D123706).

References

1. McCarthy EJ, Perreault WD, Quester PG (1990) Basic marketing: a managerial approach. Irwin, Homewood
2. Schultz DE (1992) Integrated marketing communications. J Promot Manage 1(1):99–104
3. Lauterborn B (1990) New marketing litany: four P's passe: c-words take over. Advertise Age 61(41):26
4. Constantinides E (2002) The 4S web-marketing mix model. Electron Commer Res Appl 1:57–76
5. Beaumont C (2008) Tweet, tweet, here comes twitter. Telegraph 12:21
6. Hsu CL et al (2010) Effect of commitment and trust towards micro-blogs on consumer behavioral intention. Inter J Electron Business Manage 4(8):292–303
7. Kaplan AM, Haenlein M (2011) The early bird catches the news: nine things you should know about micro-blogging. Bus Horiz 54(2):105–113
8. Li JB (2011) The construction of micro-blogs in libraries abroad and its enlightenment. Lib Inform 1:70–73
9. Yang S, Xu J, Shao S (2012) Library microblogging based on sina microblogging platform. Inform Comput Appl 702–707

Chapter 21
On Ethics and Values with Online Education

Jiayun Wang and Jianian Zhang

Abstract Education goals are introduced and applied to E-learning programs by different agents, which, ethically, is due to the various values shared. After explaining such concept as value-oriented online education, this article will firstly put forward to two ideas such as equality and harmoniousness guiding the carrying out of online education, and secondly based on that will explore the meaning of those two points.

Keywords Value of online education · Value-oriented online education · Harmoniousness · Equality

21.1 Introduction

Online education is an extension of education practice from the real world into virtual one involving kinds of agents, complicated social relationship, different interest groups, with the conflict of ideas of education, of the culture background, and of language environment, as well as of education goals and values, etc. Difference, complexity and diversity in online education reveal that all education programs, involved subjects and objects and intricate relationship, will bear obviously and definitely different ethics and values. If so, we cannot help asking ourselves that what values and ethics those agents should be observing and what those different values and ethics should be. This paper will focus on those topics invited by the characteristic of network technology, ethics and pedagogy, and based on that, such ideas as equality and harmoniousness will be advocated and observed.

J. Wang
Educational School of Huaibei Normal University, Huaibei 235000, China

J. Zhang (✉)
Huaibei Normal University, 100 Dongshan St, Huaibei 235000, China
e-mail: chzjn@126.com

S. Li et al. (eds.), *Frontier and Future Development of Information Technology in Medicine and Education*, Lecture Notes in Electrical Engineering 269,
DOI: 10.1007/978-94-007-7618-0_21,

21.2 Online Education Value and Its Connotation

21.2.1 Online Education Value

Online education is a branch of education system, so online education value can be assessed in the line with formal education values and it is an embodiment of formal education value as the form of education on the Internet. With respect to the definition of this concept, here we share [1] views that it means that the attributes, characteristic, function, effect of online education and the relationship among the involved different agents, which reveals the degree of accordance and satisfaction that all involved agents will experience, which has been influenced by the process as well as the results of education activities on the Internet. We can explain that online education value, on the one hand, can display the diversified relationship that is constructed by agents involving in all kinds of learning program; on the other hand, it can demonstrate to what extent those programs meet participators' needs or whether those programs keep in the line with what all involved expected.

21.2.2 Value-Oriented Online Education

Value-oriented online education concerns an education value. According to Liu [2], value-oriented online education can be defined as an intention held by educators who follow some views on value in order to make judgments on how to make up programs to educate. Value-oriented online education serves as a direction regulating the goal, standards and methods carried out in education assessment. From the standpoint of education on which the online education lays, value-oriented online education is a subset of education value, which means in the process of online education, agents involved who has established some relationships in terms of value will make learners' special interests as a target to pursuit of in order to meet their needs. Those agents involved comes from all works of life, who maybe a learner educated by Internet or an educator who gives his lectures on the Internet, or a designer, a developer, an agency related to online education. They can even be an organization, enterprise or government department. They share different values remarkably. Although they are quite different in terms of education values, they also can seek and share the common ground. According to Li [3], such common goal as aiming to improve people's abilities to get along with the rapid progress of the society and people's overall development can be achieved by the distance education. He took value-oriented distance education as a tool to serve to person and social development, person development in particular. If so, what is value oriented online education? We argue that equality and harmoniousness is the most valuable in orienting the distance education based on the consideration of network technology, pedagogy and ethnics.

21.3 Equality: The First Point of the Value-Oriented Online Education

Network technology dispels the big gap in terms of social hierarchy, classes and status, and advocate that everyone is equal by using and learning on the Internet. Modern education abides by such ideas as equality in education and takes it as its mission to promote all progress and advancement. Therefore, we can see that "equality" observed by online education is a project by principle such as equality on the Internet, equality in the society and equality in education field onto the education on the Internet in terms of value.

Equality of online education is an extension and embodiment of education equality in the virtual world (online environment). From the standpoint of the meaning and the processes of equality of education online, this concept covers three aspects: equality of opportunity, equality of learning process (freely) and equality of being treatment.

21.3.1 Equality of Online Education Opportunity

Simply, equality of opportunity means whether chance of being educated on the Internet is equivalent. It decides whether everybody can access to online education. Superficially, everyone can access to education on the Internet, however, there are still some prerequisites to limit some access to online education. To obtain the opportunity of online education, firstly, learners should have the network devices available in order to get access to Internet, and the basic technology to operate computer (including hardware technology and software technology), the technology of surfing on the Internet (including the technology of communication on online), as well as ability to pay. Can we say that those who have network devices to connect Internet and some skills will definitely enjoy the opportunities to learn on the Internet? Superficially, the answer is Yes. However, in the daily life, most people have been excluded, such as the disabilities and aged people.

In addition, equality opportunity should also been demonstrate that all learners should be treated undifferentiately without reference to personal character or social status (sex, age or social classes), and without reference to locations (urban or rural areas, zones or locations, native or foreign language, different nationalities or different states. etc.). From the angle of digital divide, these problems are reflections of digital divide in the area of online education.

21.3.2 Equality in the Process of Learning

After those learners get access to education on the Internet, whether they can be equally treated when carrying out their learning, whether they can freely chose what they want to learn as well as learning on their own, will be very important during the learning process. Therefore, equality in the learning process mainly means that a learner can make at his disposal the way he will be taught, the materials he wants to learn, the path he is willing to follow, the way the media present itself and the time as well as place he would like to study, etc. Equality in the learning process requires that educators on the Internet take into consideration the students' difference in learning, and that such idea as universal design be observed and run through all courses as well as curriculum when designing the learning process in order to meet the most learners' needs. Along with them, learner requirements should be viewed equally during the process of learning. Ormond [4] expressed his opinions critically on E-learning that if e-learning is effective in initially helping the educationally disadvantaged to access education, will it also be effective in retaining them in learning? Or will an apparently open door really be a revolving door?

In addition, learners share the diversified culture background, so in the process of education online, we should design the cross-cultural courses and curriculum to meet learners' needs. Reeves [5] summed up dozens of impact factors which can be taken to design the multimedia and learning environment. As far as those factors are concerned, he explained that among those learners who expects of the introduction of Web for learning, they should realize that Web-based learning should respect students' diversified ethnic and cultural background. McLoughlin [6] put that Web-centered inclusive learning should be established in the field of online education. So, the cultural background of learner as one of important aspects should be high valued.

21.3.3 The Learners by Online Education Enjoying the Same Treatment as the Graduates Do

It means that after online learning, learners should be equally assessed and respected in the following aspects such as knowledge and skills, process and method, attitude and values, as well as personal development when they are employed in the future, etc. Although learners who pursuit of their online education always coming from all works of life, they all expect of the same rights shared by the peer when they make a start of learning process on the Internet. However, this point should be stressed here that what I mean by the same rights doesn't mean Equivalence but means that all efforts should be paid during the learning process as a result of hard working, which will finally help them with equal chance to be valued in the years ahead, and promote the healthily development of their body and soul in line with what they expected. Also, it means that they will exert their influences as much as others from school education in their daily life.

21.4 Harmoniousness: The Second Point of Value-Oriented Online Education

We understand harmoniousness as a relatively steady situation between person and person, man and nature, man and society, in which equality, natural, coordination, reason, complement, inclusiveness, truth, goodness, and co-existence can be found. As far as online education is concerned, harmoniousness is also the ideal relationship between educators and the educated, and the way questions concerning education are be dealt with, as well as the high value in the line with the top primary goal of education, which the involved agents aim to achieve.

The importance of harmoniousness concerns the following aspects: firstly, the relation among the involved subjects is harmonious. Agents involving online education come from all works of life, so the key to success is to keep all involved agents being in the harmonious situation. Secondly, contradictions and conflicts in the education should be harmoniously dealt with. Online education involves kinds of interest group (organizations, or enterprisers, or individuals) with social responsibilities and economic benefits interweaved and combined. So, how to solve those complicated problems harmoniously is the key to success to online education. Thirdly, harmoniousness itself is the top primary that online education aims to realize. Harmonious development of body and soul of learners, the goal pursued by the designer, developer and operator in the line with the goal of learners, the realization of goal by the enterpriser or related organization, and the shaping of learning person, the establishment of learning organization and the society, all are closely related and consistent.

Harmonious relationship is divided into three categories (see Fig. 21.1) the harmonious relation between agents, the harmonious relationship between subjects and objects, and harmonious development of one's potential abilities. The first two serve the foundation and requirement for carrying out the online education, while the latter acts as the results and final goal. These three aspects are closely related

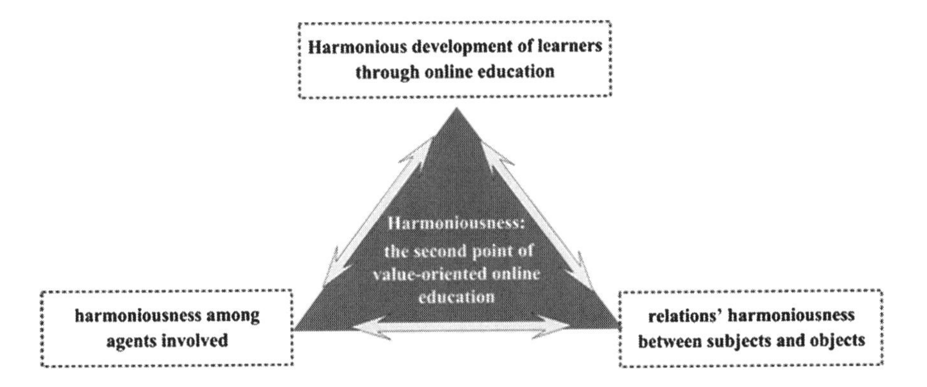

Fig. 21.1 The relationships of harmonious in online education

and complementary. For example, the harmonious and active interaction among subjects (educator and learner, between learners, learner and administer, etc.) will promote the advancement of kinds of web-learning such as learning on his own, learning by cooperation, learning by exploring, which will facilitate the active interaction between learner and his learning materials, environment, resources and tools, and will serve finally the improvement in learners' knowledge, abilities to study, the spirit of cooperation and information skills.

21.4.1 Relations' Harmoniousness Between Subjects and Objects

Relationship between a subject and an object includes teacher and materials, learners and materials, learners and environment in which online education can be carried out, learners and hardware as well as software, etc. Among of them, teachers and learners are subjects while teaching materials, resources, disciplinary level, hardware and software are objects. It's the interactive and interweaving relationship between them, among of them that make the overall development of learners possible. Exactly, it is the level of interaction that will exert significant and strong influence on the development of learners and fulfill educators' expectations.

21.4.2 Harmoniousness Among Agents Involved

Interactive process is also an organic part of online education. The interaction among of them is not face-to-face, but, according to results of research, emotional communication, answering questions put by students, and municipal influence, are indispensable to online education. Subjects involved are such persons as learners, experts on courses, teachers, designers of curriculum, developers of operation system (designer, developer and operator), related agents (organizations), etc. which facilitates the multiple and complicated social connections such as the relationship between teacher and students, students and students, experts and teachers, teachers and online curriculum designers, curriculum designers and network system designers, related agents and those subjects just mentioned, etc. Diversity in agents and complication with their social connections will be having significant impacts on the realization of the goal set by online education. As far as the social connection among those agents is concerned, harmoniousness will play an important role to achieve a success in online education, among of which harmoniousness between educator and learners, between students, between educator students and administrators do mean more.

21.4.3 Harmonious Development of Learners Through Online Education

According to Ye and Liu [7], educational objective consists of a set of clear and definite provisions for improving the quality of students, however, aiming to promote the development of students is its ultimate goal. The primary goal for any education system is to promote the overall and free advancement of the educated. So does online education. That means the harmonious growth of the educated mentally and physically, and displaying what they have learnt by taking part in E-learning programs contributing to the development of the society is the highest goal that online learning seeks. We can take this issue from two points.

- **Overall and harmonious development in terms of knowledge, skills and qualities** the growth of the educated includes the attainment of knowledge, the advancement of skills, experience in the learning process, the improvement of the methods, the development of attitudes and values. What's more, personal growth should observe and share the ethics and values of the whole society. Online education can utilize its richest resources; establish various learning channels by hypertext links, widen the ways that materials are presented, promote the connection of networks. At the same time, free in visiting and linking networks together will lay a good foundation of advancement in learners' knowledge, skills and qualities as well as their growth harmoniously.
- **Coordinated development of the two worlds** the virtual and the real one. It means the balanced and coordinated development of both two worlds. As far as this situation with online education is concerned, it refers to the situation in which online education and the traditional education have complementary teaching programs and develop harmoniously. Specifically, we should understand this harmonious situation as one that both neglect the formal differences in education and respect each other in terms of learning materials, resources, methods, functions, and assessments, etc. Harmonious situation doesn't mean that online education should follow suit of traditional education which makes the former subservient to its system. Therefore, hand in hand development harmoniously between the two education systems can combine two respective strengths and resources to realize the overall development of the educators.

Whoever wants to improve himself or herself, online education can get him or her access to what he or she wants. It doesn't mean, however, learning will be going automatically and smoothly. On the contrary, conditions and value-oriented in education are prerequisites for online to being carried out. Equality and harmoniousness are to be observed and taken as a way necessary to the realization of the ultimate goal of online education. Only the subjectivity, diversity and differences shared by all agents are respected, only the right of being education, of making a choice, of freedom are high valued, only harmonious connections among all agents are established and maintained, as well as the overall and harmonious development of learners involved are valued, can the goal set by online education be achieved.

21.5 Conclusion

Although anyone can realize what he or she want to obtain by online education, it doesn't mean that would be happened automatically. There are some corresponding conditions and premise for them. Equality and harmoniousness are the most important value of online education, and they are the choices of realizing the ultimate targets of online education. Only does it respect everyonc's subjcctivity and otherness, only does it respect learners' rights of being educated, choosing and freedom, only are all relations harmonious, the ideality of online education could be realized.

Acknowledgments This work was supported by the Humanity and Social Science Foundation of Ministry of Education of China (Grant No.: 09JYC880041) and supported by the Major Project of the College Teaching and Research Project of Anhui Province in China (Grant No.: 2012jyxm250).

References

1. Hu Z (1996) Educational laws and educational values. Educ Rev 2:14
2. Liu Z (2000) The characteristics of educational value orientation and its impact to educational review. Henan Soc Sci 6:93–95
3. Li J (2005) On transformation of value orientation in distance education. Dist Educ China 4:20–22
4. Simpson O (2005) E-learning, democracy and social exclusion. In: Carr-Chelman AA (ed) Global perspectives on e-learning: rhetoric and reality. Thousand Oaks, California
5. Reeves T, Reeves P (1997) Effective dimensions of interactive learning on the world wide web. In: Khan B (ed) Web-based instruction educational technology publications. Englewood Cliffs, New Jersey
6. McLoughlin C (1999) Culturally inclusive learning on the web. In: Martin K, Stanley N, Davison N (eds) Teaching in the disciplines/learning in context
7. Ye Z, Liu H (2009) The value orientation of personnel quality standard in open education. Mod Educ Technol 11:92–94
8. Feng W (2008) Harmoniousness between virtual world and reality in online environment. Tsinghua University Press, Beijing
9. Li B, Zhang Y (2003) Exploration of humanity and online education. e-Educ Res 10:55–58
10. Ren R (2004) Analysis of emotional communication in e-learning environment. J Open Educ Res 3:47–50
11. Wu F (2006). Basic issues in research of web-based instruction. J Beijing Norma Univ (Philos Soc Sci) 2:17–22
12. Qian X (2009) Empirical analysis of students' satisfaction degree of the service quality in online education. Chin Dist Educ 7:57–60

Chapter 22
What? How? Where? A Survey of Crowdsourcing

Xu Yin, Wenjie Liu, Yafang Wang, Chenglei Yang and Lin Lu

Abstract Crowdsourcing system recruits an undefined group of people to accomplish tasks proposed by a requester in a short time with low cost. Crowdsourcing makes great contributions in many fields. Building a crowdsourcing system faces many challenges, such as how to motivate people, how to decompose and assign tasks, how to control quality, how to aggregate contributions. In this paper, we explain what the crowdsourcing is and propose three necessary characters as criteria to judge a crowdsourcing system. Then, we introduce solutions to those challenges of crowdsourcing system. Finally, we talk about where crowdsourcing can be used and choose two fields to illustrate the usefulness of crowdsourcing.

Keywords Crowdsourcing · Survey

22.1 Introduction

At the beginning of the twenty-first century, outsourcing was popular, which meant that a company relocated a part of their business to a third-party company. Crowdsourcing, coined by Jeff Howe in 2006, leveraged a large and uncertain group of people to accomplish tasks. However, crowdsourcing assigned the work to an uncertain group of people rather than employees, which make it different from outsourcing.

Actually, the history of crowdsourcing is not that short. Charles Babbage, the earliest people who applied crowdsourcing, found that the director of Alman office decomposed the computations into subtasks and assigned those to a group of qualified individuals in 1820s. The means of communication at that time might restrict the development of crowdsourcing, and also, new computers were invented

X. Yin · W. Liu · Y. Wang (✉) · C. Yang · L. Lu
School of Computer Science and Technology, Shandong University, Jinan, China
e-mail: yafang.wangcs@gmail.com

S. Li et al. (eds.), *Frontier and Future Development of Information Technology in Medicine and Education*, Lecture Notes in Electrical Engineering 269,
DOI: 10.1007/978-94-007-7618-0_22,

to do the computations. Due to the technological advances (e.g. Internet) and limitation of computer (e.g. computers are not good at translation, visual recognition.), crowdsourcing is popular and studied by many researchers.

Crowdsourcing has four advantages comparing with assigning tasks to an individual. First, tasks can be finished faster. Crowds can finish tasks, such as adding tags to photos [1], in shorter time than single person does. Second, work can be done with low cost. It is much cheaper to recruit a group of non-expert to write captions than to hire a stenographer [2]. Third, high-quality answers can be yielded. Even though people may make mistakes, it is difficult for a group of people to produce bad answers, especially when many quality control techniques can be utilized. Finally, crowdsourcing paradigm can do some special work that a person cannot accomplish, such as prediction markets [3].

When building the crowdsourcing system, people may face a series of challenges. Doan et al. [4] proposed four challenges of crowdsourcing system, i.e. how to recruit and retain users, what contributions can users make, how to combine user contributions and how to evaluate users and contributions. In order to solve those problems, many researchers have studied the motivation of workers [5–7], the quality control techniques [8–12] and the aggregation of contributions [2, 13, 14].

In this paper, we review the definition of crowdsourcing and propose its three necessary characters. Then, we propose four challenges of crowdsourcing system and study the solutions. Finally, we illustrate where crowdsourcing can be applied.

22.2 "What" is Crowdsourcing

In 2006, Howe Jeff first proposed the term crowdsourcing [15]. Afterwards, many different definitions were given, which made it blurring. To give an integrated definition, Estells et al. [16] studied about 40 definitions of crowdsourcing. From these definitions, we summarize three necessary characters of crowdsourcing, which can provide people criteria to judge crowdsourcing system. They are:

- There should be a designated agent (or a requester) to propose tasks.
- Workers are a group of individuals with varying knowledge, skill, culture, etc.
- Both requester and workers can obtain benefits.

There are some overlaps between related concepts and crowdsourcing. However, the emphasis points on these concepts are different (see Table 22.1).

Table 22.1 The differences between related topics and crowdsourcing

Term	The gravity of term
Crowdsourcing	Focus on outsourcing tasks to an uncertain group of people
Human computation	Focus on using human to replace the computer
Social computing	Focus on the interplay between social behavior and interaction
Collective intelligence	Focus on intelligence from people working collectively

22.3 "How" to Crowdsourcing

In this section, four challenges are found out when using crowdsourcing paradigm, i.e. how to motivate and retain crowds, how to decompose and assign tasks, how to control quality and how to aggregate the results. Table 22.2 shows an overview of the challenges and their solutions.

22.3.1 How to Motivate

Generally, crowds are driven by both intrinsic and extrinsic motivations [5, 7].

22.3.1.1 Intrinsic Motivations

Enjoyment Sometimes, even if some applications are not funny anyway, people may use them as a tool to kill time when they are bored [17, 18]. However, making the tasks entertaining can effectively make workers participate and contribute. Games With A Purpose (GWAP) are designed to be full of fun in order to attract a large number of people to solve a task. For instance, ESP game [1], a game labeling image with tags, randomly paired two players to see the same image and let them type words relevant to that image in order to come up with some matching tags. Besides, GWAP can also solve complex scientific problems, e.g. Foldit [19] encouraged normal players to build a structure with the lowest Rosetta energy.

Altruism People will spontaneously give their help during disasters and emergencies. For instance, during the Haiti quake, individuals sent messages about "trapped people, needs of food", and also, experts and volunteers offered their assistance in the relief efforts [20].

Personal Improvement People prefer to take part in the crowdsourcing systems which permit their creativity and give them the feedback (result or score). When participating in such systems, people feel satisfied. Also, learning and improving skill are important reasons for people to take part in. With Duolingo.com, people can learn a language and simultaneously help to translate the contents from the web. People can improve photography skill with iStockers and assist in building stock photography at the same time [18]. With galaxyzoo.org, people study astronomy and aid in classification of large numbers of galaxies in the meantime.

Habit and Preference Wohn et al. [21] suggested that the habit was an explanation of participation and habit could make people spend more time. Moreover, if the user interface of crowdsourcing system is difficult for people to complete tasks or even annoying to some people in other cultures, workers will probably not take part in [17].

Table 22.2 An overview of the challenges and their solutions

How to motivate	Intrinsic motivation	Enjoyment	Entertaining tasks encourage workers to participate	ESP [1], Foldit [19]
		Altruism	Some people are willing to do good or help others	Helps during Haiti quake [20]
		Personal improvement	Personal improvement, such as satisfaction, learning and reputation, can also be the incentive	Duolingo.com, iStockers [18], http://www.galaxyzoo.org
		Habit and preference	The habit could make people spend more time Workers' preference may influence the participation	Habit research [21], Culture [17]
	Extrinsic motivation	Payment	Payment is the easiest method to motivate people	Amazon mechanical turk, Community Sourcing [25]
		Social	Social motivations can motivate workers to participate	Negative/positive feedback [26]
		Requirement	Some people complete tasks because of requirement	ReCAPTCHA [27]
How to assign tasks	Task decomposition	Parallel tasks	Tasks can be decomposed into parallel subtasks and be assigned to workers simultaneously	SCRIBE [2], PhotoCity [28] and ReCAPTCHA [27]
		Sequential tasks	Tasks can be decomposed into sequential subtasks and be accomplished in several steps	PlateMate [11]
		Complex tasks	Complex tasks can be decomposed by workers	Turkomatic [10]
	Task allocation	According to the character of tasks	Task allocation should take into account the character of tasks, such as difficulty and importance	MonoTrans Widgets [30]
		According to human factors	Task assignment should consider the worker's ability and worker's condition	Individual differences [30]
		According to desired tradeoff	Assign tasks to workers and machines according to desired tradeoff	Jabberwocky [33]

(continued)

Table 22.2 (continued)

How to control quality	Before-working	Task design	Tasks can be specially designed using strategies and restrictions to ensure quality	Gold standard tasks [13, 34], No copy and paste [8]
		Reputation	Reputation system can restrain cheating and encourage high-quality answers	Amazon Mechanical Turk
	During-working	Input/output agreement	The answers can only be accepted when the pair of workers reaches agreement	ESP game [1]
		Behavior trace	Workers' behavior can be used to predict quality	CrowdScape [36]
	After-working	Human check	Requesters, experts and other workers can check and evaluate the answers	Turkomatic [10], Shepherd [37]
		Computer check	Some tasks may be difficult for the computer to do, but easier for the computer to check	PhotoCity [28], FoldIt [19]
		Models and patterns	Models and patterns can reduce cheating, remove irrelevant answers and improve quality	Economical model [9], Statistical model [38] and Find-Fix-Verify [39]
How to aggregate	Algorithms		Many algorithms are designed to aggregate the results for special tasks	Genetic algorithm [75], MSA and ODSA [2]
	Wisdom of crowds		Crowds can yield more accurate answers on the average than an individual [65]	Web security [41]
	Iteration		Aggregating the results iteratively can yield a high quality result	Adrenaline [13]
	None		Some tasks need no aggregation or a little aggregation	http://www.Threadless.com

22.3.1.2 Extrinsic Motivations

Payment Payment is the easiest method to motivate people. Some crowdsourcing systems give the monetary reward when workers complete tasks, for example, Amazon Mechanical Turk give money to workers who have completed Human Intelligence Tasks (HITs). Some crowdsourcing systems pay for worker in another way, for example, Crowds in Two Seconds [13] pays money to keep workers on hold. However, financial incentives can effectively increase participation, but cannot improve quality [22, 23]. The amount of money to pay is extremely important, because too much money may cause cheating behavior, and too little money is worse than nothing [24]. Payment can be all kinds of rewards, such as monetary, snacks [25], goods and even virtual currency.

Social People play some crowdsourcing games because their friends play those games and they can have competition and cooperation with their friends. Social feedback can also influence the participation and performance. For example, people would like to contribute in Blog after getting feedbacks, and negative voting may probably increase the chances of deletion [26].

Requirement Employees can be required by their manager to do certain tasks [4]. ReCAPTCHA [27] also uses requirement as an incentive. When people want to register or login, they have to recognize the words which cannot be effectively transcribed by Optical Character Recognition (OCR).

22.3.2 How to Decompose and Assign Tasks

22.3.2.1 Task Decomposition

Parallel tasks Some types of tasks can be decomposed into parallel subtasks. For example, due to the requirement of low latency, SCRIBE [2] first cuts a sentence into smaller segments and assign them to workers. PhotoCity [28] decomposes the creating 3D model task into taking photos by a group of players. ReCAPTCHA [27] breaks down the transcribing old books task into recognizing words.

Sequential tasks Some types of tasks can be decomposed into sequential subtasks. For example, Bernstein et al. [29] proposed that a method to generate tail answers using crowdsourcing techniques and divided the task into several steps, i.e. extract tail answers, vote, proofread and title the answers. Furthermore, PlateMate [11] estimates users' food intake/composition and decomposes tasks into several subtasks, i.e. tag food, identify food and measure energy.

Complex tasks Many tasks in the real world are complex and cannot be decomposed easily. To solve that, task decomposition can be raised as a new task and be solved by the workers. For instance, Turkomatic [10] can ask workers to iteratively decompose the complex tasks into new subtasks until the subtasks cannot be decomposed. After finishing the decomposition, workers can accomplish the subtasks and finally combine the results together.

22.3.2.2 Task Allocation

Assign tasks according to the character of tasks Just like allocating tasks with high priority first in operating system, allocating tasks in crowdsourcing systems should consider the character of tasks. For example, MonoTrans widgets [30] assigned sentences to users according to the difficulty and completion time.

Assign tasks according to human factors When allocating tasks, human factors should be considered. Parent et al. [31] proposed that a "work distribution system" could be built in order to adapt tasks to workers based on between-worker and within-worker variability. Between-worker variability should be solved by adapting the difficulty of tasks to individual differences, such as allocating the initial task type to a new user in MonoTrans widgets [30]. Within-worker variability can be addressed by adapting to workers' performance.

Assign tasks according to desired tradeoff In some fields, computers can solve some parts of tasks quickly and cheaply, but with more errors. Hence, some subtasks can be distributed to computers according to desired tradeoff. For example, CrowdFlow [32] allows users to specify speed-cost-quality tradeoff and assigns tasks to humans and machines. Dormouse in Jabberwocky [33] can also manage human and machine resource.

22.3.3 How to Control Quality

Workers may make a mistake, misunderstand the tasks or deliberately cheat the system, which can cause errors or bad results. In order to obtain accurate answers, quality must be controlled by crowdsourcing system.

22.3.3.1 Before-Working

Task design Well-designed tasks can obtain high-quality answers. Le et al. [34] inserted gold standard data into questions and easily rejected bad answers to ensure quality when workers made mistakes in those gold standard data. Bernstein et al. [13] extended gold standard questions with inclusion/exclusion technique. Also, some known-answer questions can be mixed with real questions and the system can easily find out the bad answers. Moreover, Callison-Burch et al. [8] suggested that the tasks should be well-priced and make clear enough for workers to follow. They also proposed several approaches to make cheating difficult, such like using images of sentences instead of text in order to prohibit copying and pasting in translation tasks.

Reputation When cheating is detected, the reputation reduces and the system forbids low reputation workers, e.g. users who fail two tasks may be put into blacklist [25]. In Amazon Mechanical Turk, requesters can require the level of worker's HITs Approval Rate and some other qualifications, such as language skill.

22.3.3.2 During-Working

Input and output agreement Input agreement method [12] is that the system first gives input to two random workers and then asks them to describe the inputs to each other to decide whether that is the same inputs or not. The description can be regarded as correct one when both workers agree. Output agreement method [12] is that the system asks two random workers to give outputs, and the outputs can be accepted when both of them agree.

Behavior trace Workers' behavior during working on tasks can be used to predict quality, errors and cheating [35]. For example, workers who take an extremely short time glancing at image may produce worse label than workers who look carefully. CrowdScape [36] visualizes the workers' behavior and outputs to allow human to evaluate the complex tasks. For example, a worker who rapidly picks radio buttons can be easily found out and regarded as a lazy worker.

22.3.3.3 After-Working

Human check Human check includes checking by requesters, checking by experts and checking by other workers. Requesters can check the results and have an option to reject the work when cheating is detected. An expert can credibly find out that whether the results are correct. It may be cheaper to pay experts to check than to accomplish. Generally, after obtaining multiple answers, workers are enlisted to vote [10, 11, 29] or evaluate those answers. For example, in the external assessment condition of Shepherd, workers can get assessors' feedback to help them produce better results before submission [37].

Computer check Some tasks may be difficult for computers to do, but easier for computers to check. For example, FoldIt system can easily compute the Rosetta energy of the protein structure to identify the good results [19]. In order to create 3D building models, users can take and upload photos according to the PhotoCity system's instructions and the system can effectively find out whether the photo can fit into an existing model or not [28].

Models and patterns Some models and patterns can reduce the likelihood of cheating, remove irrelevant answers and improve quality. For example, economical model is utilized to catch dishonest clients by adding redundant problem assignments and the differences of global labor rates [9]. The statistical model is used to remove problematic inputs by assessing individual consistency and overall consistency of participants' judgments [38]. Find-Fix-Verify crowd programming pattern splits tasks into three stages to improve the quality [39].

22.3.4 How to Aggregate Answers

Algorithms A genetic algorithm is used to combine the workers' design and obtain more creative design results [14]. Modified multiple sequence alignment and online dynamic sequence alignment algorithms are utilized to combine the segments of caption together in a short time [2]. Modified map-reduce algorithms are also used to aggregate results in systems like CrowdForge [40] and Jabberwocky [33].

Wisdom of crowds Wisdom of crowds can aggregate all the answers from an uncertain group of people into better answers, because special crowds can yield more accurate answers and show more intelligent than an individual. The crowds show wisdom only when the crowds fulfill four criteria, i.e. diversity of opinion, independence, decentralization and aggregation. For example, the wisdom of crowds can be used to obtain a prediction by polling websites and prediction markets, or to evaluate the reputation and security of millions of websites [41].

Iteration The iteration can be utilized to aggregate the results and yield a high quality results in combining tasks. Adrenaline [13] uses crowds to find the best photo in a short video, and aggregates the results using iteration strategy. Crowds first select a part of the video which may contain the results from the entire video, and then a shorter part can be picked from the previous results. Finally, after several iterations, the right moment (final photo) can be found out.

None Some independent tasks need no aggregation at all, such as designing a T-shirt on Threadless.com. Also, some tasks need only put the results together, e.g. collecting all of the final labels of images.

22.4 "Where" Crowdsourcing can be Used

In this section, we focus on applying crowdsourcing in HCI and visualization.

VizWiz [42], a mobile crowdsourcing application, leverages a group of people to help blind people to "see". Scribe [2] provides the caption of the speech in real time with non-expert crowd workers and offers people with hearing impairment an opportunity to "hear". Also, there are many crowdsourcing translating systems to help people to understand, such as Duolingo.com and MonoTrans widgets [30]. Moreover, crowdsourcing may improve the user experience to display the tail answers directly on the result page [29]. LemonAid [43] that could provide users technical supports without leaving the website.

Crowdsourcing can provide a new approach to analyze the charts of social data. Willett et al. [44] presented a method to generate the explanations of charts using crowdsourcing paradigm. After analyst selecting a chart, crowd workers submitted their explanations of the chart, such as "why peak or valley might happen", and provided outside URLs that proved their explanations. Finally, all the explanations should be rated by other workers to evaluate the quality. In this way, diverse and high-quality explanations of the chart could be produced by crowds.

22.5 Conclusions

This paper has reviewed the definitions of crowdsourcing, concluded its necessary characters and presented the differences between crowdsourcing and the related concepts. We also studied four challenges of crowdsourcing system. The methods to motivate people, the approaches of outsourcing tasks to workers, the techniques to control the quality and the strategies to aggregate contributions were classified and introduced in detail. In the end, we selected two important fields, HCI and visualization, to illustrate where crowdsourcing could be applied.

Acknowledgments This work was partly supported by China national natural science foundation (61272243, 61202146, 61003149), Shandong Provincial Natural Science Foundation, China (ZR2010FQ011, ZR2012FQ026).

References

1. von Ahn L, Dabbish L (2004) Labeling images with a computer game. In: CHI'04, pp 319–326
2. Lasecki W, Miller C, Sadilek A, Abumoussa A, Borrello D, Kushalnagar R, Bigham J (2012) Real-time captioning by groups of non-experts. In: UIST'12, pp 23–34
3. Hankins RA, Lee A (2011) Crowdsourcing and prediction markets. http://crowdresearch.org/chi2011-workshop/papers/lee-alison.pdf
4. Doan A, Ramakrishnan R, Halevy AY (2011) Crowdsourcing systems on the world-wide web. Commun ACM 54(4):86–96
5. Kaufmann N, Schulze T, Veit D (2011) More than fun and money. Worker motivation in crowdsourcing – a study on mechanical turk. In: AMCIS'11, pp 1–11
6. Quinn AJ, Bederson BB (2011) Human computation: a survey and taxonomy of a growing field. In: CHI'11, pp 1403–1412

7. Yuen MC, King I, Leung KS (2011) A survey of crowdsourcing systems. In: Passat'11 and Socialcom'11, pp 766 –773
8. Callison-Burch C, Dredze M (2010) Creating speech and language data with amazon's mechanical turk. In: CSLDAMT'10, pp 1–12
9. Gentry C, Ramzan Z, Stubblebine S (2005) Secure distributed human computation. In: EC'05, pp 155–164
10. Kulkarni A, Can M, Hartmann B (2012) Collaboratively crowdsourcing workflows with turkomatic. In: CSCW'12, pp 1003–1012
11. Noronha J, Hysen E, Zhang H, Gajos KZ (2011) Platemate: crowdsourcing nutritional analysis from food photographs. In: UIST'11, pp 1–12
12. von Ahn L, Dabbish L (2008) Designing games with a purpose. Commun ACM 51(8):58–67
13. Bernstein MS, Brandt J, Miller RC, Karger DR (2011) Crowds in two seconds: enabling realtime crowd-powered interfaces. In: UIST'11, pp 33–42
14. Yu L, Nickerson JV (2011) Cooks or cobblers?: crowd creativity through combination. In: CHI'11, pp 1393–1402
15. Howe J (2006) The rise of crowdsourcing. Wired 14(6):1–4
16. Estells-Arolas E, Gonzlez Ladrn-de Guevara F (2012) Towards an integrated crowdsourcing definition. J Inf Sci 38(2):189–200
17. Antin J, Shaw A (2012) Social desirability bias and self-reports of motivation: a study of amazon mechanical turk in the US and India. In: CHI'12, pp 2925–2934
18. Brabham DC (June 2008) Moving the crowd at istockphoto: the composition of the crowd and motivations for participation in a crowdsourcing application. First Monday 13(6):1–22
19. Cooper S, Khatib F, Treuille A, Barbero J, Lee J, Beenen M, Leaver-Fay A, Baker D, Popovic Z, Players F (2010) Predicting protein structures with a multiplayer online game. Nature 466:756–760
20. Starbird K (2011) Digital volunteerism during disaster: crowdsourcing information processing. http://crowdresearch.org/chi2011-workshop/papers/starbird.pdf
21. Wohn D, Velasquez A, Bjornrud T, Lampe C (2012) Habit as an explanation of participation in an online peer-production community. In: CHI'12, pp 2905–2914
22. Ariely D, Gneezy U, Loewenstein G, Mazar N (2009) Large stakes and big mistakes. Rev Econ Stud 76(2):451–469
23. Mason W, Watts DJ (2009) Financial incentives and the "performance of crowds". In: HCOMP'09, pp 77–85
24. Gneezy U, Rustichini A (2000) Pay enough or don't pay at all. Q J Econ 115(3):791–810
25. Heimerl K, Gawalt B, Chen K, Parikh T, Hartmann B (2012) Community sourcing: engaging local crowds to perform expert work via physical kiosks. In: CHI'12, pp 1539–1548
26. Sarkar C, Wohn D, Lampe C, DeMaagd K (2012) A quantitative explanation of governance in an online peer-production community. In: CHI'12, pp 2939–2942
27. von Ahn L, Maurer B, McMillen C, Abraham D, Blum M (2008). ReCAPTCHA: human-based character recognition via web security measures. Science 321(5895):1465–1468
28. Tuite K, Snavely N, Hsiao D, Tabing N, Popovic Z (2011) Photocity: training experts at large- scale image acquisition through a competitive game. In: CHI'11, pp 1383–1392
29. Bernstein MS, Teevan J, Dumais S, Liebling D, Horvitz E (2012) Direct answers for search queries in the long tail. In: CHI'12, pp 237–246
30. Hu C, Resnik P, Kronrod Y, Bederson B (2012) Deploying monotrans widgets in the wild. In: CHI'12, pp 2935–2938
31. Parent G, Eskenazi M (2011) Sources of variability and adaptive tasks. http://crowdresearch.org/chi2011-workshop/papers/parent.pdf
32. Quinn AJ, Bederson BB (2011) Human-machine hybrid computation. http://crowdresearch.org/chi2011-workshop/papers/quinn.pdf
33. Ahmad S, Battle A, Malkani Z, Kamvar S (2011) The jabberwocky programming environment for structured social computing. In: UIST'11, pp 53–64
34. Le J, Edmonds A, Hester V, Biewald L (2010) Ensuring quality in crowdsourced search relevance. In: Workshop on crowdsourcing for search evaluation at SIGIR'10, pp 21–26

35. Rzeszotarski JM, Kittur A (2011) Instrumenting the crowd: using implicit behavioral measures to predict task performance. In: UIST'11, pp 13–22
36. Rzeszotarski J, Kittur A (2012) Crowdscape: interactively visualizing user behavior and output. In: UIST'12, pp 55–62
37. Dow S, Kulkarni A, Klemmer S, Hartmann B (2012) Shepherding the crowd yields better work. In: CSCW'12, pp 1013–1022
38. Chen K-T, Wu C-C, Chang Y-C, Lei C-L (2009) A crowdsourceable QoE evaluation framework for multimedia content. In: MM'09, pp 491–500
39. Bernstein MS, Little G, Miller RC, Hartmann B, Ackerman MS, Karger DR, Crowell D, Panovich K (2010) Soylent: a word processor with a crowd inside. In: UIST'10, pp 313–322
40. Kittur A, Smus B, Khamkar S, Kraut RE (2011) Crowdforge: crowdsourcing complex work. In: UIST'11, pp 43–52
41. Chia PH, Chuang J (2012) Community-based web security: complementary roles of the serious and casual contributors. In: CSCW'12, pp 1023–1032
42. Bigham JP, Jayant C, Ji H, Little G, Miller A, Miller RC, Miller R, Tatarowicz A, White B, White S, Yeh T (2010) Vizwiz: nearly real-time answers to visual questions. In: UIST'10, pp 333–342
43. Chilana PK, Ko AJ, Wobbrock JO (2012) Lemonaid: selection-based crowdsourced contextual help for web applications. In: CHI'12, pp 1549–1558
44. Willett W, Heer J, Agrawala M (2012) Strategies for crowdsourcing social data analysis. In: CHI'12, pp 227–236

Chapter 23
Hierarchical Clustering by a P System with Chained Rules

Jie Sun and Xiyu Liu

Abstract Membrane computing has been applied in broad fields such as Biological modeling, NPC problems and combinatorial problems. It has great parallelism and non-determinacy. In this paper, a new variety of P system with chained rules is first applied to the problem of the hierarchical clustering. This new model of P system is designed to solve hierarchical clustering of individuals with nonnegative integer variables. Through performance analysis, this new model of P system can reduce the time complexity of clustering process comparing with the classical clustering algorithm. And it is proved to be more concise and explicit to realize agglomerative hierarchical clustering algorithm by example verification. This is a great improvement in applications of membrane computing.

Keywords Hierarchical clustering · P system · Chained rules

23.1 Introduction

Hierarchical clustering, as an important method of clustering method, separates individuals hierarchically to obtain clusters. Membrane computing has been applied in broad fields such as biological modeling, NPC problems, graph theory and combinatorial problems. It has great parallelism and non-determinacy [2]. In this paper, a P system with chained rules is proposed to solve hierarchical clustering of individuals with nonnegative integer variables [3]. This new model of

J. Sun · X. Liu (✉)
School of Management Science and Engineering, Shandong Normal University, Jinan, China
e-mail: sdxyliu@163.com

J. Sun
e-mail: sjiezz@163.com

S. Li et al. (eds.), *Frontier and Future Development of Information Technology in Medicine and Education*, Lecture Notes in Electrical Engineering 269,
DOI: 10.1007/978-94-007-7618-0_23,

P system uses vectors of rules to describe a causal dependence relation between the executions of the rules. It is a great attempt of membrane computing in clustering problems.

23.2 Hierarchical Clustering Algorithm

Agglomerative hierarchical clustering treat each individual as a singleton cluster at first and then successively group pairs of clusters until all clusters have been grouped into a single cluster that contains all individuals. In order to obtain any clustering, we need to select the similar individuals in the same group. The less dissimilar two individuals are, the more similar they are, and so the individuals with lowest dissimilarity will be grouped together. In this paper we define a dataset set $\Omega = \{a_1, a_2, \cdots, a_n\}$ as the dataset to classify. The dataset includes N elements, as we called individuals. We work with nonnegative integer variables, so the dissimilarity function used for nonnegative integer variables is the Manhattan Distance [4] and it is defined as follows:

$$\forall a_i, a_j \in \Omega: \quad d(a_i, a_j) = \sum_{r=1}^{k} \left(|a_{ir} - a_{jr}| \right) \tag{23.1}$$

The dissimilarity between the individuals can be represented in matrix form:

$$D_{nn} = \begin{pmatrix} w_{11} & w_{12} & \cdots & w_{1n} \\ w_{21} & w_{22} & \cdots & w_{2n} \\ & & \cdots & \\ w_{n1} & w_{n2} & \cdots & w_{nn} \end{pmatrix} \tag{23.2}$$

where w_{ij} is the dissimilarity between individual a_i and a_j. Significantly, in this paper, we presume that the maximum value in D_{ij} is A^*, $\max_{i,j=1}^{i,j=n}(D_{ij}) = A^*$.

23.3 P Systems with Chained Rules

The P System is composed of membrane structure, multisets of objects and evolution rules. The evolution rules determine the reaction results of a specific P system. In general, a P system is designed with the rules executed in a precise temporal order, but not necessarily based on the resulted compounds of the execution of each individual rule. In that case, one might know that two rules are executed in sequence at two different moments, but do not know the underlying intermediate steps. For this reason, the P system with chained rules is proposed in paper [5]. This new model of P system uses vectors of rules to describe a causal dependence relation between the executions of the rules. It makes the P system more concise and explicit to solve problems.

A P system with chained rules of degree n is a construct:

$$\prod = (O, C, \mu, \omega_1, \ldots, \omega_n, R_1, \ldots, R_n, i_0) \tag{23.3}$$

where

1. O is an alphabet of objects;
2. C $\subseteq$ O is the set of catalysts;
3. μ is a structure of labeled membranes;
4. $\omega_i \in O^*$, $1 \leq$ i $\leq$ n, is the initial multisets of objects in membrane i;
5. R_i, $1 \leq$ i $\leq$ n, is the set of vectors of evolution rules. $R_i = \left\{v_{(i,1)}, \cdots, v_{(i,s_i)}\right\}$ and $v_{(i,1)} = \left(r_{(i,j,1)}, r_{(i,j,2)}, \cdots, r_{\left(i,j,t_j\right)}\right)$ where $1 \leq i \leq n$, $1 \leq j \leq s_i$, and $t_i \geq 1$. In other words, in the rule $r_{\left(i,j,t_j\right)}$, i indicates the membrane where the rule belongs, j indicates the vector from which it belongs, and finally t_j indicates the position of the rule in the vector. Each $r_{\left(i,j,t_j\right)}$ is a non-cooperative rule $u \rightarrow v$ or a catalytic rule $cu \rightarrow cv$.
6. i_0 is the output membrane.
The computation in a P system with chained rules has the following characteristics. If a vector v_i of chained rules R_i is triggered (that is, the first rule in this vector is applied), then the rest of the rules from v_i will be applied in order in consecutive steps. However, for an already started vector v_i of chained rules, if a rule from a given position in v_i cannot be applied, then the execution of v_i is dropped and the remaining rules of v_i are not executed anymore. The computation of a P system is halted, if no rule in the vectors can be applied. The result of a halting computation is objects contained in the output membrane.

23.4 A P System with Chained Rules for Hierarchical Clustering

23.4.1 Designing a P System for Hierarchical Clustering

We design a P system with chained rules for agglomerative hierarchical clustering algorithm. The structure of this P system is shown in Fig. 23.1.

The P system with chained rules for clustering is defined as follows:

$$\prod = (O, \mu, \omega_0, \omega_1, \ldots, \omega_{n-1}, \omega_n, R_0, R_1, \ldots, R_{n-1}) \tag{23.4}$$

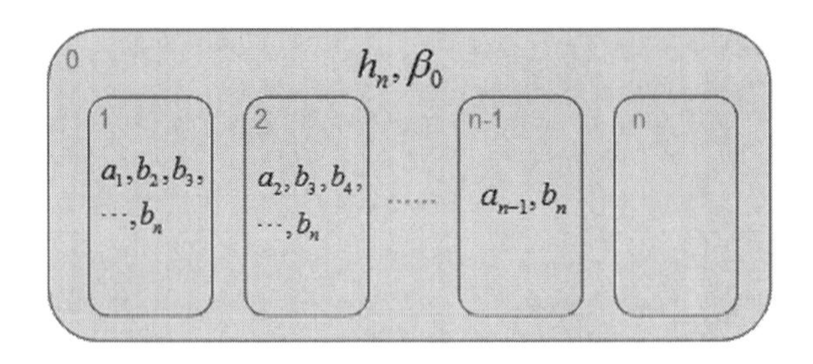

Fig. 23.1 The P system for hierarchical clustering

where

1. Working alphabet:
   $O = \{ \varepsilon, \beta_u, h_q, a_i, b_j, D_{ij}, C_{ij}, \alpha_{iju}, X_{iju} : 1 \le i < j \le n, 0 \le u \le A^*, 1 \le q \le n \}$
2. Membrane structure: $\mu = [_0 \, [_1]_1 \, [_2]_2 \cdots [_{n-1}]_{n-1} [_n]_n \,]_0$
3. Initial multisets:
   $\omega_0 = \{ h_n, \ \beta_0 \}$; ω_0 represents the set of initial objects in skin membrane;
   $\omega_i = \{ a_i, b_j : \ 1 \le i < j \le n \}$;
   $\omega_n = \{\}$; ω_n is the output membrane of this P system.
4. The set R of evolution rules consists of the following rules:

– Rules in the skin membrane labeled 0:

$$R_0 = \{ v_{(0,1)}, v_{(0,2)}, v_{(0,3)}, v_{(0,4)}, v_{(0,5)} \}$$

$$v_{(0,1)} = \{ r_{(0,1,1)} : \varepsilon\beta_0 \to \beta_1 \}$$

$$v_{(0,2)} = \left\{ \begin{array}{r} r_{(0,2,1)} : \beta_u D_{iju} \to \alpha_{iju} \ , \ 1 \le i < j \le n, 1 \le u \le A^*; \\ r_{(0,2,2)} : \beta_u \to \beta_{u+1} \ , \ 1 \le i < j \le n, 1 \le u \le A^* \end{array} \right\}$$

$$v_{(0,3)} = \left\{ r_{(0,3,1)} : h_q \alpha_{iju} \to X_{iju}^{A^*} h_{q-1} (X_{iju})_{in_n}, \ 1 \le q \le n, 1 \le i < j \le n, 1 \le u \le A^* \right\}$$

$$v_{(0,4)} = \left\{ \begin{array}{r} r_{(0,4,1)} : X_{iju} D_{ip} D_{jp} \to C_{ip} X_{iju}, 1 \le i < j < p \le n, \ 1 \le u \le A^*; \\ r_{(0,4,2)} : (X_{iju} D_{ip} \to C_{ip} X_{iju}) \cup (X_{iju} D_{jp} \to C_{ip} X_{iju}), 1 \le i < j < p \le n, \ 1 \le u \le A^*; \\ r_{(0,4,3)} : X_{iju} D_{ip} D_{pj} \to C_{ip} X_{iju}, 1 \le i < p < j \le n, \ 1 \le u \le A^*; \\ r_{(0,4,4)} : (X_{iju} D_{ip} \to C_{ip} X_{iju}) \cup (X_{iju} D_{pj} \to C_{ip} X_{iju}), 1 \le i < p < j \le n, \ 1 \le u \le A^*; \\ r_{(0,4,5)} : X_{iju} D_{pi} D_{pj} \to C_{pi} X_{iju}, 1 \le p < i < j \le n, \ 1 \le u \le A^*; \\ r_{(0,4,6)} : (X_{iju} D_{pi} \to C_{pi} X_{iju}) \cup (X_{iju} D_{pj} \to C_{pi} X_{iju}), 1 \le p < i < j \le n, \ 1 \le u \le A^* \end{array} \right\}$$

$$v_{(0,5)} = \left\{ \begin{array}{r} r_{(0,5,1)} : C_{ij} \to D_{ij}, 1 \le i < j \le n; \\ r_{(0,5,2)} : X_{iju}^{A^*} h_{q-1} \to \beta_0 h_{q-1}, \ 1 \le q \le n, 1 \le i < j \le n, 1 \le u \le A^* \end{array} \right\}$$

$$v_{(0,6)} = \left\{ r_{(0,6,1)} : h_1 \to (h_1)_{in_n} \right\}$$

– Rules in the membrane labeled$i$, $\{\ 1 \leq i \leq n-1\}$:

$$R_i = \left\{ v_{(i,1)} : a_i b_j b_{j+1} \cdots b_n \rightarrow \left(D_{ij}^{w_{ij}} D_{ij+1}^{w_{ij+1}} \cdots D_{in}^{w_{in}} \varepsilon \right)_{in_0} \delta, 1 \leq i < j \leq n \right\}$$

23.4.2 The Computations in P System

At the beginning of a computation, the membrane labeled i $(1 \leq i \leq n-1)$ contains objects a_i, b_j $(1 \leq i < j \leq n)$. The object a_i represents the ith object of the dataset and b_j represents the jth object that behinda_i. Initially in the P system the only rules that can be applied is $R_i = v_{(i,1)}$ [6] in membrane labeled i, which send the object $D_{ij}^{w_{ij}}$ $(1 \leq i < j \leq n)$ and ε to the skin membrane.

The skin membrane labeled 0 firstly contains the objects h_n, β_0. The evolution of the object h_n indicates the number of clusters produced in the P system. The execution of the rule in $v_{(0,1)}$ determines the moment that the loop starts. Afterwards the rules in $v_{(0,2)}$ is applied to select the object D_{ij} with minimum multiplicity which encoding the maximum similarity between the clusters i and j. The rules in $v_{(0,3)}$ produces the objects X_{iju} in the skin membrane and sends a copy to the output membrane. This object X_{iju} represents that the two clusters with lowest dissimilarity can be united to form a new cluster. At the same time, the object h_q is transformed in the object h_{q-1}, which indicates the number of the clusters has decreased by one. Then the rules in $v_{(0,4)}$ recalculate the dissimilarities between new cluster i and the other clusters. After the execution of the rules in $v_{(0,5)}$, this information is kept in the multiplicity of the objects D_{ip}, and the object β_0 is produced to start another loop.

So when the object h_1 appears, the rule in $v_{(0,6)}$ is triggered to send h_1 to the output membrane which determines the finish of this P system. On the whole, in hierarchical clustering there are n clusters representing n individuals and in each loop two clusters are united so we need $n-1$ loops to obtain the last cluster containing all n individuals. As a result, the loop repeats $n-1$ times.

23.4.3 Performance Analysis of the P System

In this paper, we analyze the time complexity based on the rules execution times. In order to obtain the result of hierarchical clustering, we need $n-1$ loops. In every loop, the maximum execution time of every rules vector is listed as follows.

$v_{(0,1)}$	$v_{(0,2)}$	$v_{(0,3)}$	$v_{(0,4)}$	$v_{(0,5)}$	$v_{(0,6)}$	$v_{(i,1)}, 1 \leq i \leq n-1$
$O(1)$	$O(A^*)$	$O(1)$	$O(2)$	$O(2)$	$O(1)$	$O(1)$

As we analyzed above, the time complexity of hierarchical clustering in this P system with chained rules is $O(n)$. However, the time complexity of the traditional clustering algorithms is $O(n^2)$. As a result, this P system can reduce the time complexity of clustering process and make the clustering more concise and explicit.

23.5 Test and Analysis

In order to verify the feasibility and effectiveness of the improved P system, we cluster an example of dataset to obtain the final results.

As an example, the seven points (0,0), (1,0), (1,1), (3,1), (3,2), (2,3), (2,4) is shown in Fig. 23.2.

The dissimilarity matrix D_{77} of these seven points can be obtained as follows.

$$D_{77} = \begin{pmatrix} 0 & 1 & 2 & 4 & 5 & 5 & 6 \\ 1 & 0 & 1 & 3 & 4 & 4 & 5 \\ 2 & 1 & 0 & 2 & 3 & 3 & 4 \\ 4 & 3 & 2 & 0 & 1 & 3 & 4 \\ 5 & 4 & 4 & 3 & 0 & 2 & 3 \\ 5 & 5 & 5 & 4 & 4 & 0 & 1 \\ 6 & 5 & 4 & 4 & 3 & 1 & 0 \end{pmatrix} \tag{23.5}$$

The maximum value of this matrix D_{77} is 6, so $A^* = 6$.

Operating in P system with hierarchical clustering algorithm, we can obtain the computational process of P system. It is shown in Table 23.1.

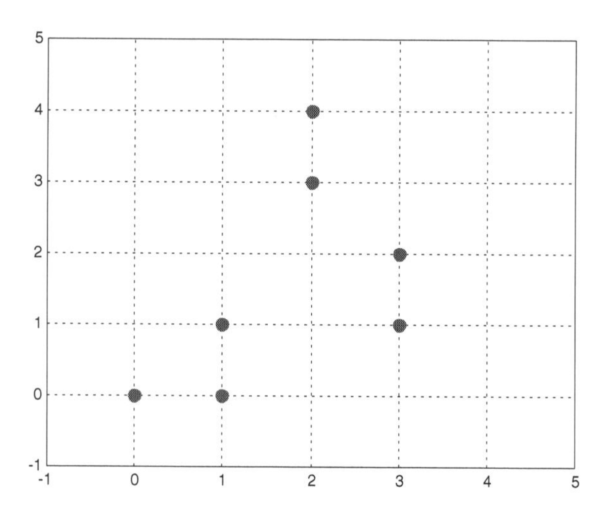

Fig. 23.2 The example of seven points

Table 23.1 The clustering process in P system

	Membrane 0	Membrane 1	Membrane 2	…	Membrane 6	Membrane 7
0	β_0, h_7	$a_1, A_2, A_3, A_4, A_5, A_6, A_7$	$a_2, A_3, A_4, A_5, A_6, A_7$	…	a_6, A_7	
	Membrane 0					Membrane 7
Steps of the first loop of the clustering						
1	$\beta_0, h_7, \varepsilon^6, \mathrm{D}_{12}^1, \mathrm{D}_{13}^2, \mathrm{D}_{14}^4, \mathrm{D}_{15}^5, \mathrm{D}_{16}^5, \mathrm{D}_{17}^6, \mathrm{D}_{23}^1, \mathrm{D}_{24}^3, \mathrm{D}_{25}^4, \mathrm{D}_{26}^4, \mathrm{D}_{27}^5, \mathrm{D}_{34}^2, \mathrm{D}_{35}^3, \mathrm{D}_{36}^3, \mathrm{D}_{37}^4, \mathrm{D}_{45}^1, \mathrm{D}_{46}^3, \mathrm{D}_{47}^4, \mathrm{D}_{56}^2, \mathrm{D}_{57}^3, \mathrm{D}_{67}^1 \left(v_{(i,1)}\right)$					
2	$\beta_1, h_7, \varepsilon^5, \mathrm{D}_{12}^1, \mathrm{D}_{13}^2, \mathrm{D}_{14}^4, \mathrm{D}_{15}^5, \mathrm{D}_{16}^5, \mathrm{D}_{17}^6, \mathrm{D}_{23}^1, \mathrm{D}_{24}^3, \mathrm{D}_{25}^4, \mathrm{D}_{26}^4, \mathrm{D}_{27}^5, \mathrm{D}_{34}^2, \mathrm{D}_{35}^3, \mathrm{D}_{36}^3, \mathrm{D}_{37}^4, \mathrm{D}_{45}^1, \mathrm{D}_{46}^3, \mathrm{D}_{47}^4, \mathrm{D}_{56}^2, \mathrm{D}_{57}^3, \mathrm{D}_{67}^1 \left(v_{(0,1)} : r_{(0,1,1)}\right)$					
3	$h_7, \varepsilon^5, \alpha_{451}, \mathrm{D}_{12}^1, \mathrm{D}_{13}^2, \mathrm{D}_{14}^4, \mathrm{D}_{15}^5, \mathrm{D}_{16}^5, \mathrm{D}_{17}^6, \mathrm{D}_{23}^1, \mathrm{D}_{24}^3, \mathrm{D}_{25}^4, \mathrm{D}_{26}^4, \mathrm{D}_{27}^5, \mathrm{D}_{34}^2, \mathrm{D}_{35}^3, \mathrm{D}_{36}^3, \mathrm{D}_{37}^4, \mathrm{D}_{46}^3, \mathrm{D}_{47}^4, \mathrm{D}_{56}^2, \mathrm{D}_{57}^3, \mathrm{D}_{67}^1 \left(v_{(0,2)} : r_{(0,2,1)}\right)$					
4	$h_6, \varepsilon^5, X_{451}^6, \mathrm{D}_{12}^1, \mathrm{D}_{13}^2, \mathrm{D}_{14}^4, \mathrm{D}_{15}^5, \mathrm{D}_{16}^5, \mathrm{D}_{17}^6, \mathrm{D}_{23}^1, \mathrm{D}_{24}^3, \mathrm{D}_{25}^4, \mathrm{D}_{26}^4, \mathrm{D}_{27}^5, \mathrm{D}_{34}^2, \mathrm{D}_{35}^3, \mathrm{D}_{36}^3, \mathrm{D}_{37}^4, \mathrm{D}_{46}^3, \mathrm{D}_{47}^4, \mathrm{D}_{56}^2, \mathrm{D}_{57}^3, \mathrm{D}_{67}^1 \left(v_{(0,3)} : r_{(0,3,1)}\right)$					X_{451}
5	$h_6, \varepsilon^5, X_{451}^6, \mathrm{D}_{12}^1, \mathrm{D}_{13}^2, \mathrm{D}_{14}^4, \mathrm{D}_{15}^5, \mathrm{D}_{16}^5, \mathrm{D}_{17}^6, \mathrm{D}_{23}^1, \mathrm{D}_{24}^3, \mathrm{D}_{25}^4, \mathrm{D}_{26}^4, \mathrm{D}_{27}^5, \mathrm{D}_{34}^2, \mathrm{D}_{35}^3, \mathrm{D}_{36}^3, \mathrm{D}_{37}^4, \mathrm{C}_{46}^3, \mathrm{C}_{47}^4, \mathrm{D}_{67}^1 \left(v_{(0,4)} : r_{(0,4,1)}\right)$					X_{451}
6	$h_6, \varepsilon^5, X_{451}^6, \mathrm{D}_{12}^1, \mathrm{D}_{13}^2, \mathrm{C}_{14}^5, \mathrm{D}_{16}^5, \mathrm{D}_{17}^6, \mathrm{D}_{23}^1, \mathrm{C}_{24}^4, \mathrm{D}_{26}^4, \mathrm{D}_{27}^5, \mathrm{C}_{34}^3, \mathrm{D}_{36}^3, \mathrm{D}_{37}^4, \mathrm{C}_{46}^3, \mathrm{C}_{47}^4, \mathrm{D}_{67}^1 \left(v_{(0,4)} : r_{(0,4,3)}\right)$					X_{451}
7	$h_6, \varepsilon^5, X_{451}^6, \mathrm{D}_{12}^1, \mathrm{D}_{13}^2, \mathrm{D}_{14}^5, \mathrm{D}_{16}^5, \mathrm{D}_{17}^6, \mathrm{D}_{23}^1, \mathrm{D}_{24}^4, \mathrm{D}_{26}^4, \mathrm{D}_{27}^5, \mathrm{D}_{34}^3, \mathrm{D}_{36}^3, \mathrm{D}_{37}^4, \mathrm{D}_{46}^3, \mathrm{D}_{47}^4, \mathrm{D}_{67}^1 \left(v_{(0,5)} : r_{(0,5,1)}\right)$					X_{451}
8	$h_6, \varepsilon^5, \beta_0, \mathrm{D}_{12}^1, \mathrm{D}_{13}^2, \mathrm{D}_{14}^5, \mathrm{D}_{16}^5, \mathrm{D}_{17}^6, \mathrm{D}_{23}^1, \mathrm{D}_{24}^4, \mathrm{D}_{26}^4, \mathrm{D}_{27}^5, \mathrm{D}_{34}^3, \mathrm{D}_{36}^3, \mathrm{D}_{37}^4, \mathrm{D}_{46}^3, \mathrm{D}_{47}^4, \mathrm{D}_{67}^1 \left(v_{(0,5)} : r_{(0,5,2)}\right)$					X_{451}
Steps of the second loop of the clustering						
9	$h_6, \varepsilon^4, \beta_1, \mathrm{D}_{12}^1, \mathrm{D}_{13}^2, \mathrm{D}_{14}^5, \mathrm{D}_{16}^5, \mathrm{D}_{17}^6, \mathrm{D}_{23}^1, \mathrm{D}_{24}^4, \mathrm{D}_{26}^4, \mathrm{D}_{27}^5, \mathrm{D}_{34}^3, \mathrm{D}_{36}^3, \mathrm{D}_{37}^4, \mathrm{D}_{46}^3, \mathrm{D}_{47}^4, \mathrm{D}_{67}^1 \left(v_{(0,1)} : r_{(0,1,1)}\right)$					X_{451}
10	$h_6, \varepsilon^4, \alpha_{671}, \mathrm{D}_{12}^1, \mathrm{D}_{13}^2, \mathrm{D}_{14}^5, \mathrm{D}_{16}^5, \mathrm{D}_{17}^6, \mathrm{D}_{23}^1, \mathrm{D}_{24}^4, \mathrm{D}_{26}^4, \mathrm{D}_{27}^5, \mathrm{D}_{34}^3, \mathrm{D}_{36}^3, \mathrm{D}_{37}^4, \mathrm{D}_{46}^3, \mathrm{D}_{47}^4, \left(v_{(0,2)} : r_{(0,2,1)}\right)$					X_{451}
11	$h_5, \varepsilon^4, X_{671}^6, \mathrm{D}_{12}^1, \mathrm{D}_{13}^2, \mathrm{D}_{14}^5, \mathrm{D}_{16}^5, \mathrm{D}_{17}^6, \mathrm{D}_{23}^1, \mathrm{D}_{24}^4, \mathrm{D}_{26}^4, \mathrm{D}_{27}^5, \mathrm{D}_{34}^3, \mathrm{D}_{36}^3, \mathrm{D}_{37}^4, \mathrm{D}_{46}^3, \mathrm{D}_{47}^4 \left(v_{(0,3)} : r_{(0,3,1)}\right)$					X_{451}, X_{671}
12	$h_5, \varepsilon^4, X_{671}^6, \mathrm{D}_{12}^1, \mathrm{D}_{13}^2, \mathrm{D}_{14}^5, \mathrm{C}_{16}^6, \mathrm{D}_{23}^1, \mathrm{D}_{24}^4, \mathrm{C}_{26}^5, \mathrm{D}_{34}^3, \mathrm{C}_{36}^4, \mathrm{C}_{46}^4 \left(v_{(0,4)} : r_{(0,4,3)}\right)$					X_{451}, X_{671}
13	$h_5, \varepsilon^4, X_{671}^6, \mathrm{D}_{12}^1, \mathrm{D}_{13}^2, \mathrm{D}_{14}^5, \mathrm{D}_{16}^6, \mathrm{D}_{23}^1, \mathrm{D}_{24}^4, \mathrm{D}_{26}^5, \mathrm{D}_{34}^3, \mathrm{D}_{36}^4, \mathrm{D}_{46}^4 \left(v_{(0,5)} : r_{(0,5,1)}\right)$					X_{451}, X_{671}
14	$h_5, \varepsilon^4, \beta_0, \mathrm{D}_{12}^1, \mathrm{D}_{13}^2, \mathrm{D}_{14}^5, \mathrm{D}_{16}^6, \mathrm{D}_{23}^1, \mathrm{D}_{24}^4, \mathrm{D}_{26}^5, \mathrm{D}_{34}^3, \mathrm{D}_{36}^4, \mathrm{D}_{46}^4, \left(v_{(0,5)} : r_{(0,5,2)}\right)$					X_{451}, X_{671}

(continued)

Table 23.1 (continued)

	Membrane 0	Membrane 1	Membrane 2	…	Membrane 6	Membrane 7
0	β_0, h_7	$a_1, A_2, A_3, A_4, A_5, A_6, A_7$	$a_2, A_3, A_4, A_5, A_6, A_7$	…	a_6, A_7	

	Membrane 0	Membrane 7
Steps of the third loop of the clustering		
15	$h_5, \varepsilon^3, \beta_1, D^1_{12}, D^2_{13}, D^5_{14}, D^6_{16}, D^1_{23}, D^4_{24}, D^5_{26}, D^3_{34}, D^4_{36}, D^4_{46}$ $(v_{(0,1)} : r_{(0,1,1)})$	X_{451}, X_{671}
16	$h_5, \varepsilon^3, \alpha_{231}, D^1_{12}, D^2_{13}, D^5_{14}, D^6_{16}, D^4_{24}, D^5_{26}, D^3_{34}, D^4_{36}, D^4_{46}$ $(v_{(0,2)} : r_{(0,2,1)})$	X_{451}, X_{671}
17	$h_4, \varepsilon^3, X^6_{231}, D^1_{12}, D^2_{13}, D^5_{14}, D^6_{16}, D^4_{24}, D^5_{26}, D^3_{34}, D^4_{36}, D^4_{46}$ $(v_{(0,3)} : r_{(0,3,1)})$	$X_{451}, X_{671}, X_{231}$
18	$h_4, \varepsilon^3, X^6_{231}, D^1_{12}, D^2_{13}, D^5_{14}, D^6_{16}, C^4_{24}, C^5_{26}, D^4_{46} (v_{(0,4)} : r_{(0,4,1)})$	$X_{451}, X_{671}, X_{231}$
19	$h_4, \varepsilon^3, X^6_{231}, C^2_{12}, D^5_{14}, D^6_{16}, C^4_{24}, C^5_{26}, D^4_{46} (v_{(0,4)} : r_{(0,4,3)})$	$X_{451}, X_{671}, X_{231}$
20	$h_4, \varepsilon^3, X^6_{231}, D^2_{12}, D^5_{14}, D^6_{16}, D^4_{24}, D^5_{26}, D^4_{46} (v_{(0,5)} : r_{(0,5,1)})$	$X_{451}, X_{671}, X_{231}$
21	$h_4, \varepsilon^3, \beta_0, D^2_{12}, D^5_{14}, D^6_{16}, D^4_{24}, D^5_{26}, D^4_{46} (v_{(0,5)} : r_{(0,5,2)})$	$X_{451}, X_{671}, X_{231}$
…		
Steps of the last loop of the clustering		
38	$h_2, \beta_1, D^6_{14} (v_{(0,1)} : r_{(0,1,1)})$	$X_{451}, X_{671}, X_{231}, X_{122}, X_{464}$
39	$h_2, \beta_2, D^6_{14} (v_{(0,2)} : r_{(0,2,2)})$	$X_{451}, X_{671}, X_{231}, X_{122}, X_{464}$
…		…
43	$h_2, \beta_6, D^6_{14} (v_{(0,2)} : r_{(0,2,2)})$	$X_{451}, X_{671}, X_{231}, X_{122}, X_{464}$
44	$h_2, \alpha_{146} (v_{(0,2)} : r_{(0,2,1)})$	$X_{451}, X_{671}, X_{231}, X_{122}, X_{464}$
45	$h_1, X^6_{146} (v_{(0,3)} : r_{(0,3,1)})$	$X_{451}, X_{671}, X_{231}, X_{122}, X_{464}, X_{146}$
46	$h_1 (v_{(0,5)} : r_{(0,5,2)})$	$X_{451}, X_{671}, X_{231}, X_{122}, X_{464}, X_{146}$
47	$(v_{(0,6)} : r_{(0,6,1)})$	$X_{451}, X_{671}, X_{231}, X_{122}, X_{464}, X_{146}, h_1$

Finally, the hierarchical clustering of these seven points is finished. According to the objects $X_{451}, X_{671}, X_{231}, X_{122}, X_{464}, X_{146}, h_1$ from output membrane, the result is shown in Fig. 23.3.

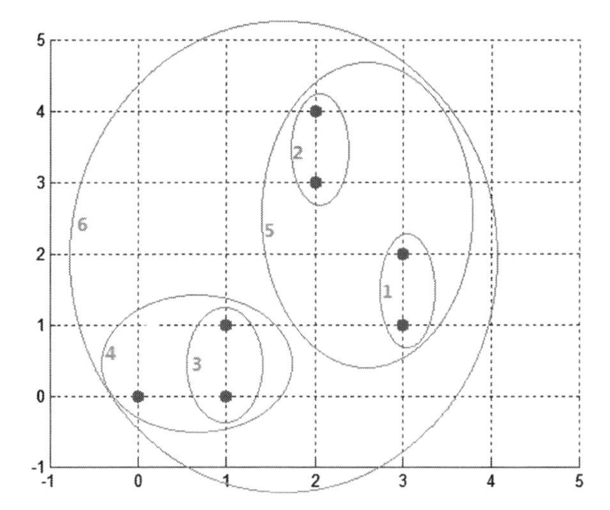

Fig. 23.3 The result of hierarchical clustering

23.6 Conclusions

In this paper, we propose a P system with chained rules to solve agglomerative hierarchical clustering of individuals with nonnegative integer variables. This new model of P system uses vectors of rules to describe a causal dependence relation between the executions of the rules. It makes the P system more concise and explicit to realize agglomerative hierarchical clustering algorithm. Then the paper provides a general example to verify the feasibility and effectiveness of this P system. Although the membrane computing is now used to solve hierarchical clustering problems, our work is basic and there is much more work for membrane computing to do. In future, we will continue to research how to using membrane computing techniques to realize more clustering algorithms.

Acknowledgments This work was supported by the Natural Science Foundation of China (No.61170038), Natural Science Foundation of Shandong Province, China (No.ZR2011FM001), Humanities and Social Sciences Project of Ministry of Education, China (No.12YJA630152), Social Science Fund of Shandong Province, China (No.11CGLJ22), Science-Technology Program of the Higher Education Institutions of Shandong Province, China (No.J12LN22).

References

1. Han J, Kambr M (2005) Data mining concepts and techniques, 2nd edn. Morgan Kaufmann, San Francisco
2. Paun G, Rozenberg G, Salomaa A (2010) Membrane computing. Oxford University Press, New York
3. Cardona M, Colomer AM, Pérez-Jiménez MJ et al (1999) Hierarchical clustering with membrane computing. Comput Inform 27:497–513

4. Jia ZW, Cui J, Yu HJ (2009) Graph-clustering method based on the dissimilarity. J Shanxi Agric Univ 29(3):284–288
5. Sburlan D (2012) P systems with chained rules. Lect Notes Comput Sci 7186:359–370
6. Zhao YZ, Liu XY, Qu JH (2012) The k-medoids clustering algorithm by a class of P system. J Inf Comput Sci 9(18):5777–5790

Chapter 24
Design and Implementation of Key Techniques in TCM Clinical Decision Support System

Mingfeng Zhu, Bin Nie, Jianqiang Du, Chenghua Ding and Qinglin Zha

Abstract This paper introduced an integrated type of TCM clinical decision support system. The components and principles of our system are illustrated. TCM CDSS are divided into eight components. They are TCM DSEMRS, TCM EMRTMS, PIMS, UIMS, IRS, UIR, PIR and KR respectively. Principles of TCM DSEMRS and principles of TCM EMRTMS are discussed in this paper. Among these components, IRS is the core of TCM CDSS. Principles of IRS are discussed in detail in this paper. In IRS, a method of heuristic reasoning is suggested. And the comparison experiment results show our method of heuristic reasoning is much faster than traditional method of full matching and the matching degrees of our method are the same as those of traditional one when using the same data.

Keywords Traditional Chinese medicine · Clinical decision support system · Heuristic reasoning · Production system

24.1 Introduction

Decision is to make a choice or make a determination which is a process of selecting the best solution in multiple candidates by analysis. And Traditional Chinese Medicine (TCM) clinical decision is a method which takes the TCM doctors' knowledge as background, determines disease names, disease situations, disease positions, disease mechanisms and disease trends, etc. in order to determine the principles and schemes of treatments, give correct prescriptions and give correct and scientific methods and measures of treatments according to the data of TCM four diagnoses. Actually, TCM clinical decision is a kind of decision mentioned above. In this process, the diagnostic information of patients and the

M. Zhu (✉) · B. Nie · J. Du · C. Ding · Q. Zha
School of Computer Science, Jiangxi University of Traditional Chinese Medicine, Nanchang 330004, China
e-mail: solarlight@163.com

S. Li et al. (eds.), *Frontier and Future Development of Information Technology in Medicine and Education*, Lecture Notes in Electrical Engineering 269,
DOI: 10.1007/978-94-007-7618-0_24,

TCM knowledge are the base of it. Studying the information and rules in the process of TCM clinical diagnoses and building Clinical Decision Support Systems (CDSS) can provide information support for TCM clinical decisions, can help the TCM clinical diagnoses and treatments, can improve the level of TCM clinical diagnoses, can reduce the influences of human actions during the diagnosis process and can improve the effects of TCM diagnoses and treatments.

At present, according to the difference of application fields, CDSS can be divided into two types. One is convergent system and the other one is integrated system. The representative convergent systems are e.g. the antepartum decision system by Andesen et al. [1], the intelligent fetal heart rate and uterine contraction diagram decision support system by Keith et al. from O&G of postgraduate school of British Plymouth medical school [2] and the intelligent expert system which can estimate gestational age through ultrasound to measure associated data of fetal heads by Besac from O&G of Turkey Hacettepe university [3] etc. The representative integrated systems are e.g. DxPlain developed by American Massachusetts state integrated hospital which can analyze 5,000 kinds of symptoms and can diagnose 2,000 kinds of diseases [4], Iliad developed by Utah state university of American Salt Lake City the data dictionary of which contains more than 1,500 kinds of integrated diseases and treatment schemes [5], QMR system developed by Pittsburgh University which can diagnose more 700 kinds of diseases [6], HELP decision support component hospital information system developed by Utah state university of American Salt Lake City [7] and EON/PROTEGE system developed by American Stanford university which contains components that can be combined with some large scale medical information systems [8], etc.

In mainland, many researchers also devoted themselves into the research of CDSS. Zhao et al. suggested a kind of obstetrics clinical decision support system [9]. Yang et al. introduced a clinical support system named Chuyi and analyzed the mode of information streaming [10]. Su et al. proposed a kind of clinical decision support system based on hospital information system [11]. Ye et al. developed a kind of clinical decision support system aiming at diagnoses and treatments of senile dementia [12]. Deng et al. designed a kind of clinical decision support system for medication of diabetes patients [13]. Deng et al. designed a kind of clinical decision support system used for neurosurgery diagnoses [14].

From the reports of current literature, in mainland, the applications of TCM clinical decision support system are seldom, but the requirements of TCM modernization are desirable. Here, we designed and implemented an integrated type of TCM clinical decision support system which is named as Jiangzhong TCM CDSS. Now, we begin to introduce the components and principles of it.

24.2 Components of TCM CDSS

Jiangzhong TCM CDSS is composed of eight parts. They are TCM dynamic structured electronic medical record system (TCM DSEMRS), TCM electronic medical record template management system (TCM EMRTMS), patient

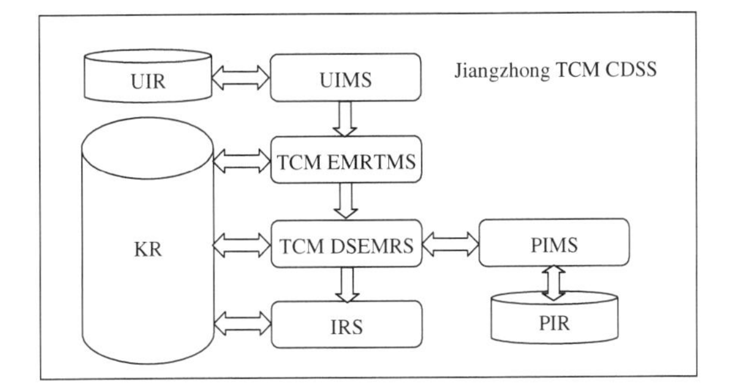

Fig. 24.1 Components of Jiangzhong TCM CDSS

information management system (PIMS), user information management system (UIMS), intelligent reasoning system (IRS), user information repository (UIR), patient information repository (PIR) and knowledge repository (KR). The component diagram is shown below Fig. 24.1.

The component of knowledge repository is divided into 4 parts. The first one is electronic medical record template database, the second one is electronic medical record database, the third one is diagnosis rule database, and the fourth one is prescription rule database.

24.3 Principles of TCM EMRTMS

Design of TCM EMR template is the start of the whole system work. To write TCM EMR, first we need to design a scientific and reasonable EMR template. The design of TCM EMR template is fully dynamic, structured and visual. Firstly, TCM EMR template can be dynamically modified under supervising. Secondly, TCM EMR template is structured which usually contains document name, document sections, data groups and data elements. One or more data groups can be embedded into one document section and one or more data elements can be embedded into one data group. Thirdly, design of TCM EMR template is fully visual. On one hand we can edit the contents of the template, on the other hand we can see the distribution of the contents on graphic user interface. Management of TCM EMR template is strictly conform to electronic work flow, which comprised of three key element i.e. authorization, modification and verification. Work flow of TCM EMR template is shown below Fig. 24.2.

Graphic user interface (GUI) of TCM EMRTMS is comprised of three parts. They are edit area which lies on the left, document view area which lies in the middle and EMR template list area which lies on the right as Fig. 24.3 shows.

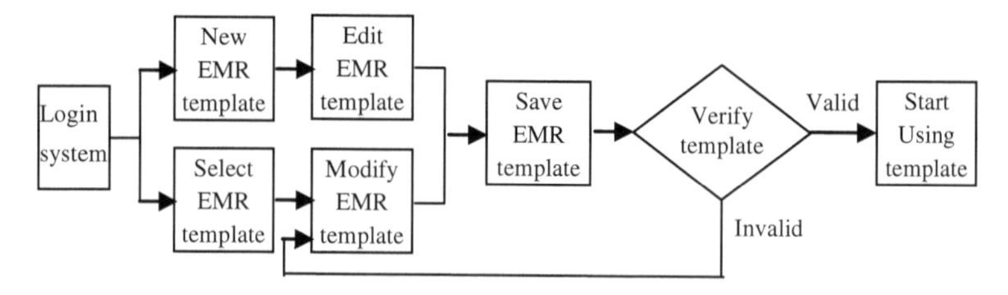

Fig. 24.2 Work flow of TCM EMRTMS

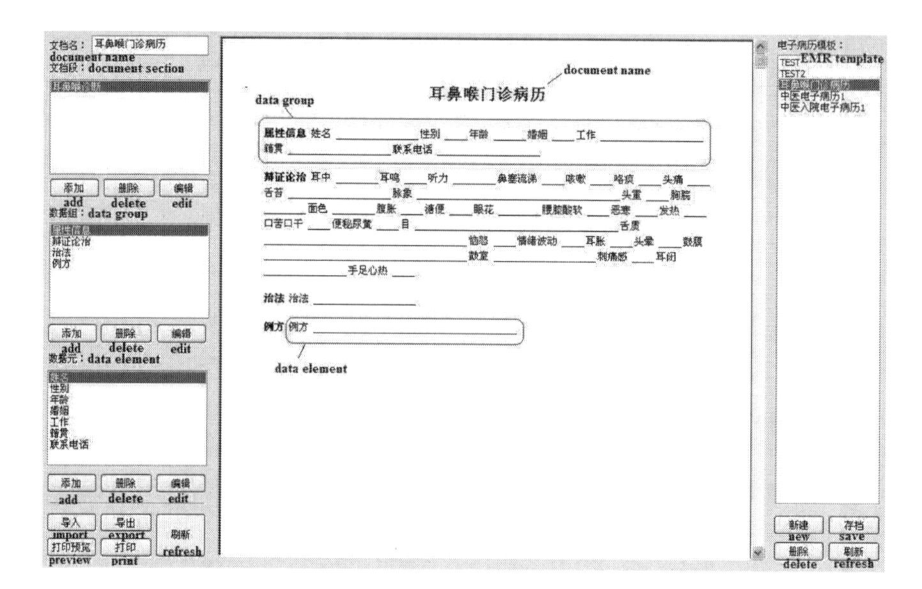

Fig. 24.3 GUI of TCM EMRTMS

24.4 Principles of TCM DSEMRS

TCM DSEMR is one important data source of disease diagnosis, reasoning and analysis. The terms of TCM DSEMR must be highly normative, structured and exact, so that the data can be the reliable base of IRS which are the guarantee of successful reasoning and analyzing of disease of patients. The main work flow is comprised of two. One is newly-build of EMR and the other is modification of EMR. Different users can only see and modify their own EMRs and before the operations on EMRs authentication is need. Then users can operate EMRs, such as write new EMR or modify existing EMR. Before EMRs are used to reason the diseases of patients the saved EMR must be verified and saved in repository. The work flow of TCM DSEMRS is shown below Fig. 24.4.

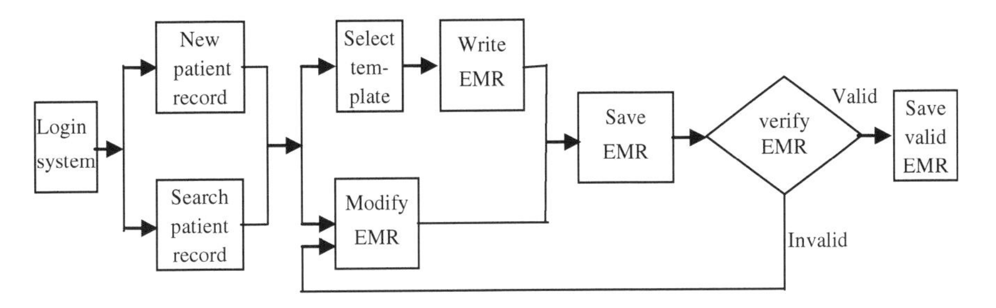

Fig. 24.4 Work flow of TCM DSEMRS

24.5 Principles of IRS

IRS is the core component of TCM CDSS. It has four main functions which are feature extraction, disease reasoning, reasoning explanation, and prescription reasoning. Feature extraction is to extract key features of EMR to match production rules. Disease reasoning is to reason the type of disease and dialectic treatment according to key features and production rules. Reasoning explanation is to explain the reason why the disease type of patient is the reasoning result. And prescription reasoning is to reason the prescription of disease according to the disease reasoning result and prescription rules. The work flow of IRS is shown as following Fig. 24.5.

Principle of disease reasoning is based on production system. A production rule usually contains several conditions and one conclusion. When features match most of conditions, we can say conclusion comes into existence. Otherwise, to match other production rules is needed. Traditional production system uses full matching of conditions to reason [15]. Our system utilizes a kind of heuristic matching method. Full matching is to match all disease production rules one by one in KR and find the best one as result. This kind of matching is accurate, but when number of disease production rules is large the matching process is relatively slow. Nevertheless, heuristic matching is fast. Principle of heuristic reasoning is to use the first key feature to filter disease production rules and then use the second and third key feature to filter disease production rules and so on. So number of rules to be matched is greatly reduced and efficiency of whole matching process is highly improved. In addition, selection and order of key features have some influences on the accuracy of heuristic reasoning.

As far as matching of rules is concerned, we utilize the method of text similarity analysis to match each condition sentence of rules. This method contains two steps. The first step is Chinese word segmentation, i.e. to segment condition

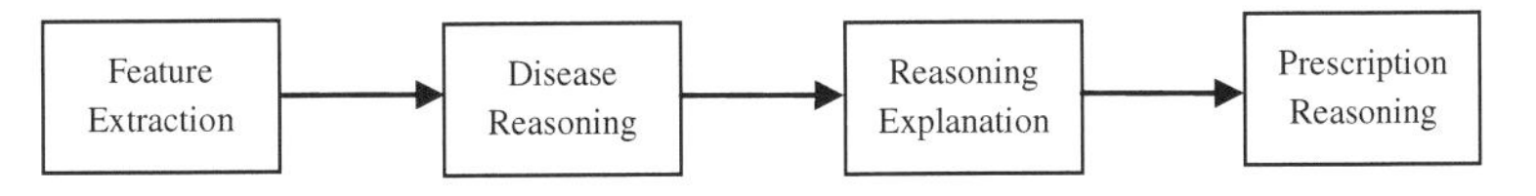

Fig. 24.5 Work flow of IRS

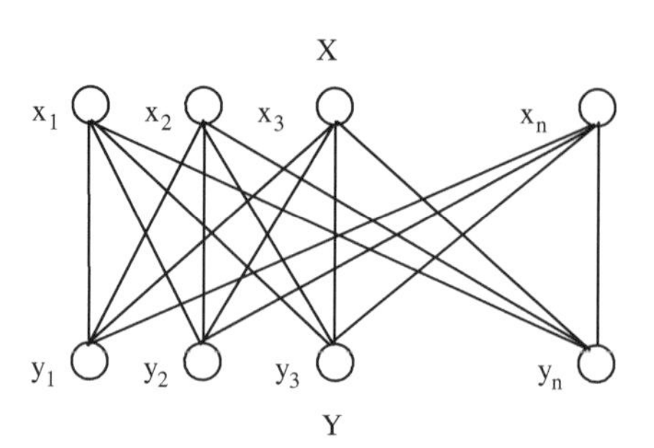

Fig. 24.6 2-part graph of two condition sentences

sentence into separate words. The second step is semantic similarity computation of words. The common word mechanic segmentation methods are positively directional maximum matching, negatively directional maximum matching, minimal syncopate, bidirectional maximum matching and so on. Here we illustrate in detail the method of semantic similarity computation of words.

In the method of semantic similarity computation of words, each condition sentence is seen as a word vector. Word vector can be expressed like $s_i(w_1, w_2, w_3, \ldots, w_n)$. We compute the similarity degree of each word in first vector and each word in the other vector using maximal weight matching method. The algorithm of maximal weight matching method is shown as following.

Step 1: take each word of s_i as one vertex x_i of X part of graph and take each word of s_j as one vertex y_i of Y part of graph.

Step 2: compute the similarity between each vertex x_i of s_i and each vertex y_i of s_j and take the similarity between x_i and y_i as the weight of them. The similarity between x_i and y_i is denoted as $x_iy_i = sim(x_i, y_i)$. Then we can get a weighted 2-part graph of two condition sentences which is shown as following Fig. 24.6.

Step 3: get the maximal weight matching of weighted 2-part graph G. To fulfill this step we need to utilize Hungary algorithm. We will introduce Hungary algorithm later.

Step 4: in the end, compute similarity of two condition sentences X and Y using following formula.

$$SIM(s_i, s_j) = \frac{\sum_{j=1}^{n} x_{i(j)}y_j \times \sqrt{w_{i(j)} \times w_j}}{n} \tag{24.1}$$

Herein, $i(j)$ is the number of word x maximally matched to word y_j.

Hungary algorithm can be denoted as following.

Step 1: create initial vertex symbol L. We utilize following formulas to compute Ls.

$$\forall x \in X, L(x) = \max\{xy\} \tag{24.2}$$

$$\forall y \in Y, L(y) = 0 \tag{24.3}$$

Step 2: let $E_L = \{xy|xy \in E(G), L(x) + L(y) = xy\}$ and find equal child graph G_L the edge set of which is E_L.
Step 3: if G_L has maximal matching M, stop the algorithm.
Step 4: if G_L doesn't have maximal matching M, modify L to get new vertex symbol L'. We use the following formula to compute L'.

$$L'(v) = \begin{cases} L(v) - \delta \quad v \in S \\ L(v) + \delta \quad v \in T \\ L(x) \qquad \textit{in other cases} \end{cases} \tag{24.4}$$

Herein, $\delta = \min\{L(x) + L(y) - xy\} \quad x \in S \quad y \in Y - T$. And S is vertex set which belongs to X in interleaving tree of M in G_L and T is vertex set which belongs to Y in interleaving tree of M in G_L. Finally, we can get maximal weight matching $M = \{x_{i(1)}y_1, x_{j(2)}y_2, x_{i(3)}y_3, \ldots, x_{i\ (n)}y_n\}$.

24.6 Comparison Experiment of Disease Reasoning

In the experiment, we collect otolaryngology experts' experience and knowledge to build 23 pieces of disease rules which contains five kinds of common ear diseases and 14 kinds of dialectic treatment methods. We used 10 groups of disease features to compare the time cost and matching degree of traditional production system and our heuristic system. The comparison data are shown below.

Traditional systems utilize full matching method to match each rule in rule repository. The accuracy of this method is high, but when it comes to large amount of rules, the efficiency of it will greatly reduce. Nevertheless, our heuristic method utilizes multi-step filtered data set to search and match rules. We needn't match each rule in rule repository, but match rules in smaller rule sets. So the efficiency of our method is highly increased. And because the filtered data set includes all possible rules in which the specified rule may reside, so the accuracy of our method remains the same as that of traditional one, i.e. our method is also of high accuracy.

From Table 24.1, we can know the efficiency of our method is much higher than the traditional one (objectively to say, our method is up to one time to seven times faster than the traditional one) and matching degrees of our method are the same as those of the traditional one.

Table 24.1 Efficiency and accuracy comparisons of two types of reasoning

No.		1	2	3	4	5	6	7	8	9	10
Traditional system	Time cost (ms)	219	140	609	156	703	360	203	265	188	453
	Matching degree (%)	77.8	70.0	77.1	87.5	88.9	91.7	85.7	88.9	88.9	88.9
Our system	Time cost(ms)	63	78	78	78	110	109	94	62	32	78
	Matching degree (%)	77.8	70.0	77.1	87.5	88.9	91.7	85.7	88.9	88.9	88.9

24.7 Conclusion

Firstly, we introduced the development situation of CDSS nowadays. Secondly, we introduced the components of Jiangzhong TCM CDSS in which there are 8 components including TCM DSEMRS, TCM EMRTMS, PIMS, UIMS, IRS, UIR, PIR and KR. Thirdly, we suggested the principle of TCM CDSS, including principles of TCM EMRTMS, principles of TCM DSEMRS and principles of IRS. And IRS is the core of TCM CDSS. Fourthly, we compared our heuristic reasoning method with traditional full matching method and the experiment results show that the efficiency of our method is much higher than the traditional one and matching degrees of our method are the same as those of traditional one.

Acknowledgments This project is supported by Youth Science Fund of Education Department of Jiangxi Province of China (No. GJJ12539). We appreciate the related departments a great deal for their support.

References

1. Andesen G, Llerena C, Davidson D et al (1976) Practical application of computer assisted decision making in an antenatal clinic: a feasibility study. Methods Inf Med 15:224–229
2. Keith RD, Beckley S, Garibaldi JM et al (1995) A multicentre comparative study of 17 experts and an intelligent computer system for managing labour using the cardiotocogram. Br J Obstet Gynaecol 102:668–700
3. Beksac MS, Odeikin Z, Egemen A et al (1996) An intelligent diagnostic system for the assessment of gestational age based on ultrasonic fetal head measurements. Technolheath Care 4:223–231
4. Barnett GO, Cimino JJ et al (1987) DXplain, an evolving diagnostic decision support system. J Am Med Assoc 258(1):67–74
5. Lincoln MJ, Turner CW et al (1991) Iliad training enhances medical students' diagnostic skills. J Med Syst 15(1):93–110
6. Miller R, Masarie FE et al (1986) Quick medical reference (QMR) for diagnostic assistance. MD Comput 3(5):34–48
7. Kuporman Giled J, Gardner Reed M et al (1991) HELP: a dynamic hospital information system. Springer, New York
8. Shortlifie EH, Wiederhold G et al (2000) Medical Informatics: computer applications in health care and biomedicine. Springer Verlag, New York

9. Zhao CW, Yan ZZ, Sun YG (2006) The design of obstetric decision support system. Beijing Biomed Eng 25(1):85–88
10. Yang HB, Fan WH, Tang YP, Cai GX (2009) The development of Chuyi TCM clinical decision support system. J Guangxi Tradit Chin Med Univ 12(4):109–110
11. Su SS, Du X (2005) The discussion of the CDSS based on HIS. Med Inf 18(12):1610–1611
12. Ye F, Zhou GG, Nan S (2009) A design and evaluation of clinical decision support system on alzheimer's disease diagnosis. Chin J Biomed Eng 28(6):873–877
13. Deng Y, Peng LF (2007) Study on clinical decision support system in drug decision. Med Inf 20(10):1746–1750
14. Deng HS, Xin JB, Mo MQ (2007) The research and design of clinical decision support system for neurosurgery. Shanghai Biomed Eng 28(4):208–212
15. Cai ZX, Xu GY (1996) Artificial intelligence: principles and applications. Tsinghua University Press, Beijing

Chapter 25
The Effect of a Simulation-Based Training on the Performance of ACLS and Trauma Team of 5-Year Medical Students

Jie Zhao, Shuming Pan, Yan Dong, Qinmin Ge, Jie Chen and Lihua Dai

Abstract *Objective* 56 5-year medical students without Advanced Cardiovascular Life Support (ACLS) and trauma management learning experience were took as the research object, to compare the efficacy of a simulation- based course versus a video plus case-based learning course in medical students on ACLS and trauma management. *Methods* This is a self-controlled randomized crossover study design with blinded assessors carried out in a university simulation center and using a high -fidelity patient simulator. Two hour simulation course or video plus case-based learning (CBL) course were taken after the theory course. The students undertook a theory test before and after the training. ACLS and trauma management skills assessment and teamwork behavior evaluation were made before and after the simulation course or video plus case-based learning course in pre- and post-assessment scenarios. *Results* We demonstrated significant improvements in scores after the simulation training for the theoretical examinations, the practical skills and the team cooperation ability. There was significant difference of improvements between simulation group and CBL group except for overall teamwork behavior in trauma teamwork. *Conclusion* Simulation-based learning or video plus case-based learning also seemed to be an effective teaching strategy. A simulation-based learning for emergency team training in medical students can improve practical ability and teamwork more.

Keywords Advanced cardiovascular life support · Trauma · Medical education · Simulation-based learning · Case-based learning · Teamwork

J. Zhao · S. Pan (✉) · Y. Dong · Q. Ge · J. Chen · L. Dai
Emergency Department, Xinhua Hospital, Kongjiang Road No. 1665, Shanghai 200092, China
e-mail: drshumingpan@gmail.com

J. Zhao
e-mail: smilejacky0707@gmail.com

S. Li et al. (eds.), *Frontier and Future Development of Information Technology in Medicine and Education*, Lecture Notes in Electrical Engineering 269,
DOI: 10.1007/978-94-007-7618-0_25,

25.1 Background

During the last decade, medical education in the world has been striving to become more practice-oriented. This is currently being achieved in many schools through the implementation of simulation-based instruction in skills labs. From flight simulation in the 1920s to the first full-body medical simulator SimOne in the 1960s, simulation technology has long been implemented to meet curricular needs. In the last decade, high-fidelity mannequins have been developed [1]. These are computer-controlled, humansized simulation mannequins that are programmed to mimic human physiology and to respond to medical interventions. Through either operator-controlled or preprogrammed scenarios, these high-fidelity mannequins are able to respond to treatments and receive procedures useful. The complexity of scenarios and algorithms can be integrated with the technology available with current high-fidelity simulators. This allows for great variations in teaching and scenario designs.

As a result of time constraints in training and the need for optimal patient safety, the use of highfidelity simulation has become integral to teaching high risk and emergency skills. Human Patient Simulation (HPS) provides learners with an opportunity to apply and integrate new knowledge in a safe, challenging environment without placing patients at risk. HPS has been used to teach pathophysiology, diagnosis and management, clinical team-building, practice remediation, and procedural-surgical skills [2, 3]. And simulation is positive for both improving knowledge acquisition and learning clinical decisionmaking [2]. In 2009, Okuda et al. conducted a meta-analysis on the utility and evidence of simulation in medical education and found that simulation has led to improvements in medical knowledge, comfort in procedures, and improvements in performance [4]. In this meta-analysis, Okuda et al. found evidence that simulation is effective in the teaching of basic science and clinical knowledge, procedural skills, teamwork, communication, and assessment at the undergraduate and graduate medical education levels. A more recent systemic review and meta analysis found that simulation training improves not only knowledge, skills, and behaviors of health care professionals but also patient-related outcomes, compared with no simulation training. As such, simulation is being incorporated into medical education at all levels of training for teaching and assessment of clinical skills [5].

In addition to technical and cognitive skills, the other crucial component of successful resuscitation is effective teamwork. Evidence suggests that teams make fewer mistakes than individuals and that good teamwork improves patient safety [6, 7]. Evidence also suggests that teamwork failures make a substantial contribution to suboptimal patient care [8, 9]. Retrospective analyses of adverse events and critical incidents have identified communication and teamwork issues as among the most common contributing factors [10]. Despite various statements regarding importance, teamwork programs have not yet gained a solid foothold in the medical culture. As in medical school, there has been limited application of teamwork training in large health care systems. Those institutions that have implemented pilot teamwork training programs report positive feedback from participants; those who used simulation to enhance their didactic teamwork curriculum also reported a positive impact on teamwork behaviors measured in the actual clinical environment [11, 12].

In this study, we evaluated the effect of a simulation-based intervention to improve clinical skills and teamwork behaviors in five-year medical students and compared the relative effectiveness of video plus case-based learning (CBL) and simulation-based learning (SBL) in trauma management and ACLS. We measured teamwork behaviors and technical components of clinical management in pre- and post-assessment scenarios.

25.2 Materials and Methods

This is a self-controlled randomized crossover study design with blinded assessors carried out in a university simulation center and using a high-fidelity patient simulator (Laerdal 2G). Ethics approval was obtained from the hospital committees. All the subjects were informed and consented. This study allowed for equivalent time on the simulator and comparable educational experiences for all teams.

25.2.1 Study Population

The study was conducted about 8 days (2 h each) at a university simulation center in 2012. We recruited all 56 5-year medical students who chose the emergency medicine elective courses. All the subjects were randomized into ACLS group (n = 28) or trauma group (n = 28). And then each four subjects made up a team.

25.2.2 Study Design

We aimed for a high degree of realism in the simulations using a recreated critical care ward, a Laerdal 2G high-fidelity human patient simulator, and real drugs, fluids, equipment, and disposable items. Before the 2 days theoretical lectures we took a written pre-test. We developed four highly standardized assessment simulations: ACLS 1 and 2 and Trauma 1 and 2. Each team undertook one ACLS and one Trauma simulation after the theoretical lectures. Teams randomized to the ACLS group underwent three CBL discussions on trauma management and three simulations (SBL) on ACLS. Teams in the trauma group underwent three simulations involving trauma management and three CBL discussions on ACLS. An instructional debrief followed each simulation addressing both behavioral and technical aspects of the team's performance. To ensure a comparable educational experience, the cases in the SBL and the CBL were the same and equal time was spent in each activity. At the end of the study, they undertook the two remaining assessment simulations and a written post-test (Fig. 25.1). Scenario order was randomly assigned to control for order and time-of-day effects.

Every assessment simulation was independently rated by two emergency expert assessors. They were experienced in simulation-based instruction and in the behavioral components of teamwork and crisis management. Assessors were not involved in any aspect of the study days and were blinded to group allocation and scenario order. Teamwork was assessed using the Teamwork Behavioral Rater (TBR). Developed from a previously published teamwork scale [13], the TBR has

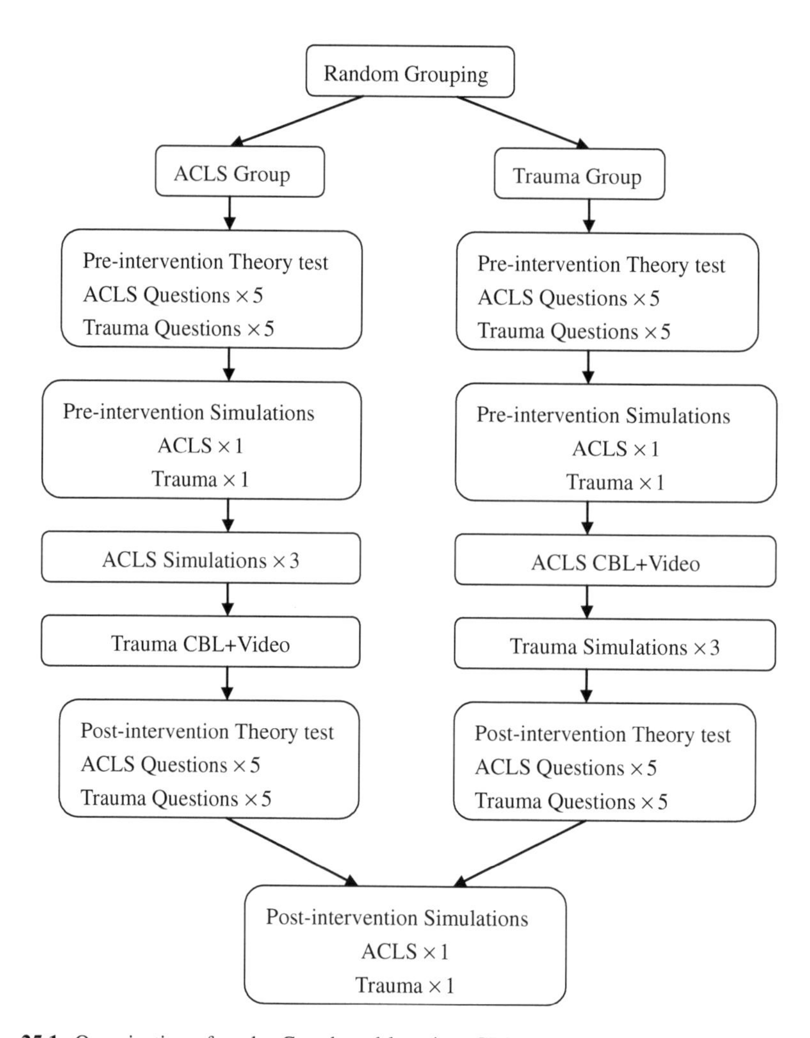

Fig. 25.1 Organization of study. Case-based learning, CBL

good reliability as an overall measure of team performance and for the factors "Leadership and Team Coordination," "Verbalizing Situational Information," and "Mutual Performance Monitoring". The TBR consists of 23 items, each of which is rated on a 7-point scale with descriptors of desirable and undesirable behaviors. The clinical management items measuring technical aspects of performance were developed from published treatment guidelines and International Trauma Life Support (ITLS) procedure which were scored against a 0–2-point rating scale (Appendix 25.1 for TBR items).

25.2.3 Statistical Procedures

Mean scores of the two pre- and two post-intervention simulations were calculated separately for each team for the following measures: Overall Teamwork Behavior; Leadership and Team Coordination; Verbalizing Situational Information; and Mutual Performance Monitoring. Similarly, pre- and post-means were calculated for written tests and clinical management of ACLS and Trauma simulations. Paired t tests were used to measure the impact of the intervention on theory master, clinical management, Teamwork Behavior and the three factors for all 14 teams. A p value of < 0.05 was considered significant. Unpaired t tests were used to compared the impact of the CBL or SBL intervention. A p value of < 0.05 was considered significant. All data were analyzed by SPSS 17.0.

25.3 Results

25.3.1 Theory Master

Mean scores of the written pretests of Trauma group and ACLS group on ACLS respectively were 25.00 ± 9.23 and 21.07 ± 7.86. There was no significant difference between the two group with $P = 0.092$, $P > 0.05$. Mean scores of the written pretests of two group on trauma management respectively were 21.07 ± 7.86 and 17.86 ± 8.33. There was no significant difference between the two group with $P = 0.143$, $P > 0.05$. We demonstrated a significant improvement in scores for ACLS theory master in both ACLS group and Trauma group, respectively were 26.43 ± 9.89 and 12.5 ± 8.44. There was a significant difference between two group with $P = 0.000$, $P < 0.05$ (Fig. 25.2). There was also a significant improvement in scores for trauma theory master in both ACLS group and Trauma group, respectively were 17.50 ± 7.52 and 22.50 ± 8.87. There was a significant difference between two group with $P = 0.027$, $P < 0.05$ (Fig. 25.3). The comparison of the scores for theory master before and after the intervention for two groups in ACLS and trauma management was shown in Table 25.1

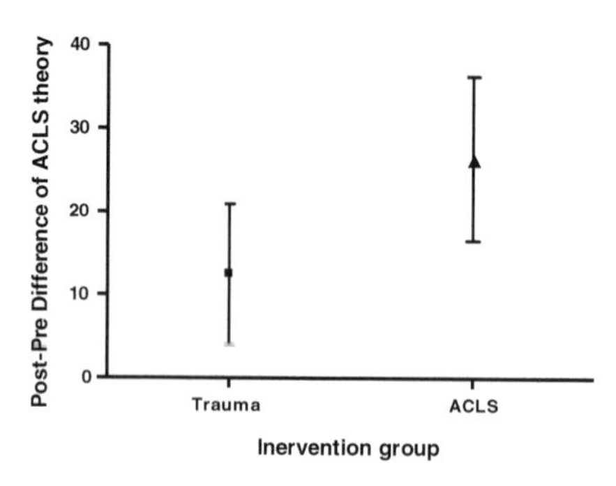

Fig. 25.2 Post-/pre-differences in written test scores of two group on ACLS

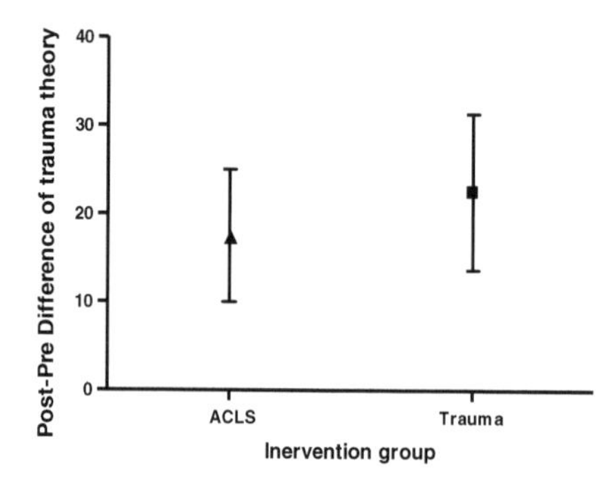

Fig. 25.3 Post-/pre-differences in written test scores of two on trauma management

25.3.2 Clinical Management Skills

Mean scores on clinical management of Trauma group and ACLS group in pre-intervention ACLS simulation respectively were 10.86 ± 1.35 and 10.57 ± 1.13. There was no significant difference between the two group with $P = 0.675$, $P > 0.05$. Mean scores on clinical management of two group in pre-intervention trauma simulation respectively were 7.14 ± 1.35 and 7.43 ± 1.27. There was no significant difference between the two group with $P = 0.690$, $P > 0.05$. Teams receiving SBL or CBL for ACLS showed a significant difference of improvement in clinical management with $P = 0.000$, $P < 0.05$ (Fig. 25.4). Teams receiving SBL or CBL for trauma also showed a significant difference of improvement in

Table 25.1 Scores for theory master before and after the intervention for two groups

Simulation type	Intervention group	Pre-intervention score	Post-intervention score	95 % confidence interval difference of improvement	*t*	*P*
ACLS	ACLS	21.07 ± 7.86	47.50 ± 4.41	22.59–30.26	14.135	0.000
	Trauma	25.00 ± 9.23	37.50 ± 6.45	9.23–15.77	7.833	0.000
Trauma	ACLS	17.86 ± 8.33	35.36 ± 5.76	14.59–20.41	12.322	0.000
	Trauma	21.07 ± 7.86	43.57 ± 6.21	19.06–25.94	13.420	0.000

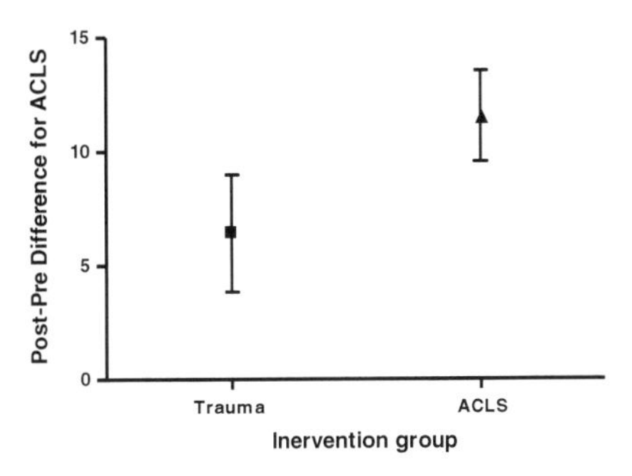

Fig. 25.4 Post-/pre-differences in clinical management scores of two group for ACLS

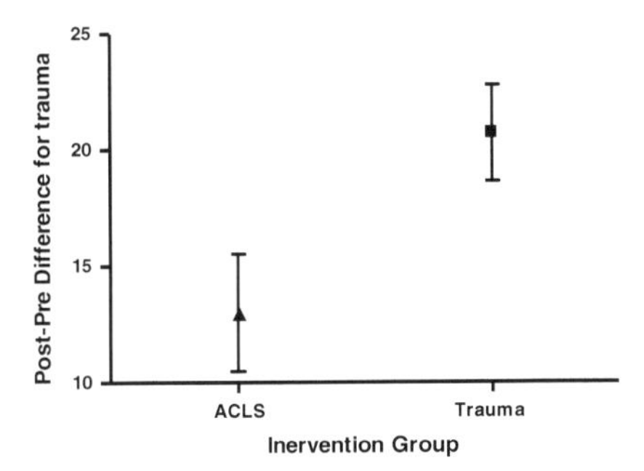

Fig. 25.5 Post-/pre-differences in clinical management scores of two trauma management

clinical management with $P = 0.000$, $P < 0.05$ (Fig. 25.5). The comparison of the scores on clinical management before and after the intervention for two groups in ACLS and trauma management was shown in Table 25.2

25.3.3 Teamwork Behaviors Assessment

We demonstrated a significant improvement in scores for teamwork from pre- to post-intervention simulations in both group (Table 25.3). There was a significant difference between two group. This in ACLS simulation included overall teamwork behavior ($p = 0.008$) and "Leadership and Team Coordination" ($p = 0.005$) and "Verbalizing Situational Information" ($p = 0.001$) and "Mutual Performance Monitoring" ($p = 0.000$). This in trauma simulation included "Leadership and Team Coordination" ($p = 0.000$) and "Verbalizing Situational Information" ($p = 0.001$) and "Mutual Performance Monitoring" ($p = 0.000$). There was no significant improvement difference between two group for overall teamwork behavior ($p = 0.056$).

Table 25.2 Scores on clinical management before and after the intervention for two groups

Simulation type	Intervention group	Pre-intervention score	Post-intervention score	95 % Confidence interval difference of improvement	*t*	*P*
ACLS	ACLS	10.57 ± 1.13	22.14 ± 1.35	9.73–13.41	15.399	0.000
	Trauma	10.86 ± 1.35	17.29 ± 1.98	4.05–8.81	6.611	0.001
Trauma	ACLS	7.43 ± 1.27	20.43 ± 1.72	10.67–15.33	13.661	0.000
	Trauma	7.14 ± 1.35	27.86 ± 1.35	18.81–22.62	26.622	0.000

Table 25.3 Scores for teamwork and components of teamwork in the two groups in ACLS and trauma simulations

Item	Simulation type	Intervention group	Pre-intervention score	Post-intervention score	95 % Confidence interval difference of improvement	*t*	*P*
LTC	ACLS	ACLS	3.04 ± 0.21	5.47 ± 0.35	2.05–2.81	15.784	0.000
		Trauma	3.06 ± 0.26	4.81 ± 0.28	1.47–2.04	14.990	0.000
	Trauma	ACLS	3.04 ± 0.25	4.26 ± 0.26	0.87–1.55	8.752	0.000
		Trauma	3.19 ± 0.37	5.59 ± 0.34	1.94–2.86	12.785	0.000
VSI	ACLS	ACLS	3.55 ± 0.27	5.36 ± 0.38	1.53–2.09	16.067	0.000
		Trauma	3.33 ± 0.27	4.38 ± 0.38	0.69–1.41	7.075	0.000
	Trauma	ACLS	3.38 ± 0.33	4.47 ± 0.23	0.83–1.36	10.107	0.000
		Trauma	3.45 ± 0.25	5.40 ± 0.42	1.54–2.36	11.603	0.000
MPM	ACLS	ACLS	3.32 ± 0.37	5.79 ± 0.57	1.94–2.99	11.500	0.000
		Trauma	3.29 ± 0.34	4.47 ± 0.23	0.93–1.45	11.329	0.000
	Trauma	ACLS	3.29 ± 0.34	4.32 ± 0.37	0.72–1.35	8.148	0.000
		Trauma	3.68 ± 0.51	5.71 ± 0.34	1.63–2.45	12.152	0.000
OTB	ACLS	ACLS	3.00 ± 0.58	5.57 ± 0.53	2.08–3.07	12.728	0.000
		Trauma	3.00 ± 0.82	4.43 ± 0.53	0.70–2.16	4.804	0.003
	Trauma	ACLS	3.00 ± 0.58	4.43 ± 0.53	0.93–1.92	7.071	0.000
		Trauma	3.00 ± 0.82	5.43 ± 0.53	1.38–3.48	5.667	0.001

25.4 Discussion

Our study showed that simulation-based learning or video plus case-based learnings also seemed to be an effective teaching strategy in ACLS and trauma management. These two teaching strategies in our study could also improve theory master and clinical management. This study provides evidence supporting the potential of such two interventions to improve teamwork behaviors in clinical teams. We demonstrated that SBL can improve theory master and clinical management more.The difference between CBL and SBL group is significant. A prior study of 3rd-year students during an internal medicine clerkship showed that although medical students are adapt at obtaining adequate history and physical exams, they have difficulty in applying the knowledge in the care of critical care patients in a simulated setting [14]. The deliberate practice of specific ACLS and trauma scenarios in the high-fidelity simulation setting is an effective means of medical education and acquisition and mastery of these skills and knowledge. We also demonstrated significant difference of the improvements in two groups in measures of teamwork in three major components of teamwork: "Leadership and Team Coordination" and "Verbalizing Situational Information" and "Mutual Performance Monitoring." But there is no significant difference between the SBL and CBL group in the improvement for overall teamwork behavior in trauma training ($p = 0.056$).

Interventions to improve teamwork in healthcare teams have been reported in increasing numbers, but as a result of the nature of the research area, robust studies are limited, and the evidence on the effectiveness of team training is moderate to poor with little evidence specifically relating to critical care unit teams. The ability of measurement tools to discriminate between the different components of teamwork has been limited. The TBR used in this study is designed to measure whole team performance, has published psychometric data supporting its reliability, and can measure components of teamwork as well as overall team performance [13].

Our study suggests that it is equally effective to use a mix of CBL and SBL. This would in fact increase feasibility of such training by reducing reliance on multiple, resource-intensive simulations. We suggest that the debriefing portion of all simulations should include a behavioral, teamwork-oriented component. Demonstrating objective, long-term improved performance in the simulated environment or the workplace, and ultimately improved patient outcome, was beyond the scope of this study but an area for future research.

25.5 Conclusion

Simulation-based learning or case-based learning also seemed to be an effective teaching strategy. A simulation-based learning for emergency team training in medical students can improve theory knowledge, practical ability and teamwork more. Results suggest that a mix of SBL and CBL is effective, which has implications for course costs and feasibility of training.

Appendix 25.1

Team behavioral rater
1. A leader was clearly established
2. The leader's plan for treatment was communicated to the team
3. Priorities and orders of actions were communicated to the team
4. The team leader showed an appropriate balance between authority and openness to suggestion
5. The team leader was able to maintain an overview of the situation
6. Plans were adapted when the situation changed
7. Each team member had a clear role
8. Instructions and verbal communication was explicit and directed
9. Team members repeated back or paraphrased instructions and clarifications
10. When directions were unclear, team members asked for repetition and clarification
11. Team members shared situation assessment information
12. Team members asked each other for assistance before or during periods of task overload
13. Team members offered assistance when other team members became task overloaded
14. Team members verbalized important clinical interventions (e.g., I am giving adrenaline)
15. Task implementation was well coordinated
16. Team members referred to written aids appropriately
17. The team sourced external assistance when appropriate
18. Team members called attention to potentially hazardous actions or omissions
19. Individual team members reacted appropriately when other team members pointed out their potential errors or mistakes
20. When statements directed at avoiding or containing potential hazards, did not elicit a response, team members persisted in seeking a response, or took action
21. Disagreements or conflicts impaired team performance
22. The team became fixated on an isolated indicator or occurrence to the exclusion of other important aspects of care
23. Team members made inappropriate assumptions about the capabilities or actions of other team members
24. Overall behavioral performance

References

1. Bradley P (2006) The history of simulation in medical education and possible future directions. Med Educ 40:254–262
2. Wittels KA, Takayesu JK, Nadel ES (2012) A two-year experience of an integrated simulation residency curriculum. J Emerg Med 43(1):134–138
3. Gordon JA (2000) The human patient simulator: acceptance and efficacy as a teaching tool for students: the Medical Readiness Trainer Team. Acad Med 75:522
4. Okuda Y, Bryson EO, DeMaria S et al (2009) The utility of simulation in medical education: what is the evidence? Mt Sinai J Med 76:330–343
5. Cook DA, Hatala R, Brydges R et al (2011) Technology-enhanced simulation for health professions education. JAMA 306:978–988

6. Manser T (2009) Teamwork and patient safety in dynamic domains of healthcare: a review of the literature. Acta Anaesthesiol Scand 53:143–151
7. Volpe CE, Cannon-Bowers JA, Salas E (1996) The impact of cross-training on team functioning: an empirical investigation. Hum Factors 38:87–100
8. Helmreich R (2000) Threat and error in aviation and medicine: similar and different. In: Special medical seminar, lessons for health care: applied human factors research. Australian Council of Safety and Quality in Health Care & NSW Ministerial Council for Quality in Health Care
9. Reader TW, Flin R, Cuthbertson BH (2007) Communication skills and error in the intensive care unit. Curr Opin Crit Care 13:732–736
10. Webb RK, Currie M, Morgan CA et al (1993) The australian incident monitoring study: an analysis of 2000 incident reports. Anaesth Intensive Care 21:520–528
11. Grogan EL, Stiles RA, France DJ et al (2004) The impact of aviation-based teamwork training on the attitudes of health-care professionals. J Am Coll Surg 199(6):843–848
12. DeVita MA, Schaefer J, Lutz J et al (2005) Improving medical emergency team (MET) performance using a novel curriculum and a computerized human patient simulator. Qual Saf Health Care 14(5):326–331
13. Weller JM, Frengley RW, Torrie J et al (2011) Evaluation of an instrument to measure teamwork in multidisciplinary critical care teams. Qual Saf Health Care 20:216–222
14. McMahon GT, Monaghan C, Falchuk K et al (2005) A simulator-based curriculum to promote comparative and reflective analysis in an internal medicine clerkship. Acad Med 80:84–89

Chapter 26
A Novel Enhancement Algorithm for Non-Uniform Illumination Particle Image

Liu Weihua

Abstract In order to improve the influence of non-uniform illumination and the measurement precision, a novel enhancement algorithm was proposed. Although bad illumination condition infection could be removed by MSR, when used in particle images, contrast enhancement effect was not been satisfactory. Then a non-linear gray transformation was introduced in image contrast extending. The experiments proved that enhanced images processed by the novel algorithm had more uniform background and higher contrast than former enhancement algorithmic. Over enhancement was avoided and it also could improve segmented efficient and ensure accurate segmented results.

Keywords Non-uniform illumination · Particle image · Multi-scale Retienx · Gray non-linear transformation

26.1 Introduction

With the development of machine vision, particle detection methods based on machine vision also have very great improvement. Then morphological parameters, which include particulate matter size, fractal dimension, shape factors and so on, can be got using image analysis. Machine vision is approach to measure micrometre particle or nanometer particle structure information, quantitative analysis of powder nature and other useful particle information, the most important is it can real-time monitor its industrial process. Make use of advantages of machine vision technique is promptly and accurately, analysis particle size

L. Weihua (✉)
School of Management Science and Engineering, Shandong University of Finance and Economics, 250014 Jinan, Shandong, China
e-mail: liuwh76@163.com

S. Li et al. (eds.), *Frontier and Future Development of Information Technology in Medicine and Education*, Lecture Notes in Electrical Engineering 269,
DOI: 10.1007/978-94-007-7618-0_26,

distribution, number concentration, and weight concentration which has important role in guiding and monitoring industrial process.

Once the images have been obtained, digital image processing techniques can be applied to extract information such as particle size distribution and absolute solids concentration and so on. The main processing challenge lies in separating the particles from the background in a consistent and repeatable manner—inconsistent image segmentation will lead to variances in measured particle size and, since other measurements such as concentration are simply arrived at through statistical analysis of particle size data, the variances will lead to cascading measurement errors [1].The simplest form of image segmentation is thresholding. This method is fast and easy to implement but, in order to provide good result, a very high contrast between particles and background must be present in the images. The quality of particle images is poor because of non-uniform illumination, and the segmentation result is also unsatisfactory when using classical grey-image enhancement algorithm such as histogram equalization. So a new method of particle image enhancement based on MSR is provided, which can firstly remove bad illumination. Then normalized incomplete Beta function B(α, β) is introduced for extending image contrast, at the same time, two parameters of Beta function is given according to simulation result. The experiment proves that enhanced images have more uniform background, higher contrast than former enhancement algorithm. This method provides a consistent repeatable segmentation result for subsequently particle processing.

26.2 Multi-Scale Retinex

The Retinex theory is designed to emulate the specific human visual ability, i.e., the ability to see the same objects under different illumination conditions, such as in direct sunlight, in shadow, or in the presence of artificial illuminations of different types. This psychophysical phenomenon is often called "brightness/lightness constancy," or more generally, "color constancy". Based on this model, the obtained environmental brightness function is slow changed image low-frequency information and reflective function includes the majority high-frequency details of the image. The basic concept in the Retinex theory is to separate the illumination and reflectance components of an image is the product between illumination and reflectance. That means the reflectance and an estimate of illumination [11].

Let the image be the result of the point-by-point product of the illumination $L(x, y)$of the scene and the reflectance $R(x, y)$ of the objects in the scene.

$$I(x, y) = L(x, y)R(x, y) \tag{26.1}$$

In the Retinex theory, the illumination component is first estimated as $L(x, y)$, Then, an estimate of reflectance is determined as the ration between the input luminance $I(x, y)$ and the estimated illumination $L(x, y)$.That is

$$R(x, y) = \log(I(x, y)) - \log(L(x, y)) \tag{26.2}$$

The idea of the Retinex was conceived by Land [2] as a model of the lightness and color perception of human vision. Retinex theory addresses the problem of separating the illumination from the reflectance in a given image and thereby compensating for non-uniform lighting. Through the years, Land evolved the concept from a random walk computation to its last form as center/surround. Then Jobson extend a previously designed single-scale center/surround Retinex (SSR) to a Multi-scale version that achieves simultaneous dynamic range compression, color constancy [3–5].

MSR is explained easily from single-scale Retinex. For SSR we have

$$R_i(x, y, c) = \log\{I_i(x, y)\} - \log\{F(x, y, c) \otimes I_i(x, y)\}\} \; i = 1, \cdots, N \tag{26.3}$$

where $R_i(x, y, c)$ is the output for channel "i", $I_i(x, y)$ is the image value for channel "i", " " denotes convolution, and is a Gaussian surround function explicitly given by:

$$F(x, y, c) = Ke^{-(x^2+y^2)/c^2} \tag{26.4}$$

where selected so that: $\iint F(x, y, c)dxdy = 1$, the constant "c" is the scale.

The MSR output is simply the weighted sum of several SSR with difference scales:

$$R_{M_i}(x, y, w, c) = \sum_{n=1}^{N} w_n R_i(x, y, c_n) \tag{26.5}$$

where $R_{M_i}(x, y, w, c)$ is the MSR result for channel "i", $w = (w_1, w_2, w_3, \ldots, w_N)$ where w_n is the weight of the nth SSR, $c = (c_1, c_2, c_3, \ldots, c_N)$, where c_n is the scale of the nth SSR, and we insist that $\sum_{n=1}^{N} w_n = 1$. The choice of scales is application dependent, but that for most applications at least three scales are required, and that scales of 15, 80 and 250 pixels, which is the set used in [6].

The result of the above processing will have both negative and positive RGB values, and the negative value will exceed the range display support. Thus a gain/offset is applied as Eq. (26.6), but this processing can cause image colors to go grey, and thus an additional processing step as Eq. (26.7) is proposed for re-map to the normal range (0–255).

$$R^{'}(x, y) = G \times R(x, y) + \mathit{offset} \tag{26.6}$$

$$f(x, y) = \frac{255}{I_{\max} - I_{\min}}(R^{'}(x, y) - I_{\min}) \tag{26.7}$$

where, G=3, *offset*=50, and $I_{\min} = \min(R_1(x,y), R_2(x,y), R_3(x,y))$
where, $R^{'}(x,y)$ is the output for $R(x,y)$, is the final output, $I_{\max}$ and $I_{\min}$ are the maximum and minimum value of $R^{'}(x,y)$ respectively. Because images processed by Retinex have similar histogram, the gain/offset parameters are usually a relatively fixed value such as $G = 3$, $offset = 50$, and they will not affect the final enhance result so much.

However MSR was usually used in colour image processing, other algorithms which have been used successfully in colour image when were used in particle images leaded to greying out and its contrast enhancement effect was not satisfactory. Then a normalized incomplete Beta function $B(\alpha, \beta)$ was introduced in image contrast extending.

26.3 Enhancement Algorithm for Non-uniform Illumination Particle Image

26.3.1 Non-Linear Gray Transformation

The purpose of image enhancement is to improve image quality, to highlight some specified features and recover the fine details in degraded images. And the commonly used method is rescales gray-scale or stretch the grayscale histogram. As for humans' visual sense, there are three states for most of the gray-level images such as image too dark or too light or grey level concentration. Accordingly, four functions are used to transform gray level of images as Fig. 26.1, which horizontal axis indicates original image grey level and vertical axis indicates transformed image grey level. (a) is to stretch dark picture areas, (b) is to stretch light picture areas, (c) and (d) are to stretch image grey level concentration.

To simulate the four kinds of transform functions stated above, Tubbs proposed a regularized incomplete Beta function [7]. With the different values of α and β, the four kinds of functions can be simulate as Eq. (26.8): if $\alpha < \beta$, the Beta function will stretch the dark areas of images; if $\alpha = \beta$, the curve of transform function is symmetric and it will stretch the middle grey value; if $\alpha > \beta$, the function will stretch the light areas of images.

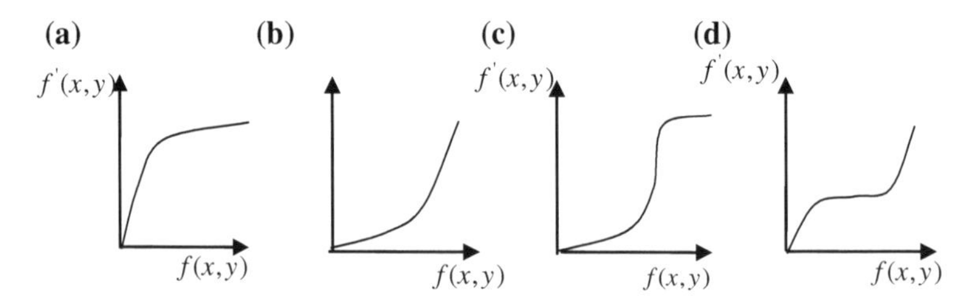

Fig. 26.1 Function of *grey* level transformation

$$F(u) = B^{-1}(\alpha, \beta) \times \int_0^u t^{\alpha-1}(1-t)^{\beta-1}dt \tag{26.8}$$

where $0<\alpha, \beta<10$, $B(\alpha, \beta)$ is the Beta function,denoted as:

$$B(\alpha, \beta) = \int_0^1 t^{\alpha-1}(1-t)^{\beta-1}dt \tag{26.9}$$

Most of papers employ optimization method to decide suitable value of α and β adaptively according to the quality of image. Because of our particle images all have the same character which is weak contrast and simple background. The main aim is to stretch lighter background and increase particle part and background part contrast. Our experiments show that the contrast is much better than in the original image and other classical gray value transformation method. The Beta function parameters are set fixed value such as $\alpha = 7.5$ and $\beta = 4$ according to our simulation experiments. Figure 26.2 shows this incomplete Beta function curve.

26.3.2 Detailed Calculating Procedure

1. Calculate grey value of $I(x, y)$;
2. MSR algorithm is employed in $I(x, y)$ using Eq. (26.5). Then $f(x, y)$is modified by using equation (26.6) and (26.7) modify;
3. $f(x, y)$ is normalized into the range [0,1] as Eq. (26.10), where $L_{\max}$ and $L_{\min}$ are the maximum and minimum values of $f(x, y)$;

$$g(x, y) = \frac{f(x, y) - L_{\min}}{L_{\max} - L_{\min}} \tag{26.10}$$

4. $F(u)$.is given by Eq. (26.8) which is a nonlinear transform function, $g(x, y)$ is the parameter and $g'(x, y)$ is the output

$$g'(x, y) = F[g(x, y)] \tag{26.11}$$

5. Then $g'(x, y)$ is anti-regularized by Eq. (26.12) and $h(x, y)$ is the finally result of our algorithm

$$h(x, y) = (L_{\max} - L_{\min})g'(x, y) + L_{\min} \tag{26.12}$$

26.3.3 Simulation Results and Conclusion

Because excellent enhanced result will provided good result for particle analysis and particle measure, we have to enhance image contrast. Figure 26.3a and Fig. 26.4a were non-uniformly illumination. In order to improve image quality,

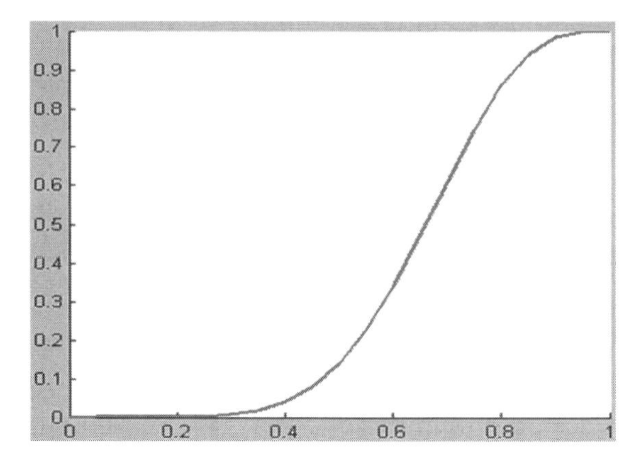

Fig. 26.2 The curve of incomplete Beta function if $\alpha = 7.5$, $\beta = 4$

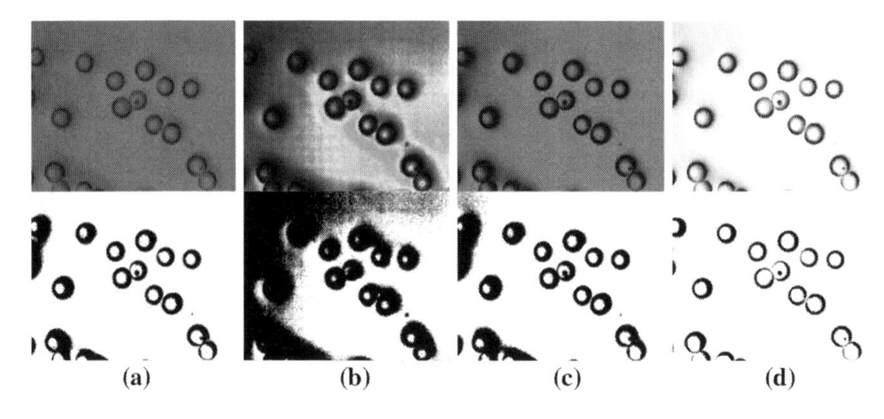

Fig. 26.3 Enhancement standard particle image and segmented result: **a** the original image; **b** the enhanced image by histogram equalization; **c** regularized incomplete Beta function; **d** the proposed algorithm

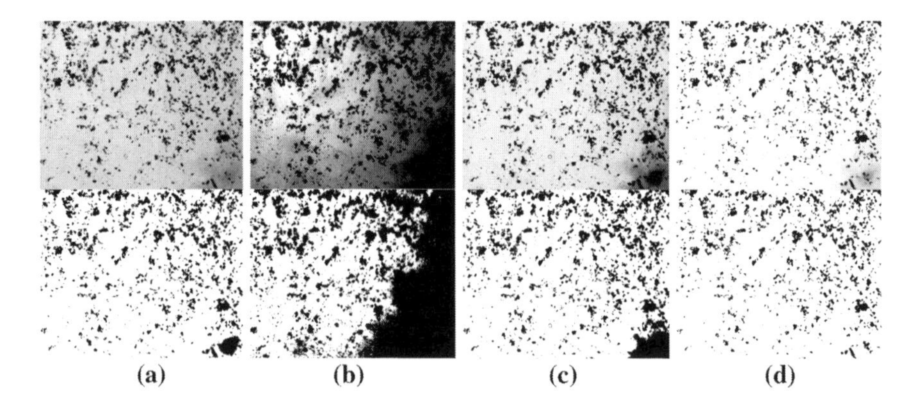

Fig. 26.4 Enhancement coal dust particle image and segmented result: **a** the original image; **b** the enhanced image by histogram equalization; **c** regularized incomplete Beta function; **d** the proposed approach

Table 26.1 Plea

Parameters	Average long diameter	Average short diameter	Average feret diameter
Diameter	71	71	71
Figure 26.3a	77.03	72.23	78.73
Absolute deviation	6.03	1.23	7.73
Figure 26.3a	72.90	69.94	74.25
Absolute deviation	1.90	1.06	3.25

those images were enhanced by different approach: histogram equalization, regularized incomplete Beta function and the proposed approach respectively, enhanced results are show in Fig. 26.3b–d and Fig. 26.4b–d.

From these images we can see that the difference is obviously among those algorithms. The first two approaches also got better enhanced result, however, some darkness areas belonged to background were over enhanced, which would be regarded as objective particle incorrectly. The experiments proved our proposed approach enhanced images had more uniform background and higher contrast than former enhancement algorithmic and over enhancement parts also had been avoided.

By comparing particles diameter and other parameters acquired from Fig. 26.3a and Fig. 26.3d. Experimental results showed that all parameters of particle measurement average deviation of our proposed approach were far less than direct measurement based on the original image.

In summary, we have proposed a new approach handling non-uniform brightness of particle micrographic image. First, MSR is applied to compensate inadequate illumination. Then, a non-linear gray level transformation was introduced to enhance image contrast. Experiments proved the processed images using our proposed approach with more uniform background and higher contrast (Table 26.1).

References

1. Carter RM, Yan Y, Lee P (2006) On-line nonintrusive measurement of particle size distribution through digital imaging. IEEE Trans Instrum meas 55(6):2034—2038
2. Land E (1986) An alternative technique for the computation of the designator in the Retinex theory of color vision. Proc Nat Acad Sci (83) 3078—3080
3. Rahman Z, Jobson DJ, Glenn A (2004) Retinex processing for automatic image enhancement. J Electron Imaging 13(1):100—110
4. Rahman Z, Jobson DJ, Glenn A,et al. (2005) Image enhancement,image quality,and noise. Photonic devices and Algorithms for Computing VII SPI, vol 590, pp 164–178
5. Ogata M, Tsuchiya T (2001). Dynamic range compression based on illumination compensation. IEEE Trans Consumer Electron 8(3):548—558
6. Jobson DJ, Rahman Z (1997) Properties and performance of a center/surround Retinex. IEEE Trans Image Process 6(3):451—462
7. Tubbs JD (1997) A note on parametric image enhancement. Pattern Recogn 30(6):617—621

8. Zhou J,Hang LV (2001) Image enhancement based on a new genetic algorithm. Chin J Comp 9(24):959—964
9. Guo X,Wu Z (2007) Radiation image contrast enhancement based on genetic algorithm. Nucl Electron Detect Technol 1(27):104–107
10. Liu W,Sui Q (2007) Image segmentation with 2-D maximum entropy based on comprehensive learning particle swarm optimization. IEEE international conference on automation and logistics. China,Jinan,pp 793–797
11. Lee S (2007) An efficient content-based image enhancement in the compressed domain using Retinex theory. IEEE Trans Circuits Syst Video Technol 11(17):199–213

Chapter 27
Research on Predicting the Number of Outpatient Visits

Hang Lu, Yi Feng, Zhaoxia Zhu, Liu Yang, Yuezhong Xu and Yingjia Jiang

Abstract *Objective* To build prediction model and provide data for the management and policy-making of the hospital by analyzing the data of outpatient visits by time series analysis. *Methods* The prediction model was built by regression equation and elimination method to perform value prediction and interval prediction about the future trend of outpatient visits. Standard value was calculated according to staff distribution. *Results* The change of the number of outpatient visits was closely related to seasonality. Error rate of outpatient visits prediction was less than 5 % except that the rate was about 10 % in 2003 and 2006. Actual number of every year was within the scope of prediction interval. The prediction value of 2013 was 549856 (497739, 601974), an increase of 7.22 % compared with that of 2012 (512852). Standard values of 2013 were 887680 and 543120, increasing by 73.09 and 5.90 % respectively compared with that of 2012 (512852). *Conclusion* Based on the prediction, we can rationally allocate resources, guide the management of outpatient departments, increase the number of outpatient visits and improve the efficiency of outpatient service.

Keywords Time series analysis · Season index · Regression equation and elimination method

The number of patients is a significant statistical index for the work of the hospital [1]. The scientific prediction can provide basis for the planning and development of hospital, setting objectives and responsibilities for president and heads of departments in hospital, performance evaluation and human resources management. It is necessary for scientific management and rational arrangement of manpower, materials and financial resources to predict the number of outpatient visits [2, 3].

H. Lu · Y. Feng · Z. Zhu · L. Yang · Y. Xu · Y. Jiang (✉)
Sichuan Provincial Hospital for Women and Children, Chengdu 610045, Sichuan, China
e-mail: jiaduo108@sina.com

S. Li et al. (eds.), *Frontier and Future Development of Information Technology in Medicine and Education*, Lecture Notes in Electrical Engineering 269,
DOI: 10.1007/978-94-007-7618-0_27,

27.1 Data and Methods

27.1.1 Sources of Data

The data came from outpatient enquiry mode of hospital information system.

27.1.2 Statistic Methods [4–9]

27.1.2.1 Calculation of Prediction Value

The number of outpatient visits varies with seasonality, and shows an increasing trend in the long term. To accurately reflect the characteristics and eliminate long-term influence, we adopted regression equation and elimination method as follows:

Firstly, calculate season index: calculate chronological average of each year, and then contrast the average with the whole average to get the seasonality ratio. Secondly, regression equation and elimination method: with month x as independent variable and the number of outpatient visits y as dependent variable, we got prediction value using least squares regression equation, then multiplied by season index and got the correction prediction value. Thirdly, calculate internal prediction: confidence level $1 - p = 0.95$, $n = 120$, standard deviation $S_y = \sqrt{\frac{\sum (y-\bar{y})^2}{n-2}}$, then the range of prediction $y = \bar{y} \pm t_{0.05,n-2} \times S_y$, which means the possibility that the actual number of outpatient visits will be with the scope is 95 %.

27.1.2.2 Calculation of Standard Value

According to the staff distribution and the operation of outpatient departments in our hospital, each doctor in outpatient departments can attend to five patients per hour (three patients in stomatology department), the daily number of outpatient visits in each department is 40 (24 in stomatology department), and the daily number of outpatient visits in each department multiplied by the number of departments and then multiplied by the number of days equals the monthly standard value in one department. The predicted standard value and actual standard value were calculated respectively, and the standard value of each department was added to get the whole standard value of the hospital.

27.2 Results

27.2.1 Analysis of Season Index

To analyze and master the variation trend from Jan. 2003 to Dec. 2012 in our hospital, season index was calculated by season average method (Table 27.1).

The curve graph shows that monthly number of outpatient visits varies with seasons. The numbers in January and February were lower than that of other months, especially in February. The number rose from the lowest in February, reaching the highest in August, and then declined from the beginning of December to February (Graph 27.1).

27.2.2 Regression Equation and Elimination Method

The number of outpatient visits has been increasing in recent years, with an year-on-year increase rate of 12.36 % (Table 27.2). Regression model was established based on the data from Jan. 2003 to Dec. 2012, with month x as independent variable and the number of outpatient visits (1000) y as dependent variable. Variance analysis shows that the model has significant difference, $F = 1368.70$, $P < 0.05$. Determination coefficient $r^2 = 0.921$, which demonstrates that independent variable x can account for the 92.1 % variation of dependent variable. Equation of linear regression is $y = 0.281x + 10.156$, through which we got the regression prediction value from Jan. 2003 to Dec. 2012, then multiplied by corresponding season index equals correction prediction value. As is shown in Graph 27.2, prediction curve based on seasonality model and long-term tendency is identical with actual curve.

27.2.3 Establishment of Interval Estimation Model

Estimation value was got by regression equation and elimination method, confidence level $1\text{–}p = 0.95$, $n = 120$ (the number of months), standard deviation $S_y = \sqrt{\frac{\sum (y-\bar{y})^2}{n-2}} = 2.216$, thus the scope of prediction value $y = \bar{y} \pm t_{0.05,n-2} \times S_y = \bar{y} \pm 1.96 \times 2.216$. Error rate of outpatient visits prediction was less than 5 % except that the rate was about 10 % in 2003 and 2006. The number of outpatient visits in 2012 was 5,12,852, fitted value was 5,09,326, and fitted error value was −0.69 %. The actual number of outpatient visits every year was within the scope of the prediction value, which is shown in Table 27.2.

Table 27.1 Season index

Month/year	Jan.	Feb.	Mar.	Apr.	May	Jun.	Jul.	Aug.	Sept.	Oct.	Nov.	Dec.	Average
2003	10988	10473	13194	13347	12831	13616	14820	14522	14157	14749	14559	12667	13327
2004	13635	14243	16544	16162	15872	16324	16834	17003	15566	15237	16290	13696	15617
2005	16280	12060	19044	17881	18815	21157	19129	18473	17781	18408	18992	18101	18010
2006	14940	15719	20732	20143	20184	20587	21821	21473	20337	21165	21790	21935	20069
2007	24330	16589	23779	23261	24472	26055	27523	28278	26984	28143	29611	27393	25535
2008	26594	22074	31974	29876	27812	28745	30446	30280	31404	34378	33560	32068	29934
2009	23674	30108	33235	33357	33379	33700	34222	36815	33530	32750	35816	33686	32856
2010	32285	23033	36484	37193	38557	36625	37726	39144	35244	35108	37131	38928	35622
2011	32751	27168	38352	37772	40314	40314	39533	40251	37267	38915	42350	42631	38135
2012	31963	41138	44992	42124	45381	45055	50052	46473	41387	39664	41963	42660	42738
Average	22744	21261	27833	27112	27762	28218	29211	29271	27366	27852	29206	28377	27184
Season ratio	0.837	0.782	1.024	0.997	1.021	1.038	1.075	1.077	1.007	1.025	1.074	1.044	12

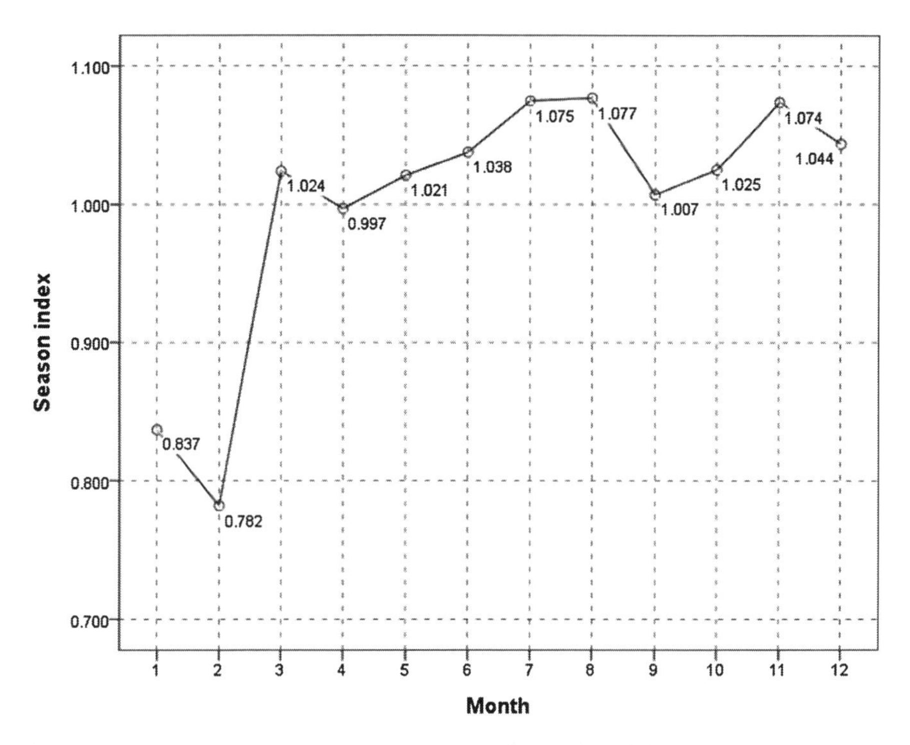

Graph 27.1 Curve of season index on the number of outpatient visits

Table 27.2 Prediction value of the number of outpatient visits from 2003 to 2012 (thousand)

Years	Actual number	Link relative ratio(%)	Prediction value	Prediction error(%)	Lower limit of prediction interval	Upper limit of prediction interval
2003	159.923	–	144.549	−9.61	92.431	196.667
2004	187.406	117.19	185.080	−1.24	132.962	237.197
2005	216.121	115.32	225.610	4.39	173.493	277.728
2006	240.826	111.43	266.141	10.51	214.024	318.259
2007	306.418	127.24	306.672	0.08	254.554	358.790
2008	359.211	117.23	347.203	−3.34	295.085	399.320
2009	394.272	109.76	387.733	−1.66	335.616	439.851
2010	427.458	108.42	428.264	0.19	376.147	480.382
2011	457.618	107.06	468.795	2.44	416.677	520.913
2012	512.852	112.07	509.326	−0.69	457.208	561.443

27.2.4 Standard Value of the Outpatient Work in 2013

The daily number of outpatient visits in each department is 40 (24 in stomatology department), and the daily number of outpatient visits in each department

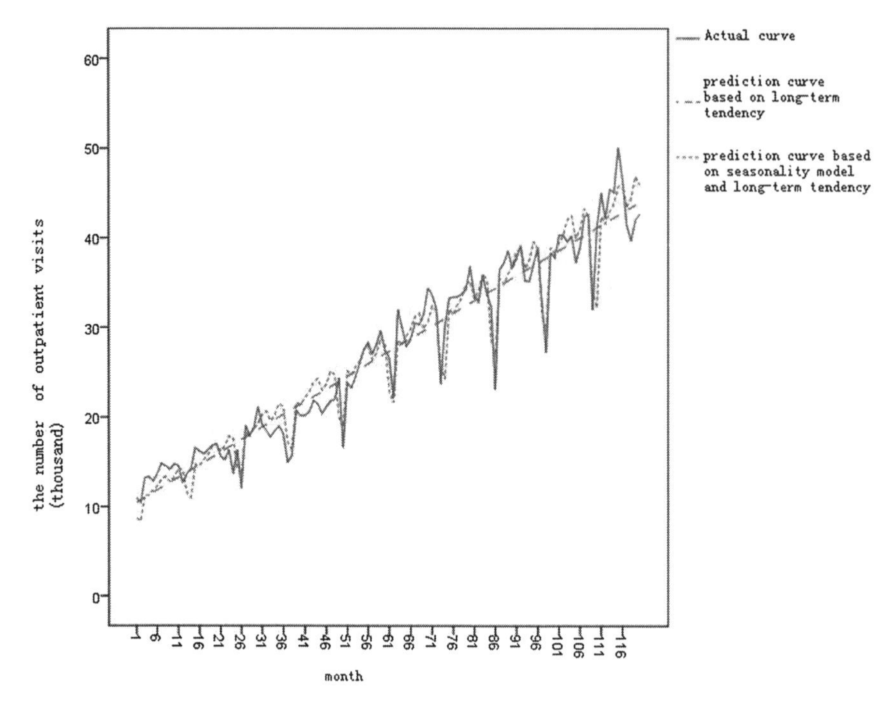

Graph 27.2 Sequence chart

Table 27.3 Prediction interval and standard value of the number of outpatient visits (thousand)

Years	Month	Prediction value	Prediction interval		Standard value	
			Lower limit	Upper limit	Based on the number of departments planned	Based on actual number of departments
2013	1	36.991	32.648	41.334	75.392	46.128
2013	2	34.798	30.455	39.142	68.096	41.664
2013	3	45.844	41.501	50.187	75.392	46.128
2013	4	44.937	40.594	49.280	72.960	44.640
2013	5	46.302	41.959	50.645	75.392	46.128
2013	6	47.355	43.011	51.698	72.960	44.640
2013	7	49.323	44.980	53.666	75.392	46.128
2013	8	49.729	45.385	54.072	75.392	46.128
2013	9	46.775	42.432	51.118	72.960	44.640
2013	10	47.894	43.551	52.237	75.392	46.128
2013	11	50.525	46.182	54.868	72.960	44.640
2013	12	49.384	45.041	53.727	75.392	46.128

multiplied by the number of departments then multiplied by the number of days equals the monthly standard value in one department. Standard value was calculated based on planned departments (66) and actual departments (41) (Table 27.3).

The results showed that the standard values in 2013 are 887,680 and 543,120, rising by 73.09 and 5.90 % compared with that of 2012.

27.3 Conclusion

The number of outpatient visits is influenced by seasons, for example, besides a spring festival break and the coldest climate, there are only 28 days in February, so the number of outpatient visits is the lowest. The newly-married couples would like to choose the wedding day on National day, New year day or Spring festival vacation, which lead to dramatic rise of pregnancy, especially in July, August, November and December. Season index can analyze the changeable factors of time series and indicate the effect of seasons exactly, which is practical and can be widely-used in outpatient management. Outpatient departments should make the following preparations for the rush period: ensure the sufficient medical supplies; strengthen the coordination of cashiers, information department and medical affairs department; guarantee the running of network; endeavor to decrease the vacation and outings of outpatient staff and shorten the waiting time of patients; with the improvement of quantity and quality of emergency and specialist clinics, much attention should be paid to general outpatient and patient-oriented to gain fine social and economic benefits through high-quality services.

The number of outpatient visits has been on the rise during the recent years, with an annual increase of 12.36 %, which is attributed to the rational application of information system. A multifunctional, fast and convenient digital information system can further optimize the treatment process, standardize medical behavior, enhance medical quality and strengthen effective hospital management.

Digital outpatient system is a complicated project, so our hospital has to quicken the construction and realize information sharing. Greater breakthrough should be achieved in optimizing procedure and improving mode to boost efficiency and enhance service level.

As a conventional analysis method, linear regression forecasting method shows development pattern and forecasts the future trend through establishing functional relation between sequence and time [10]. Prediction value of outpatients is got considering of increasing tendency of our hospital and season index. Standard value is calculated based on the formation and deployment of the hospital. The prediction value and standard value (based on actual number of departments) in 2013 increase by 7.22 and 5.90 % compared to the actual number of outpatient visits in 2012. Because the prediction is not always precise, it is necessary to make interval prediction, which requires possible scope and certainty of the scope besides detail prediction [11, 12]. The number of outpatient visits was expected to be 549,856 in 2013 by linear regression forecasting method and it is 95 % possible to be between 497,739 and 601,974, which indicates the integration of certainty and accuracy. It is valuable and practical for managing hospital, increasing outpatient visits, rationally allocating resources and better meeting the needs of patients.

Despite the accuracy and precision of time series method, there still exists some limitation: first, any model is a simplified and abstract form, so it is inevitably limited. It is hopeful to find an integrated model or a multi-analysis method to demonstrate the internal regularity of dynamic phenomena more comprehensively. Second, Random variables in medical field are related with each other, multivariate regression with a group of multidimensional correlated random variables as a whole needs to be researched in the future [13].

References

1. Shi L (1991) Analysis of multiple regression prediction on inpatients. China Health Stat 8(6):33–35
2. Lin J, Yao M, Tan J (2002) Predicting the number of outpatient visits by ratio-to-moving-average method. China Hosp Stat 9(1):9
3. Ching CH (2008) Forecasting the number of outpatient visits using a new fuzzy time series based on weighted-transitional matrix expert systems with applications. Expert Syst Appl 34(4):2568–2575
4. Chen F (2010) Medical multivariate statistical analysis method. China Statistic Press, China
5. Flores RM (1968) Simple linear regression as a means of predicting the thickness of middle allegheny stratigraphical interval in eastern Ohio. J Sediment Res 38(2):400–410
6. Pigage LC (1982) Linear regression analysis of sillimanite-forming reactions at azure lake. Can Mineral 20(3):349–378
7. Matsuda S, Kahyo H (1994) Geographical differences and time trends in the seasonality of birth in Japan. Int J Epidemiol 23(1):107–118
8. Yuefeng L (2010) Forecasting the number of outpatient visit and discharged patients by applying moving average seasonal index. China Hosp Stat 17(2):138–139
9. Cang S, Hemmington N (2010) Forecasting U.K: inbound expenditure by different purposes of visit. J Hosp Tourism Res 34(3):294–309
10. Yunxuan Z, Xuna C (2009) Prediction model based on time series method. China Hosp Stat 16(4):313
11. Examination syllabus of national statistics of professional and technical qualification (1997) Statistical work practice. China Statistic Press, Beijing, p 167–178
12. Liangwen H (1991) Social economy statistics theory. Financial and Economic Publishing House. Beijing, China p 342–349
13. Deng D, Wang R, Zhou Y (2002) The application of time series method on health. J Pharm Sci 15(5):457

Chapter 28
Acute Inflammations Analysis by P System with Floor Membrane Structure

Jie Xue and Xiyu Liu

Abstract In this paper, a new structure of P systems has been proposed which has upstairs/downstairs rules and the same floor dissolution, creation rules to solve the disease analysis by clustering technique. Up to authors' knowledge, this is the first time modifying the structure of P systems on floor. We do the Acute Inflammations data set from UCI by FS P system. All the processes are conducted in membranes. The analysis of Acute Inflammations data set is 83.3 % correct, which verifies that the proposed new P system can cluster data set accurately.

Keywords FS P system · Acute inflammations analysis · Clustering technique

28.1 Introduction

Membrane computing is initiated by Păun at the end of 1998 [1], the computation models obtained in the framework of membrane computing are usually called P systems, which are distributed and parallel computation models. Many variants of P systems are investigated [2–5], most of the variants are proved to be universal [6–8] and efficient [9–13]. An introduction to the area of membrane computing can be found in [14], while an overview of the "state-of-the-art" in 2010 can be found in [15], with up-to-date information available at the membrane computing website [16]. The obtained computing systems are proved to be so powerful that they are equivalent with Turing machines [15] even when using restricted combinations of features. A number of applications were reported in several areas: biology,

J. Xue (✉) · X. Liu
Shandong Normal University, Jinan 250014, China
e-mail: xiaozhuzhu1113@163.com

X. Liu
e-mail: sdxyliu@163.com

S. Li et al. (eds.), *Frontier and Future Development of Information Technology in Medicine and Education*, Lecture Notes in Electrical Engineering 269,
DOI: 10.1007/978-94-007-7618-0_28,

bio- medicine, linguistics, computer graphics, economics, approximate optimization, cryptography, etc. [16].

Clustering plays an important and indispensable role in data mining. Although several methods are available in these areas [17], these algorithms exhibit polynomial or exponential complexity when the number of clusters is unknown and the data set is huge, which make problems more challenging.

Acute Inflammations data set is an example of diagnosing of the acute inflammations of urinary bladder and acute nephritises. The data was created by a medical expert as a data set to test the expert system, which will perform the presumptive diagnosis of two diseases of urinary system. The basis for rules detection was Rough Sets Theory. Each instance represents an potential patient.

Inspired by the researches above, this paper focuses on the joint study of membrane computing with cluster analysis. We improve the membrane structure into floor one, let those membranes exchange objects up-down and right-left, adding objects communication directions, corresponding rules are designed for the exchange. At last, we use the new structure of P system in analysis of Acute Inflammations to get decision about disease.

28.2 P System with Floor Membrane Structure

Traditional membrane structure of N membranes is a cell-like architecture which can be expressed with parentheses expressions $[[\cdots[\,]_1\cdots]_{N-1}]_N$.

At first, we define a floor membrane structure as Fig. 28.1. In our structure, those membranes have two types of relations: Up-down stairs: if membrane σ_1 is the parent of σ_2, σ_1 is called upstairs of σ_2. On the contrary, σ_1 is downstairs of σ_2. Same floor: if membrane σ_1 is beside (sibling membrane of) σ_2, σ_1 is called the same floor membrane of σ_2.

A P system with floor structure, called a FS P system is a construct:

$$\Pi = (O, \mu_f, \omega_0, \omega_1, \cdots, \omega_N, R_0, R_1, \cdots, R_N, i_0) \tag{28.1}$$

where O is the alphabet, μ_f is membrane structure of the FS P system, $\omega_0, \cdots, \omega_N$ are initial strings over O of multiset, $R_0, \cdots, R_N$ are rules, $i_0 = 0$ is the output cell.

A upstairs/downstairs direction rule will have the following form:

$$\{\alpha \rightarrow (\delta, up_i)\}|_j, \quad \{\alpha \rightarrow (\delta, down_i)\}|_j, \tag{28.2}$$

Equation 28.2 means that α in upstairs/downstairs membrane j will change into δ and be transformed into its downstairs/upstairs membrane meantime.

A create upstairs/downstairs direction rule will have the following form:

$$\{[\alpha]_i \rightarrow [\delta]_{up_i}[\alpha]_i\}|_i, \quad \{[\alpha]_i \rightarrow [\delta]_{down_i}[\alpha]_i\}|_i \tag{28.3}$$

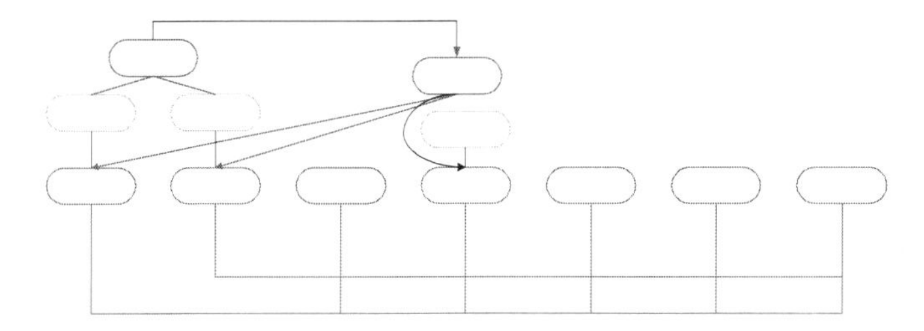

Fig. 28.1 A floor membrane structure, where *black membranes* stand for those output membrane, *yellow membrane* are upstairs of their vertically downwards membrane with *red color*

Equation 28.3 means that membrane i divides into two membranes, the first one is itself and the second one is its upstairs/downstairs, at the same time, upstairs/downstairs membrane of i have δ in. membrane i has αunchanged.

A dissolution upstairs/downstairs direction rule will have the following form:

$$[e\delta]_{up_i} \rightarrow \varepsilon, \ [e\delta]_{down_i} \rightarrow \varepsilon \tag{28.4}$$

Equation 28.4 means that upstairs/downstairs membrane of initial i dissolved into empty with their objects gone.

Other types of rules in FS P systems are evolution and communication rules of traditional P systems.

28.3 Clustering by FS P System

In this section, we use the thought in Table 28.1 to implement our clustering algorithm. The strategy is similar to PAM algorithm, where we choose k numbers of data as initial representations, compute similarities between non-representative and representative, find the nearest core for every non-representative data, in this strategy, the larger the similarity is,the nearer the data are. Then, it sum similarities and record the clustering result. Next, it select a non-representative data to instead of a representative data randomly, compute and sum similarities, compare it with above one, record the larger one. It means that if the new energy is larger, then, we

Table 28.1 Clustering algorithm

Steps	Procedures
One	Initiate a random k data as initial representations
Two	Compute the similarities of the rest of data to those k initial representations, sum them as energy
Three	Select a random non-representative data to instead of one initial representation. Compute the similarities of the rest of data to those k initial representations, sum them as new energy
Four	Find the best solution with most energy. Store and export the solution

use the new representative data to replace the old one, otherwise, the computation will not change.The process will continue until the energy will not add any more. The final result will be put out.

28.4 FS P System Designed for Clustering

The whole process of computation will conduct in membranes. FS P system designed for clustering is a construct:

$$\Pi = (O,\ \mu_f,\ \omega_0,\ \omega_1, \ldots,\ \omega_N,\ R_0,\ R_1, \ldots,\ R_N,\ i_0) \tag{28.5}$$

where O = {d, a_i, a_{i1}^{β}, $a_{i2}^{\beta}, \ldots,$ a_{in}^{β}, δ, b_{ij}, c_i, b_q, t_{ij}, c_q, e, f, h},$i \in 1,\ 2,\ 3, \ldots,\ n$, $\#(\sum i) = k$, $j \in \{\{1,\ 2,\ 3, \ldots,\ n\} - S_{etinitial\,k}\}$, $\#(\sum j) = n - k$, q is a number of every iteration from 1,2,3 to n-2,n-1,n; $\beta = \{0, 1\}$, $\omega_0 = ha_i d^k$, $\omega_i = a_{i1}^{\beta}$, $a_{i2}^{\beta}, \ldots, a_{in}^{\beta}$, every membrane i has enough numbers of $a_{i1}^{\beta}, a_{i2}^{\beta}, \ldots, a_{in}^{\beta}$. $I_0 = 0$.

Rules: $i \in 1,\ 2,\ 3, \ldots,\ n$, $\#(\sum i) = k$, $j \in \{\{1, 2, 3, \ldots, n\} - Set_{initial\,k}\}$, $\#(\sum j) = n - k$, $new \in \{\{1, 2, 3, \ldots, n\} - Set_{initial\,k}\}$, $\#(\sum new) = n - k$

$$\mathrm{r}_1 = \{da_i \rightarrow (da_i, down_i)\}|_0 \tag{28.6}$$

$$r_2 = \{[a_i]_i \rightarrow [\delta]_{up_i} [a_i]_i\}|_i \tag{28.7}$$

$$r_3 = \left\{a_i,\ a_{i1},\ a_{i2}, \ldots,\ a_{in} \rightarrow a_{i1}^{n-k},\ a_{i2}^{n-k}, \ldots,\ a_{in}^{n-k}\right\}\Big|_i \tag{28.8}$$

$$r_4 = \left\{a_{i1},\ a_{i2}, \ldots,\ a_{in} \rightarrow \left(a_{i1},\ a_{i2}, \ldots,\ a_{in},\ go_j\right)\right\}\Big|_i$$

$$r_5 = \{a_{ik}^{\beta} a_{jk}^{\beta} \rightarrow b_{ij} c_i\}|_j,\ r_{51} = \{a_{ik}^{0} a_{jk}^{0} \rightarrow b_{ij} c_i\}|_j,\ r_{52} = \{a_{ik}^{1} a_{jk}^{1} \rightarrow b_{ij} c_i\}|_j \tag{28.9}$$

$$\begin{aligned} r_{61} &= \{c_i \ldots c_l \rightarrow \lambda\}|_j, c_i \neq c_l \\ r_{62} &= \{c_i \ldots c_l \rightarrow c_i\}|_j, c_i \neq c_l \end{aligned} \quad r_{61} \succ r_{62} \tag{28.10}$$

$$r_7 = \{c_i b_{ij}^{s} \rightarrow (b_{ij}^{s}, up_i)\}|_j \quad r_5 \succ r_6 \succ r_7 \tag{28.11}$$

$$r_8 = \{b_{ij}^{s} \rightarrow 2b_{ij}^{s}\}|_{up_i} \tag{28.12}$$

$$r_9 = \{b_{ij}^{s} \rightarrow (b_q^{s}, up_0)\}|_{up_i} \tag{28.13}$$

$$r_{10} = \left\{b_{ik}^{s} \ldots b_{jm}^{s'} \rightarrow \left(t_{ik}^{s} \ldots t_{jm}^{s'},\ up_0\right)\right\}\Big|_i \tag{28.14}$$

$$r_{11} = \{b_q^{\sum^s} \rightarrow c_q^{\sum^s} b_q^{\sum^s} b_q\}|_0 \tag{28.15}$$

$$r_{12} = \left\{b_q t_{ik}^{s} \ldots t_{jm}^{s'} \rightarrow t_q t_{ik}^{s} \ldots t_{jm}^{s'}\right\}\Big|_0 \tag{28.16}$$

$$r_{13} = \{b_q^{\sum^s} \rightarrow def^{k-q}\}|_0 \tag{28.17}$$

$$r_{14} = \{he \rightarrow (e,\ down_i^{up})\}|_0 \tag{28.18}$$

$$r_{15} = \{f \rightarrow (f,\ down_j^{up})\}|_0 \tag{28.19}$$

$$r_{16} = \{da_{new} \rightarrow (a_{new},\ down_{new})\}|_0 \quad r_{14} \succ r_{15} \succ r_{16} \tag{28.20}$$

$$r_{17} = \{[e\delta]_{up_i} \rightarrow \varepsilon\}|_{up_i} \tag{28.21}$$

$$r_{18} = \{f\delta \rightarrow a_j\}|_j \tag{28.22}$$

$$r_{19} = \{c_{q_1}c_{q_2} \rightarrow \lambda\}|_0,\ \text{assume that the number of } c_{q_1} \text{ is larger than that of } c_{q2} \tag{28.23}$$

$$r_{20} = \{c_{q_1}^{|c_{q1}^{\sum^{si}} - c_{q2}^{\sum^{sj}}|} \rightarrow 2h_{q_2}b_{q_1}^{\sum^s}\}|_0 \tag{28.24}$$

$$r_{21} = \left\{h_{q2}t_{q2}t_{ik}^{s} \ldots \ldots t_{jm}^{s'} \rightarrow \lambda\right\}_0 \tag{28.25}$$

$$r_{22} = \{h_{q_2}e \rightarrow (e, down_{q_2}^{up})\}|_0 \tag{28.26}$$

$$r_{23} = \left\{\left(t_{q1}t_{ik}^{s} \ldots t_{jm}^{s'}\right) \rightarrow \left(t_{q1}t_{ik}^{s} \ldots t_{jm}^{s'}, out\right)\right\}_0 \tag{28.27}$$

28.4.1 Overview of Computation

In the initial configuration, there are enough number of $a_{i1},\ a_{i2}, \ldots,\ a_{in}$, in every membrane i ($i \in 1,\ 2,\ 3, \ldots,\ n$). At beginning, k numbers of b in membrane 0 combine with a_i(the connection of b and$a_i$is random) by r_1, which are sent down to k different membranes. Then, a_i in membrane i activates r_2 in membrane i to divide into two up-down membranes up_i and i, where δ is in up_i and $a_i$stays in i. By the help of a_i, r_3 chooses n-k multiple number of $a_{i1},\ a_{i2}, \ldots,\ a_{in}$,and r_4 sends them into n–k membranes respectively. Then, the first round of clustering begins, r_5 includes two situations: one: the same bits are 0, then r_{51} will be active and produce string $b_{ij}c_i$, otherwise, 1 are that same bits, r_{52} will produce their $b_{ij}c_i$ too. The function of rules r_5 is to find same bits of two strings(data), every time the same bits are found, one c_i will appear, after all the comparison being done, membrane i with the most number of c_i will be the nearest data to current membrane j.

If the numbers of different c_i which stands for initial represented objects are not equal, then, r_{61} will act, the rest of $c_i$represent the nearest data to current membrane j. Otherwise, we choosec_i with the smallest subscript as the nearest data to j by r_{62}. r_7 will be activated by c_i and b^s_{ij} will be sent to membrane up_i. It should be noted that r_5,r_6,r_7 have a priority that $r_5 \succ r_6 \succ r_7$,which means they must act as the order. To record the clustering result of every iteration and compare their energy,we use r_8 to duplicate b^s_{ij}.r_9 is also the preparation for comparison, b^s_{ij} is transformed into b^s_{q},where q is the serial number of iteration.r_{10} and r_{12} are used for record, r_{11} prepares strings needed afterwards. Then, $b_q^{\sum^s}$ produces def^{k-1}, which severs for r_{14},r_{15},r_{16}, r_{14},r_{15},r_{16} have a priority that $r_{14} \succ r_{15} \succ r_{16}$. r_{14} and r_{17} make one of the initial representation become empty, which means it is replaced, where h exists in the initial configuration.

The k-1 numbers of f will be sent into different j by r_{15}, where j has not been chosen as representation and r_{18} produces a_j for next iteration by the help of f and δ. As beginning, d is used for ensuring the representation, a_{new}appears. Then, the new iteration of finding nearest data to current membrane starts, $r_2 \sim r_{13}$ will work as before, here, there will be multiple number of c_{q_1} and c_{q_2},r_{19} will find the bigger one of them, and r_{20},r_{21},r_{22} will erase the representation of smaller energy. The bigger one will be output by r_{23} from membrane 0. Because there is only one h in the initial configuration, r_{20} will produce a h with subscript to activate rule r_{22}.

The process will continue until the energy will not change any more. The computation halts, the last strings which are put out by membrane 0 are the final clustering result.

28.5 Acute Inflammations Analysis

In this section, we use techniques above to do the analysis of actue inflammations [19] shown in Table 28.2. The data was created by a medical expert as a data set to test the expert system, which will perform the presumptive diagnosis of two diseases of the urinary system. Attributes are shown in Table 28.3. Data set is shown in Fig. 28.2, where we choose the second to six dimensions to do the clustering analysis, data are numbered from 1 to 120, every dimension of data is numbered from 1 to 5. Thus, abscissa stands for data, ordinate is their dimensions. The classification of actue inflammations data set is shown in Fig. 28.3, there are two classes.

Table 28.2 Description of data set: acute inflammations

Data set characteristics	Multivariate
Attribute characteristics	Categorical, integer
Associated tasks	Classification
Number of instances	120
Number of attributes	6
Missing values	No
Area	Life

Table 28.3 Attributes and classification of Acute Inflammations

Attribute	Value
Temperature of patient	{35C–42C}
Occurrence of nausea	{yes, no}
Lumbar pain	{yes, no}
Pushing (continuous need for urination)	{yes, no}
Micturition pains	{yes, no}
Burning of urethra, itch, swelling of urethra outlet	{yes, no}
Decision d_1: inflammation of urinary bladder	{yes, no}
Decision d_2: nephritis of renal pelvis origin	{yes, no}

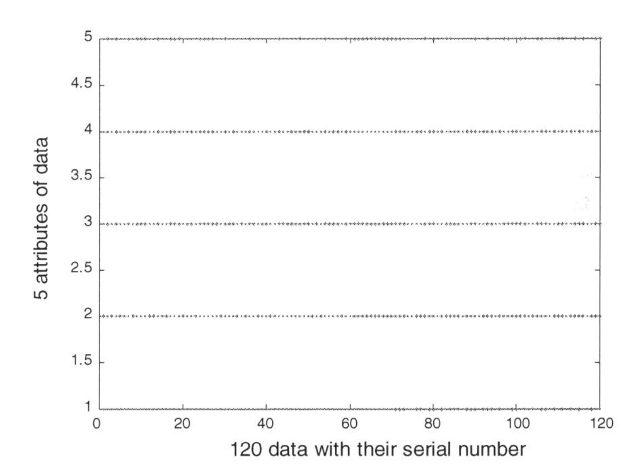

Fig. 28.2 Actue inflammations data set, abscissa stands for data, ordinate is their dimensions

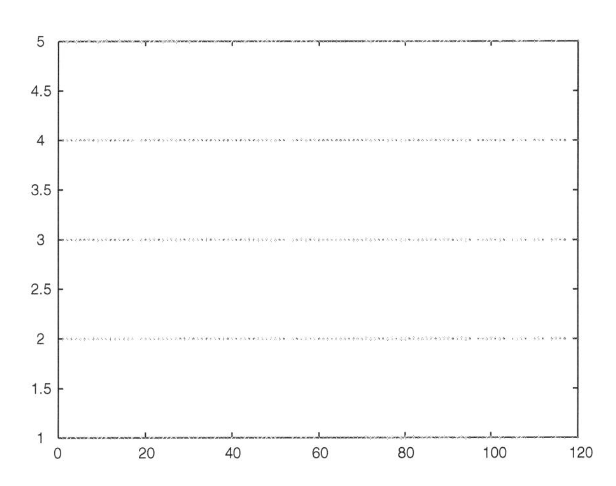

Fig. 28.3 Classification of actue inflammations data set of decision d_1

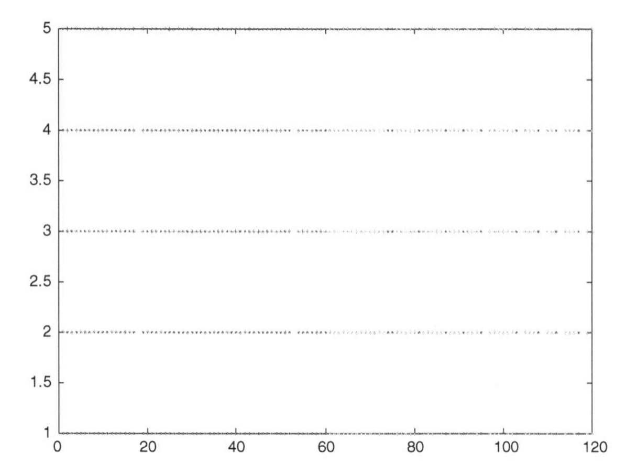

Fig. 28.4 Classification of actue inflammations data set of decision d_2

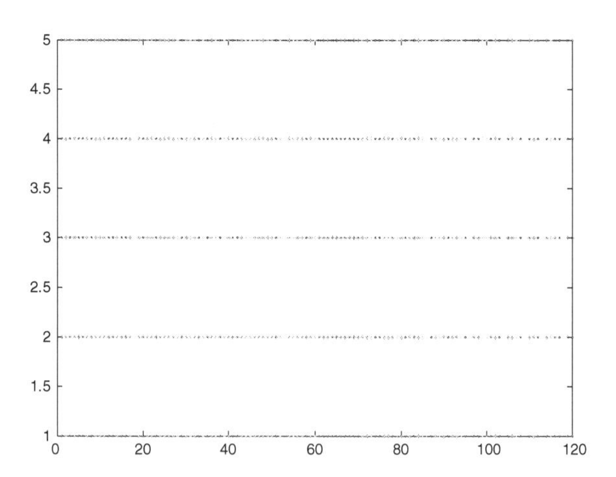

Fig. 28.5 The clustering result of decision d_1

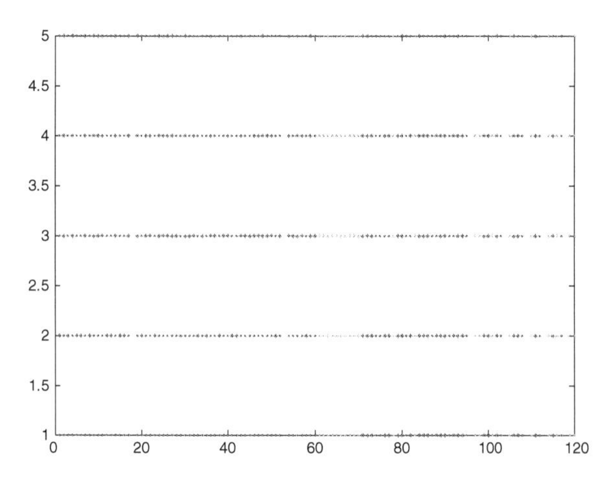

Fig. 28.6 The clustering result of decision d_2

We use dimension second to six to do the clustering analysis for decision d_1 in detail. 01000 and 00111 are chosen as initial representations. Rules execute as follows:

$\{da_1 \to (da_1, down_1)\}|_0$, $\{da_2 \to (da_2, down_2)\}|_0$, $\{[a_1]_1 \to [\delta]_{up_1}[a_1]_1\}|_1$, $\{[a_2]_2 \to [\delta]_{up_2}[a_2]_2\}|_2$

$\{a_1 a_{11} a_{12} a_{13} a_{14} a_{15} \to a_{11}^{118} a_{12}^{118} a_{13}^{118} a_{14}^{118} a_{15}^{118}\}|_1$, $\{a_2 a_{21} a_{22} a_{23} a_{24} a_{25} \to a_{21}^{118} a_{22}^{118} a_{23}^{118} a_{24}^{118} a_{25}^{118}\}|_2$

$\{a_1 a_{11} a_{12} a_{13} a_{14} a_{15} \to (a_1 a_{11} a_{12} a_{13} a_{14} a_{15}, go_3)\}|_1 \cdots$ $\{a_1 a_{11} a_{12} a_{13} a_{14} a_{15} \to (a_1 a_{11} a_{12} a_{13} a_{14} a_{15}, go_{120})\}|_1 \cdots$

$\{a_{11} a_{31} \to b_{13} c_1\}|_3$, $\{a_{12} a_{32} \to b_{13} c_1\}|_3$, $\{a_{13} a_{33} \to b_{13} c_1\}|_3$, $\{a_{14} a_{34} \to b_{13} c_1\}|_3$, $\{a_{15} a_{35} \to b_{13} c_1\}|_3$, $\{a_{21} a_{31} \to b_{23} c_2\}|_3$, $\{a_{11} a_{41} \to b_{14} c_1\}|_4$, $\{a_{21} a_{41} \to b_{24} c_2\}|_4$, $\{a_{22} a_{42} \to b_{24} c_2\}|_4$, $\{a_{23} a_{43} \to b_{24} c_2\}|_4$

$\{a_{24} a_{44} \to b_{24} c_2\}|_4$, $\{a_{25} a_{45} \to b_{24} c_2\}|_4 \ldots\ldots$ $\{c_1 c_2 \to \lambda\}|_3$, $\{c_1 c_2 \to \lambda\}|_4 \ldots\ldots$ $\{c_1 b_{13}^5 \to (2b_{13}^5, up_1)\}|_3$, $\{c_2 b_{24}^5 \to (2b_{24}^5, up_2)\}|_4 \cdots$ $\{b_{13}^5 \to (b_1^5, up_0)\}|_{up_1} \cdots$ $\{b_{1'120}^5 \to (b_1^5, up_0)\}|_{up_1} \{b_{24}^5 \to (b_1^5, up_0)\}|_{up_1}$

$\cdots$ $\{b_{2'111}^5 \to (b_1^5, up_0)\}|_{up_1}$, $\{b_{13}^5 \cdot \ldots . b_{1'120}^3 \to (t_{13}^5 \cdot \ldots . t_{1'120}^3, up_0)\}_1$ $\{b_{24}^5 \cdot \ldots . b_{2'111}^3 \to (t_{24}^5 \cdot \ldots . t_{2'111}^3, up_0)\}|_2$,

$\{b_1^{267} \to c_1^{267} b_1^{267} b_1\}|_0$ $\{b_1 t_{13}^5 \cdot \ldots . t_{1'120}^5 t_{24}^5 \cdot \ldots . t_{2'111}^3 \to t_{13}^5 t_{24}^5 t_{2'111}^3 \cdot \ldots . t_{1'120}^5\}|_0$ $\{b_1^{267} \to def\}|_0$

$\{e \to (e, down_1^{up})\}|_0 \{f \to (f, down_2^{up})\}|_0 \{da_{61} \to (a_{61}, down_{61})\}|_0 \{[e\delta]_{up_1} \to \varepsilon\}|_{up_1} \{f\delta \to a_2\}|_2$

$\{[a_{61}]_{61} \to [\delta]_{up_{61}} [a_{61}]_{61}\}|_{61}$, $\{[a_2]_2 \to [\delta]_{up_2}[a_2]_2\}|_2$, $\{a_2 a_{21} a_{22} a_{23} a_{24} a_{25} \to a_{21}^{118} a_{22}^{118} a_{23}^{118} a_{24}^{118} a_{25}^{118}\}|_2$

$\{a_{61} a_{61'1} a_{61'2} a_{61'3} a_{61'4} \to a_{61'1}^{118} a_{61'2}^{118} a_{61'3}^{118} a_{61'4}^{118} a_{61'5}^{118}\}|_{61}$

$\{a_{61} a_{61'1} a_{61'2} a_{61'3} a_{61'4} a_{61'5} \to (a_{61} a_{61'1} a_{61'2} a_{61'3} a_{61'4} a_{61'5}, go_3)\}|_{61} \cdots$

$\{a_{61} a_{61'1} a_{61'2} a_{61'3} a_{61'4} a_{61'5} \to (a_{61} a_{61'1} a_{61'2} a_{61'3} a_{61'4} a_{61'5}, go_{120})\}|_{61} \cdots$ $\{b_2^{207} \to c_2^{207} b_2^{207} b_2\}|_0$

$\{c_1^{207} c_2^{207} \to \lambda\}|_0$, $\{c_1^{60} \to h_2 c_1^{267}\}|_0 \{h_2 t_2 t_{24}^4 \cdot \ldots . t_{68'120}^{s'} \to \lambda\}_0$,

$\{t_{13}^5 t_{24}^5 t_{2'111}^3 \cdot \ldots . t_{1'120}^5 \to (t_{13}^5 t_{24}^5 t_{2'111}^3 \cdot \ldots . t_{1'120}^5, out)\}|_0 \ldots\ldots$

We shows some of the clustering computation process above, after the process of membrane computing, we can see that for decision d_1, the best similarities is 267, correct rate is 100/120 = 83.33 %, clustering core is 01000,00111; or decision d2, the best similarities is 180, correct rate is 100/120 = 83.33 %, clustering core is 01000,00111.

28.6 Conclusion

In this paper, a new structure of P systems has been proposed which has upstairs/downstairs and the same floor dissolution, creation rules to solve the spatial cluster analysis. Up to authors' knowledge, this is the first time modifying the structure of P systems on floor. We also do the Acute Inflammations data set from UCI by FS P system. All the processes are conducted in membranes. The analysis of Acute Inflammations data set is 83.3 % correct, which verifies that the proposed new P system can cluster data set accurately.

Acknowledgments Research is supported by the Natural Science Foundation of China (No. 61170038), the Natural Science Foundation of Shandong Province (No. ZR2011FM001), the Shandong Soft Science Major Project (No. 2010RKMA2005).

References

1. South J, Blass B (2001) The future of modern genomics. Blackwell, LondonGheorghe Păun, A quick introduction to membrane computing, The Journal of Logic and Algebraic Programming 79(2010):291–294
2. Pan Linqiang (2004) Tseren-OnoltIshdorj. P systems with active membranes and separation rules, Journal of Universal Computer Science 10(5):630–649
3. Linqiang Pan, Gheorghe Păun, Spiking Neural P Systems with Anti-Spikes, Int. J. of Computers, Communications & Control, IV (3)(2009), 273-282
4. Wang Jun (2010) Hendrik Jan Hoogeboom, Linqiang Pan, Gheorghe Păun, Mario J. Pérez-Jiménez, Spiking Neural P Systems with Weights, Neural Computation 22(10):2615–2646
5. Pan Linqiang, Wang Jun (2012) Hendrik Jan Hoogeboom. Spiking Neural P Systems with Astrocytes, Neural Computation 24(3):805–825
6. Pan Linqiang, Pérez-Jiménez Mario J (2010) Computational Complexity of Tissue-like P Systems. Journal of Complexity 26(3):296–315
7. Pan Linqiang (2011) XiangxiangZeng. Xingyi Zhang, Time-Free Spiking Neural P Systems, Neural Computation 23:1320–1342
8. Song Tao, Pan Linqiang, Wang Jun, Venkat Ibrahim (2012) K. G. Subramanian, Rosni Abdullah, Normal Forms of Spiking Neural P Systems With Anti-Spikes. IEEE Trans Nanobiosci 11(4):352–360
9. Pan Linqiang, Martin-Vide Carlos (2005) Solving multidimensional 0–1 knapsack problem by P systems with input and active membranes. Journal of Parallel and Distributed Computing 65:1578–1584
10. ArtiomAlhazov, Carlos Martin-Vide, and Linqiang Pan, Solving a PSPACE-complete problem by recognizing P systems with restricted active membranes, Fundamenta Informaticae, 58(2)(2003), 66-77
11. Tseren-OnoltIshdorj Alberto Leporati, Pan Linqiang, XiangxiangZeng, (2010) Xingyi Zhang, Deterministic Solutions to QSAT and Q3SAT by Spiking Neural P Systems with Pre-Computed Resources. Theoret Comput Sci 411:2345–2358
12. Xingyi Zhang, Shuo Wang (2011) NiuYunyun. Pan Linqiang, Tissue P systems with cell separation: attacking the partition problem, Science China Information Sciences 54(2):293–304
13. Pan Linqiang, Păun Gheorghe, Perez-Jimenez Mario J., Spiking neural P systems with neuron division

14. Linqiang Pan, Gheorghe Păun (2011) Perez-Jimenez Mario J., Spiking neural P systems with neuron division and budding, Science China. Inf Sci 54(8):1596–1607
15. Păun Gheorghe, Computing Membrane (2002) An Introduction. Springer-Verlag, Berlin
16. Păun G, Rozenberg G, Salomaa A (2010) Membrane Computing. Oxford University Press, New York
17. Ciobanu Gabriel, Păun Gheorghe, Pérez-Jiménez Mario J (2005) Applications of Membrane Computing. Springer-Verlag, Berlin
18. Han J, Kamber M (2002) Data Mining. Higher Education Press, Morgan Kaufmann Publishers, Beijing, Concepts and Techniques
19. http://archive.ics.uci.edu/ml/

Chapter 29
Different Expression of P_{53} and Rb Gene in the Experimental Neuronal Aging with the Interference of Cholecystokinin

Feng Wang, Xing-Wang Chen, Kang-Yong Liu, Jia-Jun Yang and Xiao-Jiang Sun

Abstract *Objective*: By using experimental neuronal aging study model, established by NBA_2 cellular serum-free culture method, we may observe the different expression of P_{53} and Rb gene in the experimental neuronal aging with the interference of cholecystokinin. *Methods*: Cells were assigned to AID and CCK group randomly, replaced with the above medium every other day, and then collected on day 0, day 5, day 10, day 15. Extraction the total mRNA of the collected cells, using the Reverse Transcription and Polymerase Chain Reaction technology, detect the different value of P_{53} and Rb. *Results*: According to the experimental neuronal aging processes, the expressions of P_{53} and Rb gene up-regulated, and the 10D group and 15D group were lower than the 0D group; With the influence of CCK_8, the expressions of P_{53} and Rb gene had little change in every group, and there were not statistically significant among those groups. *Conclusion*: According to the experimental neuronal aging processes, the expressions of P_{53} and Rb gene were up-regulated. It was speculated that P_{53} and Rb gene might be involved in the aging processes; With the influence of CCK_8, the aging has been delayed, and it could depress the expressions of P_{53} and Rb gene. A tenable hypothesis is that the genes are involved in the development of aging, and CCK can delay the aging processes through down-regulating the P_{53} and Rb gene.

Keywords CCK_8 · Experimental neuronal aging · P_{53} · Rb

F. Wang · X.-W. Chen · K.-Y. Liu
Shanghai Sixth People's Hospital Affiliated to Shanghai Jiaotong University, Shanghai, People's Republic of China

J.-J. Yang (✉) · X.-J. Sun (✉)
Department of Neurology Affiliated Sixth People's Hospital of Shanghai Jiaotong University, Yishan Road, Xuhui District, Shanghai 200233, People's Republic of China
e-mail: sunxj155@sohu.com

S. Li et al. (eds.), *Frontier and Future Development of Information Technology in Medicine and Education*, Lecture Notes in Electrical Engineering 269,
DOI: 10.1007/978-94-007-7618-0_29, © Springer Science+Business Media Dordrecht 2014

29.1 Introduction

The peptide cholecystokinin (CCK) is a neuroendocrine peptide expressed in I-cells of the small intestine and in central and peripheral neurons, and it is now generally believed to be the most widespread and abundant neuropeptide in the CNS, which is also considered as one kind of neurotransmitters [1–3]. This peptide is present in a variety of biologically active molecular forms, such as CCK_{33}, CCK_{58}, CCK_{39}, CCK_{22}, CCK_8, CCK_7, CCK_5 and CCK_4, among which CCK_8 appears to be the minimum sequence with full biological activity [4]. In the nervous system CCK is involved in anxiogenesis, satiety, feeling, neuroendocrine, pain, memory and learning processes. Furthermore, the colocalization and interaction of CCK with other neurotransmitters in some CNS areas, suggests its implication in other disorders. Meanwhile, CCK plays an important role in elevating cognition, learning and memory. More and more work has been done on its protection in the aging processes, but the precise mechanism is unknown yet.

As the world aging population is on the rising, finding the reasons of aging and the ways to postpone its processes has theoretical implications and extensive application value. Many scholars have done much work in the epidemiology, etiopathogenesis and mechanism in aging. Most of all, the research of P_{53} and Rb gene involved in this processes was the most attractive. Therefore, it may provide a new way in the development of aging through CCK delays this processes whether it has something to do with P_{53} and Rb gene or not. This study was to observe the different expression of P_{53} and Rb gene in experimental neuronal aging process and the molecular mechanism through which CCK_8 could delay the aging process in our experiment.

29.2 Materials and Methods

29.2.1 Cell Culture

29.2.1.1 Cell Line

Neuroblastoma A2 (NBA2) from American Type Culture Collection was a gift from Professor Larry Davis of University of New Mexico School of Medicine.

29.2.1.2 The Neuronal Aging Experimental Model and Reagents

Except for [Tyr-So3H27]-cholecystokinin fragment 26–33 amide (CCK_8 No. 031K12311, Sigma), all chemicals, cell line, cell culture medium, experimental equipments were just as previously described [5].

29.2.2 Reverse Transcription Reaction

(1) Application of sample: The volume of reverse transcription system is 20 μl, which contains 0.1 % DEPC ddH2O of 7 μl, total RNA of 3 μl and 100 pmol random hexamer primer of 1 μl.
(2) Before centrifuge, there should be a warm bath at 65 °C for 10 min and an ice bath for 5 min.
(3) Put the centrifuge tube on the ice and apply samples of 10 mmol/L dNTP of 1 μl, 5 x reverse transcriptase buffer of 4 μl, 0.1 % DEPC ddH2O of 2 μl, M-MLV of 1 μl and RNasin of 1 μl.
(4) Set the tube at 37 °C for 60 min.
(5) Terminate the reaction by incubation at 94 °C for 5 min,with the composite cDNA conserved at −20 °C.

29.2.3 PCR

Reagents: TRIZOL Reagent (Invitrogen company); chloroform; isoamyl alcoholdiethylpyrocarbonate (DEPC, Sigma Company); formamide(Sigma Company); ethidium bromide (Sigma Company); agarose (Agarose BIOASIA Biotechnology, BIOWEST); M-MLV, RNasin, PCR Marker (Promega Company). Real-time PCR primer sequences are given below: β-Actin forward, 5'AGC CAT GTA CGT AGC CAT CC 3'; reverse, 5'ACA TCT GCT GGA AGG TGG AC 3'. P_{53} gene forward, 5'GTA TCC GGG TGG AAG GAA AT 3'; reverse, 5'CTG TAG CAT GGG CAT CCT TT 3'; Rb gene forward, 5'ATC TAC CTC CCT TGC CCT GT 3'; reverse, 5'CAG GAA TCC GTA AGG GTG AA 3'. The primers were offered by Shanghai bo-ya biotechnology company limited.

29.2.3.1 Selection the Proportion of Primer

Two primer pairs were put into one reaction system, the β-actin primer was set as the ento-confer. The proportions between P_{53} and β-actin are listed below: 18:2 (track 1); 17:3 (track 2); 16:4 (track 3); 15:5 (track 4); 14:6 (track 5); 13:7 (track 6) (0.2 μl). The PCR system contains 10x PCR buffer of 2.5 μl, 10 mmol/L dNTP of 2 μl, 50 μmol/L P_{53} Primer, 50 μmol/L β-actin Primer, RT product of 1 μl, Taq enzyme of 1 μl (1U) and deionized water was added until the total volume reached 25 μl.Add liquid paraffin (50 μl) before the amplification of DNA followed by 25 cycles of denaturation at 94 °C for 30 s, annealing at 55 °C for 30 s and extension at 72 °C for 60 s. Electrophoresis was made on 2 % agarose gel after the amplification and the results were observed by uviol lamp after 30–45 min. The photo was shown below (Fig. 29.1).

Two primer pairs were put into one same reaction system, among which the β-actin primer was set as the ento-confer. The proportions between Rb and β-actin

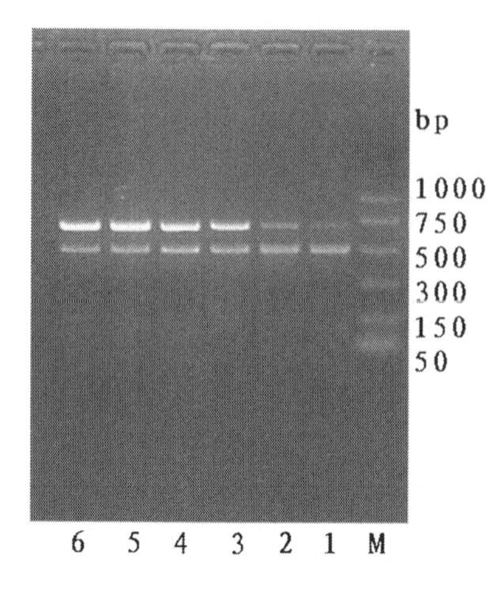

Fig. 29.1 Results of different proportions between P_{53} and β-actin

are listed below: 19:1 (track 1); 18:2 (track 2); 17:3 (track 3); 16:4 (track 4); 15:5 (track 5); 14:6 (track 6). The PCR system contains with 10x PCR buffer of 2.5 μl, 10 mmol/L dNTP of 2 μl, 50 μmol/L Rb Primer, 50 μmol/L β-actin Primer, RT product of 1 μl, Taq enzyme of 1 μl (1U) and deionized water was adder until the total volum was 25 μl. Add fluid par. Of 50 μl before the amplification of DNA followed by 25 cycles of denaturation at 94 °C for 30 s, annealing at 55 °C for 30 s and extension at 72 °C for 60 s. Electrophoresis was made on 2 % agarose gel after the amplification and the results were observed by uviol lamp after 30–45 min. The photo was listed below (Fig. 29.2).

29.2.3.2 Selection the Number of Cycles of Amplification

Two primer pairs were put into one reaction system, the β-actin primer was set as the ento-confer. The PCR system contains 10x PCR buffer of 2.5 μl, 10 mmol/L dNTP of 2 μl, 50 μmol/L P_{53} Primer of 1 μl for each strand, 50 μmol/L β-actin

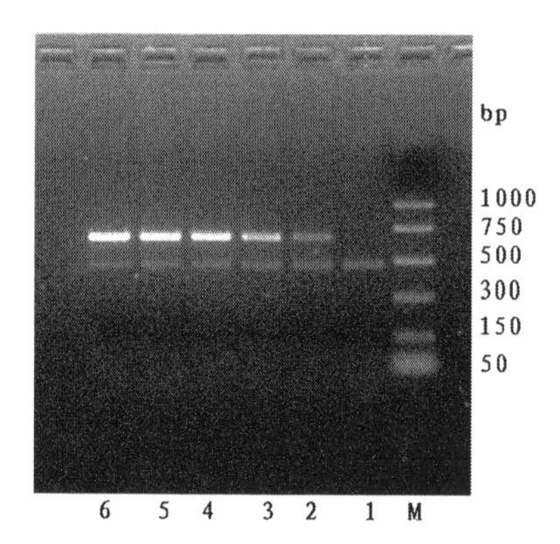

Fig. 29.2 Results of different proportions between Rb and β-actin

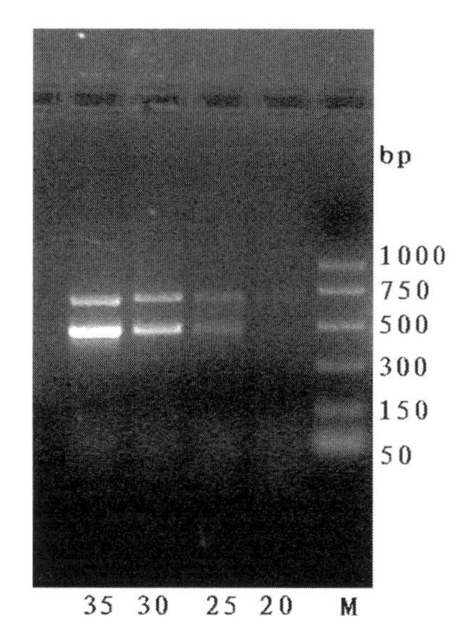

Fig. 29.3 Results of different number of cycles of amplification

Primer of 0.25 μl for each one, RT product of 1 μl, Taq enzyme of 1 μl (1U) and deionized water was added until the total volume of this system reached 25 μl. Add liquid paraffin (50 μl) before the amplification of DNA followed by 20, 25, 30, 35 cycles of denaturation at 94 °C for 30 s, annealing at 55 °C for 30 s and extension at 72 °C for 60 s. Electrophoresis was made on 2 % agarose gel after the amplification and the results were observed by uviol lamp after 30–45 min. The photo was shown below (Fig. 29.3).

Two primer pairs were put into one same reaction system, among which the β-actin primer was set as the ento-confer. The PCR system contains with 10x PCR buffer of 2.5 μl, 10 mmol/L dNTP of 2 μl, 50 μmol/L Rb Primer of 1 μl for each strand, 50 μmol/L β-actin Primer of 0.25 μl for each one, RT product of 1 μl, Taq enzyme of 1 μl(1U) and deionized water was adder until the total volume of this system was 25 μl. Add fluid par. Of 50 μl before the amplification of DNA followed by 20,25,30,35 cycles of denaturation at 94 °C for 30 s, annealing at 55 °C for 30 s and extension at 72 °C for 60 s. Electrophoresis was made on 2 % agarose gel after the amplification and the results were observed by uviol lamp after 30–45 min. The photo was listed below (Fig. 29.4).

The final PCR reaction system of P_{53} gene was combined with 10x buffer of 2.5 μl, 10 mmol/L dNTPs of 2 μl, each forward and reverse primer of 1 and 0.25 μl, cDNA of 1 μl, Taq enzyme of 1 μl and ddH2O of 16 μl. Initial denaturation was set at 94 °C for 5 min and followed by 30 cycles of denaturation at 94 °C for 30 s, annealing at 55 °C for 30 s and extension at 72 °C for 60 s. Re-extension at 72 °C for 5 min was the last step.

The final PCR reaction system of Rb gene was combined with 10x buffer of 2.5 μl, 10 mmol/L dNTPs of 2 μl, each forward and reverse primer of 1 μl and 0.125μl, cDNA of 1 μl, Taq enzyme of 1 μl and ddH2O of 16 μl. Initial denaturation

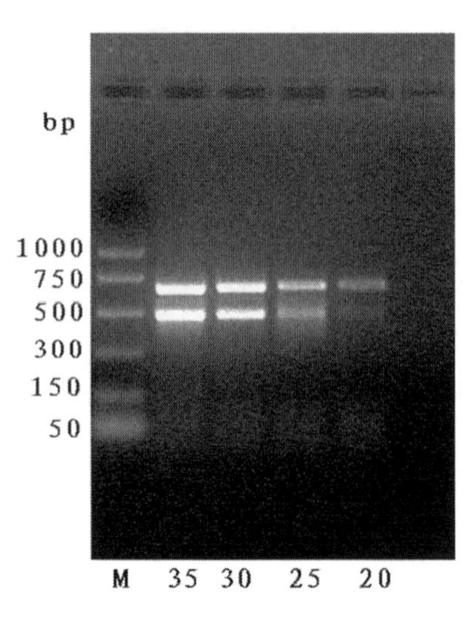

Fig. 29.4 Results of different number of cycles of amplification

was set at 94 °C for 5 min and followed by 25 cycles of denaturation at 94 °C for 30 s, annealing at 55 °C for 30 s and extension at 72 °C for 60 s. Re-extension at 72 °C for 7 min was the last step.

29.2.4 Statistical Analysis

Statistic analysis of P_{53} gene expression was based on the analysis of gel imaging system.

29.3 Results

29.3.1 Assessment of the Quality of the Total RNA

Total RNA was extracted using the TRIZOL Reagent(Invitrogen company) following the manufacture's instructions. The OD260/OD280 value of total RNA of each group was between 1.80 and 2.00 detected by ultraviolet spectrophotometer, and the potency ratio of 28 s and 18 s from the result of the agarose electrophoresis was 2, which meant that the total RNA was extracted completely and it could be used in reverse transcriptase-PCR(RT-PCR) analysis (Fig. 29.5).

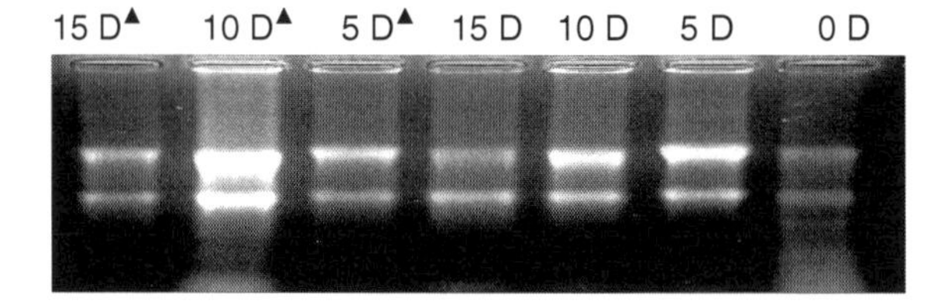

Fig. 29.5 Electrophoretic analysis of total RNA; 15 D▲, 10 D▲, 5 D▲ means CCK group; 15 D, 10 D, 5 D means control group

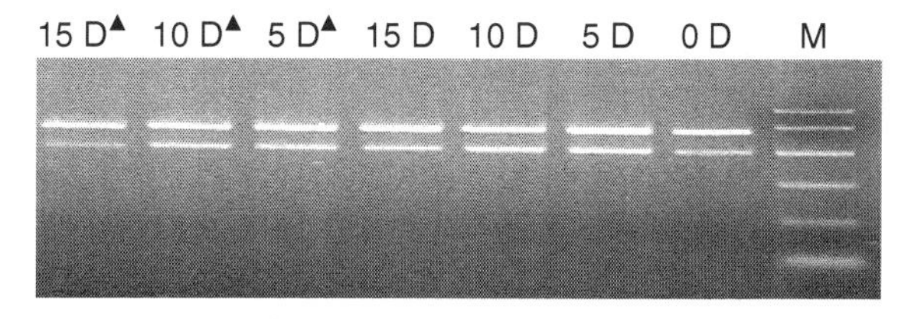

Fig. 29.6 The electropherogram of P_{53} gene expression; 15 D▲, 10 D▲, 5 D▲ means CCK group; 15 D, 10 D, 5 D means control group; M means Maker

Table 29.1 The expression of P_{53} gene ($\bar{x} \pm SD$)

Days of culture	Control group	CCK group
0	0.41 ± 0.05	0.41 ± 0.05
5	0.48 ± 0.07	0.52 ± 0.12
10	0.61 ± 0.07	0.45 ± 0.07[a]
15	0.68 ± 0.06	0.37 ± 0.04[b]

[a] $P < 0.05$ versus 10D group and 0D group
[b] $P < 0.05$ versus 15D group and 0D group

29.3.2 Effect of CCK_8 on P_{53} Gene Expression

From the electropherogram, the expression of P_{53} mRNA in the control group was increased with the extension of culture time, which meant that P_{53} gene was activated in the progress of cell aging process. In CCK group, such situation could not be observed. The up-regulation of P_{53} gene expression was inhibited in experimental neuronal aging with the interference of CCK_8 and the aging process was delayed (Fig. 29.6).

The automatic analysis of P_{53} gene expressions in different period by gel imaging system was shown in Table 29.1. According to the statistical analysis of the control group, the expression of P_{53} gene was up-regulated along with the experimental neuronal aging processes, and there was statistical significant between the 10D group,15D group and the 0D group ($P < 0.05$) (Fig. 29.7).

In the CCK group, there was no statistical significant between the 5D group, 10D group, 15D group and the 0D group, which means that the expression of P_{53} gene was inhibited by the use of CCK_8 (Fig. 29.8).

By comparing the expression of P_{53} gene of the control group and the CCK group in the same period, the up-regulation of P_{53} gene in 10D and 15D group was inhibited under the persistent effect of CCK_8. There was statistical significant between the two groups (Fig. 29.9).

29.3.3 Effects of CCK_8 on Rb Gene Expression

From the electropherogram, the expression of Rb gene's mRNA in the control group was increased with the extension of culture time, which means that Rb gene

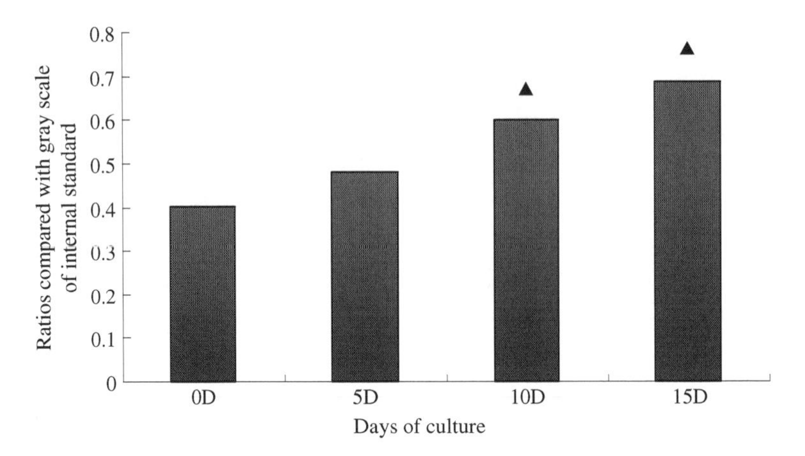

Fig. 29.7 The expression of P_{53} gene in the control group; ▲ means statistical significant between the 10D group, 15D group and the 0D group ($P < 0.05$)

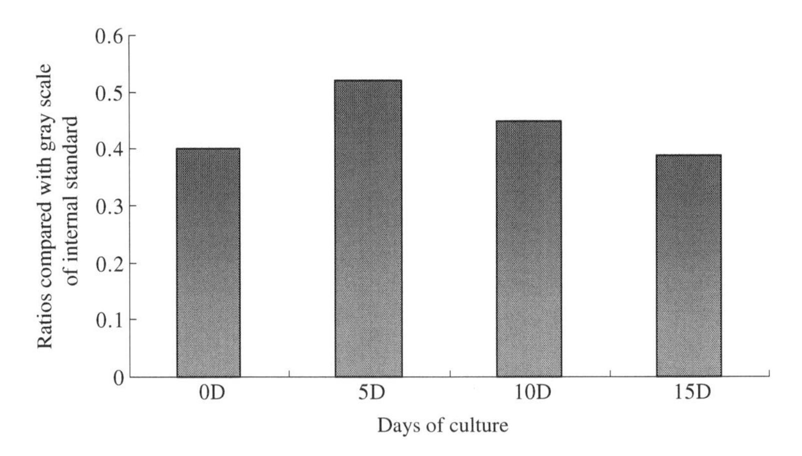

Fig. 29.8 The expression of P_{53} gene in CCK group

was activated in the progress of cell aging. While in the CCK group, such situation could not be observed, the Rb gene expression's up-regulation was inhibited in the experimental neuronal aging with the interference of CCK and the aging processes was delayed (Fig. 29.10).

The automatic analysis of Rb gene expressions in different period by gel imaging system was shown in Table 29.1. According to the statistical analysis of the control group, the expression of Rb gene was up-regulated along with the experimental neuronal aging processes, and there was statistical significant between the 10D group, 15D group and the 0D group ($P < 0.05$). Such phenomenon is speculated that Rb gene may involved in the aging process (Table 29.2, Fig. 29.11).

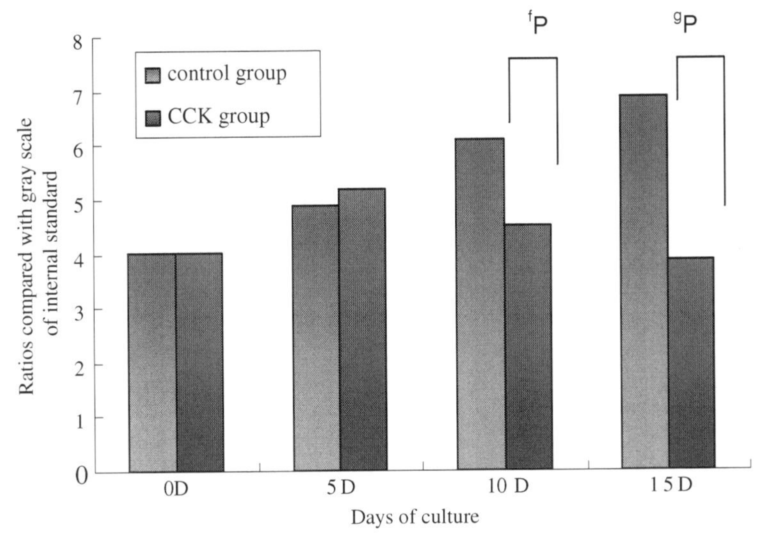

Fig. 29.9 The expression of P_{53} gene mRNA in two groups; $^{f}P < 0.05$ versus control group and CCK group on 10D; $^{g}P < 0.01$ versus control group and CCK group on 15D

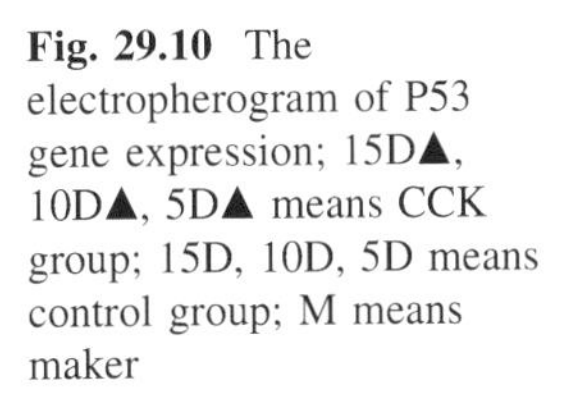

Fig. 29.10 The electropherogram of P53 gene expression; 15D▲, 10D▲, 5D▲ means CCK group; 15D, 10D, 5D means control group; M means maker

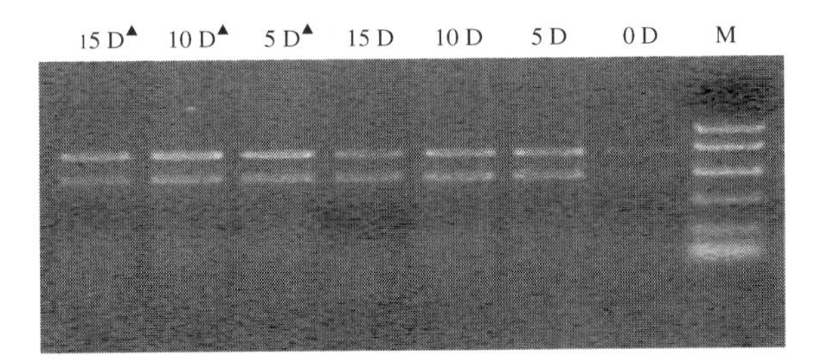

While in the CCK group, there was no statistical significant between the 5D group, 10D group, 15D group and the 0D group, which means that the expression of Rb gene was inhibited by the use of CCK_8 (Fig. 29.12).

By comparing the expression of Rb gene on the same period of the control group and the CCK group,the up-regulation of Rb gene in 10D and 15D group was inhibited under the persistent effect of CCK_8. There was statistical significant between two groups, which means that down-regulating the Rb gene may one of the molecule mechanisms that CCK_8 can delay the aging process (Fig. 29.13).

The expression of Rb gene increased with the process of aging and it could be down-regulated by using CCK, which might support the idea that the down-regulating of Rb gene expression was one of the molecule mechanisms that CCK_8 could delay the aging process.

Table 29.2 The expression of Rb gene ($\bar{x} \pm$ SD)

Days of culture	Control group	CCK group
0	0.62 ± 0.18	0.62 ± 0.18
5	0.70 ± 0.20	0.74 ± 0.06
10	0.86 ± 0.16	0.58 ± 0.13
15	1.00 ± 0.21	0.49 ± 0.11

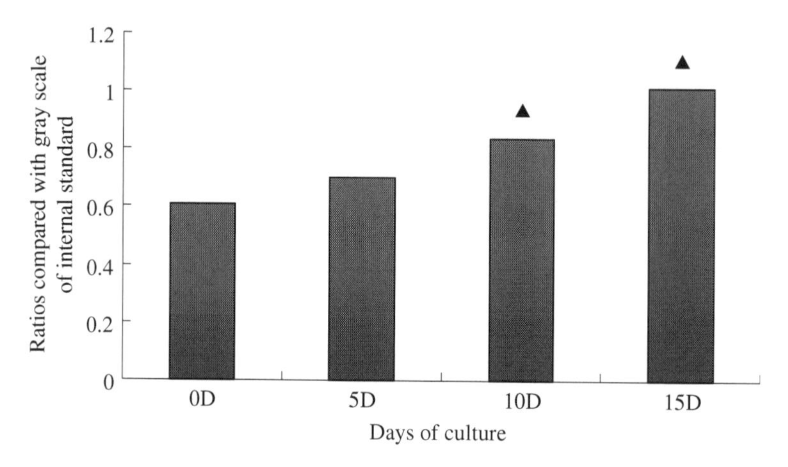

Fig. 29.11 The expression of Rb gene in the control group; ▲ means statistical significant between the 10D group, 15D group and the 0D group ($P < 0.05$)

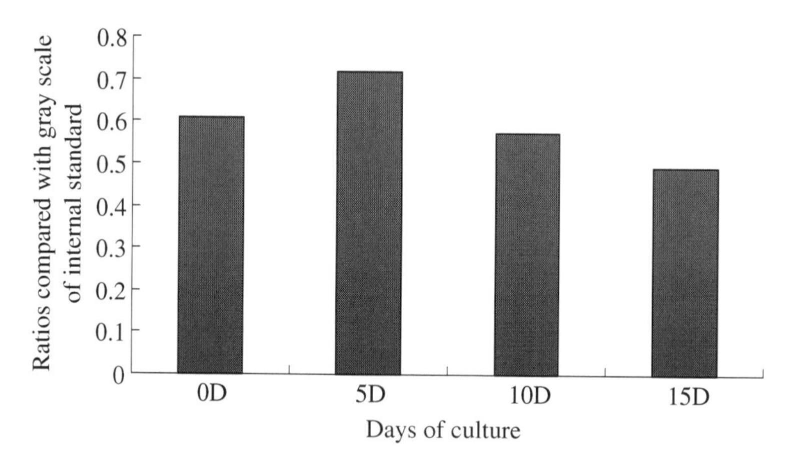

Fig. 29.12 The expression of Rb gene in CCK group

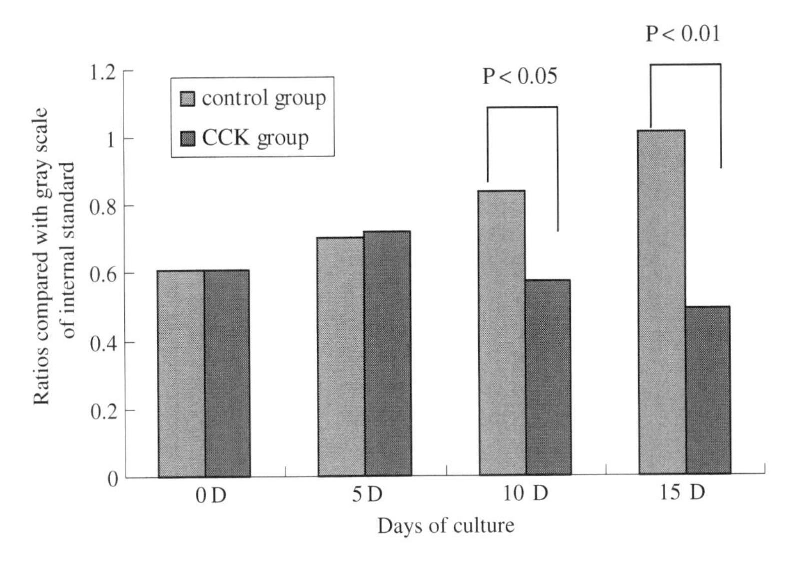

Fig. 29.13 The expression of Rb gene's mRNA in two groups. There was statistical significant in 10D group ($P < 0.05$) and 15D group ($P < 0.01$) between the CCK group and the control group

29.4 Discussion

Nowadays, regulation of aging has been extensively studied. Neuronal aging is a core subject in geriatrics. Because human life span is long, directly studying aging in humans is impractical. Fortunately, significant insights into aging can be achieved by studying experimental cell culture. Mice neuroblastoma cell culture model is widely recognized by scholars for studies of neural functions in vitro [6]. Cai et al. [7] devised an experimental neuronal aging model by culturing mice neuroblastoma cells under the condition of serum-free culture, which can avoid the influence of serum.

Our experiment adopted AID as serum-free culture medium, and as the culture time extended, differentiation appeared, which was just as the same as that we observed in our prior experiment. We have proved that CCK_8 could protect the aging process of experimental neuronal aging through cell morphous, total cellular protein, intracellular lipofusin [5]. Finding the molecular mechanisms of aging and the ways to postpone its process are what interest us and they have theoretical implications, extensive application value.

Cholecystokinin is an important gastrointestinal hormone, and it is one of the most abundant neurotransmitter peptides expressed in the brain. In the nervous system, CCK plays an important role in sensitivity [8], satiety [9], pain, memory and learning processes [10], reflection [11], adaptive development and brain plasticity [12]. Increasing work has been done on its protection of aging process.

The P_{53} tumor suppressor is activated by numerous stressors to induce apoptosis, cell cycle arrest, or senescence. Recently, mice were generated in which one allele of the P_{53} gene had a deletion of the first six exons [5]. These mice had hyperactive P_{53}, as assessed by enhanced apoptosis in response to genotoxic stress. Interestingly, these mice also displayed premature aging phenotypes [13]. Similar results were obtained in a BRCA1-P_{53} transgenic study, where it was reported that premature activation of P_{53} due to BRCA1 deficiency causes accelerated aging in vivo [14]. Another study group unexpectedly found that overexpression of the short form of P_{53} had effects on both size and life span, such mice had shortened health and life spans, and had reduced cellular proliferation with increased cellular senescence [15]. On the other hand, mice carrying one extra copy of the normal P_{53} gene did not show any indication of premature aging [16]. These observations suggest that while normally regulated P_{53} can provide enhanced tumor suppression, uncontrolled P_{53} activity generates phenotypes that mimic in vivo aging. Indeed P_{53} activity is high in senescent cells [17]. These findings also indicate that P_{53} gene is accompanied with aging process and it needs further investigation to identify such phenomenon in our experimental neuronal aging model.

It is generally believed that cellular senescence reflects some of the changes that occur during the aging of organisms, and specific genes have been identified that regulate aging. Several lines of evidence support the idea that cellular senescence suppresses tumorigenesis and at the molecular level, cellular senescence is controlled by Rb [18]. Rb is an important tumor suppressor that acts to restrict cell proliferation in response to DNA damage or deregulation of mitogenic oncogenes, by leading to the induction of various cell cycle. The tumor suppressor pathways controlled by Rb are necessary for the cellular senescence program [19]. Rb is found at senescence in its active, hypophosphorylated form, in which it binds to the E2F protein family members to repress their transcriptional targets [18].

In recent researches, it was reported that CCK might play an important role in learning and memory by influencing dendritic development [20]. This might be one of the causes to delay the aging processes. Another report showed that CCK could protect noradrenergic neurons and involved in ERK 1/2-Akt/PKB-PKA-dependent pathways. CCK markedly induced expression of neuronal survival markers [21]. The expression of P_{53} and Rb gene was up-regulated in the experimental neuronal aging process in our trial. With the influence of CCK_8, the aging process was delayed and the expression of P_{53} and Rb gene was depressed. Combined with the results that CCK could delay the aging processes and the fact that P_{53} and Rb play important roles in suppressing tumor, the theory that aging is one special way to depress tumor might be proved in our trial and the P_{53} and Rb had important effect on experimental neuronal aging process. By adding CCK, the expression of P_{53} and Rb gene was down-regulated and the aging process was postponed.

In conclusion, P_{53} and Rb gene might be involved in the aging processes of experimental neuronal aging model with the influence of CCK_8. A tenable hypothesis is that the P53 and Rb gene involved in the development of aging, and CCK could delay the aging processes through down-regulating the P_{53} and Rb gene. If the specific molecular pathway controlling the aging rate could be modulated genetically, it is modulated pharmacologically. These insights might ultimately have an important impact on the discovery and development of therapies and drugs to prevent and treat the diseases related to senescence.

References

1. Rehfeld JF, Lindberg I, Friis-Hansen L (2002) Increased synthesis but decreased processing of neuronal proCCK in prohormone convertase 2 and 7B2 knockout animals. J Neurochem 83(6):1329–1337
2. Sohal VS, Cox CL, Huguenard JR (1998) Localization of CCK receptors in thalamic reticular neurons: a modeling study. J Neurophysiol 79(5):2820–2824
3. Fratucci De Gobbi JI, De Luca LA Jr et al (2001) Interaction of serotonin and cholecystokinin in the lateral parabrachial nucleus to control sodium intake. Am J Physiol Regul Integr Comp Physiol 280(5):R1301–1307
4. Noble F, Wank SA, Crawley JN et al (1999) International union of pharmacology. XXI. structure, distribution, and functions of cholecystokinin receptors. Pharmacol Rev 51(4):745–781
5. Sun XJ, Lu QC, Cai Y (2005) Effect of cholecystokinin on experimental neuronal aging. World J Gastroenterol 11(4):551–556
6. Hamprecht B (1984) Cell culture as models for studying neural functions. Prog Neuropsychopharmacol Biol Psychiatry 8(4–6):481–486
7. Cai Y, Shen JK, Lu RH (1985). An experimental model for the study of the aging of neurons: serum-free culture of mouse neuroblastoma cells. Shi Yan Sheng Wu Xue Bao 18(4):453–461
8. Manni L, Lundeberg T, Tirassa P et al (2000) Cholecystokinin-8 enhances nerve growth factor synthesis and promotes recovery of capsaicin-induced sensory deficit. Br J Pharmacol 129(4):744–750
9. Plagemann A, Rake A, Harder T et al (1998) Reduction of cholecystokinin-8S-neurons in the paraventricular hypothalamic nucleus of neonatally overfed weanling rats. Neurosci Lett 258(1):13–16
10. Matsushita H, Akiyoshi J, Kai K et al (2003) Spatial memory impairment in OLETF rats without cholecystokinin—a receptor. Neuropept 37(5):271–276
11. Funakoshi K, Nakano M, Atobe Y et al (2001) Selective projections of cholecystokinin-8 immunoreactive fibers to galanin immunoreactive sympathetic preganglionic neurons in a teleost, stephanolepis cirrhifer. Neurosci Lett 316(2):111–113
12. Pisu MB, Conforti E, Scherini E et al (2000) Gastrin-cholecystokinin immunoreactivity in the central nervous system of Helix aspersa during rest and activity. J Exp Zool 287(1):29–37
13. Tyner SD, Venkatachalam S, Choi J et al (2002) p53 mutant mice that display early ageing-associated phenotypes. Nature 415(6867):45–53
14. Cao L, Li W, Kim S, Brodie SG et al (2003) Senescence, aging, and malignant transformation mediated by p53 in mice lacking the Brca1 full-length isoform. Genes Dev 17(2):201–213
15. Maier B, Gluba W, Bernier B et al (2004) Modulation of mammalian life span by the short isoform of p53. Genes Dev 18(3):306–319
16. Garcia-Cao I, Garcia-Cao M, Martin-Caballero J et al (2002) "Super p53" mice exhibit enhanced DNA damage response, are tumor resistant and age normally. EMBO J 21(22):6225–6235
17. Itahana K, Dimri GP, Hara E, Itahana Y et al (2002) A role for p53 in maintaining and establishing the quiescence growth arrest in human cells. J Biol Chem 277(20):18206–18214. Epub 2002 Mar 5

18. Narita M, Nunez S, Heard E et al (2003) Rb-mediated heterochromatin formation and silencing of E2F target genes during cellular senescence. Cell 113:703–716
19. Serrano M, Lin AW, McCurrach ME et al (1997) Oncogenic ras provokes premature cell senescence associated with accumulation of p53 and p16INK4a. Cell 88:593–602
20. Zhang LL, Wei XF, Zhang YH et al (2013) CCK-8S increased the filopodia and spines density in cultured hippocampal neurons of APP/PS1 and wild-type mice. Neurosci Lett 542:47–52
21. Hwang CK, Kim DK, Chun HS (2013) Cholecystokinin-8 induces brain-derived neurotrophic factor expression in noradrenergic neuronal cells. Neuropeptides. pii: S0143–4179(13)00025–5

Chapter 30
Attitudes Toward and Involvement in Medical Research: A Survey of 8-year-Program Undergraduates in China

Jie-Hua Li, Bin Yang, Jing-Xia Li, Yan-Bo Liu, Hui-Yong Chen, Kun-Lu Wu, Min Zhu, Jing Liu, Xiao-Juan Xiao and Qing-Nan He

Abstract *Background* The implementation and expansion of an 8-year program is among the most important reforms in medical education in China within the past 10 years. In an effort to cultivate world-class medical professionals, there has been a significant movement toward engaging 8-year-program students in scientific research within the medical school curriculum. However, attitudes of these students toward and their involvement in undergraduate medical research have not been adequately addressed. This study aims to assess attitudes toward and participation in medical research of 8-year-program undergraduates in China. *Methods* A cross-sectional survey using an anonymous, self-report questionnaire was designed and implemented with 8-year-program students in their third to eighth years at the Xiangya School of Medicine at Central South University between March and April 2012. *Results* Among the 583 students targeted in our study, 415 responded, yielding an overall response rate of 71 %. Though most of the respondents had generally positive attitudes toward undergraduate medical research, only 47 % of them had been involved in research activities by the time of our survey. The principal barriers to research participation were inadequate experimental facilities and funding, high pressure to study, ineffective management structure, and limited availability of research supervisors. *Conclusions* The results of our study outline current attitudes toward and involvement in research of 8-year-program medical students in China. Though the necessity and importance of undergraduate medical research have been recognized, there is still much work needed to increase the participation of students in research and to improve the quality of research training.

J.-H. Li · B. Yang · H.-Y. Chen · K.-L. Wu · M. Zhu · J. Liu (✉) · X.-J. Xiao
Molecular Biology Research Center, School of Life Science, Central South University, 110# Xiangya Road, Changsha 410078, Hunan, People's Republic of China
e-mail: jingliucsu@hotmail.com

J.-H. Li · B. Yang · J.-X. Li · Y.-B. Liu · Q.-N. He
Xiangya School of Medicine, Central South University, 172# Tongzipo Road, Changsha 410083, Hunan, People's Republic of China
e-mail: heqn2629@163.com

S. Li et al. (eds.), *Frontier and Future Development of Information Technology in Medicine and Education*, Lecture Notes in Electrical Engineering 269,
DOI: 10.1007/978-94-007-7618-0_30,

Keywords: 8-year-program undergraduates · Attitudes · Involvement · Medical research

30.1 Background

Health is a permanent theme in human society. Medical education has drawn worldwide attention because it influences the quality of health care services provided to the public [1–5]. With progress in science and technology, development of the economy, and improvements in human living conditions, the need for health care services is continuously expanding. Thus, it is necessary for medical education to be reconfigured in response to the changing scientific, economic, and social circumstances [6]. Improving the quality of medical education, cultivating a sufficient number of qualified health professionals, and guaranteeing the health of the public are common topics explored by medical educators worldwide [7].

In China, the implementation and expansion of 8-year programs are among the most significant and important reforms in medical education [8, 9]. In 2001, the Ministry of Health and the Ministry of Education jointly issued the 'Outline of China's National Plan for Medium and Long-term Education Reform and Development', which clearly established that China would gradually expand medical education with a longer period of schooling. Seven key medical schools in China piloted 8-year programs in 2004, and to date, the number of medical schools providing 8-year programs has increased to 16.

Compared with 5-year programs, which currently represent the majority in China's medical schools, the 8-year program is an elite education that aims to cultivate high quality, internationally competitive clinical expertise by extending the duration of schooling and reforming the medical school curricula. Students in 8-year programs receive an MD degree after graduation, and 5-year-program students receive a bachelor's degree. Students of 8-year programs are expected to possess a sound knowledge of clinical medicine as well as demonstrate actively innovative thinking, excellent research capabilities, and a strong exploratory spirit toward medical science.

With the rapid development and updating of medical knowledge, and increasing emphasis on evidence-based medicine and translational medicine, it is becoming increasingly important for health professionals to gain a sound understanding of scientific principles and methodology, and to be skillful at acquiring and appraising new information [10, 11]. Therefore, scientific research experience has been recognized as an important and essential component in the modern undergraduate medical curriculum [12–14]. Encouraging medical students to engage in scientific research is suggested as one possible strategy to improve the quality of medical education [15]. Several authors, who studied the relationship between research participation and medical education, indicated that among academic physicians, career success is independently associated with having conducted research as a student [16], and that exposure to research activities during medical school leads to greater scientific output after graduation [17].

The value and necessity of undergraduate medical research have been recognized in China. Many medical schools have established a series of programs to provide students with opportunities to participate in scientific research, such as innovative experimental projects, experimental design competitions, and early scientific research training. Students in 8-year programs are highly encouraged to engage in research activities. However, how medical students perceive such research as well as the degree of their involvement in these activities are not clear. In this study, we investigated the general attitudes of 8-year-program students toward scientific research, their research-specific competence and research experience, their expectations regarding mentors, possible barriers to their participation, and their understanding of molecular medicine.

30.2 Methods

The research was conducted at the Xiangya School of Medicine at Central South University (CSU) in Changsha, Hunan Province, China. Xiangya is one of the most prestigious medical schools in China and was among the first seven key medical schools to pilot an 8-year program in 2004.

Our study surveyed 8-year-program students enrolled at Xiangya. The questionnaires were completed between March and April 2012. Students in their third, fourth, fifth, sixth, seventh, or eighth year were invited to participate in this survey. Students in their first or second year were excluded because these years focus on "general education" or "pre-medical education", which consist primarily of courses in the natural and social sciences, and offer little opportunity to be involved in medical research. Participation was completely voluntary, and confidentiality was maintained at all times as no identifying information was collected from the participants. The students were contacted between lectures and invited to participate in the survey by each class monitor. An explanation of the objectives of the study and assurances of confidentiality were distributed to students responding to the survey, and oral informed consent was obtained from each. All investigation procedures were approved by the Central South University Ethics Committee.

The first part of the questionnaire assessed demographic information (age, gender, grades) for all study subjects. For senior students (those in their 7th or 8th year), their medical specialty was also required. The primary part of the questionnaire was developed with 41 items focusing on attitudes toward undergraduate medical research, research-specific competence, research experience, expectations regarding mentors, factors that influence research participation, and attitudes toward molecular medicine. The final item was an open question offering the respondents an opportunity to comment and give more extensive replies. The questionnaire was made available in Chinese and took 5–10 min to complete, on average. And minor modifications were made to further refine the questionnaire after we piloted it with a small group of students. All responses were entered into a Microsoft Excel file, and each completed questionnaire was assigned an identifying number to prevent duplicate data entry. The data were analyzed using a version of Microsoft Excel statistical software (Microsoft Office Excel 2007 for Windows) and SPSS 13.0. ANOVAs, t-tests, and Pearson's Chi-square test were used to examine some of the data in this study, and $p < 0.05$ was considered to be of significance.

30.3 Results

30.3.1 Demographic Information and Response Rate

Of the 583 8-year-program students targeted in our study, 415 responded, with an overall response rate of 71 %. The response rates were 82 % (n = 80), 89 % (n = 89), 91 % (n = 90), 69 % (n = 68), 37 % (n = 33), and 55 % (n = 55) for students in their third through eighth years, respectively. At the time of our survey, the seventh and eighth year students were on their internships or preparing for their graduation theses in laboratories. Thus, their attendance at large group lectures was lower, which resulted in lower response rates for these two groups. Therefore, we combined the results of these groups who had relatively homogenous demographic backgrounds when we compared responses between students in different years of study. The mean age of respondents was 23.1 years (SD 4.6 years, range 20–28 years); 56 % were female, and 44 % were male. Table 30.1 summarizes the demographic information of the respondents. All entered the university with high school backgrounds and had finished two years of "general education" or "pre-medical education" at CSU (see Table 30.1).

30.3.2 Attitudes Toward Medical Research

Over half of the 415 respondents (60 %) stated that they were interested or very interested in participating in research activities; only 6 % of them expressed no interest in research. In our survey, male students showed more interest in research than female students (119 out of 181, 66 % vs. 130 out of 234, 56 %, $\chi^2 = 4.42$, $p < 0.05$). And the students who have experience of research showed more interest in research than those who don't (though the difference was not significant enough) (123 out of 195, 64 % vs. 126 out of 220, 57 %, $\chi^2 = 1.45$, $p > 0.20$). However, we discovered a decreasing interest in research from third-year students to eighth-year students (Fig. 30.1). The overwhelming majority (91 %) of respondents agreed that it was necessary for 8-year-program students to participate in research activities, and 60 % of them planned to publish SCI research papers

Table 30.1 Demographic information of respondents

Variables	Number of students	%
Gender		
Male	181	44
Female	234	56
Student year		
Third year	80	19
Fourth year	89	22
Fifth year	90	22
Sixth year	68	16
Seventh year	33	8
Eighth year	55	13
Interest in research		
Not interested	23	6
Somewhat interested	143	34
Interested	185	45
Very interested	64	15
Research experience		
Yes	195	47
No	220	53

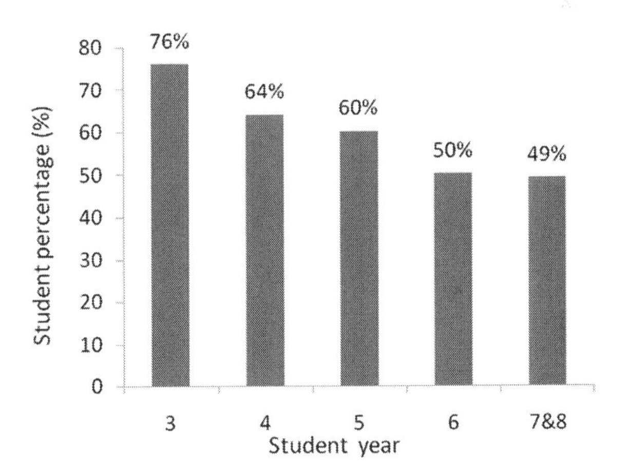

Fig. 30.1 Interest in medical research of students from different academic years

before graduating, even though it was not mandatory at the time. Eighty-eight percent of the students responded positively to the idea that research training should be a compulsory part of medical school curricula, and 55 % agreed that engaging in laboratory-based scientific research would be beneficial for clinicians desiring to improve their clinical practice. Additionally, 60 % of the respondents planned to be involved in scientific research throughout their medical careers. All of these findings showed that 8-year-program students generally had positive attitudes toward medical research. Table 30.2 summarizes the students' responses to several statements designed to evaluate their attitudes toward such research.

Table 30.2 Respondents' attitudes toward medical research

Statements	Affirmative (%)	Neutral (%)	Negative (%)
It is necessary for 8-year program students to participate in research activities	91	5	4
I plan to publish an SCI research paper before graduating even though it is not mandatory	60	23	17
Research training should be a compulsory part of the medical school curriculum	88	8	4
Engaging in laboratory-based research is beneficial for clinicians to improve their clinical practice	55	29	16
I plan to be involved in scientific research throughout my medical career	60	30	10

30.3.3 Research-Specific Competence

We designed five items in our questionnaire to measure self-reported research-specific competence: familiarity with the general process of research activities, competence in designing a study, ability to search for and appraise information, competence in writing a paper, and frequency of reading scientific literature. Each item was scored on a four-point scale with 1 = low, 2 = moderate, 3 = relatively high, and 4 = high, for a potential total score of 20. We obtained the total measurement of research-specific competence by tallying the scores for each item. The mean score was somewhat lower than what we had expected, which might have been owing to the modest character of our respondents. However, the means differed greatly among students in different years ($p < 0.01$) (Fig. 30.2) and showed a number of interesting points. The mean score of third-year students was the lowest (7.24); seventh- and eighth-year students had the highest mean score

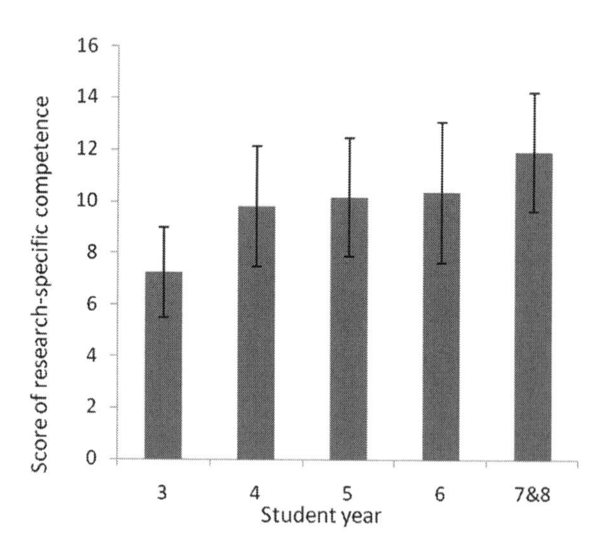

Fig. 30.2 Measured research-specific competence of students from different academic years

(11.91). Male students scored higher in research-specific competence than did female students (10.32 vs. 9.61, $t = 2.63$, $p < 0.01$), and students who had been involved in research activities scored significantly higher than those who had not (11.15 vs. 8.82, $t = 9.66$, $p < 0.01$). However, there was no significant difference in the mean score between students who were interested in medical research and those who were not (9.95 vs. 9.87, $t = 0.31$, $p > 0.75$). Overall, 54 % of respondents reported that they were not satisfied with the current level of their research-specific competence, and 78 % were either "unaware" or "totally unaware" of their teachers' research projects.

30.3.4 Research Experience

Of the 415 respondents, 195 (47 %) reported having been involved in research activities during medical school, and 59 (14 %) had published research papers. For eighth-year students, research activities related to graduate theses were excluded from this study. Only 5 % of 3rd-year students were involved in research activities because they had been exposed to medical courses for less than one year at the time of this survey. Upon exclusion of the third-year students from these data, students with research experience increased to 58 %. Undergraduate research participation rates did not vary greatly from the fourth-year students to those in their eighth year, though there was a slightly increasing trend (Fig. 30.3). In this study, male students were slightly more active in research activities than female students, though this difference was not significant (90 out of 181, 50 % vs. 105 out of 234, 45 %, $\chi^2 = 0.97$, $p > 0.30$). The most common reason for participating in research was "to improve research ability and enhance competitiveness" (66 %). In addition, designing a study was considered to be the most challenging

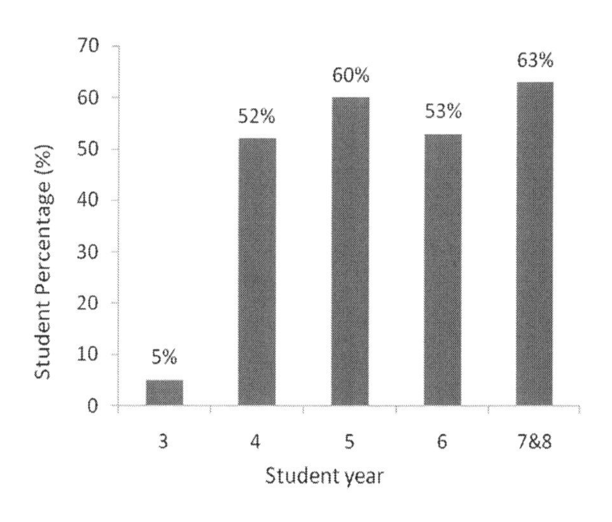

Fig. 30.3 Percentage of students with undergraduate research experience from different academic years

part of research by 66 % of students. Sixty-eight percent of respondents preferred clinical projects, and only 28 % were interested in basic medical research.

30.3.5 Expectations Regarding Mentors

The most desirable characteristics of mentors reported by our respondents were scientific erudition (83 %), sufficient time available to mentor students (71 %), and personal charm (57 %) (see Fig. 30.4). Additionally, most students hoped that research mentors would be able to help them in regard to scientific thinking and research methodology (79 %) as well as with financial support (51 %).

30.3.6 Factors That Influenced Involvement in Research

To determine the most significant factors that hinder student involvement in research, we designed a multiple-choice question that presented six possible barriers to research participation. The most frequently reported barriers were inadequate experimental facilities and funding (75 %), high pressure to study (63 %), ineffective management structure (56 %), and limited availability of research supervisors (53 %) (see Fig. 30.5). To obtain even more specific results, we designed another four single-choice questions. Only 30 % of respondents felt that there was adequate time set aside for research endeavors during school, and as many as 66 % stated that it was very difficult or relatively difficult to find a research mentor. Over half of the respondents (57 %) reported that there were not enough research programs for students to participate in, and the majority (87 %)

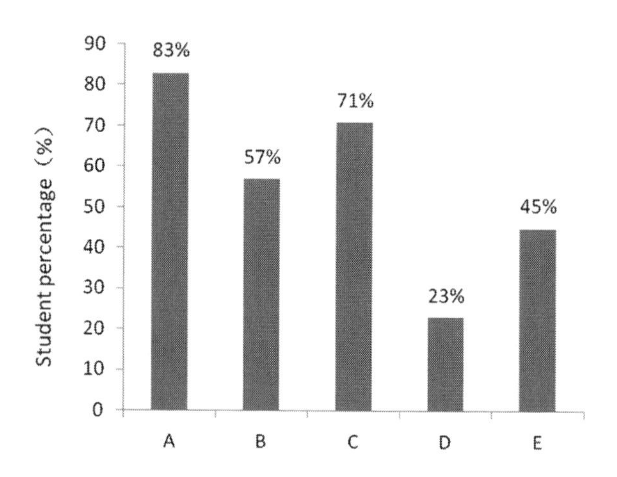

Fig. 30.4 Desirable characteristics of mentors. *A* scientific erudition *B* personal charm *C* enough time available to mentor students *D* social experience *E* international contacts

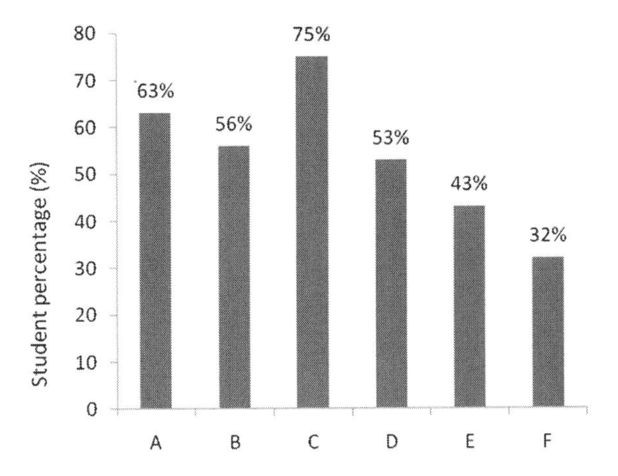

Fig. 30.5 Perceived barriers to research participation. *A* high pressure to study *B* ineffective management structure *C* inadequate experimental facilities and funding *D* limited availability of research supervisors *E* lack of research-specific ability and skills *F* lack of interest

answered that there was a lack of exploratory experiments in experimental teaching courses. All these factors may influence the degree of student participation in scientific research during medical school.

30.3.7 Attitudes Toward Molecular Medicine

We also investigated the attitudes of 8-year-program students toward molecular medicine. Eighty-five percent of them realized the importance of molecular biology in the development of modern medicine. However, over half of them (53 %) felt that molecular medicine was not incorporated thoroughly enough in the current curriculum, and 55 % expressed a lack of proficiency in some of the basic molecular biology technology that may be needed in medical research. The overwhelming majority of students (94 %) answered that it was necessary to enhance training in the experimental skills of molecular biology in the preclinical curriculum, and 92 % reported that it would be helpful to implement a clinical molecular biology course in the clinical curriculum.

30.4 Discussion

To the best of our knowledge, this is the first comprehensive study to address attitudes toward and involvement in medical research of 8-year-program students in China. Our study indicates that these students are highly interested in medical research and have generally positive attitudes toward it. However, only 47 % had participated in any kind of research activity by the time of this survey. Male students showed more interest in research than did female students, which was similar with other studies published before [18, 19]. There was decreasing interest in research from third-year to eighth-year students. This finding may reflect senior students being more immersed in clinical training and ignoring basic medical research [20]. What's more, the government and schools have placed increasing emphasis on undergraduate medical research and created more opportunities in recent years, which may be why junior students perceived more benefits and were more motivated than senior students.

Inadequate experimental facilities and funding, high pressure to study, ineffective management structure, and limited availability of research supervisors were the most frequently cited barriers to undergraduate involvement in scientific research activities. These barriers must be considered if we want to increase the participation of 8-year-program students in research. It is noteworthy that 54 % of the students reported that they were not satisfied with their current level of research-specific competence. Therefore, they may need more research training to improve their skills. Additionally, over half of students (57 %) reported that there were not enough research programs for students, indicating that the school should provide more research opportunities. Furthermore, 78 % of the students were either "unaware" or "totally unaware" of their teachers' research projects, even though most of the school's staffs were actively engaged in scientific research. This finding implies that teachers should introduce more of their own research experience in their lectures or seminars. In addition, as the majority of our respondents noted, training in molecular medicine should be enhanced to enrich the undergraduate curriculum and better prepare 8-year-program students for medical research opportunities.

China's medical education system is perhaps the largest and most complicated in the world because of the country's huge population, great cultural diversity, and uneven economic development. Medical curricula vary greatly, from 3 years at secondary medical schools to 5–8 years at universities; a stepwise system also exists in which students progress from a bachelor's to master's degree in 3 years and then to MD or PhD programs for another 3 years [9]. The 3-year diploma primarily prepares staff to serve in rural areas, the 5-year program aims to supply competent clinicians, and the 8-year program and the stepwise system aspire to produce world-class academic researchers and practitioners [8]. Much is expected of the 8-year-program students. They comprise only 7–8 % of the total students in medical schools that provide this program. The importance and necessity of engaging these students in scientific research activities through their medical course work has been recognized by most key medical schools in China.

It has been proposed that successful clinicians should be able to understand research and the research process, even if they are not actively engaged in research themselves [21]. Research-specific capability can help clinicians integrate new knowledge into clinical practice and make professional decisions more effectively and accurately as well as investigate scientific problems found in clinical practice, thus promoting the development of medical science. By being involved in research activities, medical students can learn how to appraise literature, design a study, analyze data and present results, and grasp the basic technical skills for research, which is beneficial in developing an appreciation for research methodology [22, 23]. In addition, undergraduate research exposure leads to enthusiasm for exploring the unknown, interest in academic and research careers, and greater scientific output after graduation [17, 18]. There has been a significant movement toward providing medical students with early research experience within the medical school curriculum in China and around the world [24].

Many medical schools in China are attempting to incorporate research training into medical curricula. At CSU's Xiangya School of Medicine, for example, research-specific courses such as Research Designing, Bioinformatics, Information Retrieval, and Laboratory Animal Science are among the compulsory courses. Students are encouraged to complete innovative experimental projects and to take part in experimental designing competitions, both of which require them to design a study in a specific area based on their own innovative ideas and with the guidance of their mentors. In addition, there is a special research training course called Early Scientific Research Training for 8-year-program students in their third or fourth year, which is usually implemented over summer vacation and lasts approximately 8 weeks. This training aims to educate students in basic parameters of research beginning early in their undergraduate years and cultivate their research capability, innovation ability, interest in academic medicine, and enthusiasm for exploration.

Though the benefits of participating in research as an undergraduate are well documented for graduates, institutions, and the academic community as a whole, there are still some objections [25, 26] because involving undergraduates in research creates challenges for both students and mentors. On the one hand, intense projects may increase the students' study burdens and disrupt the progress of the normal medical curriculum. On the other hand, supervision requirements may distract mentors from their own clinical and research commitments while proffering few tangible benefits. However, highly motivated students should be mentored by highly enthusiastic and research-enabled staffs [19], and good student-faculty contact and communication are vital to ensuring the quality of research training. It may be helpful to put more effort into funding undergraduate research and develop new methods of performance evaluation for both students and faculty members.

With the rapid developments in science and medicine today, more and more emphasis is being placed on translational medicine, an integrated concept based on a multidirectional understanding of research and medicine embedded in a socioeconomic environment [27]. Fostering a supportive undergraduate research environment is essential to cultivating physician investigators with the competence and enthusiasm for research who can translate the progress in basic research into clinical practice and continuously improve the quality of health care delivered to the public. It is encouraging that, in our study, a significant majority of respondents (91 %) recognized the importance and necessity of involving 8-year-program students in scientific research. Over half of students (55 %) appreciated the relevance of laboratory-based research to clinical practice, and 60 % planned to be involved in research throughout their medical careers. It is important for schools to provide a variety of opportunities and sufficient research funds to increase the participation of 8-year-program students in scientific research in an effort to prepare internationally competitive medical professionals in China.

Our study has several limitations that need to be considered when interpreting the results. First, the data presented in this paper are derived from a self-report survey and are thus based solely on the students' own perceptions. A comparison with objective data from faculty staff and a similar survey of other stakeholders in medical education such as educators would be more informative. Second, the study only targeted 8-year-program students from a single medical school. Thus, the results may not be representative of students in other programs or those from other medical schools. Third, although we attempted to obtain responses from all 8-year-program students in their third to eighth years, we were only able to obtain a total response rate of 71 %, and response rates between students in different years of study varied significantly. Finally, the method we used to analyze research-specific competence of students has not been formally standardized, and we only considered five measurement items. However, notwithstanding these limitations, our study provides valuable information about attitudes toward and participation in research of 8-year-program medical students in China.

30.5 Conclusions

Our study reveals high levels of interest in research among medical students in 8-year programs, and indicates that most students have generally positive attitudes toward undergraduate research. The principal barriers to research participation reported by our respondents were inadequate experimental facilities and funding, high pressure to study, ineffective management structure, and limited availability of research supervisors. Medical educators must constantly and systematically determine better ways to prepare future physicians as the field of medicine rapidly evolves. Involving undergraduates in research is one curricular innovation worthy of further exploration and investigation [28]. For China and other developing countries, increasing the participation of medical undergraduates in scientific research may be vital to cultivating world-class medical professionals who can improve the international competitiveness of the country's entire medical system and the quality of health care delivered to the public.

30.6 Competing Interests

The authors declare that they have no competing interests.

30.7 Authors' Contributions

Li Jie-Hua, Yang Bin, Li Jing-Xia, Liu Yan-Bo, Chen Hui-Yong, Wu Kun-Lu, Zhu Min, and Xiao Xiao-Juan performed research and analyzed the data. Liu Jing and He Qing-Nan designed the study and analyzed the data. Li Jie-Hua and Liu Jing wrote the paper. All authors read and approved the final manuscript.

Acknowledgments This work was supported by grants from New Century Excellent Talents in University (NCET-11-0518), Fundamental Research Funds for the Central Universities (No. 2011JQ015), the Hunan Education Reform Project (2011), the Project of Undergraduate Education and Teaching Reform of Central South University (2012), the National Program of Web-Delivery for Elaborate Courses (2008, Medical Molecular Biology).

References

1. Ferguson E, James D, Madeley L (2002) Factors associated with success in medical school: systematic review of the literature. BMJ 324(7343):952–957
2. Lempp H, Seale C (2004) The hidden curriculum in undergraduate medical education: qualitative study of medical students' perceptions of teaching. BMJ 329(7469):770–773
3. Woollard RF (2006) Caring for a common future: medical schools' social accountability. Med Educ 40(4):301–313
4. Hauer KE, Durning SJ, Kernan WN et al (2008) Factors associated with medical students' career choices regarding internal medicine. JAMA 300(10):1154–1164
5. Dzau VJ, Ackerly DC, Sutton-Wallace P et al (2009) The role of academic health science systems in the transformation of medicine. Lancet 375(9718):949–953
6. Cooke M, Irby DM, Sullivan W et al (2006) American medical education 100 years after the Flexner report. N Engl J Med 355(13):1339–1344
7. Frenk J, Chen L, Bhutta ZA et al (2010) Health professionals for a new century: transforming education to strengthen health systems in an interdependent world. Lancet 376(9756):1923–1958
8. Xu D, Sun B, Wan X et al (2010) Reformation of medical education in China. Lancet 375:1502–1504
9. Lam TP, Wan XH, Ip MS (2006) Current perspectives on medical education in China. Med Educ 40(10):940–949
10. Hren D, Lukic IK, Marusic A et al (2004) Teaching research methodology in medical schools: students' attitudes towards and knowledge about science. Med Educ 38:81–86
11. Byrne E (2004) The physician scientist: an endangered breed? Intern Med J 34(3):75
12. General Medical Council UK (2009) Tomorrows Doctors, outcomes and standards for undergraduate medical education
13. Scottish Deans Medical Education Group (2009) The Scottish Doctor: learning outcomes for the medical undergraduate in Scotland: a foundation for competent and reflective practitioners, 3rd edn. Scottish Deans Medical Education Group, Edinburgh
14. Illing J (2007) Thinking about research: frameworks, ethics and scholarship. ASME, Edinburgh
15. de Oliveira NA, Luz MR, Saraiva RM et al (2011) Student views of research training programmes in medical schools. Med Educ 45(7):748–755
16. Brancati FL, Mead LA, Levine DM et al (1992) Early predictors of career achievement in academic medicine. JAMA 267:1372–1376

17. Reinders JJ, Kropmans TJB, Cohen-Schotanus J (2005) Extracurricular research experience of medical students and their scientific output after graduation. Med Educ 39:237
18. Remes V, Helenius I, Sinisaari I (2000) Research and medical students. Med Teach 22(2):164–167
19. Burgoyne LN, O'Flynn S, Boylan GB (2010) Undergraduate medical research: the student perspective. Medical Educ Online 15:5212
20. Hyde S (2007) Australian medical students' interest in research as a career. Focus Health Prof Educ 9(2):27–38
21. Deborah ME, Sarah D, Sarah E et al (2010) What do medical students understand by research and research skills? Identifying research opportunities within undergraduate projects. Med Teach 32:152–160
22. Lloyd T, Phillips BR, Aber RC (2004) Factors that influence doctors' participation in clinical research. Med Educ 38(8):848–851
23. Frishman WH (2001) Student research projects and theses: should they be a requirement for medical school graduation? Heart Dis 3(3):140–144
24. Fang D, Meyer RE (2003) Effect of two Howard Hughes Medical Institute research training programs for medical students on the likelihood of pursuing research careers. Acad Med 78(12):1271–1280
25. Metcalfe D (2008) Involving medical students in research. J R Soc Med 101(3):102–103
26. Siemens DR, Punnen S, Wong J et al (2010) A survey on the attitudes towards research in medical school. BMC Med Educ 10:4
27. Sonntag KC (2005) Implementations of translational medicine. J Transl Med 3:33
28. Parsonnet J, Gruppuso PA, Kanter SL et al (2010) Required vs. elective research and in-depth scholarship programs in the medical student curriculum. Acad Med 85(3):405–408

Chapter 31
Study the Effect of Different Traditional Chinese Medicine Treatment which to the Elasticity Modulus of Asthma Rats' Lung

Zhao-xia Xu, Xue-liang Li, Na Li, Peng Qian, Jin Xu, Yi-qin Wang and Jun-qi Wang

Abstract Elasticity modulus is the most important and most characteristic of the mechanical properties which express the degree of materials. The work aimed to explore the changes of elasticity modulus in asthma rats lung and the effect of different Traditional Chinese Medicine (TCM) treatment, such as lung-diffusing therapy, body resistance-strengthening therapy, integrated therapy of lung-diffusing and body resistance-strengthening, to them. We copied rat asthma model using ovalbumin, then gavaged treatment with three Chinese medicine, After 4 weeks, we researched the changes of modulus elasticity in asthma rats lung based on the biological elasticity modulus detection system, and researched the impact of three TCM treatment to them. We found the elasticity modulus of rats lung in normal group is less than those in other groups, and there is statistically significant difference between normal group and model group, prednisone group, body resistance-strengthening group. There also is statistically significant difference between prednisone group and the combination of lung-diffusing and body resistance-strengthening group. TCM treatment can improve the elastic modulus of asthmatic rats lung, and it probable is one of the mechanisms of the treatment of asthma.

Keywords Asthma · Elasticity modulus · Traditional Chinese medicine treatment · Mechanism of effect

31.1 Introduction

The mechanical factors play a role in the process of life, people pay more and more attention to it. There are lots of domestic and overseas research that how mechanical factors affect the remodeling of revascularization. The domestic

Z. Xu · X. Li · N. Li · P. Qian · J. Xu · Y. Wang (✉) · J. Wang
Shanghai University of Traditional Chinese Medicine, 63#, No.1200 Cailun Road 201203 Shanghai, People's Republic of China
e-mail: zhaoxia7001@126.com

S. Li et al. (eds.), *Frontier and Future Development of Information Technology in Medicine and Education*, Lecture Notes in Electrical Engineering 269,
DOI: 10.1007/978-94-007-7618-0_31,

research for how mechanical factors affecting airway remodeling has only just begun. In recent years, the studies also found that the mechanical environment was as important as biochemical environment living. The research has become a hot topic of current medical research that the structural and functional changes (remodeling) of heart and lung in which adapting to the mechanical environment. Modulus of elasticity is the most important and most characteristic of the mechanical properties which express the degree of material. The limit of curving and intensity from the lung tension experiments can express affordability which force acts on the alveolar wall. The affordability which the limit volume acts on the isolated lung tissue can express the elasticity of the lung tissue biomechanics. Our study group has studied experiments based on the three traditional Chinese medicine such as lung-diffusing therapy, body resistance-strengthening therapy, integrated therapy of lung-diffusing and body resistance-strengthening [1–4].

This study investigated the elastic modulus changes of asthma rats alveolar, and analyzed the influence of three TCM treatment affect to them. In order to explore the role and mechanism of the three TCM treatment methods, at the same time, we hope that can provide some basis to elucidate the pathogenesis of asthma.

31.2 Materials and Methods

31.2.1 Animal Grouping

Sixty healthy SD male rats (purchased from Shanghai SLAC Laboratory animal co.LTD, License No.SCXK Hu 2007-0005) with the weight of 200 ± 20 g were randomly divided into six groups, which are the normal group (group A), model group (group B), prednisone group (group C), lung-diffusing therapy group (group D), body resistance-strengthening group (group E), the combination of lung-diffusing and body resistance-strengthening group (group F).

31.2.2 Modeling Method

The modeling method was modified as the method introduce in the Ref. [5, 6]. Asthma rat models were prepared by injecting ovalbumin (OVA) into the abdominal cavity and inhalation of aerosol based on the modeling method described in the reference. On the first day after animal grouping, each rat of group B, C, D, E and F was injected intraperitoneally 1 mL of solution (containing of OVA 100 mg, Aluminum hydroxide 100 mg), after fourteen days, aerosol inhalation of 1 % OVA for 20 min with the flowing rate of 2 mL·min^{-1}, and continued for 28 days. Rats in group A were injected 1 mL of 0.9 % Sodium Chloride solution and aerosol inhalation of 0.9 % Sodium Chloride solution with the flowing rate of 2 mL·min^{-1}, and continued for 28 days.

31.2.3 Treatment Intervention

Dexamethasone tablets (Shanghai Xinyi Pharmaceutical Factory Co., Ltd. No.: H3120793-01) were made into the suspension of 0.32 mg·mL^{-1} with 0.9 % Sodium Chloride solution.

Prescription of body resistance-strengthening is made of *Shengdihuang(Rehmanniae)* 10 g, *Shudi(Rehmannia)* 10 g, *Dangshen(Salvia)* 10 g, *Fuling(Poria)* 9 g, *Huangjing (Polygonatum)* 9 g, *Yuzhu(Odoratum)* 9 g, *Xianlingpi* (Epimedium) 9 g, and so on. Prescription of lung-diffusing is made of *Mahuang(Ephedra)* 4 g, *Banxia (Pinellia)* 9 g, *Dilong (lumbricus)* 9 g, *Chaihu(Bupleurum)* 9 g, *Huangqin (Scutellaria)* 9 g, *Tinglizi* 9 *(Tinglizi)* g, and so on. Prescription of the combination of lung-diffusing and body resistance-strengthening is made of *Shengdihuang* 10 g, *Shudihuang* 10 g, *Dangshen* 10 g, *Zexie (Alisma)* 10 g, *Huangjing* 10 g, *Xianlingpi* 10 g, *Nanshashen (Adenophorae* 9 g, *Beishashen (Littoralis)* 9 g, *Banxia* 9 g, *Dilong* 9 g, *Huangqin* 9 g, and so on. Herbs of three prescriptions were soaked in water for 1 h, respectively. Ten times of water were added for the first time cooking. Four times of water were added for the second time cooking. Then, prepared decoction from both times were collected, evaporated and concentrated into the solution of 3 g·mL^{-1} crude drug concentration.

The first day after asthma induced, rats of group A and group B were given normal saline by gavage; rats of group C were given Dexamethasone by gavage; rats of group D, E, and F were given decoction of lung-diffusing, body resistance-strengthening and the combination of lung-diffusing and body resistance-strengthening prescription by gavage, respectively. The administration was 10 ml/kg·bw, once a day. After 4 weeks, materials were collected for the detection of relevant indicators.

31.2.4 Establishing the Detection System of Elasticity Modulus

In this study, we used the multi-channel physiological acquisition and processing system (NO.RM6240C, made from Chengdu Factory of Instrument.) and the syringe pump (NO. LINZ-6-B, made from Shanghai Leien Medical Equipment Co.,Ltd.) to establish the detection system of elasticity modulus based on the principle of pressure sensors.

After the rats were anesthetized, their complete tracheal and lung tissue were isolated, then weighed. Transtracheal, uniform(500 ml/h) injected saline. We recorded the pressure of each rat lung tissue(kPa), at the same time, the volume change(Δv) of each rat lung tissue was observed and recorded. Then the elasticity modulus (kPa/Δv) of lung tissuewas compared.

31.2.5 Statistically Analysis

All the experimental data were analyzed statistically by SPSS18.0 statistical software. ANOVA was used for the analysis of difference between groups. The inspection level was $\alpha = 0.05$. And the $P < 0.05$ was considered as statistically significant difference.

31.3 Results

31.3.1 Comparison of the Biggest Pressure of Rat Lung Tissue

The result about the comparison of the biggest pressure of rat lung tissue is showed in Table 31.1. We can find that the greatest pressure of rat lung tissue in group A is greater than those in other five groups, and there is statistically significant difference between group A and group B, group C, group D. There also is statistically significant difference between group B, group C and group F.

31.3.2 Comparison of the Elasticity Modulus of Rats Lung

Comparison of the elasticity modulus of rats lung in Table 31.2. We can find that the elasticity modulus of rats lung in group A is less than those in other groups, and there is statistically significant difference between group A and group B, group C, group E. There also is statistically significant difference between group C and group F.

Table 31.1 The comparison of the greatest pressure of rat lung tissue ($\overline{x} \pm SD$)

Groups	n	The greatest pressure of rats' lung tissue (kPa)
Group A	10	6036.80 ± 533.79
Group B	10	5048.96 ± 613.71^{a}
Group C	9	5351.78 ± 640.22^{a}
Group D	9	5234.18 ± 820.99^{a}
Group E	10	5587.96 ± 920.73
Group F	10	$6018.36 \pm 686.2^{a,\ b}$

Compared with groupA, ^{a} $P < 0.05$; Compared with groupB, ^{a} $P < 0.05$; Compared with groupC, ^{b} $P < 0.05$

Table 31.2 Comparison of the elasticity modulus of rats lung ($\bar{x} \pm SD$)

Group	n	Elasticity modulus of rats lung (kPa/cm3)
Group A	10	516.05 ± 57.65
Group B	10	650.93 ± 98.43[a]
Group C	9	697.22 ± 122.91[a]
Group D	9	607.17 ± 128.98
Group E	10	707.32 ± 158.89[a]
Group F	10	576.29 ± 104.32[b]

Compared with group A, [a] $P < 0.05$; Compared with group C, [b] $P < 0.05$

31.4 Discussion

The organ, tissue, cell and molecular levels of Stress-Growth rule research is still forefront of the international biomechanical study. People now pay more attention on the mechanical factors and role in the life process. There are a lot of researches on mechanical factors how to affect on vascular reconstruction. Domestic only just begun to study about the mechanical factors how to affect on air passage reconstruction,. Recent studies have found, mechanics environment and biological environment are equally important, the changes (RE) of tissue structure and function of the mechanical environment which has become a hot point of current medical research [7–11].

Modulus of elasticity, also known as the elasticity coefficient, Young's modulus, which is one of the most important, most features of the mechanical properties of material elastic degree, which is also the object deformation characterization of the degree. The yield limit and ultimate strength of pulmonary tension experiment, which reflects the alveolar wall on the force bearing capacity, which also reflects the elastic pulmonary tissue biomechanics in the affordability of lung tissue in vitro to limit the small volume. In this experiment, using mechanical system to detects the stress of rat alveolar surface. Comparison of the lung maximum pressure, normal group was greater than the other groups, and the treatment group was significantly better than the model group and the dexamethasone group (with statistical significance). Comparative biology of elastic modulus in the lung tissues, normal group was significantly less than those in the other groups, and the traditional Chinese medicine group was significantly lower than that in the model group and the dexamethasone group, normal group lung tissue elasticity than other groups, and the treatment group was better than that of the model group and the dexamethasone group. These indicators, reflect to some extent the occurrence of asthma in the process, existing mechanical changes and Chinese medicine intervention effect on the lung tissue.

Traditional Chinese Medicine believes, stage involving the lung spleen kidney three dirty asthma in remission, more performance for the deficiency of Qi and Yin and Yang, treatment when invigorating lung and kidney, warming yang and replenishing essence. In this study, the main effect of lung-diffusing prescription is freeing lung and relieving asthma, eliminating phlegm and stopping cough, clearing the lung spasmolysis, can effectively relieve asthma attacks, is an effective prescription asthma attack. Retention of this side effect is the lung spleen kidney three tonic, Qi Yin and yang balance, focusing on regulation of body immunity. Lung-diffusing prescription can both supplementation and attack. We on the basis of this, in the overall concept of thinking, further integration of treatment, will integrated lung-diffusing and body resistance-strengthening, lung-diffusing and body resistance-strengthening treatment were compared, to select more effective asthma therapy.

Application and development of asthma animal model plays an important role in human and investigate the pathogenesis of asthma control and asthma, the lesion development process and human asthma etiology, pathological process of rats are similar to the human. Rat model of asthma sensitized replication using egg albumin similar to asthma status, which belongs to which Chinese medicine syndrome types needs further study. Previous studies confirmed, "body resistance-strengthening", "lung-diffusing", "integrated lung-diffusing and body resistance-strengthening" three kinds of treatment on inflammation and air passage remodeling in asthmatic rats has improved, but the three groups of Chinese medicine groups, no significant difference. Investigate its reason, may be associated with the pathogenesis related asthma. The ancient physicians think phlegmatic retention in lung for asthma is the fundamental reason, the remission of asthma to lung, spleen, kidney deficiency, but there still exist the air passage inflammation and air passage hyperresponsiveness, air passage obstruction phenomenon [12]. This deficiency is the main pathogenesis of this disease, "body resistance-strengthening", "lung-diffusing", "integrated lung-diffusing and body resistance-strengthening" three therapies of traditional Chinese medicine on asthma have improved, but also that of asthma treatment, and not a single, but can be a variety of ways. In order to explore the pathogenesis of asthma and the effect of different TCM therapy for more similar clinical conditions, further research should be expanded sample size, multiple comparison, analysis of TCM syndrome attribute rat asthma model.

Acknowledgments This study is supported by the National Natural Science Foundation of China (No.81072787), the National Natural Science Foundation of Shanghai (No.10ZR1429900) and Key Discipline of State Administration of Traditional Chinese Medicine (Chinese diagnostics).

References

1. Wang Y, Tang W, Li F et al (2001) The zero-stress state of trachea. J Med Biomech 16(1):5–9
2. Xu Z, Li X, Qian P et al (2012) Influence of three kinds of traditional Chinese therapies on airway remodeling in asthmatic rats. Modernization Tradit Chin Med Materia Medica-World Sci Technol 14(4):1853–1856
3. Xu Z, Li X, Qian P et al (2013) Expression of NF-κBmRNA in asthma rats lung based on the effect of different TCM treatment. J Investig Med 61(4):7

4. Xu Z, Li X, Qian P et al (2012) Change of TGF-β1 and smad3, smad7 in lung of asthma rats and the effect of different TCM treatment to them. Glob Tradit Chin Med 5(12):900–904
5. Wasemmn S, Olivenstein R, Renzi PM (1992) The relationship between late asthma tic responses and antigen-specific immunoglobulin. J Allergy Clin Immunol 90:661–669
6. Xu S, Xu Y, Zhang Z et al (2006) Pathological features and mechanisms of airway remodeling in asthmatic rats. Acta M ed Univ Sci Technol Huazhong 35(4): 465–472
7. Teng Z, Wang Y, Li F, Yan H, Liu Z (2008) Tracheal compliance and limit flow rate changes in a murine model of asthma. Sci China C Life Sci 51(10):922–931
8. Liu Z, Wang Y, Teng Z, Xu G, Tang W (2002) Opening angles and residual strains in normal rat trachea.Sci China C Life Sci 45(2):138–148
9. Jiang Z, Yang X, Ji K et al (2001) Effect of endothelin on zero-stress state of arteries in spontaneously hypertensive rats. Chin J Biomed Eng 20(4):289–292
10. Cai S, Lu X, Wang Y et al (2003) Study the relationship between stress and growth: cell, brace medium and interaction. In: The sixth national biomechanics academic conference workshop
11. Liu Z, Teng Z, Qin (2002) On determination of circumferential stress in arteaial-wall using P–V exponential. Relationship. Chinese J Theoret Appl Mech 34(1):87–95
12. Yin J, Shen K, Liu S et al (2004) Relationship between brondfim hyperresponsiveness and the peripheral obstruction in stable asthmatic children. Chin J Pediatr 42(2):87–89

Chapter 32
Cloning and Characterization of Two cDNA Sequences Coding Squalene Synthase Involved in Glycyrrhizic Acid Biosynthesis in *Glycyrrhiza uralensis*

Ying Liu, Ning Zhang, Honghao Chen, Ya Gao, Hao Wen, Yong Liu and Chunsheng Liu

Abstract *Glycyrrhiza uralensis* are widely used in Chinese medicine for the functions of relieving cough, clearing heat and detoxicating. They are also used as food additives and industry materials. There are various components with different pharmacological activities in *G. uralensis*, among them glycyrrhizic acid is believed as an indicator component to characterize the quality of this herb. In the present study, two cDNA sequences coding squalene synthase (SQS1 and SQS2) involved in glycyrrhizic acid biosynthesis in *G. uralensis* were cloned and expressed in *Escherichia coli* as fusion proteins, which showed the similar activity as SQS isolated from other species to catalyze farnesyl diphosphate (FPP) into squalene (SQ). Because SQS is a key enzyme in glycyrrhizic acid metabolic pathway in *G. uralensis*, this work is significant for further studies concerned with exploring the molecular mechanism of biosynthesis of glycyrrhizic acid and improving the quality of *G. uralensis*.

Keywords Glycyrrhiza uralensis · Squalene synthase · cDNA · Glycyrrhizic acid · Cloning · Characterization

Abbreviations

SQS Squalene synthase
SQ Squalene
FPP Farnesyl diphosphate
ORF Open reading frame

Y. Liu (✉) · N. Zhang · H. Chen · Y. Gao · H. Wen · Y. Liu · C. Liu
School of Chinese Pharmacy, Beijing University of Chinese Medicine, No. 6 South Wangjing Zhonghuan Road, Beijing, China
e-mail: max_liucs@263.net

S. Li et al. (eds.), *Frontier and Future Development of Information Technology in Medicine and Education*, Lecture Notes in Electrical Engineering 269,
DOI: 10.1007/978-94-007-7618-0_32,

32.1 Introduction

The roots of licorice (*Glycyrrhiza uralensis* Fisch, Gancao in Chinese and Kanzo in Japanese) are widely used in Chinese herbal compound prescriptions to nourish qi, alleviate pain, tonify spleen and stomach and to relieve coughing [19, 22]. In addition, it is also used as health food, flavoring agent and tobacco additives. There are various components with different pharmacological activities in *G. uralensis*, among them glycyrrhizic acid is believed to be the major effective constituent and treated as an indicator component to characterize the quality of this herb, which has various biological properties, such as anti-inflammatory, anticancer and strengthening immunity [1, 4, 5, 17, 21].

In recent years, the irresponsible overcollection of wild *G. uralensis* has resulted in the decrease and extinction of the wild resources of *G. uralensis*. Therefore, the Chinese government prohibited the collection of wild *G. uralensis* plants in 2000. As a result, cultivars became the main resource of this herb. However, the content of glycyrrhizic acid in cultivars of *G. uralensis* is low, which can not meet the requirements of Chinese pharmacopoeia. So improving the quality of cultivars has become the key problem of the sustainable development.

Up to now the biosynthesis pathway for forming glycyrrhizic acid has been revealed. Squalene synthase (SQS) is considered to play an important role. It is situated in a branch point and may play a role as an up-regulator for production of triterpenoids [7, 8, 13, 16]. SQS gene belongs to a multigene family, up to now two kinds of SQS gene with different expressing activity has been found in many plants, such as *Arabidopsis thaliana* [6, 14] and *Glycyrrhiza glabra* [3]. This work described the cloning and biochemical characterization of a SQS1 cDNA and a SQS2 cDNA from *G. uralensis* (*Gu*SQS1 cDNA, *Gu*SQS2 cDNA). These findings and investigations will provide an efficient route for improving the quality of cultivar of *G. uralensis* and revealing the molecular mechanism of the biosynthetic pathway of glycyrrhizic acid.

32.2 Materials and Methods

32.2.1 Plant Material and RNA Extraction

The roots of *G. uralensis* were collected from the herb garden in Beijing University of Chinese Medicine, Beijing, China. Samples were immersed in liquid nitrogen during the field collection and identified by Professor Chunsheng Liu (Beijing University of Chinese Medicine). Total RNA of *G. uralensis* was extracted from approximately 1 g fresh tissue using the "Trizol" reagent (Beijing MeiLaiBo medical technology Co., LTD), following the manufacturer's instructions. Final RNA concentrations were determined by spectrophotometry and their integrity was examined by electrophoresis in 1 % (w/v) agarose gel.

32.2.2 Molecular Cloning of the GuSQS cDNA

Single-stranded cDNA was synthesized from 1 μg of total RNA using the primers oligo (dT) and reverse transcriptase M-MLV (Takara) in 10 μL reactions, following the manufacturer's instructions. Based on the SQS cDNA sequences recorded in Genbank (AM182329 and D86409), the primers were designed using conserved regions (Table 32.1). RT-PCR was used to obtain the *Gu*SQS cDNA and the cycling parameters were as follows: 94 °C for 5 min; 35cycles of 94 °C for 30 s, annealing at 57 °C for 30 s, extension at 72 °C for 90 s; a final extension at 72 °C for 10 min. The SQS cDNA was obtained and sequenced. The open reading frame (ORF) was determined by ORF finder of NCBI. *Gu*SQS deduced amino acid sequence was aligned with the publicly available SQS groups using ClustalX and MEGA version 4.0 and a neighbor-joining tree was constructed.

32.2.3 Heterologous Expression of G. uralensis *SQS in* E. coli

*Gu*SQS1 ORF and *Gu*SQS2 ORF were amplified using primer pairs SQS-1F′, SQS-1R′ and SQS-2F′, SQS-2R′ (Table 32.1) respectively, which contained restriction enzyme cutting sites (EcoR I and Sal I) that marked by underline. The PCR procedure for *Gu*SQS1 was as follows: 94 °C for 4 min; 35 cycles of 94 °C for 30 s, annealing at 57 °C for 30 s, extension at 72 °C for 90 s; a final extension at 72 °C for 10 min. The PCR procedure for *Gu*SQS2 was as follows: 94 °C for 4 min; 35cycles of 94 °C for 30 s, annealing at 60 °C for 30 s, extension at 72 °C for 90 s; a final extension at 72 °C for 10 min.The amplified fragments were subcloned into pMD19-T (Takara, Japan), and then digested with EcoR I and Sal I (3 h at 37 °C). After digestion, the fragments were ligated into the cloning site of EcoR I- Sal I digested pET-32a plasmid for expression of recombinant His-tag fusion protein (Novagen). The resulting recombinant pET-SQS1 plasmid and pET-SQS2 plasmid were transferred into disarmed *E.coli* BL21, and sequenced to check for correct insertion. Individual correct colonies were transferred to 8 mL of

Table 32.1 Primer pairs used in this paper

Gene	Primer	Sequence (5′-3′)
SQS1	SQS-1F	ATGGGGAGTTTGGGAGCGAT
	SQS-1R	CGTGTTTGACCATTCGTTTC
	SQS-1F′	GCAGAATTCATGGGGAGTTTGGGAGCGAT (*Eco*RI)
	SQS-1R′	CACGTCGACCGTGTTTGACCATTCGTTTC (*Sal*I)
SQS2	SQS-2F	ATGGGGAGTTTGGGAGCGAT
	SQS-2R	CTAGTTATTTTGGCGGTTGGCAG
	SQS-2F′	GCAGAATTCATGGGGAGTTTGGGAGCGAT (*Eco*RI)
	SQS-2R′	CACGTCGACCTAGTTATTTTGGCGGTTGGCAG (*Sal*I)

Luria-Bertani medium supplemented with ampicillin (50 mg/mL) and cultured overnight at 37 °C and 150 rpm. Both supernatant and pellet were examined by SDS-PAGE (12 % resolving gel, 5 % stacking gel) using Coomassie brilliant blue staining. Negative controls used comparable preparations possessing a void vector.

The fusion proteins were purified as follows: The recombinant *E.coli* BL21 containing pET-SQS1 and pET-SQS2 respectively was collected by centrifugation and resuspended with PBS after inducing, which was frozenthawed three times using liquid nitrogen. Then the target proteins were released from the cells by sonication (6 times, 10 s each time, interval was 10 s, voltage was 100–300 V). Centrifugation was carried out for 20 min at 4 °C, 10,000 rpm. Supernatant was purified by flowing through the Ni^{2+}-NTA column (using wash buffer to elute the impurity proteins, using elution buffer to elute the target protein with 6-His).

32.2.4 Enzyme Assay and Product Analysis of GuSQS

For enzymatic assay of *Gu*SQS, 200 μL of a reaction mixture containing a certain amout of K_2HPO_4 (1 mol·L^{-1}, PH = 7.2), 7.7 μL FPP (1 %, V/V), 10 μL $MgCl_2$ (0.25 mol·L^{-1}), 6 μL *β*-mercaptoethanol (10 %, V/V), 10μL NADPH (0.1 mol·L^{-1}), and 17.12 μL *Gu*SQS1 protein (the amount of the final was 5 μg) or 21.46 μL *Gu*SQS2 protein (the amount of the final was 5 μg) were used. Reactions were initiated by crude extract addition, incubated at 35 °C for 50 min, and terminated by adding 100 μL 6 M HCl. Negative control was performed under the same conditions but using the extract form *E. coli* carrying an empty vector. 100 μL normal hexane was used to extract and GC–MS (Trace GC and Trace DSQ) was used to qualitatively analyse the reaction products. The chromatographic column was DB5-MS column (Agilent, 30 m × 0.25 mm × 0.25 μm). Temperature procedure was as follows: standing at 120 °C for 3 min, warming up to 180 °C at 15 °C·min^{-1}, warming up to 260 °C at 25 °C·min^{-1} and standing for 25 min. Inlet temperature was 260 °C, carrier gas was high purity helium, flow rate of carrier gas was 1 mL·min^{-1}, sampling injection mode was splitless sampling and the sample size was 1 μL. Mass spectrum conditions were as follows: GC–MS interface temperature was 260 °C, ion source temperature was 230 °C, ionization way was EI, and ionization voltage was 70 eV. The structure of production was searched using NIST 2.01.

32.3 Results

32.3.1 Molecular Cloning of the GuSQS cDNA

Using a pair of primers, SQS1-F and SQS1-R (Table 32.1), a 1,421 bp fragment was amplified. Using a pair of primers, SQS2-F and SQS2-R (Table 32.1),

Table 32.2 Physical and chemical properties of the amino acid sequences of *Gu*SQS1 and *Gu*SQS2

Items	*Gu*SQS1	*Gu*SQS2
Number of amino acid	413	412
Molecular weight (Da)	47284.1	47026.1
Isoelectric point	8.36	8.39
Instability index	42.39	36.36
Aliphatic index	97.29	94.25
Total average of hydrophobicity	−0.063	−0.080

a 1,239 bp fragment was amplified. After Blast analysis in NCBI, the two fragments were determined to be cDNA sequences of *Gu*SQS1 and *Gu*SQS2. Due to the primer pairs used in the experiment, the 1,421 bp fragment of *Gu*SQS1 (GQ266154) only included a 1,242 bp ORF and a 179 bp 3′-UTR, and the 1,239 bp fragment of *Gu*SQS2 (GQ266153) only included a 1,239 bp ORF. The ORF of *Gu*SQS1 had 3 more bases comparing with the ORF of *Gu*SQS2.

Using BlastX to analyse the cDNA sequences of *Gu*SQS1, *Gu*SQS2 and other publicly available SQS sequences, such as *G. glabra* (D86409, D86410), *Lotus japonicus* (BAC56854.1), *Panax notoginseng* (ABA29019.1), *Nicotiana tabacum* (AAB08578.1), *Artemisia annua* (AF302464.2) reveals that the most closely related sequence to *Gu*SQS1 is a sequence from *G. glabra* (D86409), with which it shares 98 % similarity, and the most closely related sequence to *Gu*SQS2 is a sequence from *G. glabra* (D86410), with which it shares 98 % similarity.

32.3.2 Analysis of Amino Acid Sequences of GuSQS1 and GuSQS2 and the Comparison with Other Species

The amino acid sequences of *Gu*SQS1 and *Gu*SQS2 were analysed (Tables 32.2, 32.3 and 32.4), the results showed that the physical–chemical properties, amino acid composition and secondary structure of *Gu*SQS1 and *Gu*SQS2 were close to each other. In the secondary structure of *Gu*SQS1 and *Gu*SQS2, the frequency of occurrence of α-helix was highest and the frequency of occurrence of β-pleated

Table 32.3 Analysis of amino acid composition

Amino acid	*Gu*SQS1		*Gu*SQS2	
	Number	Frequency of occurrence (%)	Number	Frequency of occurrence (%)
Charged amino acid (RKHYCDE)	140	33.90	137	33.25
Acidic amino acid (DE)	48	11.62	47	11.41
Basic amino acid (KR)	52	12.59	51	12.38
Polar amino acid (NCQSTY)	101	24.46	100	24.27
Nonpolar amino acid (AILFWV)	156	37.77	155	37.62

Table 32.4 Prediction of secondary structure

		*Gu*SQS1	*Gu*SQS2
α-helix	Number	344	359
	Frequency of occurrence (%)	83.30	87.14
β-pleated sheet	Number	3	3
	Frequency of occurrence (%)	0.73	0.73
Random coil	Number	66	61
	Frequency of occurrence (%)	15.98	14.81

sheet was lowest, which revealed that the structure of *Gu*SQS1 and *Gu*SQS2 was conservative.

Analysis of transmembrance domain of *Gu*SQS1 and *Gu*SQS2 (Fig. 32.1) showed that there were two transmembrance helix in *Gu*SQS1 and *Gu*SQS2 and they were transmembrance protein. The prediction of signal peptide sequence of *Gu*SQS1 and *Gu*SQS2 using SignalP2.0 showed the mean S-score was 0.47, less than 0.5, which revealed they were not secretory protein (Fig. 32.2).

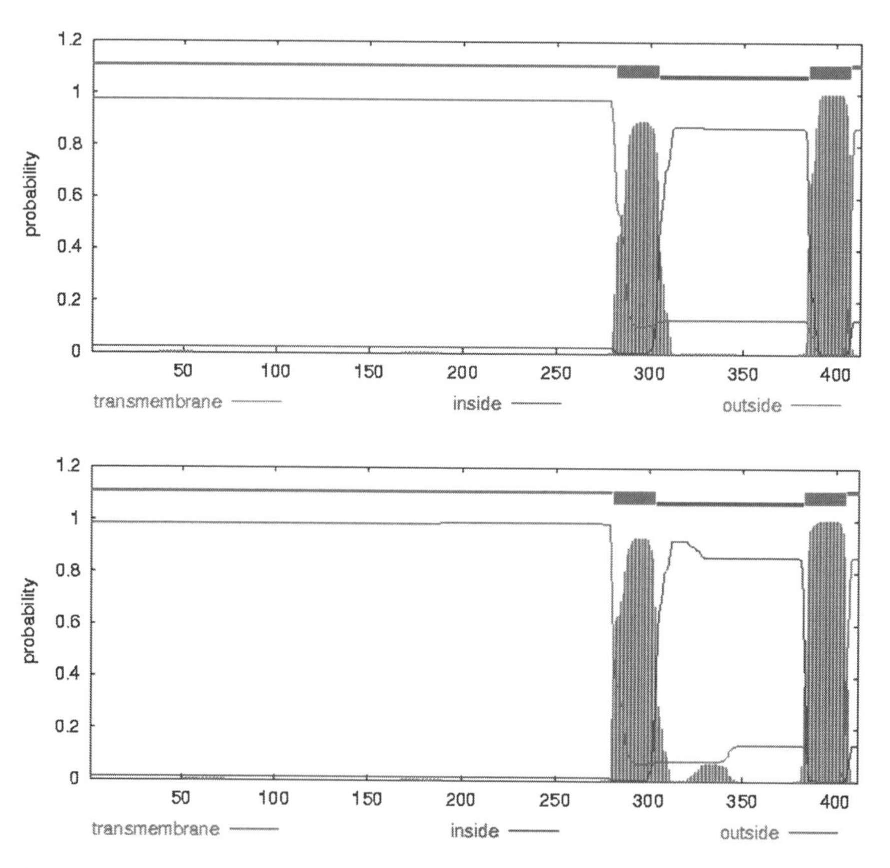

Fig. 32.1 Prediction of transmembrance domain of *Gu*SQS1 (*the upward figure*) and *Gu*SQS2 (*the downward figure*)

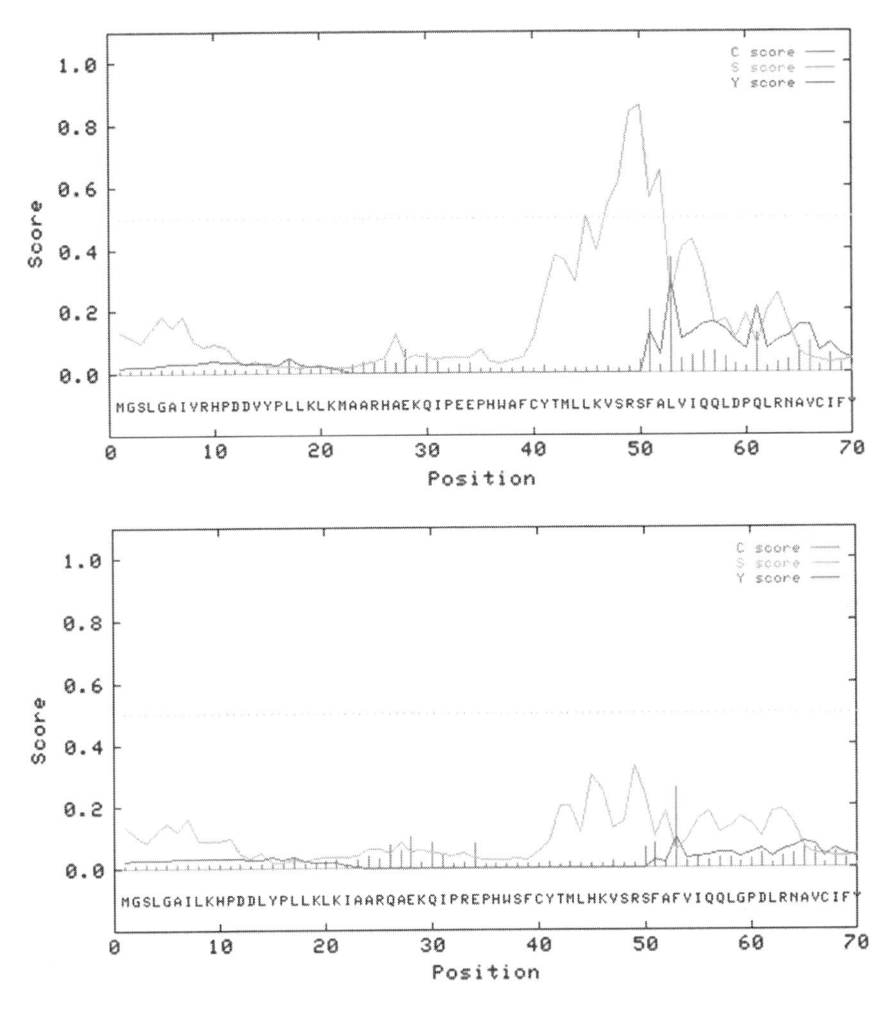

Fig. 32.2 The prediction of signal peptide sequence of *Gu*SQS1 (*the upward figure*) and *Gu*SQS2 (*the downward figure*)

Comparing amino acid sequences of *Gu*SQS1, *Gu*SQS2 and seven other species registered in Genbank (Fig. 32.3), 6 domains (I to VI) closely related to catalytic function were revealed [15]. Among them III, IV and V were more conservative than I and II. The conservative sequence containing a lot of aspartic acid (DXXDD) was present in II and IV, which would influence the combination of FPP and Mg^{2+} [2, 20]. The similar sequences were present in other isoprene synthetase, such as FPP synthetase [18], was typical structure of terpene synthetase. III could influence the production of intermediate product PSPP, and V was

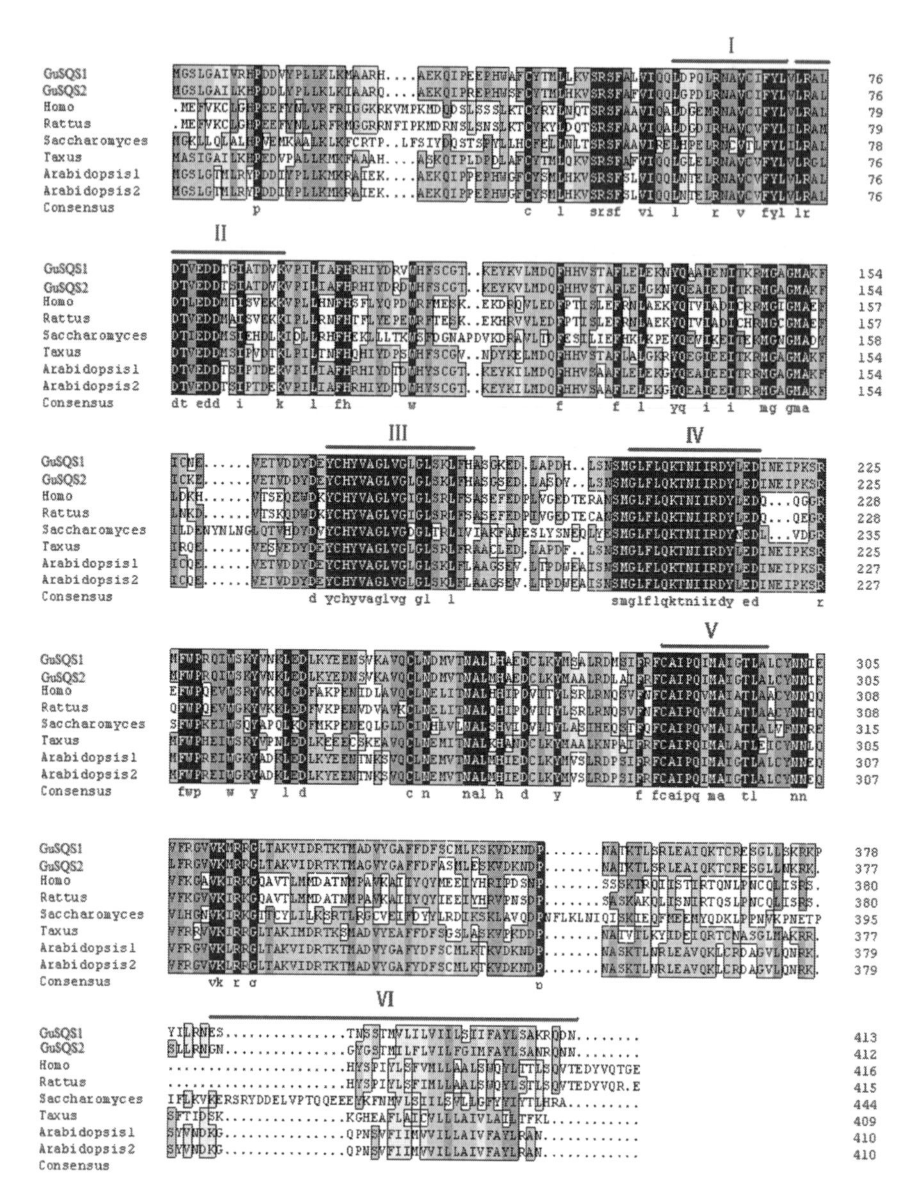

Fig. 32.3 Comparing of amino acid sequences of *Gu*SQS1, *Gu*SQS2 and seven other species (*Homo* (S76822), *Rattus* (M95591), *Taxus* (DQ836053), *Arabidopsis* 1 (U79159), *Arabidopsis* 2 (AF004396), *Saccharomyces* (NP_014175), *Gu*SQS1 (GQ266154), *Gu*SQS2 (GQ266153))

the binding domain of NADPH controlling the transformation from PSPP to squalene [20]. VI was present at the end of C-terminal, it was a highly hydrophobic region and considered as the anchoring signal of biological membrane [15].

32.3.3 Molecular Evolution Analysis of SQS

The molecular phylogenetic tree (Fig. 32.4), constructed by the neighbor-joining method in MEGA version 4.0, based on aligning publicly available SQS amino acid sequences, showed that there were two subgroup clades, SQS1 and SQS2 from *A. thaliana* clustered to one clade and all the other SQS clustered to the other clade. So it was considered that in the evolution of SQS the divergence of *A. thaliana* might be earlier than other species. Furthermore, SQS from the same family clustered to the same branch, for example *C. annuum*, *N. tabacum* and *S. tuberosum* all came from *Solanaceae*, *B. falcatum* and *C. asiatica* both came from *Umbelliferae*, *P. ginseng* and *P. notoginseng* both came from *Araliaceae*, *G. max*, *L. japonicus*, *G. glabra* and *G. uralensis* all came from *Leguminosae*. These

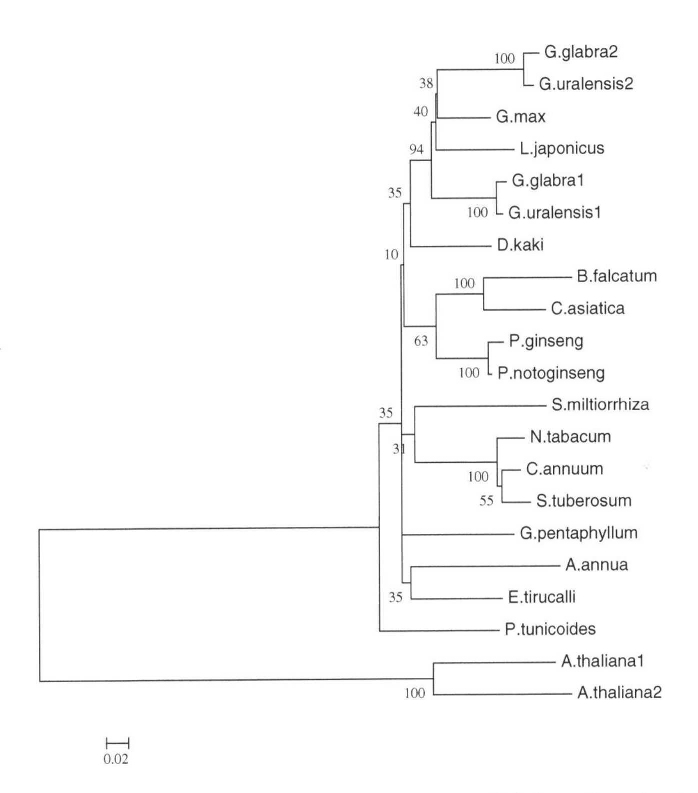

Fig. 32.4 Phylogenetic tree showing the relationship between SQS from *G. uralensis* and some other species retrieved from the Genbank. (*A. annua* (AF302464); *A. thaliana* 1 (U79159); *A. thaliana* 2 (AF004396); *B. falcatum* (AY964186);*C. annuum* (AF124842); *C. asiatica* (AY787628); *D. kaki* (FJ687954); *E. tirucalli* (AB433916); *G. glabra* 1 (D86409); *G. glabra* 2 (D86410); *G. max* (AB007503); *G. pentaphyllum* (FJ906799); *G. uralensis* 1 (GQ266154); *G. uralensis* 2 (GQ266153); *L. japonicus* (AB102688); *N. tabacum* (U60057); *P. ginseng* (AB115496); *P. notoginseng* (DQ18663); *P. tenuifolia* (DQ672339), *P. tunicoides* (EF585250); *S. miltiorrhiza* (FJ768961); *S. tuberosum* (AB022599))

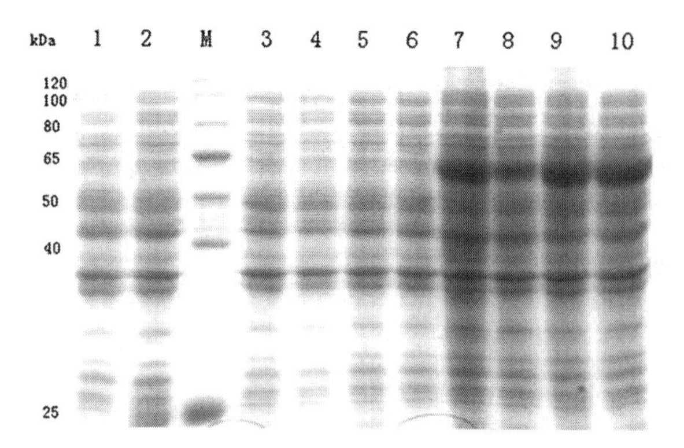

Fig. 32.5 SDS-PAGE results of pET-SQS fusion protein M: marker; 1: pET-32a (no induction); 2: pET-32a (after 4 h induction); 3, 4: pET-SQS1 (no induction); 5, 6: pET-SQS2 (no induction); 7, 8: pET-SQS1 (after 4 h induction); 9, 10: pET-SQS2 (after 4 h induction)

revealed that the evolution of amino acid sequences of SQS was according to the genetic relationship. Furthermore, in the evolutionary timeline the appearance of *Gu*SQS1 was earlier than *Gu*SQS2. All the SQS proteins came from the same ancestor and processed the similar function.

32.3.4 Heterologous Expression of G. uralensis *SQS in* E. coli

We expressed the isolated cDNA in *E.coli* as fusion proteins. SDS-PAGE analysis demonstrated the presence of a recombinant protein of apparent molecular mass 67 kDa (consistent with the predicted size of the translation product). This protein was absent from the cultures of bacteria carrying a void vector (Figs. 32.5 and 32.6).

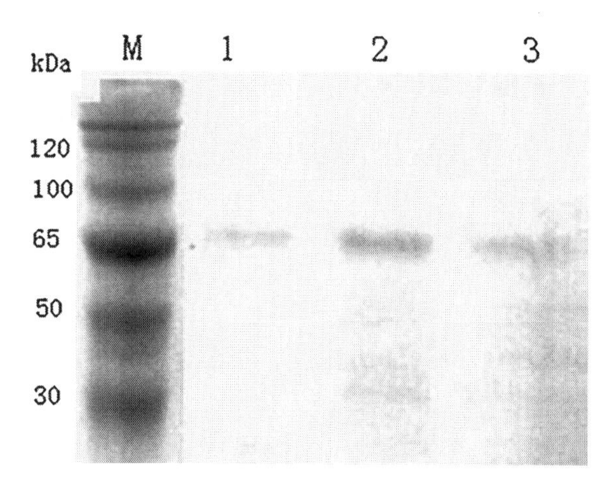

Fig. 32.6 SDS-PAGE rusults of pET-SQS fusion protein after purification (1 ~ 3: fusion protein after purification; M: marker)

32.3.5 Enzyme Assay and Product Analysis of G. uralensis *SQS*

To examine the activity of the recombinant SQS protein, the crude extract from induced *E. coli* with recombinant pET-SQS plasmid was used for the squalene synthesis reaction. The reaction carried out with the extract from *E. coli* with a void vector was treated as a negative control. TLC analysis demonstrated that a new product was produced in the synthesis reaction, while it was not present in the negative control carrying an empty vector. A standard sample of squalene and the peak present in the *E. coli* transformed with pET-SQS but absent when transformed with empty pET32a were analyzed by GC–MS (Fig. 32.7). In total ion chromatorgraphy of GC–MS, retention time of production squalene was 18.48. In MS spectrogram, the results revealed that the characteristic peaks (*m/z*: 41, 69, 81, 137) of the novel product were the same as that of the authentic squalene. All the above revealed that the recombinant SQS could catalyze FPP to form squalene.

32.4 Discussion

In conclusion, in these experiments two cDNA sequences coding squalene synthase involved in glycyrrhizic acid biosynthesis in *G. uralensis* has been obtained and characterized. As a result, a 1,421 bp cDNA sequence encoding a 413-residue protein and a 1,239 bp cDNA sequence encoding a 412-residue protein were obtained. The amino acid sequences of *Gu*SQS1 and *Gu*SQS2 were analysed, the results showed that the physical–chemical properties, amino acid composition and secondary structure of *Gu*SQS1 and *Gu*SQS2 were close to each other. And it was speculated that they were transmembrance protein but secretory protein. We compared the amino acid sequences of SQS from *G. uralensis* and other species. 6 domains (I to VI) were found. The conservative sequence containing a lot of aspartic acid (DXXDD) was present in domain II and IV, which would influence the combination of FPP and Mg^{2+}, was typical structure of terpene synthetase. Domain III could influence the production of intermediate product PSPP, and domain V was the binding domain of NADPH controlling the transformation from PSPP to squalene. Domain VI was present at the end of C-terminal and considered as the anchoring signal of biological membrane.

Both TLC analysis and GC/MS demonstrated that a new product was produced in the synthesis reaction, while it was not present in the negative control carrying an empty vector. So we could come to a conclusion that the expression products of the genes isolated in this study could catalyze FPP to form squalene.

In recent years excessive collection of wild *G. uralensis* have led to the exhaustion of this Chinese herb. Many researchers tried to solve this problem in a variety of different ways. It is interesting and meaningful to improving the accumulation of glycyrrhizic acid in cultivars of *G. uralensis* using metabolic

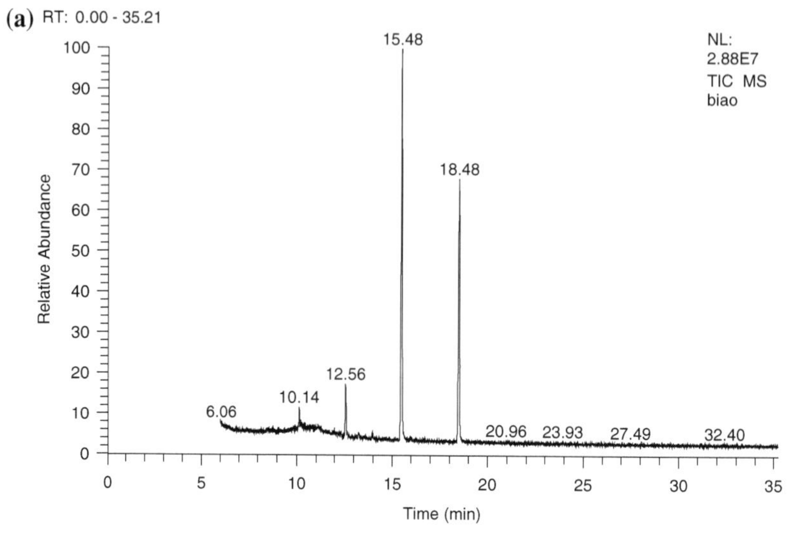

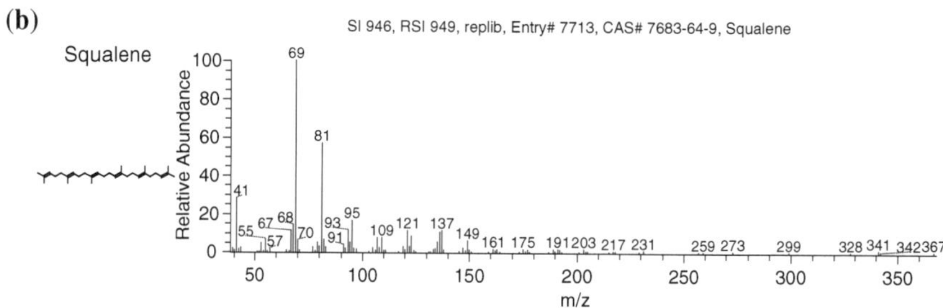

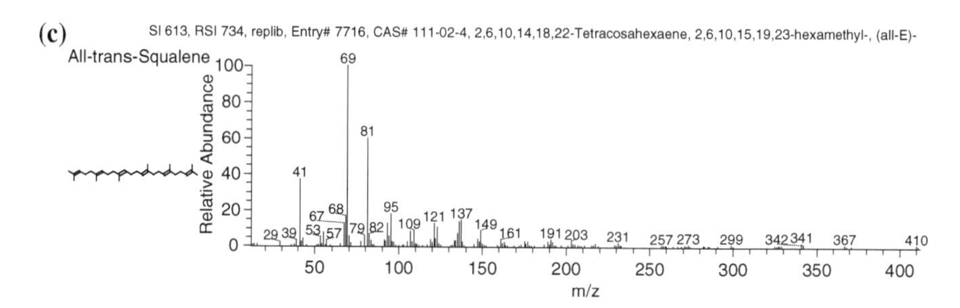

Fig. 32.7 The results of GC–MS **a** Total ion chromatorgraphy of standard solution, **b** Mass spectrogram and structure of standard substance squalene, **c** Mass spectrogram and structure of production squalene

engineering method. In our other studies we have found that there are different copies of functional genes in different *G. uralensis* plants [9–12]. And it is well known that the differences in dose of genes can cause the differences in the content of the relative enzyme and finally result in the differences in the content of products. Meanwhile we have also revealed the polymorphism of 3-hydroxy-3-methylglutary-coenzyme A reductase gene in different *G. uralensis* plants, which can

also influence the production of relative metabolites [9–12]. Therefore the cloning and characterization of functional genes are very important. This study can be used as an significant basis for further work on improving the efficacy of *G. uralensis* by means of a higher glycyrrhizic acid content, and exploring the biosynthesis of glycyrrhizic acid in vitro.

References

1. Cherng JM, Lin HJ, Hsu YH, Hung MS, Lin JC (2004) A quantitative bioassay for HIV-1 gene expression based on UV activation effect of glycyrrhizin. Antiviral Res 62:27–36
2. Devarenne TP, Shin DH, Back K, Yin S, Chappell J (1998) Molecular characterization of tobacco squalene synthase and regulation in response to fungal elicitor. Arch Biochem Biophys 349:205–215
3. Hiroaki H, Pengyu H, Kenichiro I (2003) Up-regulation of soyasaponin biosynthesis by methyl jasmonate in cultured cells of *Glycyrrhiza glabra*. Plant Cell Physiol 44(4):404–411
4. Hoever G, Bzltina L, Michaelis M (2005) Antiviral activity of glycyrrhizin derivatives against SARS-coronavirus. J Med Chem 48:1256–1259
5. Hyung KK, Yoonkyung P, Hee NK et al (2002) Antimicrobial mechanism of b-glycyrrhetinic acid isolated from licorice, *Glycyrrhiza glabra*. Biotechnol Lett 24:1899–1902
6. Kribii R, Arro M, Arco AD, Gonzalez V, Balcells L, Delourme D, Ferrer A, Karst F, Boronat A (1997) Cloning and characterization of the *Arabidopsis thaliana* SQS1 gene encoding squalene synthase involvement of the C-terminal region of the enzyme in the channeling of squalene through the sterol pathway. Eur J Biochem 249:61–69
7. Lee MH, Jeong JH, Seo JW, Shin CG, Kim YS, In JG, Yang DC, Yi JS, Choi YE (2004) Enhanced triterpene and phytosterol biosynthesis in Panax ginseng overexpressing squalene synthase gene. Plant Cell Physiol 45:976–984
8. Liu DJ (2011) Researches on the correlation between CNVs of HMGR, SQS1, β-AS gene and origin and morphology of *Glycyrrhiza uralensis*. Master Dissertation of Beijing University of Chinese Medicine. Beljing, pp 8–11
9. Liu Y, Liu DJ, Liu CS, Liao CL, Cheng XL (2012) Mechanism of genuineness of liquorice *Glycyrrhiza uralensis* based on CNVs of SQS, SQS1 and β-AS gene. Acta Pharmaceutica Sinica 47(2):250–255
10. Liu Y, Xu QX, Wang XY, Liu CS, Chen HH (2012) Researches on the influence of 3-hydroxy-3-methylglutary-coenzyme A reductase gene polymorphism on catalytic efficiency of its encode enzyme in *Glycyrrhiza uralensis*. China J Chin Materia Medica 37(24):3784–3788
11. Liu Y, Xu QX, Wang XY, Liu CS, Chen HH (2012) Analysis on correlation between 3-hydroxy-3-methylglutary-coenzyme A reductase gene polymorphism of *Glycyrrhiza uralensis* and content of glycyrrhizin. China J Chin Materia Medica 37(24):3789–3792
12. Liu Y, Zhang N, Wang XY, Liu CS, Chen HH, Wen H (2012) Researches on influence of squalene synthase gene polymorphism on catalytic efficiency of its encode enzyme in *Glycyrrhiza uralensis*. C J Chin Materia Medica 37(24):3777–3783
13. Lu HY, Liu JM, Zhang HC, Yin T, Gao SL (2008) Ri-mediated transformation of *Glycyrrhiza uralensis* with a squalene synthase gene (GuSQS1) for production of glycyrrhizin. Plant Mol Biol Rep 26:1–11

14. Mirjalili MH, Moyano E, Bonfill M, Cusido RM, Palazon J (2011) Overexpression of the *Arabidopsis thaliana* squalene synthase gene in *Withania coagulans* hairy root cultures. Biol Plant 55(2):357–360
15. Robinson GW, Tsay YH, Kienzle BK, Smith-Monroy CA, Bishop RW (1993) Conservation between human and fungal squalene synthetases: similarities in structure, function, and regulation. Mol Cell Biol 13:2706–2717
16. Seo JW, Jeong JH, Shin CG, Lo SC, Han SS, Yu KW, Harada E, Han JY, Choi YE (2005) Overexpression of squalene synthase in Eleutherococcus senticosus increases phytosterol and triterpene accumulation. Phytochemistry 66:869–877
17. Shibata S (2000) A drug over the millennia: Pharmacognosy, chemistry, and pharmacology of licorice. Yakugaku Zasshi 120:849–862
18. Song L, Poulter CD (1994) Yeast farnesyl-diphosphate synthase: site-directed mutagenesis of residues in highly conserved prenyltransferase domains I and II. Proc Natl Acad Sci USA 91:3044–3048
19. State Pharmacopoeia Committee (2010) Pharmacopoeia of China, Part 1. Chemical Industry Press, Beijing, pp 80–81
20. Tansey TR, Shechter I (2001) Squalene synthase: structure and regulation. Prog Nucleic Acid Res Mol Biol 65:157–195
21. Van Rossum TG, Vulto AG (1999) Intravenous glycyrrhizin for the treatment of chronic hepatitis C: a double blind, randomized, placebo-controlled phase I/II trial. J Gastroenterol Hepatol 14:1093–1099
22. Zeng L, Li SH, Lou ZC (1988) Morphological and histological studies of Chinese licorice. Acta Pharm Sin 23:200–208

Chapter 33
Ontology-Based Multi-Agent Cooperation EHR Semantic Interoperability Pattern Research

Jian Yang and Jiancheng Dong

Abstract EHR semantic interoperability problems have long been academic and industrial research hotspots and difficulties. By using Description Logic-based semantic web knowledge representation, first it gets a semantic interoperability document for EHR and packages it into a communicational message structure of agent communication language named KQML which support semantic.Then satisfy two aspects of semantic EHR interoperability requirements with a multi-agent cooperation model: Semantic integration and transparent query of heterogeneous EHR data sources, semantic interoperability of Heterogeneous EHR systems.

Keywords Ontology · Multi-agent Semantic interoperability · EHR

33.1 Introduction

The rapid development of the Internet makes massive data growth which dispersed throughout the network. It brings some difficulties when people analyze the data. How to integrate dispersed heterogeneous data sources in the network, so that the heterogeneous information systems which have different information representation and protocol could achieve interoperability becomes a research focus [1]. Heterogeneity of electronic health records data source, complexity of regional health network and the health system, is ideally suited to show the ability of multi-agent collaboration in semantic interoperability [2, 3].

J. Yang (✉) · J. Dong
Deptartment of Medical Informatics, Nantong University, Qixiu Road #19, 226001 Nantong, China
e-mail: dongjc@ntu.edu.cn

S. Li et al. (eds.), *Frontier and Future Development of Information Technology in Medicine and Education*, Lecture Notes in Electrical Engineering 269,
DOI: 10.1007/978-94-007-7618-0_33,

33.2 Multi-Agent Semantic Communication Mechanism

33.2.1 Agent Communication Language KQML

The universal communication language of smart subject is KQML (Knowledge Query and Manipulation Language), which is proposed by Knowledge Sharing Effort Plan of United States [4]. KQML contains three levels that are communication layer, message layer and the content layer. Subject package and send the content which is a semantic document in the content layer to achieve semantic sharing and interoperability.

Set sending agent is A, accepting agent is B, semantic document is X and the domain ontology is identified as URI,then a typical KQML message like :(tell :sender A :receiver B :ontology URI :content :(X)). The KQML message built-in carries the knowledge of domain ontology identity, that multi-agent collaborative uses KQML for semantic communicating becoming possible.

33.2.2 DL-Based Domain Ontology Knowledge Expression

The basis of semantic interoperability needs the identical understanding of the concepts and knowledge in the same knowledge universe, and the semantic interoperability of electronic health records, for example, that heterogeneous health information systems in domain need to comply with the same ontology [5]. As the development of semantic web technology, description logic gradually becomes the principal tool of knowledge expression. Description logic has not only effective expression skills, but also has decidability. Description logic is a formal tool based on objective knowledge representation and knowledge-based reasoning. It is the decidable subset of the first-order predicate logic, and its principal motivation is to provide a formal foundation to semantic network [6]. Currently, W3C recommended OWL as ontology description language in the hierarchical system architecture. The corresponding relationship of OWL constructor operator, axiom and Description Logic SHIQ is shown in Table 33.1.

According to the classification and hierarchy of domain experts on regional health information in Chinese standards "Basic Framework and Data Standards of Health Records (Trial)" and "Health Information Data Metadirectory", the article selects hypertension follow-up of hypertension patients management in the disease management dataset as a case,the dataset number is HRB04.01.Hypertension patients follow-up include symptoms, signs, medications and other components, these subjects include a number of follow-up data [7].

Knowledge universe of electronic health records is set to I. The concept collection of TBox is set to CI, the collection of concept relationship is set to PI.

Let CI = {FOLLOWUPSERVICE, SYMPTOM, SIGNS, MEDICATION, ITEMMEDICATION, LEVEL}, respectively corresponding to the concept of

Table 33.1 The correspondence of OWL DL and description logic SHIQ

OWL DL class constructor operator			
OWL element	DL grammar	OWL element	DL grammar
intersectionOf	$C1 \cap \ldots \cap Cn$	allValuesFrom	$\forall P.C$
unionOf	$C1 \cup \ldots \cup Cn$	someValuesFrom	$\exists P.C$
complementOf	$\neg C$	maxCardinality	$\geq nP$
oneOf	$\{x1\ldots xn\}$	minCardinality	$\leq nP$
hasValue	$\exists P.\{x\}$	inverseOf	P^-
OWL DL Axiom			
Axiom	DL grammar	Axiom	DL grammar
subClassOf	$C1 \subseteq C2$	equivalentProperty	$P1 \equiv P2$
equivalentClass	$C1 \equiv C2$	inverseOf	$P1 \equiv P2^-$
disjointWith	$C1 \sqsubseteq \neg C2$	TransitiveProperty	$P^+ \sqsubseteq P$
sameAs	$\{x1\} \equiv \{x2\}$	FunctionalProperty	$T \sqsubseteq \leq 1P$
differentFrom	$\{x1\} \sqsubseteq \neg \{x2\}$	InverseFunctionalProperty	$T \sqsubseteq \leq 1P^-$
subPropertyOf	$P1 \sqsubseteq P2$	SymmetricProperty	$P \equiv P^-$

follow-up services, symptoms, signs, medications, medication entry privilege level.And the confidential level of hypertension patients follow-up service value of opening to all(0), opening to doctor(1), only opening to the responsible doctor(2).

Let PI = {hasComponent, hasItem, hasLevel}, hasComponent means "composed of parts", hasItem means "contain entry", hasLevel means "have confidential level".

The formal semantics of the domain ontology model of hypertension patients follow-up (Hypertension Followup Ontology Model, HFOM) are as follows:

$\text{FOLLOWUPSERVICE} \equiv ((\geq 1\ \text{hasComponent.SIGNS}) \leq 1\ \text{hasComponent.SIGNS}) \cup (\geq 1\ \text{hasComponent.MEDICATION}) \leq 1\ \text{hasComponent.MEDICATION}) \cup (\geq 1\ \text{hasComponent.SYMPTOM}) \leq 1\ \text{hasComponent.SYMPTOM})) \cap \neg \exists \text{hasLevel}.\{0\}$

$\text{SYMPTOM} \equiv (\exists\ \text{hasItem}.\{x_{HR51.01.178}\}) \cap \neg \exists \text{hasLevel}.\{0\}$

$\text{SIGNS} \equiv ((\geq 1\ \text{hasComponent}.\{x_{HR51.02.004}\} \cap \leq 1\ \text{hasComponent}.\{x_{HR51.02.004}\}) \cup \ldots \cup (\geq 1\ \text{hasComponent}.\{x_{HR51.02.035}\} \cap \leq 1\ \text{hasComponent}.\{x_{HR51.02.035}\})) \cap \neg \exists \text{hasLevel}.\{0\}$

$\text{MEDICATION} \equiv (\exists\ \text{hasItem.ITEMMEDICATION}) \cap \neg \exists \text{hasLevel}.\{0\}$

$\text{ITEMMEDICATION} \equiv ((\geq 1\ \text{hasComponent}.\{x_{HR53.01.002}\} \cap \leq 1\ \text{hasComponent}.\{x_{HR53.01.002}\}) \cup \ldots \cup (\geq 1\ \text{hasComponent}.\{x_{HR55.02.030}\} \cap \leq 1\ \text{hasComponent}.\{x_{HR55.02.030}\})) \cap \neg \exists \text{hasLevel}.\{0\}$

According to the formal description of the hypertension patient follow-up, agent can extract semantics as follows: hypertension patient follow-up is composed of one symptom, one sign and one drug use; drug use includes at least one medication entry component, medication entry is composed of individuals which identified by data element numbers that are HR53. 01.002 (drug name) to HR55. 02.030 (adverse drug reactions); symptom is composed of at least one individuals which identified by data element number that is HR51.01. 178; sign is composed of individuals which identified by data element numbers that are HR51. 02.004 (weight) to HR51. 02.035 (diastolic pressure). These components and hypertension patient follow-up are not open to everyone.

With a common understanding of the knowledge representation, it provides support for semantic interoperability and can generate semantic interoperability entity content. Extensible Markup Language (XML) released in February 1998 by the W3C is a standard that separates the content, structure and form of data. The self-describing nature of XML has a satisfactory performance of representing many complex data relationships. Nowadays, XML has gradually become one of the standard mechanisms for data and document exchange. Modeling by HFOM meta model mentioned above, there is an example of semantic document, semantic document packages into KQML then the complete semantic interoperability message is as follows:

```
（Tell
  ： sender A
  ： receiver B
  ： ontology http://www.chinaehr.org/owl/hypertension_followupservice#
  ： content （
  <FollowUpService>
        <Symptom><HR51.01.178>Headache</HR51.01.178>
                <HR51.01.178>Tinnitus</HR51.01.178></Symptom>
        <Signs><HR51.02.004>75</HR51.02.004>……
                <HR51.02.035>60</HR51.02.035></Signs>
        <Medication>
                <MedicationItem><HR53.01.002>Hydrochlorothiazide</HR
53.01.002>……<HR53.01.002>False</HR53.01.002></MedicationItem>
                <MedicationItem><HR53.01.002>Spironolactone</HR53.01.
002>……<HR53.01.002>False</HR53.01.002></MedicationItem>
        </Medication>
  </FollowUpService>)
  )
```

Compliance the same HFOM ontology model, multi-agent agreed semantic consensus, with semantic document carried by KQML achieves semantic transfer, cooperation with performative of KQML achieves semantic interoperability. The above clearly shows the concept and the concept of has_a relations, cardinality constraint. Through extended SWRL language as well as the ability of SHOIQ(D), it can be further extended knowledge representation. Combined with health information data element value domain code standards, it can take the value range of data type and inference rules into the knowledge element model. It can be achieved Deep semantic interoperability through agent collaboration by tagging, parsing, reasoning, verification.

33.3 Semantic Interoperability Model Based on MAS

33.3.1 Model Introduction

Figure 33.1 shows two abilities of semantic interoperability: the interaction of heterogeneous information systems, and the integration of heterogeneous resources [8]. Semantic interoperability of heterogeneous systems is achieved through information semantic annotation by converting agent, sending information to target heterogeneous system and the target system extract semantic info by converting agent; the model also provides transparent data integration capabilities of heterogeneous systems by querying and integrating the data pieces by query agent and sending back the results to user by coordinating agent.

Ontology based Multi-Agent Cooperation Interoperability Model contains Facilitator Agent (FA), User Agent (UA), Query Agent (QA), Query Agent Cluster (QAC), Exchange Agent (EA), Exchange Agent Cluster (EAC), System Agent (SA). With cooperation of these agent, the model can achieve transparent semantic integration and query of heterogeneous data sources and semantic interoperability of heterogeneous systems.

UA and SA resides in the terminal, UA provides retrieval interface to users, SA provides semantic interoperability interface to information systems. UA assists users to semantic query needs and submit the needs to FA.FA maintains a state list of QAC and EAC, addition, FA also maintains a routine list of intelligent agents. FA can choose the most appropriate QA and EA based on a certain decision rule and according to the two lists.

33.3.2 Model Operation Mechanism

The semantic interoperability of heterogeneous systems: After received interoperability request from SA, FA chooses appropriate EA according to state list and then obtain an address from routine table according to the target heterogeneous system which the interoperability request, FA send request content and target address to EA. EA extracts semantic info by domain ontology and send it to the target system SA. The target SA makes corresponding operation according to the content and operation type and send result back.

The semantic integration and transparent query of heterogeneous data sources: After received query request from UA, FA chooses appropriate QA according to QAC state list, QA is instanced as Main Query Agent (MQA), MQA construct several Cloned Query Agent (CQA) according to the number of required data source.CQA send query request to corresponding SA according to the responsible data source address, the target SA executes local search with query content and send result back to CQA, then CQA return data to MQA, at last, MQA collects and integrates information from several CQA and gives information to FA which is responsible for sending result to users.

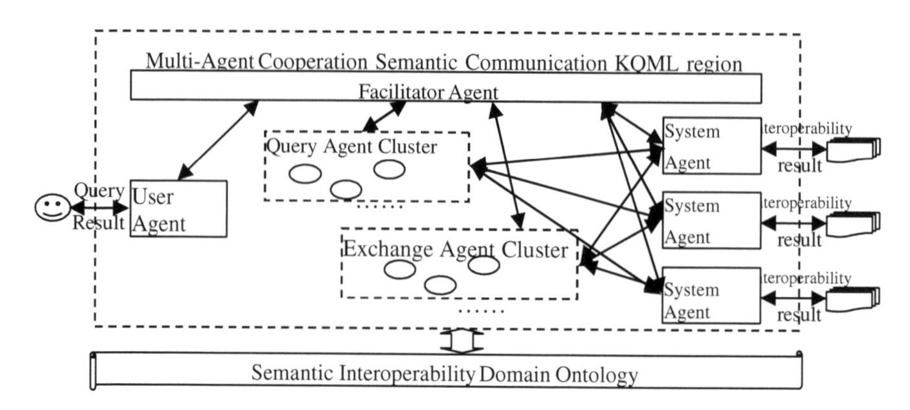

Fig. 33.1 Ontology based multi-agent cooperation interoperability model

33.4 MAS-Based Health Records Semantic Interoperability Model Implementation

According to above semantic interoperability model based on multi-agent cooperation, can achieve semantic interoperability of complex systems in an EHR environment, specific structure shown in Fig. 33.2. Agents are provided as SOA in the semantic interoperability framework of EHR and are deployed in a cluster server which contains agent container to support agents running. The corresponding framework of intelligent agents in the model is as follows:

Implementation of FA is deployed in regional health information cooperation layer HIAL and is provided as SOA, by which providing the health data interaction.The state service and routine service in the basic service component provide agent running state, server parameters, URI of servers and components in the cluster servers. Implementation of QA and EA provides SOA services as EHR cooperation component, which is the core semantic interoperability feature. Implementation of SA is deployed in the front-end machine of heterogeneous systems in hospital information integration platform and community platform. UA implemented as plug-and-play EHR browser mode. The browser can be used as a plug-in for desktop software or web systems, including embed into hospital information integration platform or community health platform.

33.4.1 The Core Implementation of Interoperability

There are two core aspects of regional health information semantic interoperability: the interoperable XML document definition based on the EHR ontology, automatically generating and parsing interoperable XML document. The definition of interoperable XML document is generated mainly based on HL7 RIM

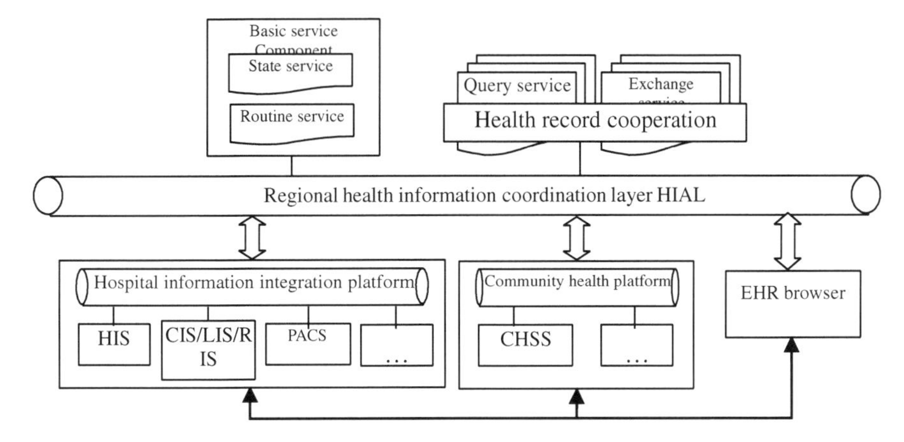

Fig. 33.2 Semantic interoperability implement framework of EHR

(Reference Information Model), the steps are as follows: select interoperable document domain model DMIM, crop based on business specifications, generate corresponding HMD files and produce XSD schema file of interoperable XML document by using HL7 V3 generator tool.

The schema file of interoperable document is accessible through the whole interoperable network environment, agent using the schema file generate and extract messages. The program of building and resolving interoperable is deployed as a web service, such as http://ip:8000/services/DocumentExport_Service represents the interface of generating interoperable document, the generated interoperable XML document fragment is shown in Fig. 33.3. The mode of web service

```
L(X) DTD/Schema(D) Schema 设计(M) XSL/XQuery(Q) 直观视图(A) 转换(C) 视图(V) 浏览器(B) WSDL(S) SOAP(O) 工具(
69  <relatedDocument typeCode="APND">
70      <parentDocument classCode="DOCCLIN" moodCode="EVN">
71          <id root="SD.1.1.4" extension="D2011000000"/>
72          <setId xsi:type="II" root="1.2.345.6789.33" extension="S001"/>
73          <versionNumber value="1"/>
74      </parentDocument>
75  </relatedDocument>
76  <component>
77      <structuredBody>
78          <!--随访事件章节 -->
79          <component>
80              <section>
81                  <code nullFlavor="UNK" displayName="随访事件"/>
82                  <entry>
83                      <observation classCode="CASE" moodCode="EVN">
84                          <!--活动代码（随访）-->
85                          <code code="DE06.00.108.00" codeSystem="SD.6.2" codeSystemName="城乡居民健康档案基本数据
86                          <!--随访时间（数据元）-->
87                          <effectiveTime value="20110212"/>
88                          <value codeSystem="SD.11.1.183" codeSystemName="随访方式代码表
89 " xsi:type="CD" displayName="门诊随访"/>
90                      </observation>
91                  </entry>
92              </section>
93          </component>
94          <!--症状章节-->
95          <component>
96              <section>
97                  <code code="11450-4" displayName=" PROBLEM LIST " codeSystem="2.16.840.1.113883.6.1" codeSystemNa
```

Fig. 33.3 Semantic interoperable XML document fragment

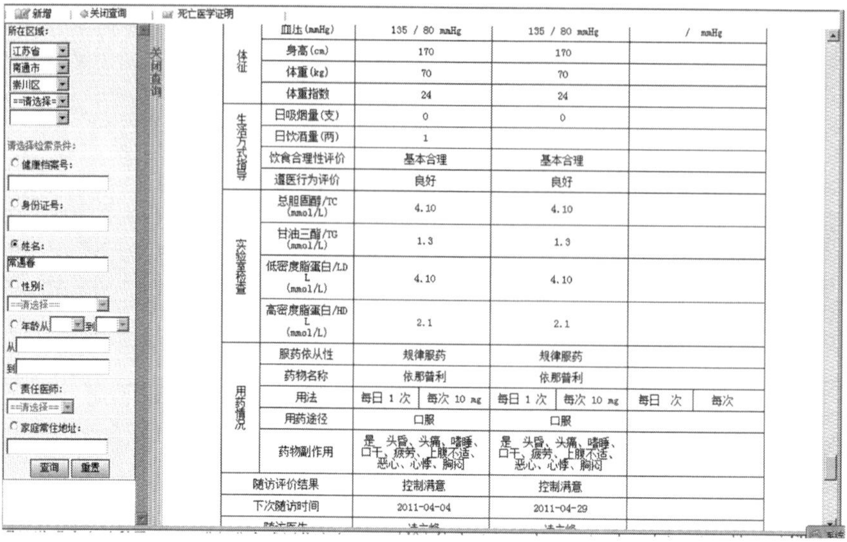

Fig. 33.4 The transparent query result returned by User Agent

open interface provides convenience that the agent can be easily moved to the various business systems in a distributed environment and handling interoperable requirements.

33.4.2 Experimental Results and Analysis

The semantic interoperable architecture based on multi-agent model can achieve EHR data share in heterogeneous systems.By EHR browser, it can provide transparent query on the heterogeneous health medical systems. Figure 33.4 shows that an embedded EHR browser displays a transparent query result of community diabetes follow-up about a resident.

33.5 Conclude

The semantic interoperability model based on multi-agent cooperation has the ability to integrate heterogeneous data sources and provide transparent query, as well as to support semantic interoperability requirement of heterogeneous systems. The model maintains the state list and routine list by facilitator agent, achieve agent cooperation, establish semantic interoperability domain ontology which is the consensus complied with agents. EHR semantic interoperability as a case study, the model is implemented to solve semantic integration, transparent query of heterogeneous data sources and semantic interoperability of heterogeneous systems.

References

1. Paepcke A, Change CCK, Garcia-Molina H et al (1998) Interoperability for digital libraries worldwide. Commun ACM 41(4):33–43
2. Weiss G (ed) (2000) Multi-agent system:a modern approach to distributed artificial intelligence. MIT Press, Cambridge
3. Costa CM (2011) Clinical data interoperability based on archetype transformation. J Biomed Inf 44(5):869–880
4. Batres R, Asprey SP et al (1999) A KQML multi-agent environment for concurrent process engineering. Comput Chem Eng 23(1)
5. Aquin M, Noy NF (2012) Where to publish and find ontologies? A survey of ontology libraries. Web Semantics Sci Ser Agents World Wide Web (11)
6. Xu GH,Xu F et al (2008) Ontology error correction reasoning research based on description logic–KMT-CPC cooperation domain ontology for example. J Libr Sci China 1:79–84
7. Yang J, Zhang ZM (2012) Research on health information document sharing specification of China based on HL7 and IHE. China Digital Med 12:50–55
8. Vallejo D, Albusac J et al (2011) A multi-agent architecture for supporting distributed normality-based intelligent surveillance. Eng Appl Artif Intell 2(24):325–340
9. May W, Behrends E et al (2008) Integrating and querying distributed XML data via XLink. Inf Syst 6(33):508–566

Chapter 34
Visual Analysis on Management of Postgraduate Degrees

Chen Ling and Xue-qing Li

Abstract In recent years, the pressure in the management of university degrees is larger and larger with the growing number of college graduates. At the same time, the phenomenon that a large number of students can't graduate on time arises. But now there are no effective methods to solve these problems. In order to solve problems above effectively, we treat each student's graduation process as a process of state changes and analyses of data created during the process of degree management. Then by visually analyzing of the process of the degree management, we can get a comprehensive grasp of the whole procedure and find out methods for optimizing and controlling the entire process; by visually analyzing cases of students' failing to obtain degrees, we can find out the main reason why they can't graduate on time and meanwhile provide convincing suggestions on how to solve these problems; by visually analyzing data created during anomalistic procedures, we can identify the implicit defects and deficiencies in the process; by visually analyzing the failing rates of different types of students over the years, we succeed in investigating the causes of their failing to graduate. All the works we do above make it have a deep and comprehensive understanding of degree managements which provides theoretical supports for the decisions of the leadership.

Keywords Degree management · Data analysis · Data visualization

C. Ling (✉) · X. Li
Department of computer science and technology, Shandong University,
Shandong 250101, People's Republic of China
e-mail: cy_446_ab@163.com

X. Li
e-mail: xqli@sdu.edu.cn

S. Li et al. (eds.), *Frontier and Future Development of Information Technology in Medicine and Education*, Lecture Notes in Electrical Engineering 269,
DOI: 10.1007/978-94-007-7618-0_34,

34.1 Introduction

In recent years, with the expansion of university enrollment, the annual number of graduates has been growing which virtually burden universities with degree management problems. At the same time, the number of students failing to graduate on time has been increasing. Facing such a long and complicated graduation process, how to effectively control and optimize it so that it can run in a smoother way? How to propose targeted solutions to raise graduation rates? How to find out the defects existing in the process so that we can make the whole progress better runny? Although many universities have already issued many policies such as and masters who postpone graduation have to pay tuition and so on, but it do not work as intended, failing to fundamentally solve problems. Based on this fact, the article do visual analysis of graduation data on four aspects, which are respectively degree management procedures, cases of students' failing to obtain degrees, anomalistic procedures and failing rates of different types of students over the years, so that we can finally find out the problem existing in the degree management process and the main factor influencing the graduation rate. Thus we can discuss the main reason why students cannot graduate smoothly and put forward the solving solution to these problems. As a consequential result, we provide theoretical support for the leadership's decision-making and make the graduation process run more smoothly so as to increase the rate of graduation.

The first part of this article shows a brief introduction of the present situation of the degree management and its problems. The second part mainly shows how we handle the data created during the degree management process. The third part carries out visual analysis on four aspects based on the results we get before, and the last part gives the conclusion.

34.2 Data Analysis on Degree Management Process

Every year there are a large number of students in Universities needed to graduate. With the passage of time, a large amount of students' graduate data has been stored in the database.

34.2.1 Introduction of Data Analysis Process

We treat each student's graduation process as a process of states changes and records the changes in each state and their corresponding time. Each student's status change situation is not exactly the same with others and a state may be repeated several times during the entire process. In order to show different aspects of the whole process, it is need to count daily students number of each state. So firstly we should remove the duplicate states of each student and then count students number according to state and time.

34.2.2 Remove the Duplicated State

For each student's repetitive states, the article only considers the first one of these states. The following state, if the same with it, should be removed and we continue to take the next state. If different, should be defined a new state and we use the function $h(y_i)$ to indicate whether this state makes sense. Assume that the state makes sense (that is to say it is a new state which not existing in the student's previous states) take $h(y_i) = 1$, otherwise take $h(y_i) = 0$. Thus the function $h(y_i)$ can be expressed as follows:

$$h(y_i) = \begin{cases} 1 & i = 0 \\ |y_i - y_{i-1}| & y_i = y_{i-1} \\ \dfrac{|y_i - y_{i-1}|}{|y_i - y_{i-1}|} & y_i \neq y_{i-1} \end{cases} \tag{34.1}$$

In the expression above y_{i-1} represents the previous state of y_i.

34.2.3 Counting Up Number

Counting up daily number of each state on the basis of gets rid of the repetitive states of each student. The specific method we use is as following: for each student, taking each state and the corresponding time, if the state and time has already existed then we add one to the number of this case; if not, adding this new case and set its initial value as 1. Function $F(y, z)$ represents the statistical result of the case of state y and time z, which is described as:

$$F(y,z) = \begin{cases} \sum f(y,z) & y,z \quad exist \\ 1 & y,z\ not\ exist \end{cases} \tag{34.2}$$

According to the function $F(y, z)$ we can get the number of students at any time of each state.

34.2.4 Statistical Results Sorting

We cannot know the daily number of each state because the statistical results we get before are disordered so it needs to sort according to status and time. New statistical results after sorting are showed in Table 34.1.

Table 34.1 Sorting results table

y, z	f(y, z)
7(2012-09-15)	6
7(2012-09-16)	4
…	…
8(2012-09-24)	66
…	…
22(2012-12-21)	4

Table 34.2 Statistical results table

Time	Submit an application for graduates	College approved	Graduate school approved	Pumping trial	College agreed to graduation	College agreed to grant degrees
First day	6	2	82	28	1	5
Second day	4	11	1	8	1	3
Third day	6	3	40	38	6	71
…	…	…	…	…	…	…
Day 27	27	4	0	0	0	0

Take 7(2012-09-15) as an example, 7 represents the state of students submitting their graduation application while 2012-09-15 represents the date, that is to say the key word is composed of two parts: state and time.

34.2.5 Counting Up Daily Number of Each State

Count up the daily number of each state according to the statistical results of above. Final results are shown in Table 34.2.

34.3 Visual Analysis

34.3.1 Visual Analysis of Degree Management Process

We can get both daily number and total number of each state through the data analysis of Sect. 34.2. This part we focus on using line chart to show the entire change situation of the total number of each state. Time distinguished by color, states marked by the abscissa, and quantity marked by the ordinate, we draw the process chart of degree management as Fig. 34.1.

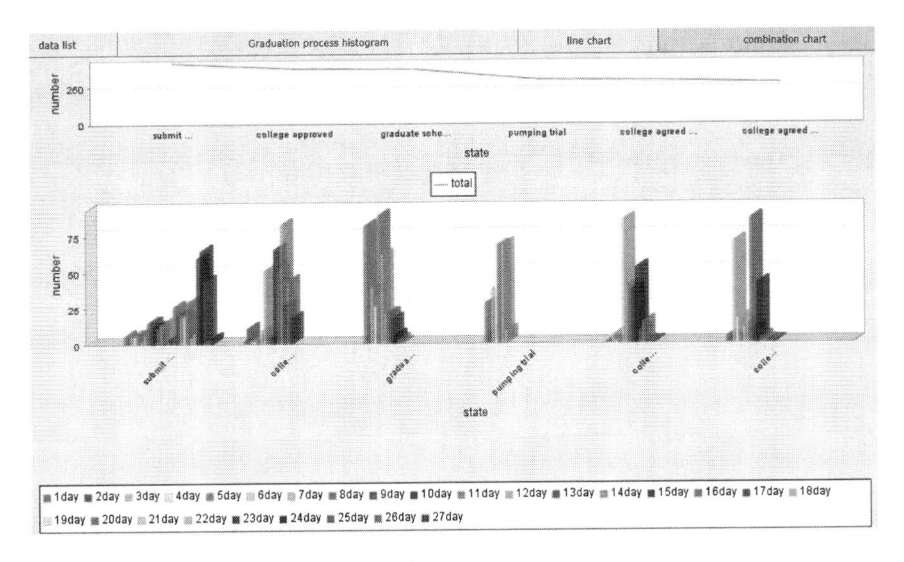

Fig. 34.1 Graduate management process figure

Overall, as the graduation process proceeds, the total number of students is declining, which indicates that at each stage there are students who do not conform to the requirements thus cannot graduate on time. Then let us focus on the histogram below. Firstly, it is easy for us to find out that the stage that students submit their graduation applications lasts especially for a long time. This fact indicates that this stage is most time-consuming and contains the most problems. So this phase is the key point for us to optimize the whole process. Why does this phenomenon happen? Is it because the students are not timely informed? Or is it because the students themselves can not submit their graduate application on time? Or is it the system problems that have affected the submission schedule? To solve this, managers should first find out the main problem, then based on the main problem, optimize this phase so as to save more time for the following phases. Secondly, as for the audit stages, only the audit stage of Graduate School concentrates on the front few days of the phase, while others on the middle even the end of the period. What is the reason? Is it because the managers' unskilled operations delay the progress? Or is it because of people's laziness and lacking of enthusiasm? Whatever the reason, it shows that these phases can be optimized. All of these above provide the theoretical support for leadership on how to control and optimize the whole process, so that it can run more smoothly.

34.3.2 Visual Analysis on Students' Failing in Gaining Degrees

34.3.2.1 Failed to Pass States Proportion

We have already count up the daily number of each state in Sect. 34.2. Summing up the daily data of each state, we get the total students number of each state. Then we can calculate the proportion of every state in all the failed to pass state. The result is shown in Table 34.3.

34.3.2.2 Failed to Obtain Degree Reasons Proportion

Find out reasons why some students are not allowed to graduate, and count up the proportion of each reason. The statistical result is shown in Table 34.4.

34.3.2.3 Graphics Display and Analysis

This part, we use pie charts to show the statistical results we have get in Sects. 34.3.2.1 and 34.3.2.2, with different colors representing different states. The pie chart is shown as Fig. 34.2.

First of all, it can be seen from the first chart that the states students failing to pass college audit, college not granting degrees and college not agree their graduation account for high percentages, totally above eighty percent. On the contrary, the proportion of graduate school disagreeing is low. This result approximately agree with the circumstance that the requirements of college be higher than school. Secondly, it can be seen from the second chart that the main reasons for students failing to obtain their degrees are students giving up the application themselves, not passing the paper review and getting cancelled the respondent eligibility because of their academic misconduct. These aspects account for more than ninety percent of all the reasons. Why the reason students themselves giving up the application rank NO. 1 of all the reasons? Is it because students do not meet the requirements for graduation? Or should the school be blamed for this? This question must be paid high attention by both school and students. As for the other two reasons, not only do they indicate that at present many students can't restrain themselves, as a result of fail to finish the work within their duties, but also many students' attitude towards academic is not right Table 34.5.

Table 34.3 Failed to pass states proportion table

State name	Proportion (%)
College audit not pass	23.1
Graduate school audit not pass	5.3
College not agree graduation	44.4
College not agree to grant degrees	14.8
Graduate school not agree graduation	8.3
Graduate school not agree to grant degrees	4.1

Table 34.4 Failed to obtain degree reasons proportion table

Reason	Proportion (%)
Cancel respondent eligibility because of academic misconduct	18
Fail to pass paper review	26.8
Oral defense failed	4.8
Waiver of the application	45.6
Fail to meet the requirements of fostering proposal	4.8

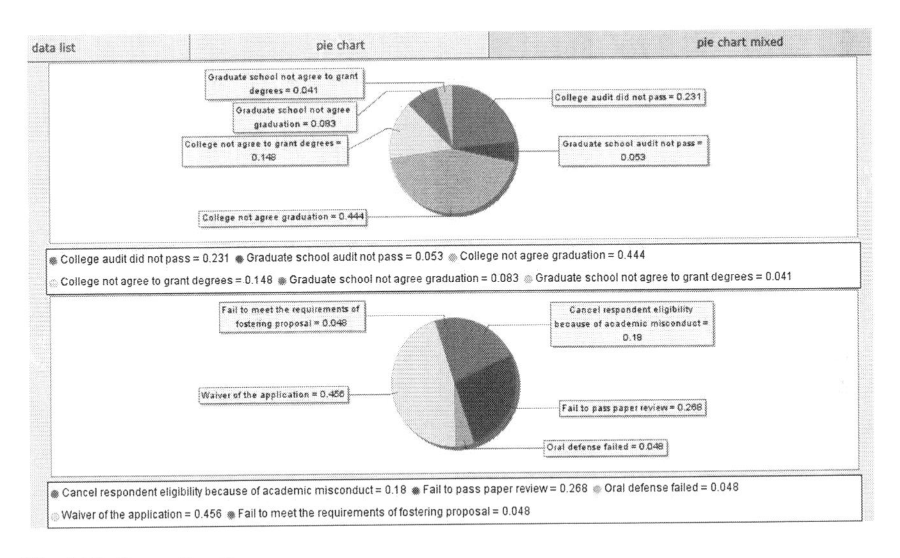

Fig. 34.2 Proportion figure

Table 34.5 Different-type students failing rates table

Time	Ordinary Dr.	Ordinary master	Ordinary profession master	Job application for master	Dr-service professional	Master of-service professional	University teachers
2011-06	0.079	0.0102	0.0314	0.079	0.087	0.1145	0.151
2011-12	0.0739	0.0023	0.0042	0.2368	0.087	0.25	0.1096
2012-06	0.062	0.0049	0.1569	0.1316	0.1304	0.19	0.082
2012-12	0.0118	0	0	0.026	0.0217	0	0

34.3.3 Visual Analysis of Abnormal Data

34.3.3.1 Abnormal Data Processing

Here, we get the data of abnormal process of students' and analysis states change in this situation.

34.3.3.2 Graphics Display and Analysis

In the line graph below, the abscissa represents time, the ordinate represents state. The graph shows the students' state changing process as time goes on, which is show as Fig. 34.3.

Normally, the change of a student's state should be a gradual increase in the graph and each state only show one time. However, the abnormal state changing process of the student, which shown in the line graph, is quite irregular and very unusual. We can see that the status of the student change from state ten (pass the graduate school audit) to five (allowed to submit graduate application), which means, with time passing, the student changes into a previous state which is not allowed in theory. Why does this phenomenon happen? Is it a man-made wrong

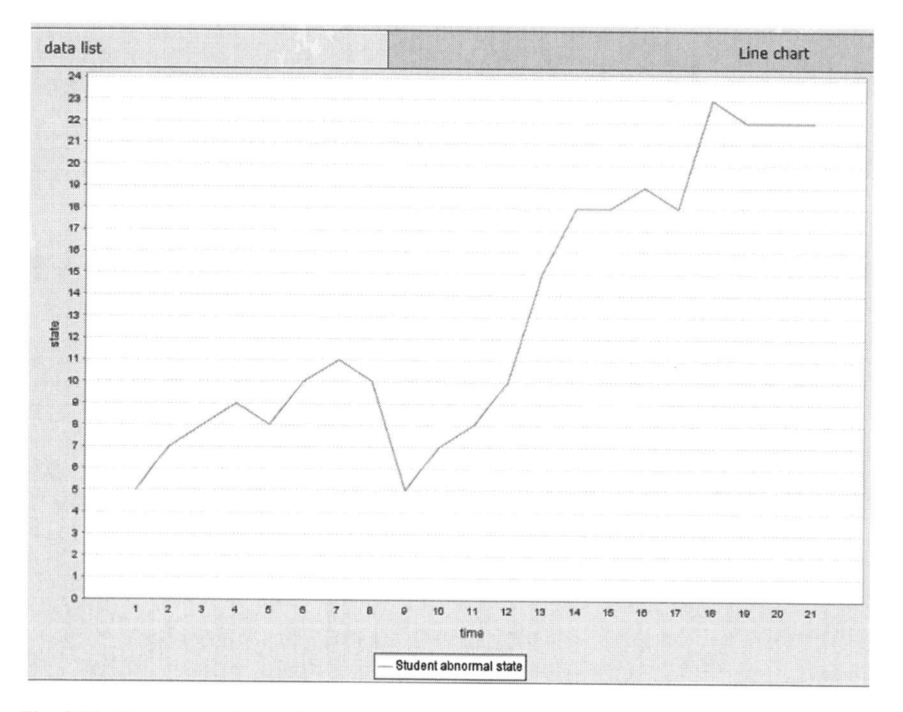

Fig. 34.3 The abnormal state figure

operation? Or are there loopholes in the policy? Whatever the reason, it reflects that the program design is not fully taken into account. In addition, it can also be seen that some states have appeared more than one time in a row, such as in the last few days state 22, repeat many times which should appear only one normally. The reason may be the college secretary's multiple operations, but the defect of system design is also possible. So it is necessary to improve the design of the system and strengthen the training of operating personnel as far as possible which conducive to prevent wrong operation.

34.3.4 Visual Analysis on Students' Failed Graduation Rates

34.3.4.1 Count Up the Failing Rates of Different Student Type Over the Years

For a certain student type and certain graduation time, count up its total number of students failed to obtain degrees and applied for graduation, then calculate the proportion of students failed to graduate over the years. Statistical results are shown in the table below:

34.3.4.2 Graphics Display and Analysis

According to the statistical results, the abscissa represents the type of student, the vertical axis represents the proportion, with colors representing different graduation time. As shown in Fig. 34.4.

From the perspective of ordinary and on-the-job, we can see that on-the-job students' proportion is much higher than ordinary which is consistent with students' attitude towards study and their study time. What's more, their desire to study is also less than ordinary students, which illustrate again that "Attitude is everything". From the perspective of doctor and master, we can see doctors' proportion is much higher than master, which is consistent with the fact that doctors are required of high-level papers and faced with higher percentage of papers blind review. Meanwhile, it also suggests that the scientific research ability of doctor is much higher than that of masters and that doctor have reached pretty high attainment in some particular area. From the perspective of time, on 2012-12-30, the proportion of students failing to pass is relatively low, which is closely associated with the policies of school about students delay graduation. From all the above, we can conclude that students' attitude towards their schoolwork and the school's policy for graduation can make a big difference to the graduation rate.

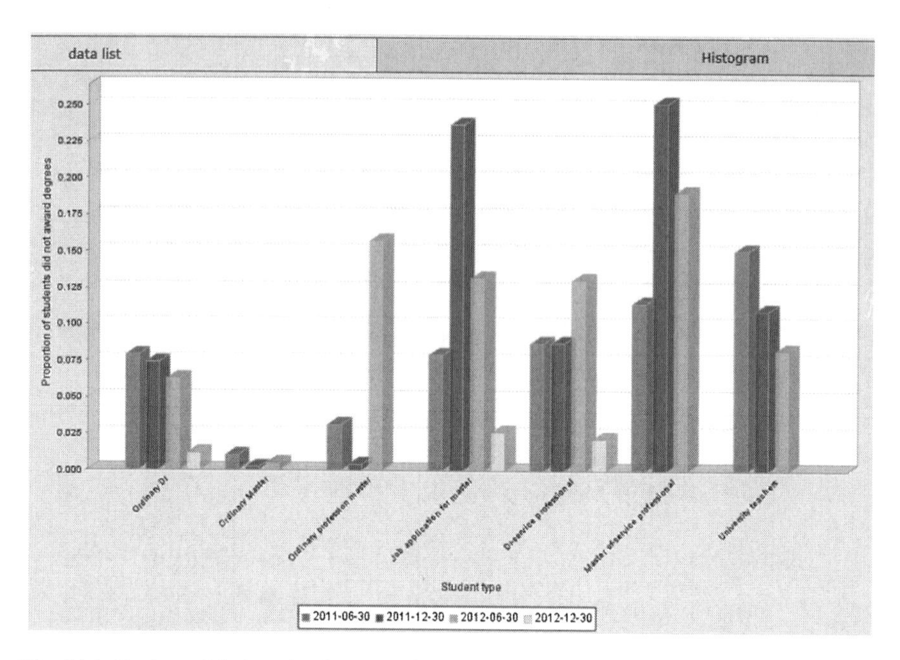

Fig. 34.4 Students failed graduation rates figure

34.4 Conclusion

This paper starts with the process of data handling, and then does a series of visual analysis on the process of degree management, the failing rates of students in different graduation phases, abnormal data created in the process and the failing rates over the years, thus providing a comprehensive and deep understanding of degree management process for us. At the same time, by doing the analysis, we finally find out the potential problems existing in the system and the management process and the main reason why some students cannot graduate, which are provide strong theoretical support for leadership on how to control and optimize the whole process, and put forward targeted policy to reduce the failing rate.

References

1. Yu P, Yan H (2008) Application of Jfreechart in network performance management system. Comput Eng Des 29(16)
2. Wang Y, Ding Y, Sun Y, Zhao Z (2007) Research on data visualization implementation methods. Mod electr technol 4
3. Liu K, Zhao X, Zhao D (2002) Data visualization research and development. Comput Eng 28(8)
4. Gao J, Ding K (2009) Analysis through visualizing the patent research articles. J intell 28(7)

5. Chen J, Yu Z, Zhu Y (2001) Data visualization and its applications. Infrared Laser Eng 30(5)
6. Zhang W, Li X (2002) Research and implementation of web-based visualization. Comput Eng Sci 24(3)
7. Wang R, Zhang N, Wan X (2005) A kind of web statistic chart based on Jfreechart. Microcomput Dev 15(3)

Chapter 35
An Energy-Saving Load Balancing Method in Cloud Data Centers

Xiao Li and Mingchun Zheng

Abstract With the development of virtualization technology, data center virtualization in Cloud Computing gradually become a hot topic. In the premise of ensuring users' SLA, this paper considers the utilization of server resources, whose objective is to minimize the number of opening servers. We propose an energy-saving strategy based on live virtual machines migration. Our ARMA-based load forecasting reduces the occurrence of virtual machines' migration caused by instantaneous load peaks. Then we select migration virtual machines and destination servers based on our proposed algorithms. Finally, the data center reaches a load balancing state. The experiments show that the strategy can improve server resource utilization and reduce energy consumption.

Keywords Cloud computing · Virtual resource scheduling · Virtual machine migration · Energy-saving

35.1 Introduction

Cloud computing is a hot technology [1]. In recent years, a large number of major companies' Cloud Computing business applications are emerging. i.e. Amazon's EC2 [2], and Microsoft's Azure [3]. Using virtualization technology, cloud computing maps physical machines' resources to a virtual machine layer, in which

X. Li (✉) · M. Zheng
School of Management Science and Engineering, Shandong Normal University, 250014 Ji'nan, China
e-mail: sdnulixiao@126.com

M. Zheng
e-mail: zhmc163@163.com

S. Li et al. (eds.), *Frontier and Future Development of Information Technology in Medicine and Education*, Lecture Notes in Electrical Engineering 269,
DOI: 10.1007/978-94-007-7618-0_35,

virtual machine perform users' tasks. With the growing number of data center servers, resource scheduling problem is becoming a hotspot [4].

Cloud data center resource scheduling is divided into static scheduling and dynamic scheduling. In static resource scheduling, we decide each virtual machine running on which server. The advantage of this strategy is that the implementation is simple and reliable. However, the static scheduling scheme is not flexible. Dynamic resource scheduling is achieved by using live virtual migration. When a server is overloaded, one or some virtual machines (VM) are migrated to another server to ensure users' SLA; When a server resource utilization is very low, we migrate all the virtual machine on it and shut down the server to achieve the purpose of saving resources. It is flexible.

Dynamic resource scheduling includes four strategies, that is, load measurement strategy, information strategy, trigger strategy and migration operations strategy. Load measurement strategy is to determine the load measurement indicators. In this paper, we select CPU and memory as load measurement indicators. Information strategy determine when and how to collect the resources utilization information. In general, we collect information in the physical server and virtual machine periodically. Trigger strategy determines when the virtual machine migration is triggered. We consider multi-threshold method. Migration operations strategy select which server is the destination server. We design a classification algorithm to select the appropriate destination server, which is aiming to minimum the open number of servers and reduce the energy consumption in cloud data centers.

35.2 Related Work

There are lots of researches about load balancing in Cloud Computing data centers based on live VM migration.

Sandpiper system [5] proposed a data center resource monitoring method which is based on black box and gray box. It can monitor and detect hotspot automatically. Then, it completes the mapping from physical resource to virtual resource. [6] is the first green computing using virtual machine migration, but in general, the algorithm in this paper is not a real scheduling algorithm as it did not consider the performance of the whole system. Using AR (p) model to predict workload, [7] proposed a resource load balancing method. However, it only takes CPU utilization into consideration. In fact, there are other resource like memory and network bandwidth.

Zhou et al. [8] implemented a load balancing scheme based on dynamic resource allocation principles in a virtual machine cluster mode. It real-time monitored resource usage of virtual machine and physical machine, then re-allocated resources to the virtual machine running in the same physical machine. Also, using live virtual machine migration between physical machines, they achieved global balancing of virtual machine cluster. Liu et al. [9] proposed a live virtual machine migration frame, which realized real-time monitor in the cloud computing. Also, it can complete the migration progress on different type of virtual machine monitor to improve the migration flexibility. Meanwhile, it ensured the VM' SLA in the migration progress.

In recent years, the study about cloud computing energy consumption showed that, the energy consumption of an opening free server is 70 % of the full server averagely [12]. The fact proved, it is correct to close the free server to sleep mode to reduce the total system energy.

35.3 Dynamic Resource Scheduling

35.3.1 Load Measurement Strategy

We consider virtual and physical machines' CPU utilization and memory utilization as load indicators. Virtual machine's CPU and memory utilization is denoted as V_{cpu} and V_{mem}. Physical server's CPU and memory utilization is expressed H_{cpu} and H_{mem}. The maximum and minimum load threshold of Physical server's CPU and memory is $H_{cputhre}$, $L_{cputhre}$, $H_{memthre}$, $L_{memthre}$.

Now, we define three states of physical server. When $H_{cpu} > H_{cputhre}$ or $H_{mem} > H_{memthre}$, we say the physical server in overloading state; When $H_{cpu} < L_{cputhre}$ or $H_{mem} < L_{mem}$, we say the physical server in hungry state; Otherwise, we say the physical server in normal state. We define a parameter $heat = \frac{V_{cpu}}{V_{mem}}$, the larger the CPU utilization, and the smaller the memory utilization, we have a larger *heat*.

35.3.2 Load Prediction Based on ARMA

Now, we introduce the load prediction mechanism. When the load of a physical server exceeds the threshold at some point, we will not immediately migrate VM on it. Only when we predict the load on this sever is still high in several subsequent time points, we migrate one or some virtual machine. Therefore, we reduce the number of unnecessary virtual machine migration.

According to the dynamic change regulation of server load, [10] proposed a server load prediction method based on time series. In this paper, we use its experimental results and predict the load of physical server based on ARMA [7, 8] model. The model is as follows:

$$\hat{y} = \varphi_1 y_{t-1} + \varphi_2 y_{t-2} + \ldots + \varphi_8 y_{t-8} + u_t - \theta_1 u_{t-1} - \theta_2 u_{t-2} - \ldots - \theta_7 u_{t-7} \tag{35.1}$$

Using the model, we can predict the n time points' load in the future. If k load value is greater than the max threshold value, we say the physical server is a hotspot. Then we start the virtual machine migration operation. Similarly, if k load value is lower than the min threshold value, we say all the VM in the physical server needing to migrate.

35.3.3 Virtual Machine Migration Strategy

With real-time monitoring data, we determine the state of every physical server. For different state of servers, we take different strategies.

- When a physical server in a overloading state
  Through the ARMA model, we decide whether the physical server is a hotspot. If it is not a hotspot, we do nothing in this period. Otherwise, we need to observe $H_{cpu} > H_{cputhre}$ or $H_{mem} > H_{memthre}$. If $H_{cpu} > H_{cputhre}$, we say this is a CPU-triggered migration. Then, we need to select the virtual machine which has the maximum *heat* to migrate; If $H_{mem} > H_{memthre}$, we say this is a memory-triggered migration. Then, we need to select the virtual machine which has the maximum V_{mem}.

- When a physical server in a hungry state
  Through the ARMA prediction, we decide whether it have k load value lower than threshold. If it has, we need to migrate all the VM on this physical server. Otherwise, we do nothing in this period.

- When a physical server in a normal state

  we do nothing in this period.

The overloading servers' virtual machine migration strategy flow is in Fig. 35.1.

35.3.4 Destination Server Selection Strategy

35.3.4.1 Describe the Problem

Firstly, we consider the following case. Now there are 4 physical server in a data center. Each server's virtual machine distribution and resource usage is shown in Fig. 35.2. We set the maximum threshold of physical server 75 %, and the minimum threshold 20 %.

As can be seen from Fig. 35.2, PM1 and PM2 are in a overloading state. We assume that from our ARMA (8,7) model, PM1 and PM2 need to migrate some

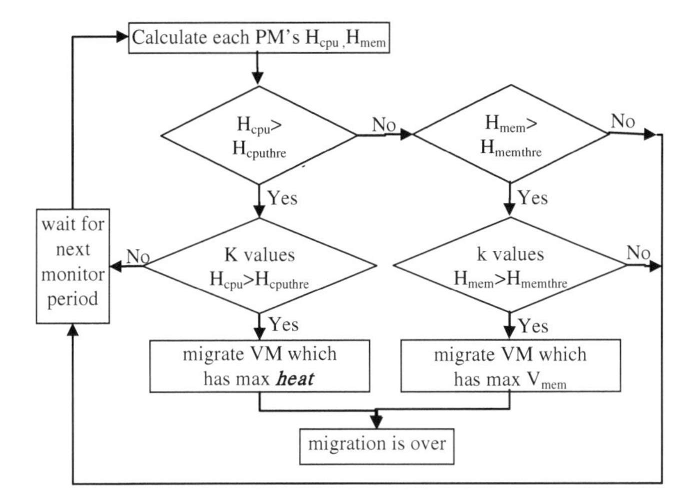

Fig. 35.1 Overloading servers' VM selection process

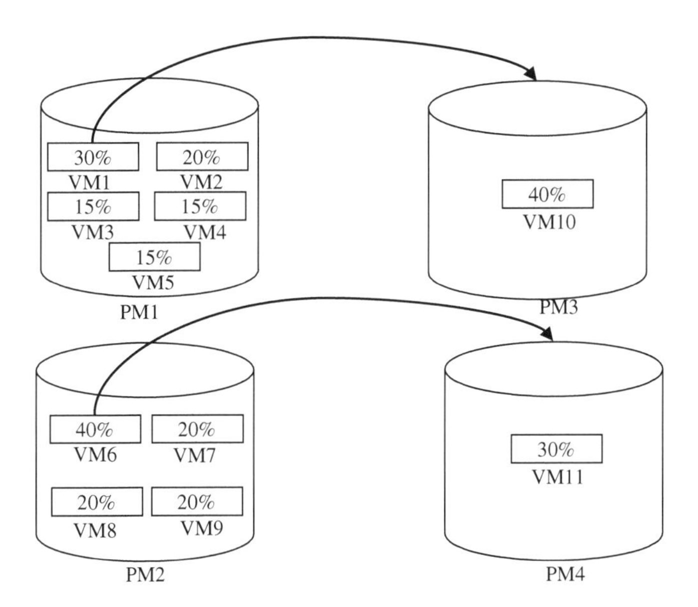

Fig. 35.2 Virtual machine distribution and resource usage in a data center

VM to ensure users' SLA. So, we select the VM which has the maximum resource usage to migrate. Then, VM1 and VM6 have been chosen. Next, we need to select the destination server. We assume VM1 is prior to VM6. For VM1, based on the traditional method, we should choose the server which has the maximum remaining resource every time, we choose PM4 as the destination server. Next, for VM6, we need to open a new server as we have not an optimal server.

However, we have an ideal solution, that is, moving VM1–PM3, and moving VM6–PM4. In this way, we can improve the resource utilization and save energy. From this case, we can see that, if we choose the server which has the maximum remaining resource every time, the resource utilization of the whole system is not the best. So we need to choose an optimal server for every migration VM.

Response to this case, we design a classification algorithm, to maximum the resource utilization of the whole data center. In accordance with the usage of resource, we classify physical servers. Using this algorithm, we migrate the VM to the most suitable server. In this way, the whole system can reach a load balancing. Moreover, it can improve the servers' resource utilization and save energy.

35.3.4.2 Algorithm Design

We assume the VM migration is CPU-triggered. The idea of our algorithm is as follows. Firstly, when we monitor one server needing to migrate their VM, we make classification for other servers according to servers' remaining resources. Secondly, based on the necessary resources which the migration VM needs, we choose the suitable class for the migration VM. Thirdly, if there are several servers which can satisfy the migration VM, we choose one server as a destination server randomly.

We need to define some parameters. Based on the monitor data, the requisite CPU of migration VM j is v^j_{cpu}, and the requisite memory of j is v^j_{mem}. The remaining CPU and memory resource of physical server i is $S^i_{cpu} = k_1 \cdot H^i_{cputhre} - H^i_{cpu}$ and $S^i_{mem} = k_2 \cdot H^i_{memthre} - H^i_{mem}$. We adjust servers' load balance level by weight coefficient k_1 and k_2. If $k_1 < H^i_{cpu} / H^i_{cputhre}$, we say the physical server i has no remaining CPU resource.

The algorithm process is as follows.

1. Physical servers are divided into m class averagely based on the interval $\lfloor 0, k \cdot H_{cputhre} - t \cdot L_{cputhre} \rfloor$, where k and t is the weight coefficient. Then, every server find their respective class based on S^i_{cpu}. We mark classes from class 1 to class m, in a descending range sequence.
2. Find the suitable class for j from class 1 to class m. If there is no suitable class for j, we open a new physical server and move i into it. Otherwise, the suitable class is marked as f.
3. VM j sends request messages to all servers in class f.
4. Every physical server who receives request message need to check their S^j_{mem}. If $v^j_{mem} < S^i_{mem}$, server i send a response message to VM j. At the same time, server i is locked, avoiding other VM to migrate into it. Otherwise, if it does not exist servers satisfying the VM j, then skip 7.
5. After VM j receive the response message, it starts to migrate.
6. After the migration is over, physical server i is unlocked. The algorithm is over.

7. Find class $f-1, f-2, \ldots, 1$ successively. Then skip3.

The memory-triggered VM migration is similar to the above algorithm.

35.4 Experimental Analysis

We use the Cloud Sim [11] as the simulation platform. We simulate a Cloud Computing data center which contains 100 isomorphic physical nodes and 290 VM on them. Each node has one CPU core, whose processing performance is equivalent to 1,000, 2,000 or 3,000 MIPS, 8G RAM and 1T capacity. Each VM needs 250, 500, 750 or 1,000 MIPS, 128 M RAM and 1G capacity.

Based on [12], the energy model we used as follows.

$$P(u) = \alpha \cdot P_{\max} + (1-\alpha) \cdot P_{\max} \cdot u \tag{35.2}$$

$P_{\max}$ denotes the maximum energy consumption when a server is fully utilized. α is the proportionality coefficient of the free server energy consumption. u is the CPU utilization. Here, we set $P_{\max} = 250W$, which is a common value of the modern server. The total energy E of a server is the integral of energy consumption function in a certain period of time. The formula is as follows.

$$E = \int_{t_0}^{t_1} P(u(t))dt \tag{35.3}$$

In order to get the standard experimental results, we compare our algorithm with Non-energy Aware Strategy (NPA), in which, all of the host runs in 100 % CPU utilization and consumes the maximum power. The second strategy we used is DVFS algorithm. Another standard we compared is the VM migration strategy with Single Threshold (ST). And we use different thresholds to check our algorithm.

We donate our algorithm as ES. The experimental result is in Table 35.1.

The experimental results show that, VM migration strategy can save lots of energy. Based on this simulation scheme, the ES (45–90 %) strategy will reduce 0.897 kWh than ST 55 % in the similar SLA. Meanwhile, the number of the VM migration reduce more than 10 times.

From the simulation experiment, we can drow the conclusion, that our algorithm is the best strategy to reduce the energy. The number of the migration VM is minimum in the lowest SLA violation efficiency. Also, the result shows our algorithm has good flexibility. Our threshold value may be adjusted according to the SLA. As a result, we can improve resource utilization, at the same time, reduce the energy consumption of the system.

Table 35.1 Simulation result comparison

Algorithm	Energy, kwh	SLA violation	VM migrations	Average SLA
NPA	9.147	–	–	–
	(9.033, 9.260)			
DVFS	4.385	–	–	–
	(4.350, 4.420)			
ST 55 %	2.038	5.5 %	35230	79.4 %
	(2.028, 2.048)	(5.4, 5.6 %)	(35142, 35318)	(78.9, 79.9 %)
ST 65 %	1.621	7.50 %	34510	84.1 %
	(1.618, 1.623)	(7.4, 7.6 %)	(34428, 34592)	(83.2.0, 85.0 %)
ES (25–75 %)	1.479	1.20 %	3359	57.0 %
	(1.470, 1.488)	(1.1, 1.4 %)	(3329, 3389)	(56.2, 57.8 %)
ES (35–85 %)	1.265	2.9 %	3233(3188, 3278)	65.8 %
	(1.260, 1.270)	(2.8, 3.0 %)		(65.2, 66.4 %)
ES (45–90 %)	1.141	6.6 %	3118(3048, 3188)	75.7 %
	(1.132, 1.150)	(6.5, 6.8 %)		(74.8, 76.5 %)

35.5 Conclusions

In this paper, we propose a live VM migration strategy which can improve the resource utilization of physical servers and reduce the energy consumption of the whole system. Our strategy can realize the migration trigger, and select the migration VM and destination physical server. The experiments show that our strategy can reduce the energy consumption. However, our strategy mainly focus on CPU and memory resources, lack of some other factors, such as network bandwidth and the disk storage. And in the future, we will extend our strategy on WAN.

References

1. Group of virtualization and cloud computing (2009) Virtualization and cloud computing. Publishing House of Electronics Industry, Beijing
2. Amazon web services introduction [EB/OL]. http//aws.amazon.com
3. Microsoft (2008) Azure service platform overview. INSIGHT (Microsoft) 2:1–23
4. Qian Q, Li C et al (2012) Virtual resources review of cloud data center. Appl Res Comput 29(7):2411–2415
5. Wood T (2007) Black-box and gray-box strategies for virtual machine migration. In Proceedings of the 4th international conference on networked systems design and implementation. [S. 1.]: IEEE (in press), pp 229–242
6. Nathuji R, Schwan K (2007) Virtual power. Coordinated power management in virtualized enterprise systems. In: Proceedings of twenty-first ACM SIGOPS symposium on operating systems principles, vol 21, pp 265–278
7. Liu Y, Gao Q, Chen Y (2010) A load balancing method of virtual machine resource in virtual computing environments. Comput Eng 36(16):30–32

8. Zhou W, Yang S et al (2010) VMC Tune a load balancing scheme for virtual machine cluster based on dynamic resource allocation. In: Proceedings of the 9th international conference on grid and cloud computing, pp 81–86
9. Liu S, Quan G, Ren SP (2011) On-line preemptive scheduling of real-time services with profit and penalty. In: Proceedings of IEEE southeast conference, pp 287–292
10. Yang W, Zhu Q et al (2006) Servers load prediction based on times series. Comput Eng 32(19):143–145, 148
11. Buyya R, Ranjan R, Calheiros RN (2009) Modeling and simulation of scalable cloud computing environments and the cloudsim Tkklkit. Challenges and opportunities. In: Proceedings of international conference on high performance computing and simulation, Kochi
12. Liu Y, Wang X, Wang Z et al (2012) Virtual machine resource scheduling driven by energy efficiency and trust. Appl Res Comput 29(7):2479–2483

Chapter 36
Application of a New Association Rules Mining Algorithm in the Chinese Medical Coronary Disease

Feng Yuan, Hong Liu and ShouQiang Chen

Abstract The paper deals with efficient mining association rules in large data sets of TCM clinical data of the coronary disease. Aiming at the problems that TCM clinical data exist a great deal of data and high association characteristics, which lead to the problem of low efficiency, slow convergence and omission rules, a new combined method is proposed based on genetic algorithm and particle swarm optimization. The method designs the fitness function, uses particle swarm optimization to finish evolution and integration, and combines with genetic manipulation the advantage of simple and robust. The medical treatment records of coronary disease were verified by the experiments. Experimental results show that compared with traditional association rules mining method, combined algorithm performs better in terms of diversity of population and discovering more effective association rules. The mining result has reference value in TCM treatment of the coronary disease.

Keywords Association rules mining · Traditional chinese medicine · Genetic algorithm · Particle swarm optimization

F. Yuan (✉) · H. Liu
School of Information Science and Engineering, Shandong Normal University, Jinan 250014, China
e-mail: yuanfeng623@163.com

F. Yuan
School of Information Engineering, College of Shandong Labour Union Administrators, Jinan, China

S. Chen
Center of Hear,The Second Affiliated Hospital of Shandong University of Traditional Chinese Medicine, Fujian, China

S. Li et al. (eds.), *Frontier and Future Development of Information Technology in Medicine and Education*, Lecture Notes in Electrical Engineering 269,
DOI: 10.1007/978-94-007-7618-0_36,

36.1 Introduction

Data mining refers to extracting or "mining" useful knowledge from large amount of data. These knowledge is impliedly, unknown before and potential useful information [1]. As a very useful knowledge model of data mining, association rules mining has received a great deal of attention and research. The key and core of the algorithm is to generate frequent item sets, so how to efficiently generate frequent item sets is a quite promising research. Genetic Algorithm (GA) and Particles Swarm Optimization (PSO) are both population based algorithms that have been proven to be successful in data mining. However, both models have strengths and weaknesses [2].

Mining genetic association rules which is one of the data mining is reconstructed and invested widely as an useful knowledge model. But there are still some abuses in service use of genetic association rules algorithm [3]. GA is a population-based evolutionary algorithm which is random, robustness and implicit parallelism, it can search for global optimization quickly and efficiently, and is a effective method of processing large set of data items [4]. Compared with GA, PSO has a much more profound intelligent background and can be performed more easily. Given that particle optimization mainly evolves via the comparison of the self position, the surrounding positions, and the global positions of all the particles as a singleton pattern, PSO may prematurely converge [5].

Due to the problems of low efficiency, slow convergence and omission rules in mining Traditional Chinese Medical (TCM) clinical data, a new combined method is proposed based on GA and particle swarm optimization. Using particle swarm optimization finish evolution and integration and combine with genetic manipulation the advantage of simple and robust to solve the problem of algorithm premature and redundancy rules. Fitness function, crossover and mutation operators are designed. At last the concrete realization process of algorithm is given through mining the case of coronary disease of TCM with association rules.

36.2 Basic Concept

36.2.1 Association Rule

Let $I = \{i1, i2,\ldots in\}$ is the collection of data items, $D = \{T_1, T_2, \ldots T_m\}$ is the transaction database, and every transaction Tj ($j = 1, 2,\ldots,m$) which has a identifier called *TID*,and is a subset of data items. Support S is the percentage of the transaction that how much D included $A \cup B$, describing the probability of the transaction that how often the union sets of item sets A and item sets B appear in all of the transactions, that is $S = P(A \cup B)$, The item sets meeting the minimum support is called frequent item sets. Confidence C is the percentage of transaction that transaction database D contains the item sets A also includes item sets B, that is the probability $P(B|A)$, i.e. $C = P(B|A)$. The rule that satisfy the minimum support degree threshold and minimum confidence threshold at the same time is named strong association rule [6].

36.2.2 Particle Swarm Optimization

Particle swarm optimization aim at producing computational intelligence by exploiting simple analogues of social interaction. In the process, each particle is moved by two elastic forces, one attracts it to the best location encountered by the particle, and the other attracts to the best location encountered by any one of the swarm. Each particle has velocity, which is called V [7].

$$V_{id}^{l} = \omega V_{id} + \eta_1 rand()(P_{id} - X_{id}) + \eta_2 rand()(P_{gd} - X_{id}) \tag{36.1}$$

The value of V_{id} is the velocity of ith particle's and the $d$thcomponent's. ω is inertia weight. η_1 and η_2 are two learning rates, and control the relative proportion of cognition and social interaction in the swarm. P_{id} is the best point visited by the ith particle. P_{gd} is the best point visited by the swarm. The position of a particle is updated every time step using the equations:

$$X_{id}^{l} = X_{id} + V_{id} \tag{36.2}$$

36.3 Transaction Matrix Design

Mining association rules algorithm needs to repeatedly scan the database which makes that it is not efficiency in practical applications. To solve this problem, transaction matrix should be set up on a scan to the database, on which mine association rule using GA.

Transaction data matrix G is designed as follows:

Order item sets $I = \{i_1, i_2, \ldots i_n\}$, collection of transaction $D = \{T_1, T_2, \ldots T_m\}$, every element of the matrix is defined as follows: If item j of transaction i appears, gij is 1, otherwise is $0(i = 1,2,\ldots,n\ j = 1,2,\ldots, m)$. The number of rows in the matrix designed is the number m of transactions in the database, while the number of rows is the number n of item sets in the database, every row of the matrix represents a transaction in the database.

To describe the algorithm, the transaction database is shown in Table 36.1, and assign an integer to each project, Szechuan lovage rhizome-1, Chinese angelica-2, Cortex moutan-3, Hooked uncaria-4, Golden thread-5, Baical skullcap root-6.

Table 36.1 Transaction database

TID	Item list
$T1$	Szechuan lovage rhizome, chinese angelica, cortex moutan
$T2$	Szechuan lovage rhizome, chinese angelica, cortex moutan, hooked uncaria, golden thread
$T3$	Szechuan lovage rhizome, cortex moutan, hooked uncaria, golden thread
$T4$	Cortex moutan, hooked uncaria, golden thread
$T5$	Chinese angelica, cortex moutan
$T6$	Szechuan lovage rhizome, cortex moutan, hooked uncaria,
$T7$	Hooked uncaria, golden thread
$T8$	Cortex moutan, hooked uncaria, golden thread
$T9$	Golden thread, Baical skullcap root
$T10$	Hooked uncaria, golden thread, baical skullcap root

36.4 Design of a New Algorithm Based on GA and Particle Swarm Optimization

36.4.1 Design of Chromosome Coding

Using the form of binary encoding, let's take the transaction matrix shown in Fig. 36.1 for example. As the number of items I is 6, so a 6-bit binary string is considered as the chromosome coding. Defining the order of chromosomal gene is $i1$, $i2$,…$i6$, Numerical 1 represents the item in the transaction is existed, while Numerical 0 does not exist.

36.4.2 Design of Fitness Function

In association rule mining, the support and confidence are the vital measure criterion. $f(i)$ is defined as follow.

$$f(i) = \begin{cases} spt(i) - \partial(l) \times \min\_spt + (cnf(i) - \min\_cnf) \\ \text{If } (spt(i) - \min\_spt) > 0 \text{ and } (cnf(i) - \min\_cnf) > 0 \\ 0 \\ \text{If} (spt(i) - \min\_spt) \leq 0 \text{ or } (cnf(i) - \min\_cnf) \leq \text{C} \end{cases} \tag{36.3}$$

The variable $\partial(l)$ is penalty coefficient which plays the role of increasing value with the increase in the length of item sets. $\partial(l)$ is defined as follow. $\partial(l) = \frac{l}{2^{l-1}}$, l is the length of item sets, $spt(i)$ is the support, and $cnf(i)$ is the confidence.min_spt is the threshold of minimum support, and min_cnf is the threshold of minimum confidence.

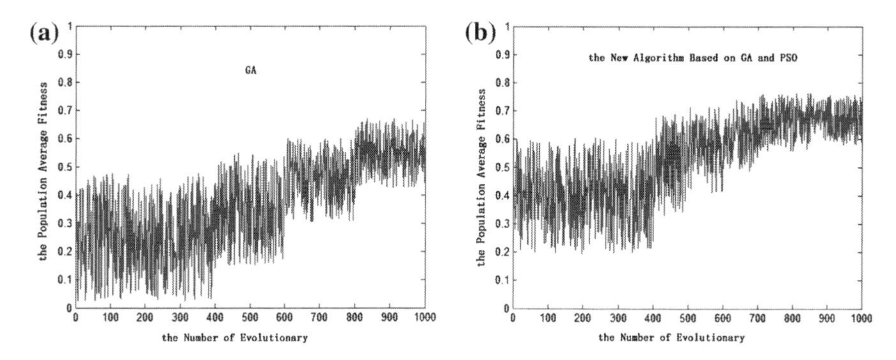

Fig. 36.1 The comparison of population average fitness (**a**) Genetic Algorithm, (**b**)The new Algorithm based on GA and PSO

36.4.3 Design of Genetic Manipulation

The diversity of the particles is increased by introducing crossover operation and mutation operation.

36.4.3.1 Crossover Operator

Single-point crossover is used, according to crossover probability *Pc*, randomly selected two rules in the pairing library to cross, and exchange part of chromosome in the two rules of at the junctions, thus produce two new rules [8]. *Pc* is defined as follows:

$$Pc = \begin{cases} Pc * \dfrac{f\max - f}{f\max - favg}, f \geq favg \\ Pc, f < favg \end{cases} \tag{36.4}$$

And f is the rule of which the fitness function value is larger in the two rules that participate in the manipulation. $f\max$ is the maximum fitness value while $f\max$ is the average fitness value.

36.4.3.2 Mutation Operator

The improved method for uniform mutation is used, mutation rule is selected randomly in the population by the probability *Pm* of mutation, and then make mutation to every locus in this rule. Every locus is valued one by one in allowing range. Mutating can increase the diversity of the population. *Pm* is defined as follows:

$$Pm = \begin{cases} Pm * \dfrac{f\max - f}{f\max - favg}, f \geq favg \\ Pm, f < favg \end{cases} \quad (36.5)$$

And f is the fitness function value of the mutation rule, $f\max$ is the maximum fitness value while $favg$ is the average fitness value.

36.4.4 Description of the New Algorithm

Input: ① transaction database: D
② minimum support: $s_{\min}$
Output: ① strong association rules

Algorithm flow is as follows:
Transaction database should be converted to transaction matrix;
An initial particle swarm will be generated randomly;
Calculate the support $s(j)$ of every particle swarm by the Bit-matrix of transaction database. If it meets $s(j) > s\min$, the individual is put into candidate rule set, otherwise, this rule is removed from the particle swarm;
While (Whether meet the conditions for the termination or not)
{
Calculating the fitness function of every particle by formula 1.3;
For every particle, it can store the best solution, which is called P_{id};
The other "best" value that is tracked by the particle swarm optimizer is the best value obtained so far by any particle in the population which is called P_{gd};
Sorting particles by its fitness value;
The half of better particles directly enters into the next generation; using formlua1.4 and formula 1.5, others take crossover operation and mutation operation; P_{id} and P_{gd} are also changed;
According to formula 1.1 and formula 1.2, the velocity and the position of particle are adjusted;
Calculate the fitness of every rule in the new population and the condition that satisfy the constraints;
Implement elitist strategy;
}
Generate frequent k item sets Lk;
Output strong association rules.

36.5 Application of the New Algorithm in Mining Diagnosis and Treatment of Traditional Chinese Medicine to Coronary Disease

36.5.1 Data Preparation

Considering the reliability, accuracy and completeness of the initial data, choose 736 TCM records as data sources, which come from professor Ding Shuwen treated patients with Coronary heart disease at the out-patient clinic (OPD) of cardiovascular in Affiliated Hospital of Shandong University of TCM from 2008 July to 2010 October. These medical records recorded the patient's name, gender, age, symptoms (for symptomatic analysis), classification type (for dialectical analysis), diagnosis (analysis for identifying diseases) and drug use etc. It is made up that is the transaction database with the diagnosis and drug use in processing of specific data.

36.5.2 Strong Association Rules

When analysis the Coronary disease Medical Records, the frequency of 12 Chinese crude drugs is founded that they are higher than the others : Szechuan lovage rhizome(343), Salvia miltiorrhiza bunge (311), Borneol (305), Panax notoginseng(300), radix rehmanniae(288), astragalus mongholicus(235), radix ophiopogonis(218), sculellaria barbata(196), wild puerarin (188), Cortex moutan (177), stir-baked Semen ziziphi spinosae (175), Raidx astragali (175). Using the mining algorithm of genetic association rules, the result is showed as Table 36.2:

Modern pharmacological studies shows that Szechuan lovage rhizome can inhibit the vasomotor center directly and reflexively and block sympathetic and ganglion because of what can make the peripheral vascular expansion and reduce vascular resistance; Salvia miltiorrhiza bunge can dilate the blood vessel, increase the antihypertensive effect of acetylcholine and block the sympathetic; Puerarin the main active ingredients of wild puerarin has retardation to β receptor that can lower blood pressure by reducing the sympathetic nerve function; Szechuan lovage rhizome and Chinese angelica are with the role of calcium channel blocking which can lower blood pressure by peripheral vascular expansion. Raidx astragali acts on center and vascular receptor which can lower blood pressure reflexively and has a sedative and diuretic effect; Oriental water plantain rhizome has significant diuresis, so that lower blood pressure [9, 10]. There are 6 Chinese crude drugs of strong association rules whose support are 0.34 were included in the Hooked uncaria recipe (this recipe contains 10 Chinese crude drugs) which Professor Ding commonly used in the treatment of coronary disease.

Table 36.2 Strong association rules in case of traditional chinese medicine in coronary disease

Strong association rules	Support
Qi stagnation and blood stasis⇒(radix bupleuri, rhizoma cyperi, szechuan lovage rhizome, salvia miltiorrhiza bunge, rhizoma corydalis, wild puerarin, borneol)	0.34
Qi deficiency and blood stasis⇒(astragalus mongholicus, radix rehmanniae, szechuan lovage rhizome, salvia miltiorrhiza bunge, rhizoma corydalis, panax notoginseng, borneol)	0.31
Yin deficiency and blood stasis⇒(radix ophiopogonis, radix rehmanniae, szechuan lovage rhizome, salvia miltiorrhiza bunge, rhizoma corydalis, wild puerarin, borneol)	0.30
Phlegm and blood stasis ⇒(rhizoma coptidis, fructus trichosanthis, radix rehmanniae, szechuan lovage rhizome, salvia miltiorrhiza bunge, rhizoma corydalis, panax notoginseng, borneol)	0.27
Noxious heat with blood stasis ⇒(rhizoma coptidis, sculellaria barbata, radix rehmanniae, szechuan lovage rhizome, salvia miltiorrhiza bunge, rhizoma corydalis, panax notoginseng, borneol)	0.25

36.5.3 The Performance Comparison of Apriori Algorithm, GA and the New Algorithm

Make comparative experiment using Apriori algorithm and genetic association rule mining algorithm to the strong association rules of which the minimum support were 0.2 and 0.1 respectively, the consequence of performance comparison as Table 36.3 shows.

The experimental results indicated that the running time of the new algorithm based on GA and particle swarm optimization is even less than one-tenth of the original Apriori algorithm under the same experimental conditions which improved the work efficiency greatly and saved lots of storage space.

By the comparison of average fitness of GA and the new algorithm, there is gradual increase in average fitness with the evolution. In the evolution to a larger number of, the average fitness gradually is stabilized. The average fitness of the new algorithm is 67.5 %, which is higher than the average fitness of the GA, which is 55.6 % of. The comparison of population average fitness is shown in Fig. 36.1.

Table 36.3 The Consequence of performance comparison

Minimum support	The time needed for apriori algorithm (s)	The time needed for genetic algorithm (s)	The time needed for the new algorithm(s)
0.2	461	360	32
0.1	2803	1230	121

36.6 Conclusions

In this paper the new algorithm which is based on GA and particle swarm optimization was applied to the extraction of association rules and then proposed a algorithm for mining association rules based on GA that was used in the analysis of medical records of coronary disease. Compared with the traditional association rule mining algorithm (Apriori algorithm) and the GA, the improved algorithm increased the efficiency of the frequent item sets extract parts in systems effectively. The algorithm is great reference to the application of data mining techniques used in traditional Chinese medicine.

References

1. Karaboga NA (2009) New design method based on artificial bee colony algorithm for digital IIR filters[J]. J Franklin Inst, 346(4):328–348
2. Na D, Chun-Ho W, Wai-Hung I (2012) An opposition-based chaotic GA/PSO hybrid algorithm and its application in circle detection.Comput math appl. 64(6):1886–1902
3. Xu CF, Duan HB (2010) Particle swarm optimission (PSO) optimized edge potential function(EPT) approach to target recognition for low altitude aircraft. Pattern Recogn Lett 31(13):1759–1772
4. Wang Z, Cheng D (2009) Method and application of mining association rules based on improved genetic algorithm. J Chongqing Insts of Technol. 23(4)
5. Shiwei Y, MingWei Y, Wang K (2012) A PSO–GA optimal model to estimate primary energy demand of China. Energy Policy 42(8):329–340
6. Riget J, Vesterstrm JS, Krink K (2002) Division of labor in particle swarm opimisation. July 11
7. Poli R, Langdon WB (2008) Extending particle swarm optimisation via genetic programming. Springer Verlag, 292–300
8. Xiaoshuang Y, Minghua J (2009) Method of association rules mining based on genetic algorithm. Softw Guide 8(10):64–66
9. Huang C (2000) TCM diagnosis and treatment Of cardiovascular division diseases. Beijing: People's medical publishing house, 128–168
10. Zeyu C (2002) Advanced studies on the puerarin radix. J Chongqing Inst Technol 18(3):105–107

Chapter 37
Design and Development of a Clinical Data Exchange System Based on Ensemble Integration Platform

Wang Yu, Guo Long, Tian Yu and Jing-Song Li

Abstract With the pace of China's New Medical Reform, medical information systems have been rapidly developing, thus generating tremendous clinical data that contain large amount of information. Clinical data exchange is one of the most important foundations to make full use of clinical data. Under the whole background of Global Dolphin (an international data exchange system between China and Japan), this paper demonstrates a method of achieving standardized clinical data exchange based on Ensemble Integration Platform and using Health Level Seven International (HL7) as the data exchange standard. HL7 helps to standardize the data exchange process; Ensemble Platform contributes to the loose coupling of medical information systems and constructing a unified data management layer in logic, ultimately achieving the goal of sharing clinical data between a data center and medical institutions.

Keywords Clinical data exchange · HL7 · Ensemble · Interoperability · Web service

37.1 Introduction

Hospital information construction in China has been developing since 30 years ago. In 2007, the National Statistical Information Center of the Ministry of Health launched a survey on the 3,765 hospitals nationwide; the results showed that the hospital information systems basically were still management information systems or clinical information systems [1]. Due to the current domestic hospital systems are from different manufactures, using different information standards and

W. Yu · G. Long · T. Yu · J.-S. Li (✉)
Healthcare Informatics Engineering Research Center, Zhejiang University, 310027 Hangzhou, China
e-mail: ljs@zju.edu.cn

S. Li et al. (eds.), *Frontier and Future Development of Information Technology in Medicine and Education*, Lecture Notes in Electrical Engineering 269,
DOI: 10.1007/978-94-007-7618-0_37, © Springer Science+Business Media Dordrecht 2014

different data format, information and resources cannot be shared between community healthcare centers and hospitals, resulting in isolated islands of information. Patients' clinical information (including text, data, images) during visits in different medical institutions cannot be transferred or reuse, leading to a waste of medical resources. Therefore, an effective way is needed to achieve the safe, efficient and flexible data exchange and sharing [2].

Furthermore, with the continuous development of global trade, floating population across countries keep growing, so the exchange of clinical data only in a country within a certain region will be unable to meet the needs. If you can imagine, a foreigner travelling to China, unfortunately had a traffic accident or acute onset. But the Chinese doctors didn't know any of his allergy history or congenital diseases, the treatment was likely delayed. If you can access to the medical information of electronic medical records (EMRs) in his own country immediately, the chance of patient survival will be greatly increased. Therefore, the establishment of an international medical data exchange is urgent. However, during the process of data exchange between two different countries will often encounter such as different languages, different storing formats of EMRs, hindering the development of international clinical data exchange.

In October 2006, Zhejiang University, Kyoto University and the University of Miyazaki launched an international clinical data exchange cooperation projects—Global Dolphin [3, 4]; in the end of 2007, as a basis for international data exchange, Xizi Regional Clinical Information Center (XRCIC, equivalent in Kyoto and Miyazaki Regional Clinical Information Center), Zhejiang University, Hangzhou, was established.

Under the framework, this paper demonstrates a method of achieving a clinical data exchange system based on Ensemble Integration Platform and Health Level Seven (HL7) on the basis of implementation of hospital information systems integration. HL7 helps regulate the data exchange process; Ensemble helps maximize the integration of a data center and systems of medical institution.

37.2 Architecture of the Clinical Data Exchange System

The entity structure of the clinical data exchange system has three parts: a data center, medical institutions, and individual users. Once patients as individual users finish their clinical examinations, relevant health information are generated and uploaded to the data center, where relevant information is packaged according to the Enterprise Master Patient Index (EMPI). Individual users can view their own health information through the web interface, as shown in Fig. 37.1.

Medical institutions are the main providers of healthcare data; they transform the clinical data in the local database into HL7-standard data files and upload the data files to the data center through FTP, the protocol of transmitting files between two computers in the TCP/IP network. Data Center interprets the received HL7-standard data files into the data schema that can be saved in the local database.

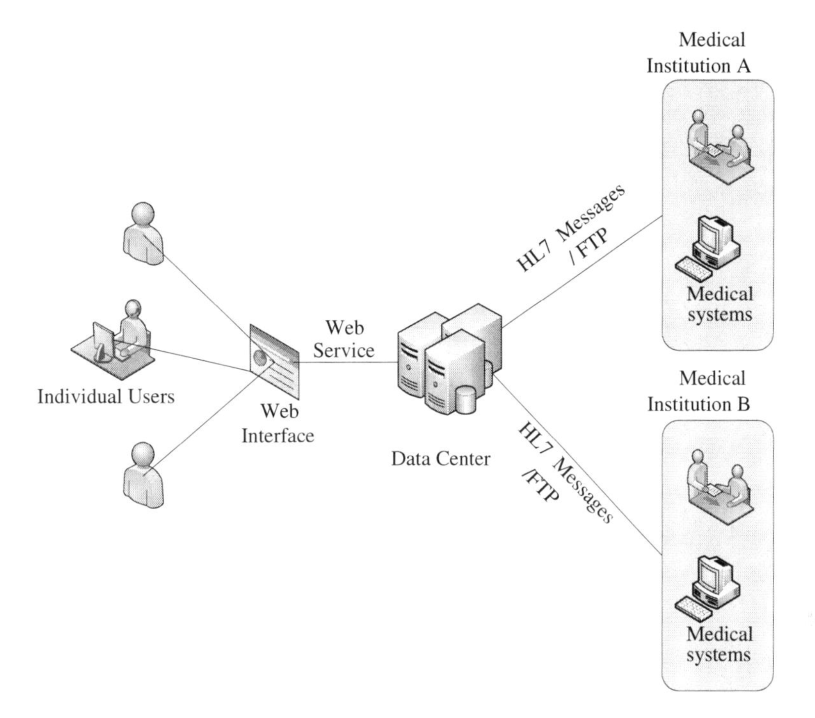

Fig. 37.1 EHR system entity architecture

Clinical data and files can be downloaded from the data center using the same exchange mechanism. All the data exchange processes described above are accomplished within Ensemble platform. Data center publishes relative web services and web site through IIS server. Individual users can access their authorized health information and view them on the website [5], as shown in Fig. 37.2.

Data Center stores the assembled healthcare information, and administrates the system users and their authorizations. Connected medical institutions and authorized individual users can download healthcare information in the data centers and view the information on the website. Saving the necessary minimum amount of clinical information in the data center benefits the storage, management, and data sharing between medical institutions [6]. The data center provides data mining and analysis services through which users can make full use of the stored medical data. The auxiliary parts of the functional modules of data centers include authority setting, privacy control, patient index, and medical terminology libraries [7]. The data center exchanges data with medical institutions through data bus and interacts with individual users through its website, as shown in Fig. 37.3

The data center publishes the patient information query, examination reports searching and viewing as web services. Users who are authorized can log in the website and call the web services, thus view corresponding authorized health information. The website has a three-tier structure that is convenient for modification and management.

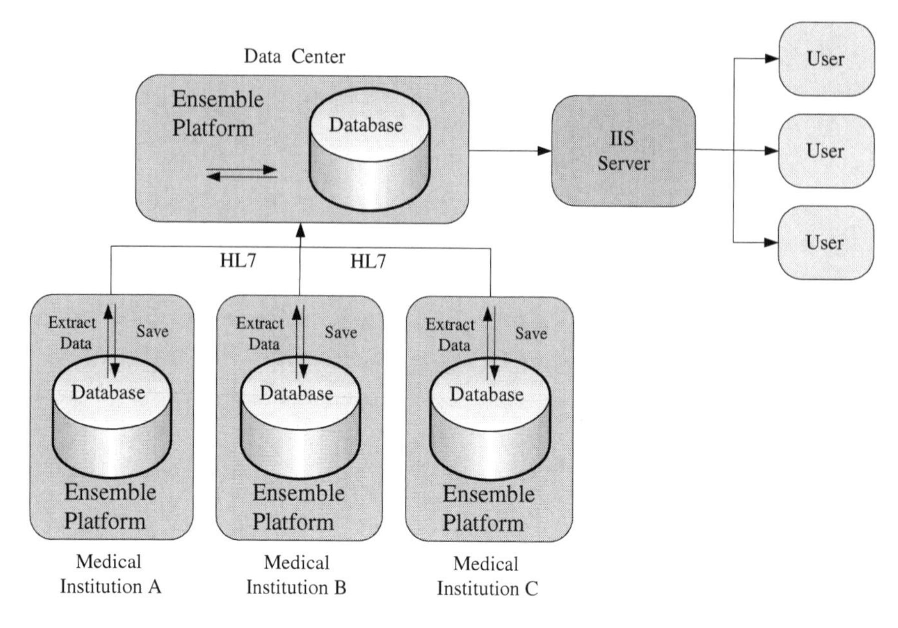

Fig. 37.2 System architecture

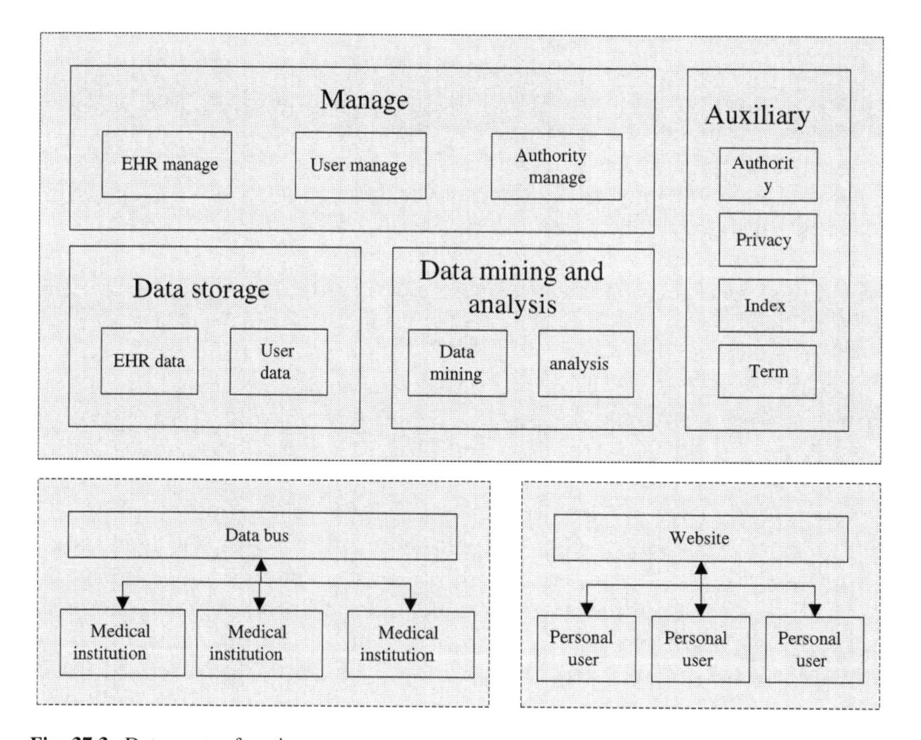

Fig. 37.3 Data center functions

37.3 Interoperability of Clinical Data Exchange System

Healthcare information should be exchanged and shared through heterogeneous-medical institutions in region. The clinical data exchange system based on Ensemble uses HL7, with good interoperability, as its data exchange standard. HL7 is the standard for data exchange among different applications in the medical field [8], and the objective of HL7 is to promote communication in the medical service field. HL7 can facilitate data exchange among systems in different technological environments and can be used with different programming languages and operating systems. Hence, information messages standardized by HL7 can be exchanged in heterogeneous systems. Ensemble platform can process HL7 information at high speed, and Ensemble's HL7 adapters can efficiently develop HL7-formatdata interfaces.

As data schema of a certain medical institution's local database differs from HL7-standard form, the healthcare record data in the local database should be converted to HL7-standard messages through Ensemble HL7 interfaces. Each HL7 message consists of a message header and message body. The information in the message header is directly assigned by medical institutions, and the information in the message body comprises the clinical data stored in the local database of medical institutions. Ensemble creates a matching model for HL7 messages and data form of the local database, as shown in Fig. 37.4 so that the local data can be converted to HL7-format messages rapidly and efficiently.

After the clinical data are converted to HL7-format messages, corresponding HL7 files are generated. At the receiving end, the received data files are then converted to HL7-format messages and imported to Ensemble through Ensemble's

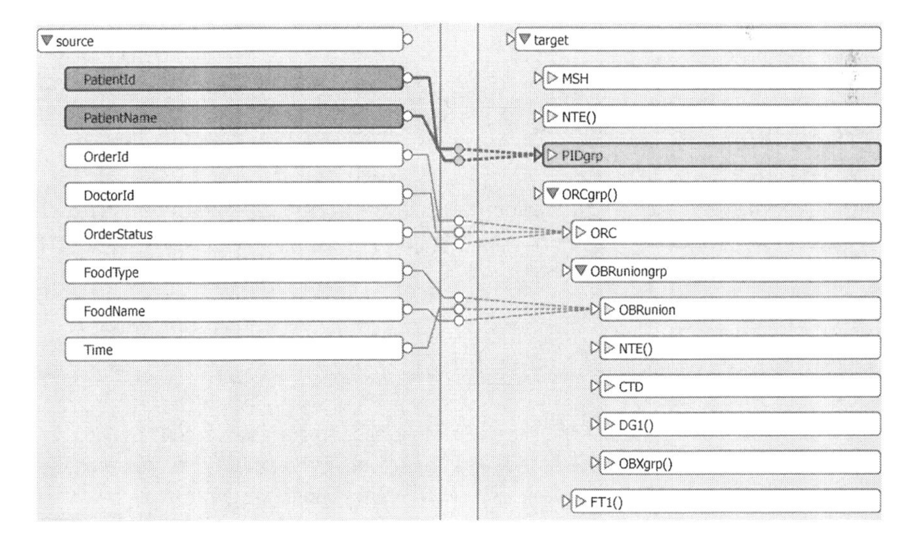

Fig. 37.4 Message transformation model

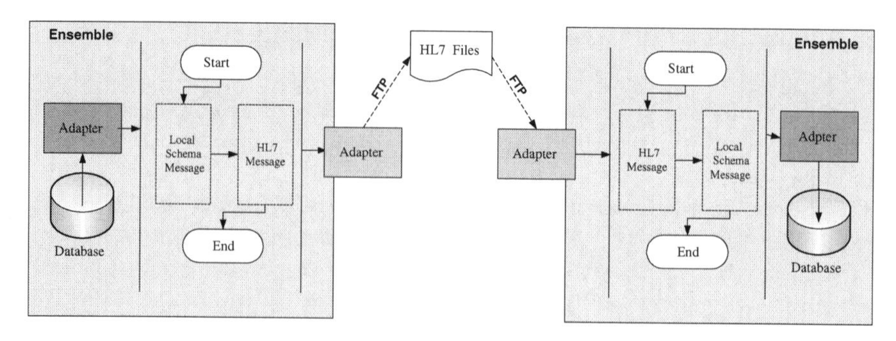

Fig. 37.5 Data interoperability process

HL7 adapter. Properties of HL7 messages are matched with the data stored in the center database, and the HL7-format messages are converted to "center-format" messages that are suitable for the center database and saved.

The detailed process of healthcare data interoperating between different systems is shown in Fig. 37.5. When the database of medical institutions or data centers produce data that require transmission, Ensemble will trigger the information transmission process. Afterwards, the data are imported to Ensemble in the form of messages through the database adapter. Data messages are then converted to HL7-format messages using a data transformation module in Ensemble. Once the transformation is completed, HL7-format messages are produced into data files and automatically transmitted to the recipient through FTP. When the recipient receives the data files through FTP, Ensemble will import the data files into the file adapter of Ensemble and convert HL7-format messages to local-format data messages, which are suitable for the local database through the data transformation module in Ensemble. Finally, the converted data messages are stored in the local database through the SQL adapter.

37.4 Results

Our system processes and transforms data using Ensemble, which contains database adapters and HL7 adapters. The database adapter connects to the local database, and the HL7 adapter outputs HL7-format files. The system uses FTP to transmit data files. Data centers use a post-relational cache database that utilizes multidimensional arrays to store data and has superior speeds suitable for large amounts of data. The interface of the data center's website is presented in Fig. 37.6.

The websites of the data centers were developed through ASP.NET using the developer tool Visual Studio 2008. The websites of data centers use dynamic link library files to call the database function. ASP.NET is the programming framework that is built in the common language library and is used to generate web applications on the server. Websites are published by the IIS, a web service component.

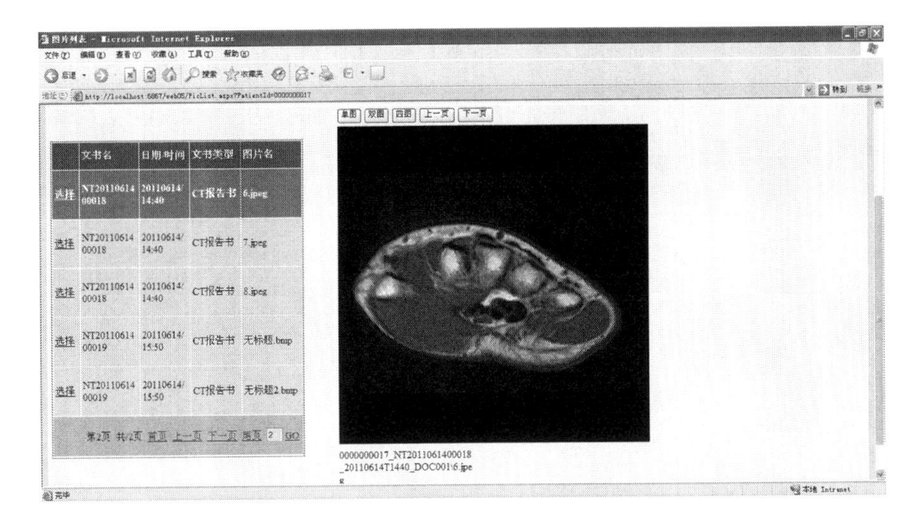

Fig. 37.6 Data center website interface

37.5 Conclusions and Discussion

Clinical data exchange has been identified as an essential strategy for addressing quality and safety all over the world. Communication, standardization, funding, and interoperability are the four common barriers that hinder the implementation of clinical data exchange system. As the extension of Global Dolphin, we use HL7 as data exchange standard instead of Medical Markup Language (MML). MML, born in Japan, adapts to Japan's national conditions [9]; HL7, as an international standard, has more compatibility, expansibility and portability. So the system described in this paper can be used in more situations, even in other international data exchange cases. In the clinical data exchange system architect proposed by this paper, various medical institutions can convert their own healthcare record data to HL7-format data files and upload data files to the data center. Medical institutions can also download HL7-format healthcare record data from the data center and save them in their local database, thus accomplishing the exchange process and solving the problem of interoperability. The system processes HL7 messages quickly and efficiently using Ensemble. Moreover, the clinical data exchange system based on Ensemble reduces the complexity of system design and implementation, improves the system's scalability, and makes maintenance easier.

Acknowledgments This work was supported by the National Natural Science Foundation (Grant No. 61173127) and Zhejiang University Top Disciplinary Partnership Program (Grant No. 188170*193251101).

References

1. Fu Z, Liang MH (2009) Introduction to digital medicine. People's Health Publishing House, Beijing
2. Xu HF, Wang WP, Zheng JH, Wen CX (2007) Research about information exchange platform based on HL7 and web services between region medical institutions. Comput Appl Softw 24(3):88–90
3. Li JS, Zhou TS, Chu J, Araki K, Yoshihara H (2011) Design and development of an international clinical data exchange system: the international layer function of the dolphin project. J Am Med Inform Assoc 18:683–689
4. Guo JQ, Takada A, Tanaka K, Sato J, Suzuki M, Suzuki T, Nakashima Y, Araki K, Yoshihara H (2002) The development of MML (Medical Markup Language) version 3.0 as a medical document exchange format for HL7 messages. J Med Syst 28(6):523–533
5. Jang BM, Kim JI, Yang KH, Han DH, Cho HM, Jung H, Kim HJ (2007) Design and implementation of the system architecture for sharing medical information based HL7-CDA among hospitals by the XDS model of IHE. In: Proceedings of international federation for medical and biological engineering. pp. 460–463
6. Gu XH (2010) Design and implementation of community electronic health record system. J Med Inform 31:8–12
7. Wu RM, Xin XX (2011) The network and information technology center. J Med Inform 32:19–23
8. Wang Y, Yao ZH, Liu L (2010) Electronic health record standard—CDA and openEHR. J Press China Med Devices 25:11–21
9. MedXML Consortium (2009) MML version 3.0 specification [EB/OL]. http://medxml.net/ E_mml30/ mmlv3_E_index.htm

Chapter 38
The Management and Application of a Radio Frequency Identification System in Operating Rooms

Jun-Der Leu, Yu-Hui Chiu and Hsueh-Ling Ku

Abstract Radio frequency identification (RFID) systems are currently employed for a wide range of health care procedures. To prevent incidents of medical negligence and occurrences of adverse events, information technology (IT) systems that facilitate instantaneous delivery of relevant information to support and remind medical professionals may provide an appropriate solution. This study focuses on the use of RFID systems for surgical patients, which involves patients wearing an RFID wristband throughout the processes of admission, preoperative examination, operation, postoperative recovery, to discharge. Subsequently, by integrating RFID and the Internet, patient information can be promptly accessed, which not only eliminates the need for manually documenting the steps throughout the operation flow, but also enables medical staff to monitor and perform relevant medical tasks, enhancing the accuracy, completeness, and success of each operation. In addition, RFID enables operating room (OR) managers to promptly and quickly obtain accurate and complete patient information (basic patient data, department, surgical procedure, time of surgery, anesthesia type, time of anesthesia, blood transfusion rate, number of surgical instruments, OR utilization time, and surgical team data) and related quality indicators to facilitate decision making.

Keywords Radio frequency identification · Surgical patient flow · Operating room management

J.-D. Leu
National Central University, Zhongli, Republic of China

Y.-H. Chiu
Wan Fang Hospital, Taipei Medical University, Taipei, Republic of China

H.-L. Ku (✉)
Cathay General Hospital, Ching Kuo Institute of Management and Health, Zhongli, Republic of China
e-mail: 201385@cgh.org.tw

S. Li et al. (eds.), *Frontier and Future Development of Information Technology in Medicine and Education*, Lecture Notes in Electrical Engineering 269,
DOI: 10.1007/978-94-007-7618-0_38,

38.1 Introduction

The operating room (OR) is a key unit for surgical patients during their inpatient stay. ORs are equipped with delicate and expensive devices and professional medical teams, and are associated with high costs; however, they also generate substantial revenue for a hospital. In addition, ORs are the core of a health care institution's operations because they facilitate emergent care, inpatient services, and intensive care and account for over half of the service volume [1]. Currently, RFID systems are widely employed in numerous health care fields, such as hospital management [2], medication safety management [3], monitoring and managing surgical dressings inventory [4], postoperative infection control associated with breast cancer operations (Allen 2007), tracheal tube position tracking [5], and intrahospital patient transportation safety [6].

RFID employs high-tech barcodes based on microchips that are integrated with radio frequencies and a scanner to track objects. Compared to traditional barcodes, the advantages of RFID include the ability to read information without contact, update data, repeated use, and simultaneous identification of various tags. Furthermore, RFID systems possess a substantial data storage capacity and sufficient data security. When an RFID reader transmits a signal to a tag, the tag reports its barcode to the reader for processing. The reader then either transfers the information to the Internet or actively transmits signals of a specific frequency. RFID offers considerable convenience by actively reading information to track patient location and monitor patient data. RFID is also effective for intrahospital medication monitoring, thereby indirectly improving patient safety by reducing dispensing errors, surgical mistakes, and nosocomial infections.

Quality health care activities and management are fundamental for excellent health care services. Health care quality can be evaluated from the following three perspectives: structure, process, and outcome. These three quality indicators are highly correlated because structure affects processes and processes influence outcomes. Thus, errors in any of these aspects cannot be tolerated. By integrating existing resources and systems, the study hospital adopted the latest information technology (IT) applications, including a health information system (HIS), a wireless environment, mobile devices, and RFID, to establish a seamless surgical patient management system for providing safe, efficient, and high-quality surgical services.

38.2 Study Materials and Methodology

38.2.1 Introduction to the Study Hospital

The case study hospital was a medical center located in Taipei, Taiwan, with 742 beds and 1,600 employees. The hospital features 14 ORs that are shared by 11 departments, including General Surgery, Plastic Surgery, Urology, Orthopedics,

Neurosurgery, Obstetrics and Gynecology (OBGYN), Otolaryngology, Ophthalmology, Cardiac Surgery, Rectal Surgery, and Oral Surgery. The annual number of operations conducted at this hospital is 22,000, of which outpatient, inpatient, and emergency operations account for 42, 52, and 6 %, respectively.

38.2.2 Implementation of RFID for Surgical Patients

Using Microsoft SQL Server 2005 as the back-end operating platform, the RFID system database combined basic patient data from the HIS with operation scheduling information, laboratory test data from the Laboratory Information System, and nursing care information from the Nursing Information System. The database was then integrated with active RFID wristbands (Fig. 38.1), RFID readers (Fig. 38.2), ultra-mobile personal computers, and laptop computers (Fig. 38.3). The system was integrated with the HIS scheduling program, and surgical data were updated every 3 min. This RFID system could display surgical patient information upon request.

38.2.3 Integration of RFID Hardware and Software

The hospital installed 15 RFID readers (Fig. 38.4) in the emergency department, ORs, recovery room, and OBGYN and surgical wards. After an inpatient is assigned an RFID wristband during preoperative preparations in the surgical ward, the system identifies the patient and begins to document the duration of each step, including the time the patient leaves the ward, registers at the OR front desk, and enters/leaves the operating/recovery room.

Fig. 38.1 Active RFID tag

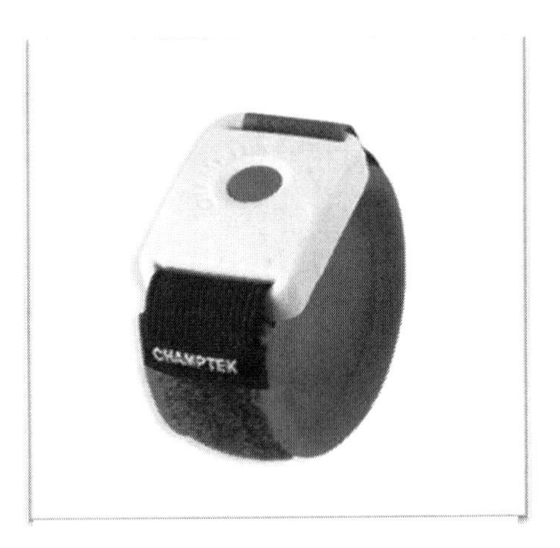

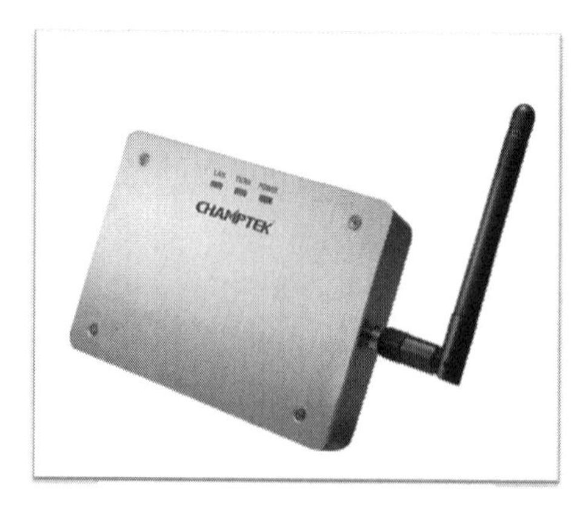

Fig. 38.2 RFID reader

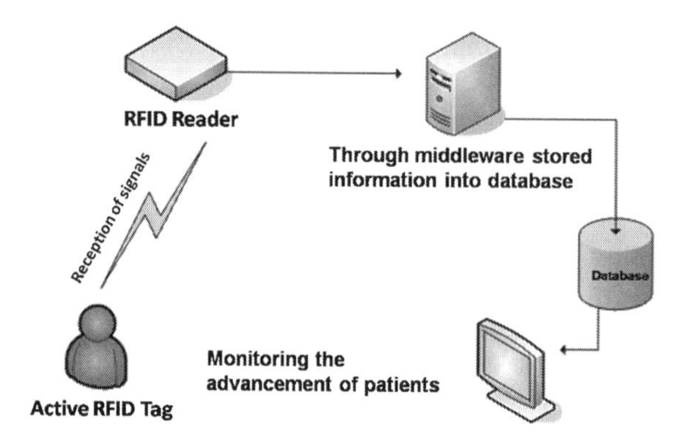

Fig. 38.3 RFID system framework

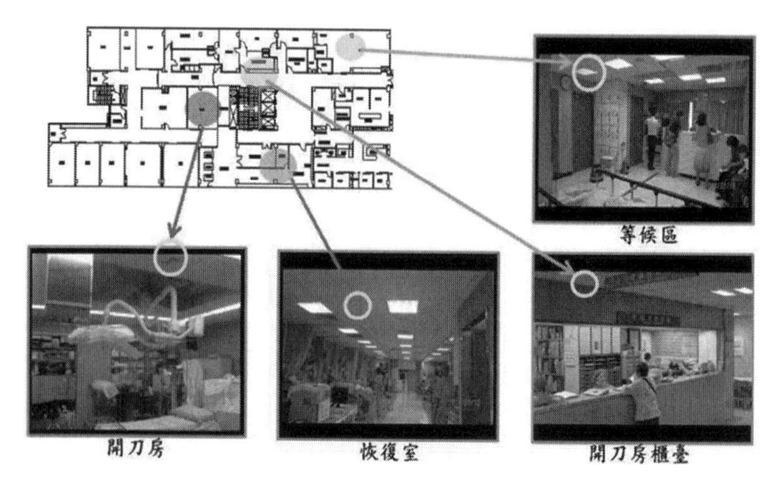

Fig. 38.4 Location of RFID readers in the OR area:waiting area; OR; recovery room; and OR front desk

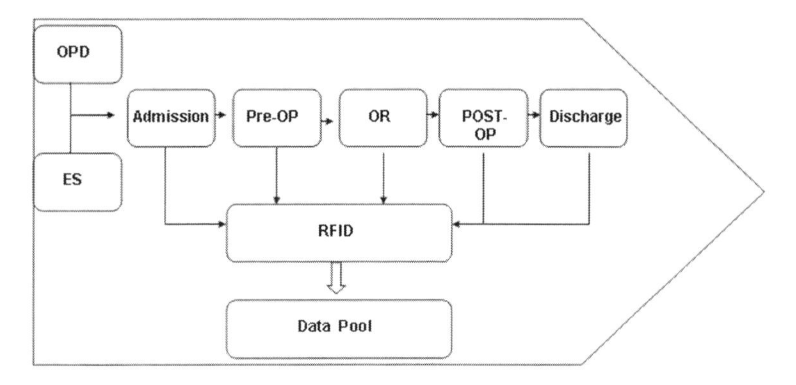

Fig. 38.5 Conceptual framework of the standardized flow for applying the RFID system

38.2.4 Standardized Flow for Applying the RFID System

After a patient agrees to undergo an operation and the operation is successfully scheduled, a series of follow-up and interacting procedures involving checking and documenting are conducted by several units. When a patient is registered following admission, his/her data are entered into the RFID system database for data integration and subsequent tracking. Subsequently, when the patient wearing the active RFID wristband passes the RFID readers located in specific areas, his/her position is documented and entered into the database. The patient information is then displayed on a front-end webpage for health care staff, who can then identify and monitor the patient status. Personnel from the Department of General Surgery, Department of Nursing, Operating Room, Department of Anesthesia, Recovery Room, Emergency Department, OBGYN wards in East five, general surgical wards in East six, 25 general surgical wards, Inpatient Center, Department of Strategic Planning in the IT Division, and Quality Management Center participated in implementing the RFID system. The conceptual system framework is shown in Fig. 38.5.

38.3 Results

38.3.1 Safety

Following the implementation of the RFID system, serious adverse events, such as wrong-site, wrong-procedure, and wrong-patient errors, have seldom occurred. Health care professionals' consideration of patient safety and the implementation of the RFID monitoring technology have reassured the hospital's surgical patients and their families.

38.3.2 *Volume of Operations*

Number of operations: The number of operations increased from 21,696 in 2009 to 21,993 in 2010, and reaching 12,291 between January and July 2011. Shown in Fig. 38.6.

38.3.3 *Quality of Operations*

The hospital regularly monitored several performance indicators for various medical procedures, such as the rates of prophylactic antibiotics administration, unscheduled returns to the OR, operative mortality, and wound infection. International literature suggests that the administration of prophylactic antibiotics 1 h pre-operation can effectively reduce nosocomial infection rates. In the study hospital, the rate of prophylactic antibiotic administration 1 h pre-operation reached 100 % for numerous surgical procedures (Fig. 38.7), demonstrating the surgical team's emphasis on maintaining health care quality. In addition, regarding surgical outcomes, the rate of unscheduled OR returns was approximately 0.5 % (Fig. 38.8), indicating that the surgical team provides outstanding health care services.

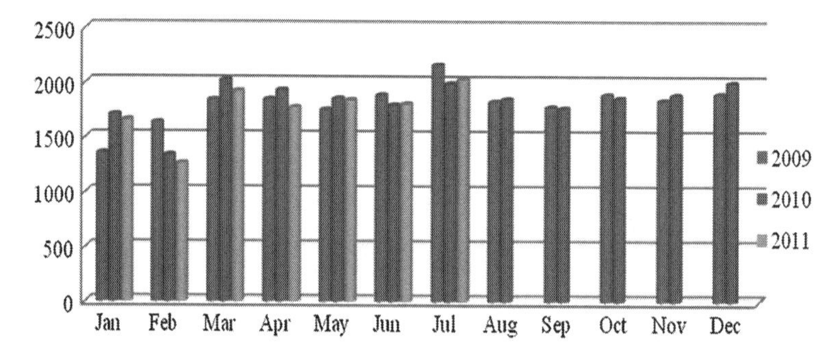

Fig. 38.6 Volume of operations

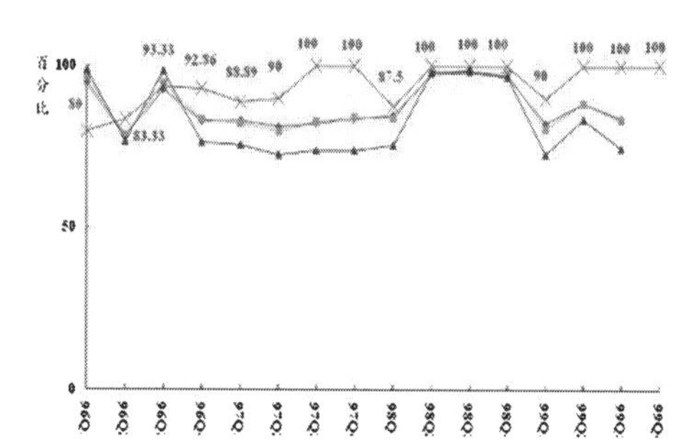

Fig. 38.7 Rate of prophylactic antibiotic administration

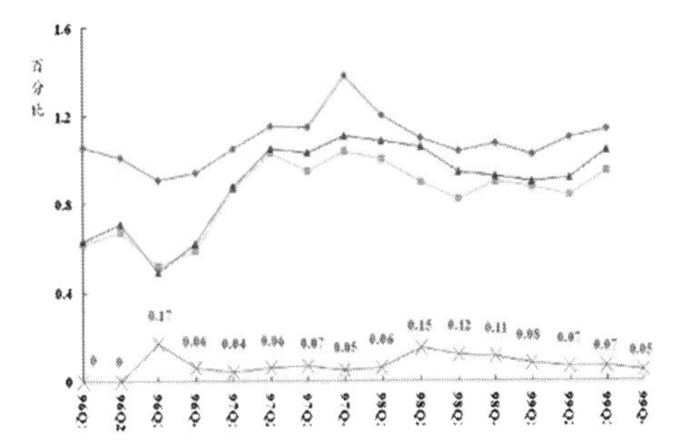

Fig. 38.8 Rate of unscheduled OR returns

38.3.4 Surgical Patient Satisfaction

The satisfaction of surgical patients at the study hospital increased from 84.0 points in 2008, 86.7 points in 2009, to 87.9 points in 2010, as shown in Fig. 38.9.

38.3.5 The Surgical Team's Acceptance of the Innovative System

The technology acceptance model was used to evaluate users' acceptance of the RFID system. The results showed that during the initial system go-live stage, users reported more positive intentions to use and attitudes, although they displayed less positive acknowledgement of the system's ease of use and usefulness. Because users were unfamiliar and tended to resist the new system when it was initially launched, the study hospital organized several training sessions, collected user feedback, and modified the user interface to effectively familiarize users with the system. The survey results regarding the system are listed in Table 38.1.

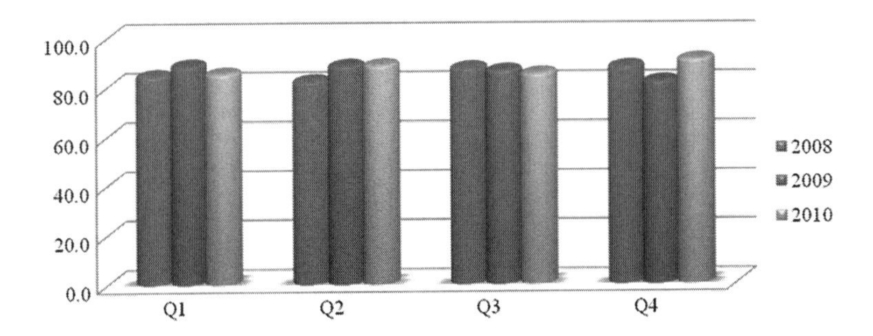

Fig. 38.9 Satisfaction of surgical patienst

Table 38.1 Evaluation of user acceptance of the new system

Item	Positive Response	
	Initial stage of system i mplementation (%)	Mature stage of system implementation (%)
Perceived usefulness	37.5	64
Perceived ease of use	20	75
Intention to use	80	85
Attitude	74.5	81

38.4 Discussion

Appropriate surgical flow management not only enhances the efficiency of OR utilization but also increases the safety of surgical patients. The research team applied RFID to ORs to establish a Patient Advancement Monitoring System. Compared to the passive mode, which necessitates the implementation of scanners at each step for data input and manual scanning of wristbands, active RFID devices offer considerable time savings. In addition to the basic locating function, the RFID system integrates existing health care management systems, producing excellent service quality and outcomes as well as a strong operation management system.

Patricia et al. suggested that before the induction of anesthesia (i.e., sign-in), before skin incision (i.e., time-out), and before the patient leaves the OR (i.e., sign-out) checklists should be used to achieve patient safety and the comprehensiveness of care. Several checklists were employed to conduct assessments of quality indicators for the services provided to surgical patients. The staff implementation rate of checklists for procedures that include checking the operating status at several steps before and during operations; monitoring surgical instruments and gauze inventory; checking the completeness of operative nursing documentation; preoperative checking; sign-in, time-out, and sign-out check; and the monitoring of each identification point for surgical safety was satisfactory.

During the system planning and implementation stage, the Quality Management Center collaborated with the IT Division to understand user needs through interviews. After building and integrating the system software and hardware, functions related to the emergency department, wards, general surgery, ORs, intensive care units, the Department of Anesthesia, and the patient transportation unit were incorporated, with the entire surgical team participating in this process. During system implementation, 88 meetings and 22 on-the-job education and training sessions were organized, incurring high manpower, time, and facility costs.

With automated data collection, the system can generate information regarding safety, management, and quality performance indicators in a timely manner. Furthermore, the system fully monitors the completion of safety procedures during each surgical operation to ensure surgical patient safety. Data regarding OR utilization and efficiency, such as the utilization rate, average time between operations, and more importantly, surgical quality and performance, including operative mortality, returns to the OR, and prophylactic antibiotic administration, are also routinely collected by the system. In the past, the data listed above were compiled in paper records; thus, data collection and output for identifying performance indicators required substantial manpower and retrospective research, rendering timely and effective management impossible. Since the implementation of the RFID system, health care professionals have additional time to spend caring for and interacting with patients. Back-end management tasks that previously necessitated considerable manpower and resources to complete have been replaced by IT, which provides extremely convenient, accurate, and comprehensive data to OR managers for timely decision making.

38.5 Conclusion

In addition to RFID technology, mobile devices, and a wireless environment, various HISs available in the hospital should be continually integrated, and the WHO Surgical Safety Checklist should also be incorporated in the information system flow to generate additional positive outcomes. Furthermore, the technical problems encountered when implementing RFID technology in actual space and practical flow should be addressed and resolved. This experience of system implementation can provide an important reference for the future promotion and development of RFID systems.

Regarding management functions, the RFID system enables OR managers to access complete surgical patient information (basic patient data, department, surgical procedure, time of operation, anesthesia type, time of anesthesia, blood transfusion rate, number of surgical instruments, OR utilization time, and surgical team data) instantly and conveniently. Managers can also readily obtain complete data for OR management indicators (number of operations; OR utilization rates; operation cancelation rates; pathological sample testing rates; and the operation consent form, preoperative and postoperative evaluation, preoperative preparation, and explanation of disease information completion rates) and for International Quality Indicator Project indicators (rate of prophylactic antibiotics administration 30, 60, and 120 min pre-operation, and the rate of unscheduled returns to the OR) through the system, which increases their job satisfaction. Thus, the study results can serve as a reference for peer hospitals when implementing a health care technology system.

Acknowledgments The researchers appreciated the assistance provided by hospital President Mr. Lin, Vice President Mr. Huang, the Quality Management Center, the Health Care Information Center, and the surgical and anesthesia teams.

References

1. Viapiano J, Ward DS (2000) Operating room utilization:the need for data. Int Anesthesiol Clin 38:127–140
2. Al NH, Deogun JS (2007) Radio frequency identification applications in smart hospitals. In: IEEE symposium on computer-based medical systems, pp 337–342
3. Sun PR, Wang BH, Wu F (2008) A new method to guard inpatient medication safety by the implementation of RFID. J Med Syst 32:327–332
4. Rogers A, Jones E, Oleynikov D (2007) Radio frequency identification (RFID) applied to surgical sponges. Surg Endosc 21:1235–1237
5. Reicher J, Reicher D, Reicher M (2007) Use of radio frequency identification (RFID) tags in bedside monitoring of endotracheal tube position. J Clin Monit Comput 21:155–158
6. Ohashi K, Kurihara Y, Watanabe K et al (2008) Safe patient transfer system with monitoring of location and vital signs. J Med Dent Sci 55:33–41

Chapter 39
Exploiting Innovative Computer Education Through Student Associations

Wei Hu, Daikun Zou, Wenfei Li, Hong Guo and Ning Li

Abstract Computer education faces with new challenges for the emerging new technologies such as multi-core/many-core technology. Practice is one way to solve this problem. However, practice is limited in the course. Other ways should be provided for students' practice. In this paper, a novel approach is described to exploit innovative computer education through student associations. Students organize themselves into a variety of associations where they conduct various activities spontaneously under the guidance of teachers. They are more actively engaged in the practice and take the initiative to learn new content. Our investigation also shows that students have a high acceptance on such associations.

Keywords Computer education · Practice · Student association

39.1 Introduction

Computer technology is developing very rapidly in recent years [1]. There are also many other new advances in computer technology. Embedded computing systems are also widely used than before. How to develop programs for mobile devices is very important. It requires new actions [2]. As the above shows, new requirements are emerging for computer education. And these are new challenges for universities.

According to the reported works, there are many different approaches to solve such new issues [3–6]. The main concerns are how to provide the solutions through the reforms, re-designs and improvements to related courses or curriculum

W. Hu (✉) · D. Zou · W. Li · H. Guo · N. Li
College of Computer Science and Technology, Wuhan University of Science and Technology Hubei Province Key Laboratory of Intelligent Information Processing and Real-time Industrial System, Wuhan, 430065 Hubei, China
e-mail: huwei@wust.edu.cn

S. Li et al. (eds.), *Frontier and Future Development of Information Technology in Medicine and Education*, Lecture Notes in Electrical Engineering 269,
DOI: 10.1007/978-94-007-7618-0_39,

architecture. For example, many universities have provided new courses as an important method to introduce multi-core technology to students [7, 8]. These courses are designed based on the research experiences in multi-core and they can provide the detail information of multi-core. So the corresponding new technologies can be introduced into the courses directly through such approaches.

Practice is very important in computer education [9]. Students should be provided enough activities to master what they have learned in computer related courses. In this paper, we describe how to provide such practice activities in a different point of view. In our consideration, students will organize themselves into different student associations. These students associations have different concerns with each other. Teachers will guide the students in these associations to construct the technology framework. The students can have different practice activities under the guidance of teachers. The students will have initiative to complete the projects and study autonomously. According to our investigation, the student associations can improve students' practical abilities and welcomed by the students.

The rest of this paper is organized as follows. Section 39.2 describes the motivation of our work. Section 39.3 provides the detail description of student associations. And the investigation and related analysis is offered in Sect. 39.4. At last, we draw the conclusions and give the future work in Sect. 39.5.

39.2 Motivations

According to the feedback from the students, we find that hands-on labs in class are still limited compared with the actual requirements of practice from the students. Hands-on labs are the common practice activities in class and they are designed according to the requirements of different courses [10–13]. The main limitations are described as the follows.

- The credit hours in class are limited. Though student can learn the principles, the advance topics will be restricted. For example, mobile application development on Android can be introduced to students in class. And hands-on labs are also provided. However, the advanced topics are difficult to cover subject to the time constraints.
- Hands-on labs are designed labs which are different from the cases in real world. Hands-on labs can be taken as propositional projects. Real cases are also difficult to complete in class which are very important to students to master what they have learned.
- Students are passive participation in hands-on labs. They complete the hands-on labs and then master the skill. This is not enough to cultivate the students' innovation. They need more practice activities for both of their innovation and skills.

Therefore, the traditional hands-on labs are provided to students. And a new approach with high flexibility is required to provide different practice out of class. This paper exploits innovative computer education through student associations which will be described in detail in the following sections.

39.3 Practices in Student Associations

39.3.1 Overview

Practice plays a critical role in computer education [14]. Hands-on labs are taken as the main practice in different courses [15–19]. Extracurricular practice is more flexible compared with hands-on labs in class. In our design, the extracurricular practice is implemented in student associations. The students associations are not directed by teachers. They are organized by the students who are interesting in different computer technologies. The students will discuss on the hot topics and have some projects as the practice. Students can have more practical projects through their own designs and innovations. Teachers will help them from different levels. Students will obtain more practice experiences through the associations.

39.3.2 Organization

The students have organized themselves into different groups according to the different technology concerns. There are two types of groups of the associations as shown in Fig. 39.1. There are two main types of the student associations.

Technical Associations and Groups. Such associations and groups focus on some special technology. The students have the same interests will join the technical associations and groups. Each association or group has a special topic. Now there are four associations/groups including embedded system association,

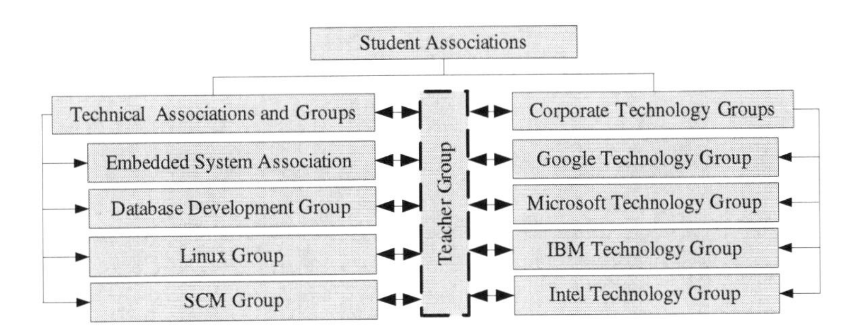

Fig. 39.1 Organization of student associations

database development group, Linux group and SCM (Single-Chip Machine) group. Embedded system association focuses on embedded system technology and development. The students gathered in database development group learn and have practice on database technology. Linux group tracks the development of Linux operating system and tries to develop to or for this system. SCM group provides the students the training and projects to master the related knowledge and develop innovative works.

Corporate Technology Groups. Such groups are for the special technology provided by some leading companies because such companies provide popular technology and development tool kits. The organized groups include Google Technology Group, Microsoft Technology, IBM Technology Group and Intel Technology Group. The students can learn the basic theories and fundamentals in different courses. And then they can learn and master more knowledge and technology. The lectures, discussions and practice can help the students understand what the real requirements are from the industry. Members of Technical Associations and Groups and Corporate Technology Groups may be overlapped for the crossing technology and tools.

There is still a special group called Teacher Group which have some teachers as the mentors for the student associations and groups. They help the students to explore the design and implementation and solve the problems. However, they will never provide the answers and solutions directly. And the teachers will not be participated in the management of the associations and groups.

39.3.3 Invited Lectures

The student associations will provide invited lectures according to the development of the technology. The invited lecturers include the engineers, the teachers from the companies and the other universities. Such invited lectures cover many topics in related topics. The contents in the invited lectures cover the corresponding theories and the experiences in different point of view. The invited teachers will provide complementary contents. The engineers from the industry will share their experiences from the real cases. It will help the students understand the requirements from the companies.

39.3.4 Training on Special Topics

The regular courses will cover the different areas. However, they rarely discuss a special topic deeply. When the students have some in-depth understanding and development, they will have to resort to some support for further study. The student associations will collect such requirements from their members. Special trainings will be organized according to the investigations. Each association or group has its training plan and provides the trainings to its members. The lecturers of the special trainings can be the teachers from the Teacher Group, the senior members of the student associations or invited engineers. Such trainings will discuss on specific topics even only a small special subject and help the students learn more knowledge and solve the problems.

39.3.5 Innovative Projects

Projects are useful practice for the students. The student associations will provide different types of the projects to their members. One of most important feature of the projects is that they are innovative projects. The members can organize themselves into different teams and select projects as the team's subjects. Open contests are the natural source of the projects. However, the main objective of the participation of the contests is how to provide innovative ideas and implement them rather than the contests themselves. And the student associations provide optional project titles for their members. Teacher Group will also provide project titles to the student associations. Such projects are called "micro-project", which are small parts of the research projects of the teachers'. The members will think carefully about what they will do.

39.4 Investigations and Analysis

39.4.1 Investigations

The student associations have been organized for some years. Investigations have been done to obtain the feedback from the members of the associations and groups, which will help us to improve the management and organization. The following table (Table 39.1) shows the total members of the student associations.

The following questions are provided in the investigations to collect the feedbacks from the members:

- Q1: where did you learn the associations from? There are four answers: C (related courses), S (students), T (teachers) and O (others).

Table 39.1 Total member number in 4 years

Years	Total member number
2010	47
2011	63
2012	82
2013	97

- Q2: Why do you want to be a member of the associations? There are four answers: Study (I want to learn more knowledge), Skill (I want to improve my skills), Interest (I am interesting in some technology), and Others (I have some other reasons). This is a multiple choice question.
- Q3: Did you participate in a project? And how many have you participated in? There are five answers: 0, 1, 2, 3-4 and more than 5 ($\geq$5).
- Q4: Have you attended a lecture? And how many lectures have you attended? There are five answers: 0, 1, 2, 3-4 and more than 5 ($\geq$5).
- Q5: Have you attended training? And how many trainings have you attended? There are also five answers: 0, 1, 2, 3-4 and more than 5 ($\geq$5).
- Q6: How much is your satisfaction? There are also five answers: unsatisfied, neutral, satisfied, very satisfied.

The following figures (Figs. 39.2, 39.3, 39.4, 39.5, 39.6 and 39.7) shows the results of the six questions respectively.

39.4.2 Analysis

Figure 39.2 shows us that most students know the student associations from their friends who are also students. The students associations themselves will attract the students' attention. When the student associations can provide good opportunities to the students for their learning and practice, the students will be actively to be a member of the associations. As Fig. 39.3 shows, most students want to learn more knowledge and have practice in the student associations. When learning goals and interests are consistent, the students have more positive learning motivations.

As we can see from Figs. 39.4, 39.5 and 39.6, many students have attended the activities provided by the student associations. The associations provide enough activities including the lectures, trainings and projects. Actually there are tens of lectures and trainings and close to 100 project titles for the students. At the same time, plentiful resources are provided by the associations. These activities make

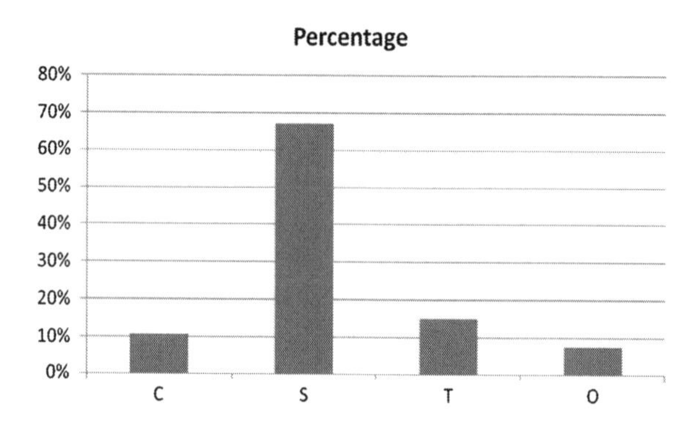

Fig. 39.2 Normalized results of Q1

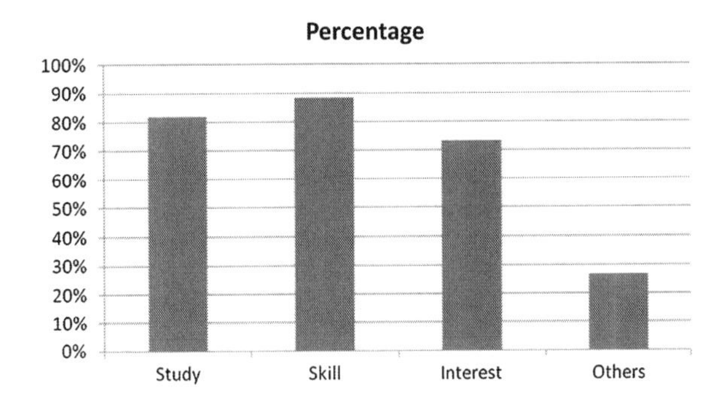

Fig. 39.3 Normalized results of Q2

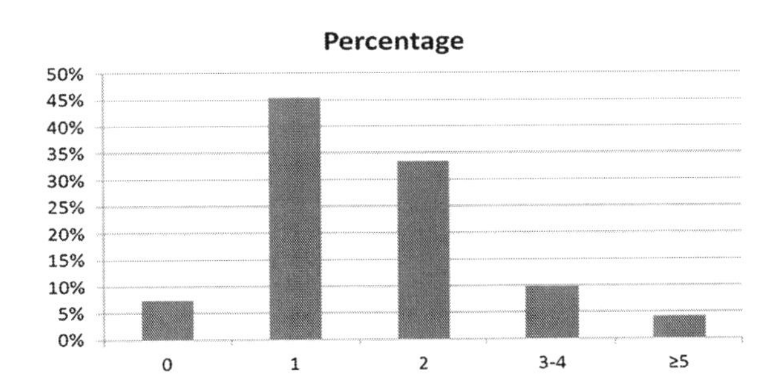

Fig. 39.4 Normalized results of Q3

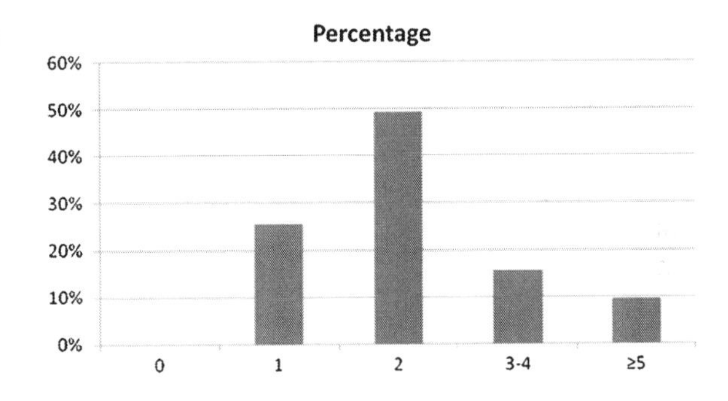

Fig. 39.5 Normalized results of Q4

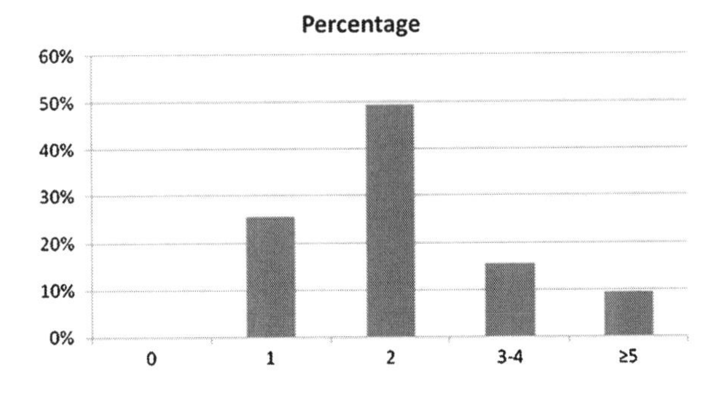

Fig. 39.6 Normalized results of Q5

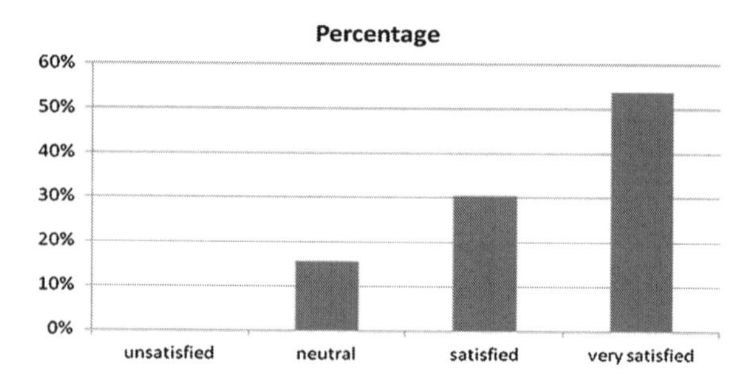

Fig. 39.7 Normalized results of Q6

the students think, discuss and work. During such processes, they win the unceasing progress. Figure 39.7 shows that the students are satisfied with the associations.

39.5 Conclusions and Future Work

Computer and related technology is developing rapidly. The courses and related hands-on labs can provide the basic theories and practice. However, the students need more opportunities for both the study and practice, which is a new challenge. In this paper, we describe a novel approach that can solve the problem. The student associations can help the students to organize themselves better for their learning. The students can find the colleagues who have a common interest in the same technology in the associations and groups. And the activities will help them to make constant progress. In the future, more investigations will be taken and the feedbacks will be used to improve the associations.

Acknowledgments This work was supported by Education Research Project from Wuhan University of Sci.&Tech. under Granted No. 2011x026 and Google Innovation Plan.

References

1. Nayfeh BA, Olukotun K (1997) A single-chip multiprocessor. IEEE Comput 30(9):79–85
2. Cardoso JMP (2005) New challenges in computer science education. In: Proceedings of the 10th annual SIGCSE conference on innovation and technology in computer science education (ITiCSE '05), Caparica, Portugal, pp 203–207
3. Hazzan O, Gal-Ezer J, Blum L (2008) A model for high school computer science education: the four key elements that make it!. In: Proceedings of the 39th SIGCSE technical symposium on computer science education (SIGCSE '08), Portland, pp 281–285
4. Murphy L, Thomas L (2008) Dangers of a fixed mindset: implications of self-theories research for computer science education. In: Proceedings of the 13th annual conference on innovation and technology in computer science education (ITiCSE '08), Spain, pp 271–275

5. Plane JD, Venter I (2008) Comparing capacity building frameworks for computer science education in underdeveloped countries: an Asian and African perspective. SIGCSE Bull 40(3):306–310
6. Aşkar P (2010) Computer science education in Turkey. In: Proceedings of the fifteenth annual conference on innovation and technology in computer science education (ITiCSE '10), Bilkent, Ankara, pp 328–328
7. Karsten S, Ada G et al (2006) Multi-core curriculum development at Georgia Tech: experience and future steps Intel Multi-Core Curriculum Conference (MCCC) 2006, http://educationforums.intel.com
8. Chen T, Yan L, Chen L, Wang J (2007) Multi-core curriculum at Zhejiang University. In: Proceedings of education and information systems, technologies and applications (EISTA'07), Orlando, 12–15 July 2007, pp 165–170
9. De Corte E, Verschaffel L, Masui C (2004) The CLIA-model: a framework for designing powerful learning environments for thinking and problem solving. Eur J Psychol Educ 19:365–384
10. Yingbing Yu. (2007) Designing hands-on lab exercises in the network security course. J Comput Small Coll 22(5):105–110
11. Trabelsi Z (2011) Hands-on lab exercises implementation of DoS and MiM attacks using ARP cache poisoning. In: Proceedings of the 2011 information security curriculum development conference (InfoSecCD '11), Kennesaw, pp 74–83
12. Qian K, Liu J, Tao L (2011) Teach real-time embedded system online with real hands-on labs. SIGCSE Bull 41(3):367–367
13. Wenliang Du (2011) SEED: hands-on lab exercises for computer security education. IEEE Secur Priv 9(5):70–73
14. Ma J, Nickerson JV (2006) Hands-on, simulated, and remote laboratories: a comparative literature review. ACM Comput Surv 38(3):1–24, Article 7
15. Lawrence KR, Chi H (2009) Framework for the design of web-based learning for digital forensics labs. In: Proceedings of the 47th annual southeast regional conference (ACM-SE 47). Clemson, Article 76, p 4
16. Qian K, Dan Lo C-T, Hu X (2010) Portable labs in a box for embedded system education. In: Proceedings of the fifteenth annual conference on innovation and technology in computer science education (ITiCSE '10), Bilkent, pp 318–318
17. Qian G (2012) Designing and implementing unsupervised online database labs. J Comput Sci Coll 27(4):30–36
18. Yuan V, Zhong J (2010) Developing and evaluating a network curriculum to meet ABET accreditation and IT industry needs. J Comput Small Coll 26(2):256–262
19. Brown B, Aaron M (2001) The politics of nature. In: Smith J (ed) The rise of modern genomics, 3rd ed. Wiley, New York

Chapter 40
Traditional Chinese Medicine Literature Metadata: A Draft Technical Specification Developed by the International Organization for Standardization

Tong Yu, Meng Cui, Haiyan Li, Shuo Yang, Yang Zhao and Zhang Zhulu

Abstract Currently, there is a lack of international standard for literature metadata in Traditional Chinese Medicine (TCM) domain, which becomes a major obstacle for the indexing and retrieval of TCM literature. In 2013, the International Organization for Standardization (ISO) finished the draft technical specification (DTS) "Traditional Chinese medicine literature metadata", which will play an important role in the preservation and utilization of TCM literature resources. In this paper, we articulate the content and characteristics of this DTS, compare it with other related ISO standards, and explain the creativity and necessity of this DTS.

Keywords Traditional Chinese medicine · Literature · Metadata · International Organization for Standardization · Technical specification · Standardization

40.1 Introduction

Traditional Chinese Medicine (TCM) is an important form of traditional medicine in practice for thousands of years. Ancient TCM practitioners have left us with a large quantity of medical classics. How to collect, classify, manage, and retrieve this massive amount of documents becomes an important and difficult problem during the process of TCM preservation and modernization. In recent years, document indexing and retrieval technologies played an important role in the digitalization, preservation, and utilization of TCM literature. However, there is currently a lack of international technical specification for literature metadata in TCM domain, which causes the heterogeneity of literature retrieval systems, and hinders the indexing and retrieval of TCM literature.

T. Yu (✉) · M. Cui (✉) · H. Li · S. Yang · Y. Zhao · Z. Zhulu
Institute of Information on Traditional Chinese Medicine, China Academy of Chinese Medicine Sciences, Beijing 100700, China
e-mail: cui@mail.cintcm.ac.cn

S. Li et al. (eds.), *Frontier and Future Development of Information Technology in Medicine and Education*, Lecture Notes in Electrical Engineering 269,
DOI: 10.1007/978-94-007-7618-0_40,

Metadata is commonly defined as "data about data" [1]. Currently, the Dublin Core Metadata Element Set (DC for short) is the most widespread metadata standard worldwide [1]. DC defines a set of core terms that can be used to describe various resources, and serves as the foundation for various domain-specific metadata standards. In addition, there are metadata standards for various domain, such as eGMS [2] for government information resources, EAD [3] for digital archival repositories, and IEEE LOM [4, 5] for e-learning.

There has been a set of metadata standards for health resources, such as MCM [6], CISMeF [7], EBM metadata [8], and NLM metadata [9]. These standards have been used in the making of online directory and indexing of medical resources, enhancing the organization of medical resources.

TCM literature has many unique characteristics, which cannot be fully captured by generic literature metadata standards such as the Dublin Core. We need a TCM-specific standard that articulates these unique characteristics, in service of the collection, storage, retrieval, and use of TCM literature resources. In 2008, to fill this void, Institute of Information on Traditional Chinese Medicine, China Academy of Chinese Medicine Sciences, on behalf of China, presented a proposal for "Traditional Chinese Medicine Literature Metadata" to International Organization for Standardization's (ISO) Technical Committee (TC) on health informatics (ISO/TC 215) [10]. In 2012, this proposal was approved, and a project for an ISO technical specification named "Traditional Chinese Medicine Literature Metadata" (numbered [ISO/DTS 17948], TCMLM for short) was initiated [11]. With the efforts of experts from multiple countries such as China, Korea, UK, and USA, the draft of TCMLM was finished in March 2013. In this paper, we will explain the technical characteristics and major content of TCMLM, and compare it with related standards in order to highlight the creativity and uniqueness of TCMLM.

40.2 Technical Characters and Major Content of TCMLM

TCMLM is currently a Draft Technical Specification (DTS) that is specialized for TCM literature, and specifies the basic principles and methods for the standardization of TCM literature metadata. TCMLM was made based on DC, and in reference with ISO standards such as "ISO 13119 Health informatics—Clinical knowledge resources-Metadata", "ISO 19115 Geographic information-Metadata". In addition, TCMLM is related to or depends on terminological systems such as "Traditional Chinese Medicine Subject Headings". Architecturally speaking, the metadata model of TCMLM contains four layers:

- *Metadata section* is defined as Subset of metadata that defines a collection of related metadata entities and elements;
- *Metadata entity* is defined as Group of metadata elements and other metadata entities describing the same aspect of data;

- *Metadata element* is defined as Discrete unit of metadata;
- *Metadata element refinement* is defined as a property of a resource which shares the meaning of a particular element but with narrower semantics.

TCMLM retains the metadata elements, and also contains TCM-specific metadata element. The TCMLM has the following design rationales: (1) Reuse the DC metadata elements, such as Type, Format, Language, Description, Relation, Identifier, Title, Creator, Date, Rights; (2) Redefine the DC metadata elements according to TCM domain logics, e.g. DC Title is further refined by "Title on Fore-edge"; (3) Add TCM-specific metadata elements as required, e.g., Syndrome Differentiation is a unique property in TCM literature metadata.

As shown in Fig. 40.1, TCMLM contains 24 metadata elements, of which 15 elements are from DC, and nine elements are newly added. The TCMLM elements are divided into seven sections: Identification section, Content section, Distribution section, Quality section, Constraint section, Maintenance section, and Relation section:

- *Identification Section*. The Identification Section is identifying the TCM literature resource, its originator(s) and conditions for accessing it.
- *Content Section*. The Content Section describes the nature or genre of the content of the TCM literature resource, as well as its provenance information.
- *Distribution Section*. The distribution section describes the information about the storage, distribution and access of the TCM literature resource.
- *Quality Section*. The quality section describes the quality management system for TCM literature, which facilitates the preservation and use of TCM literature resources.

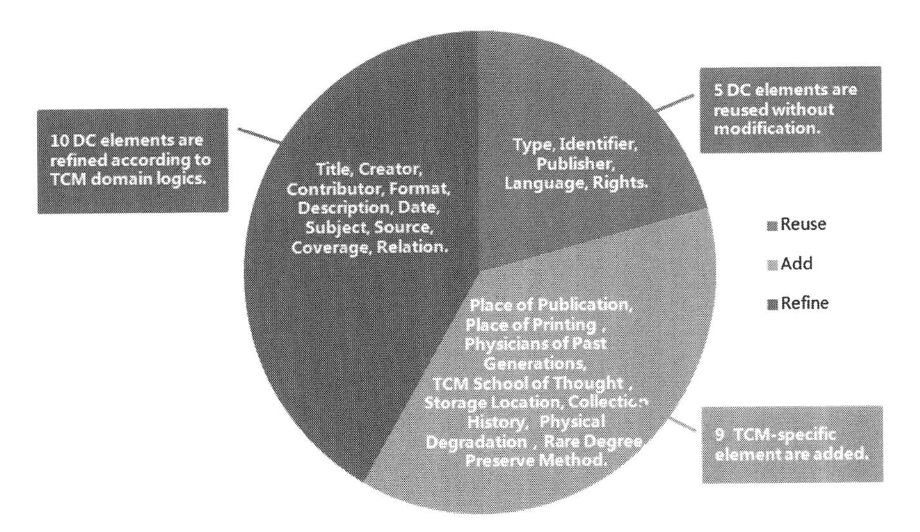

Fig. 40.1 The 24 TCMLM metadata elements and their relationships with DC metadata elements

- *Constraint Section.* The constraint section describes constraint information regarding the access and use of the TCM literature resource.
- *Maintenance Section.* The Maintenance section describes the information about the maintenance of TCM literature resources.
- *Relation Section.* The Relation section describes the types of relations between TCM literature resources, such as Inherit from, Subsequent, Substitute for, Be Replaced By, Translated From, and Contain.

40.3 A Comparison between TCMLM and Related Standards

In this section, we make a comparison between TCMLM and related ISO metadata standards. The Dublin Core Metadata Element Set (DC for short) is one of the most widely-used metadata standards recognized by the International Organization for Standardization (ISO 15836: 2003). DC is a vocabulary of fifteen properties for use in resource description, including contributor, coverage, creator, date, description, format, identifier, language, etc. In addition, "ISO 13119 Health informatics—Clinical knowledge resources—Metadata"(CKRM for short) is a new International standard that is intended for both health professionals and patients/citizens [12]. CKRM defines a number of metadata elements that describe documents containing medical knowledge, primarily digital documents provided as web resources, accessible from databases or via file transfer, but can be applicable also to paper documents, e.g. articles in the medical literature. It is a simple and flexible metadata standard which can be used in almost all domains of networked electronic resources.

Here, we make a comparison between TCMLM, DC, and CKRM. As shown in Fig. 40.2, TCMLM works for the TCM domain, CKRM works mainly for Western medicine domain, and DC is a general purpose standard that is widely adopted. Both TCMLM and CKRM adopt all of DC elements, and add domain-specific metadata elements as required. The intersection of the two standards also consists of relations such as Replaces and is replaced by.

As shown in Table 40.1, TCMLM contains elements or element sets with obvious TCM characteristics, which shows the originality and contribution of this draft technical specification. Table 40.2 is a more detailed table that compares the 24 TCMLM elements with the elements of DC and CKRM, and describes the meaning and differentiating characteristics of each TCMLM element in detail. To summarize this table, 10 TCMLM elements are adopted from DC with further refinements and tcm-specific specialization, nine TCMLM elements are added, and five TCMLM elements are directly reused without modification. Therefore, this standard has five elements that is directly borrowed from DC, and 19 items with TCM characteristics.

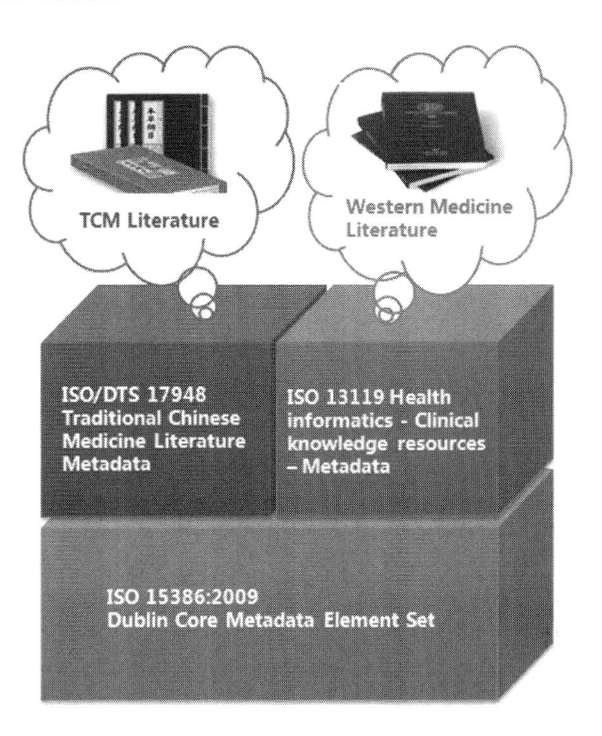

Fig. 40.2 The relationships between DC, TCMLM, and CKRM

Table 40.1 This table highlights elements/element sets with obvious TCM characteristics

Elements/ element sets	In DC	In CKRM	Description
Title	Y	Y	TCM domain has special ways to put titles. This standard specifies different titles such as "title on fore-edge"
Format	Y	Y	TCMLM defines TCM-specific formats, such as "binding and layout", "paragraph style", and "printing instructions"
Description	Y	Y	TCMLM defines TCM-specific descriptions, e.g., preface or postscript, in addition to general descriptions, e.g., Abstract
Subject	Y	Y	TCMLM specifies standards on TCM subjects, such as MeSH subject headings, TCM thesaurus, Chinese Library Classification, the Ministry of Education disciplines classification, classification standards and code of the TCM data resources
Distribution section	N	N	TCM domain has special methods for the storage and distribution of literature. This standard defines the related properties (e.g. Storage location, library information, and collection history) in the distribution section
Quality section	N	N	TCM domain has a special system of quality control. This standard defines related properties (e.g., Worn-out grading, rare degree) in the quality section
Relation	Y	Y	TCMLM defines special relations between TCM documents

Table 40.2 This table shows a comparison between TCMLM, DC, and CKRM

Section	Element	Also in CKRM	Also in DC	Description
1. Identification section	1.1 Title	√	√	TCM specific specialization: translated title, title on fore-edge, title on the inside cover, title on the book cover, title on the first page of text, etc.
	1.2 Creator	√	√	TCM specific specialization for creator description, e.g., reign dynasty dating is recorded by the order: dynasty, the emperor, and annals
	1.3 Contributor	√	√	In TCM domain, specify the relationship between a contributor and the literature resource: translate, engrave, record, photograph, calligraphy, compile, repair, annotate, edit, collect, paint, sort, modify, manufacture, etc.
	1.4 Type	√	√	Reuse DC element
	1.5 Format	√	√	TCM specific specialization: binding and layout, printing instructions, edition of ancient books, paragraph style, etc.
	1.6 Identifier	√	√	Reuse DC element
	1.7 Description	√	√	TCM specific specialization: preface or postscript
	1.8 Publisher	√	√	Reuse DC element
	1.9 Place of publication			In TCM domain, the place of publication is of special importance.
	1.10 Place of printing			In TCM domain, the place of printing is of special importance.
	1.11 Date	√	√	TCM specific specialization: creation date; update date; publication date; printing date; available date
2. Content section	2.1 Subject	√	√	TCM specific specialization: TCM thesaurus, Chinese Library Classification, The Ministry of Education disciplines classification, etc.
	2.2 Physicians of past generations			"physicians of past generations" is a crucial character of TCM literature
	2.3 TCM school of thought			Reuse DC element
	2.4 Source	√	√	TCM specific specification: ways of obtaining the data within the literature resource
	2.5 Coverage	√	√	TCM specific specification: the location and era of the literature resource
	2.6 Language	√	√	Reuse DC element

(continued)

Table 40.2 (continued)

Section	Element	Also in CKRM	Also in DC	Description
3. Distribution section	3.1 Storage location			In TCM, we need to specify the information about the storage location of a resource, e.g., library information, collection number
	3.2 Collection history			In TCM, we need to specify the information about the collection history of a resources, e.g., collection shift, obtain-way, inscriptive writings and signet
4. Quality section	4.1 Physical degradation			In TCM, the standards of ancient books worn-out grading need to be specified
	4.2 Rare degree			In TCM, the wear degree of literature resources is important for making policies regarding its preservation
5. Constraint section	5.1 Rights	√	√	Reuse DC element
6. Maintenance section	6.1 Preserve method			In TCM, we need to specify the information about the preservation methods for a literature resource, such as temperature, humidity, storage carrier
7. Relation section	7.1 Relation	√	√	TCM specific specification: inherit from, subsequent, replaces, is replaced by, translated from, collection series, fascicle, parallel, additional, annotations, missing words annotations, appendix

40.4 Conclusions

We have introduced Traditional Chinese Medicine Literature Metadata, an ISO DTS that captures the unique characteristics of TCM literature. DC defines a set of general purpose metadata elements, serving as the basis for domain-specific standards. Whereas CKRM is such a specialization for the Western medical domain, TCMLM is a specialization for the TCM domain. In this sense, they are both quite useful for their own domain. TCMLM will serve the collection, storage, retrieval, and use of the TCM literature, and contribute to the preservation and utilization of TCM knowledge assets.

Acknowledgments This work is supported by "the Fundamental Research Funds for the Central public welfare research institutes (NO. ZZ070804, NO. ZZ070311, NO ZZ060808, NO. ZZ070314)", "the China Postdoctoral Science Foundation funded project (NO. 2012M520559)".

References

1. Weibel S (1997) The Dublin core: a simple content description model for electronic resources. Bul Am Soc Info Sci Tech 24(1):9–11
2. Alasem A (2009) An overview of e-government metadata standards and initiatives based on Dublin core. Electron J e-Govern 7(1):1–10
3. Carpenter B, Park JR (2009) Encoded archival description (EAD) metadata scheme: an analysis of use of the EAD headers. J Libr Metadata 9(1–2):134–152
4. IEEE P1484.12.1 (2002) Draft standard for learning object metadata. http://ltsc.ieee.org/doc/wg12/LOM_WD6_4.pdf. Accessed on Aug 2002
5. Vargo J, Nesbit JC, Belfer K, Archambault A (2003) Learning object evaluation: computer-mediated collaboration and inter-rater reliability. Int J Comput Appl 25(3):198–205
6. Malet G, Munoz F, Appleyard R, Hersh W (1999) Model formulation: a model for enhancing internet medical document retrieval with “medical core metadata”. J Am Med Inform Assoc 6(2):163–172
7. Darmoni S, Thirion B, Platel S, Douyère M, Mourouga P, Leroy JP (2002) CISMeF-patient: a French counterpart to MEDLINEplus. J Med Libr Assoc 90(2):248–253
8. Sakai Y (2001) Metadata for evidence-based medicine resources. In: Oyama K, Gotoda H (eds) Proceedings of the international conference on Dublin core and metadata applications 2001 (DCMI ‘01). National Institute of Informatics, Tokyo, pp 81–85
9. NLM metadata: U.S. National Library of Medicine, National Institutes of Health. http://www.nlm.nih.gov/tsd/cataloging/metafilenew.html
10. Li HY, Cui M, Ren GH et al (2011) Progress of the standardization efforts for traditional medicine informatics in ISO/TC215. Int J Tradit Chin 33(3):193–195 (In Chinese)
11. Tong Y, Cui M, Yang S (2013) Investigating traditional Chinese informatics standards under the development of ISO/TC 215. Chin Dig Med 8(2):46–49 (In Chinese)
12. Klein GO (2011) Metadata-an international standard for clinical knowledge resources. Stud Health Technol Inform 169:839–843

Chapter 41
A Visualization Method in Virtual Educational System

Guijuan Zhang, Dianjie Lu and Hong Liu

Abstract We present a visualization-based knowledge expression approach for virtual educational system in this paper. Our method allows teachers and students to understand complex algorithms and procedures more intuitively and conveniently during the process of teaching and learning. We take the decision tree and the random forest algorithm in the field of Data mining as examples in this paper. In our method, the decision tree is represented by a virtual 3D tree model that both the structure and the classification results can be showed clearly. In addition, random forest is represented by a group of virtual 3D trees and their positions denote the similarity between the decision trees. We also provide several user-interaction tools in our system. The tools help users to browse the forest, select a tree, delete a tree and even see the detail information of the decision tree. The effective and understandable results show the feasibility of applying visualization method in virtual educational system.

Keywords Visualization · Virtual education · Decision tree

41.1 Introduction

In recent years, Computer-based Instruction (CBI) has become one of the most important techniques in education [1–3]. A typical CBI system includes hardware, software and the means of knowledge expression. Recent developments in technology have provided us with many types of software and hardware in CBI. Typical hardware includes audio or video tape, satellite TV, CD-ROM.

G. Zhang (✉) · D. Lu · H. Liu
School of Information Science and Engineering, Shandong Normal University,
Shandong Provincial Key Laboratory for Novel Distributed Computer Software Technology
Shandong University, Jinan, China
e-mail: guijuanzhang@gmail.com

S. Li et al. (eds.), *Frontier and Future Development of Information Technology in Medicine and Education*, Lecture Notes in Electrical Engineering 269,
DOI: 10.1007/978-94-007-7618-0_41, © Springer Science+Business Media Dordrecht 2014

The hardware can deliver text, audio, images, animation, streaming video and so on. The above various forms of CBI and multimedia instruction provide an available mode of teaching [3]. As a result, the most essential task in virtual educational system of CBI is to study knowledge expression.

Traditional methods often rely on courseware tools (e.g., the PowerPoint, AUTHORWARE) to express knowledge. In applications, knowledge is often expressed by text. However, it is difficult for students to understand the complex algorithms or processes via text. Researchers have proved that graph is more intuitive than text to represent complex algorithms and concepts [4, 5]. In [4], the authors show that the visualized fluid flows are intuitive enough for students to understand. In [5], visualization method also helps to provide intuitive geometrical information. Therefore, knowledge expression via graphs is a potential and effective method in virtual education.

Visualization method is to provide graphically illustrate result to enable scientists to understand, illustrate, and glean insight from the complex data [6]. According to the structure of the data to be visualized, visualization methods can be divided into two categories: Scientific visualization and Information visualization [7]. Since the visualization method can express the knowledge and data intuitively, it has been extensively used in the field of big data, data analysis and visual analysis. In this paper, we explore the potential of the visualization method in knowledge expression and introduce it into virtual educational system in CBI.

We take decision tree algorithm and random forest algorithm in the field of Data mining as examples in this paper. We will show how the visualization method is applied in visualizing decision tree and random forest. We also provide interaction tools in our system to help teachers and students to understand the complex algorithms. Experimental results show that the visualization approach inspires student interest, attract their attention and facilitates their understanding.

41.2 Related Work

In CBI, virtual educational system uses technologies of computer, communication, simulation and artificial intelligence to provide a teaching model. There are several successful virtual educational systems. For example, Physics Department of Dalhousie University developed a laser virtual laboratory and showed how to operate a real time dangerous laser laboratory with the help of commanding equipment through the Internet [8]. In addition, remote teaching system is also a typical virtual educational system. The famous educational expert Desmond Keegan describes the remote virtual educational system as “Face to face teaching at a distance”. In China, many universities have developed projects about virtual education [9]. For example, the smart classroom of Tsinghua University introduces the notion of space interaction in virtual educational system. Tongji University adopts virtual reality technology to build a virtual lab that simulates architectural landscape and structure. Southwest Jiaotong University develops virtual educational system that can show urban planning and can offer driver training courses.

As we know, students of computer sciences must understand a variety of algorithms and theorems that involve primarily knowledge-based learning. Current virtual educational system could not effectively illustrate these algorithms and theorems effectively. We will introduce visualization method into this process to address this problem.

41.3 System Overview

In this paper, we introduce visualization method in virtual educational system. The visualization method allows us to produce intuitive expression of knowledge that improves the teaching and learning efficiency significantly. The framework of this paper is shown in Fig. 41.1.

In virtual educational system, teachers as well as students are often required to understand complex algorithms and procedures. We take the decision tree and random forest algorithm for example. Decision tree is the most famous classification algorithm in Data mining. In addition, random forest that composed by decision trees is also used for more accurate prediction. We present visualization method for decision trees and random forest. In addition, the interaction tools will also be provided for understanding the two algorithms more conveniently. In fact, the visualization method in Data mining can also be extended to the other areas and helps to improve effectiveness of the knowledge expression in virtual educational system.

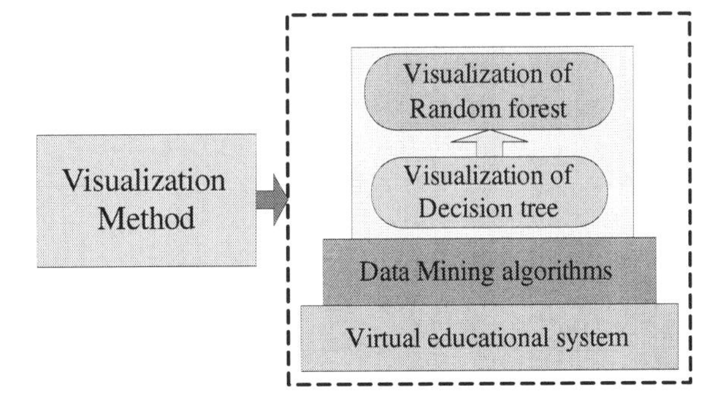

Fig. 41.1 The framework of this paper

41.4 Visualization of the Decision Tree

41.4.1 Decision Tree

Decision tree is one of the most powerful classification algorithms in Data mining. To complete the classification task, a decision tree is composed by root, nodes, branches and leaves. When constructing a decision tree, the process will start from a root node and then moves downward until the leaf node. As for each internal node, two or more branches are extended. In the decision tree, each node denotes a feature and each branch represent a range of values. Therefore, we can branch the samples with the features according to the partition points from the set of values.

Classification with decision tree requires building the tree first and then executing the task based on the given data set. We use the famous ID3 algorithm to build the decision tree in this paper. ID3 algorithm constructs the decision tree according to a top–down and greedy search approach. The notions of entropy and information gain are introduced into ID3 algorithm to select the most useful attributes that divide the data set. Thus, the information gain provides us a good function to get a most balanced splitting.

After building the decision tree, we get a prediction model that can be used to predict the class of the new record. The process is completed by following a path of the tree where for each attribute the split condition is evaluated in the decision tree.

41.4.2 Visualization Algorithm

Tree Structure. We use a 3D tree model in a virtual environment to represent the decision trees as shown in Fig. 41.2a. The root node is denoted as the root of the 3D tree. The tree is branched at the position of the internal node. The branches of an internal node will be represented as branches of the tree. The leaf node in the decision tree is denoted as leaves in the virtual tree model.

Control Parameters. In order to make the decision tree be more similar to a real tree, several parameters are required to specify. As shown in Fig. 41.2b–d, we need to define the ramify angles, growth height and the thickness of limb. In the virtual decision tree model, the height of the trunk H is related to the strength value of the tree

$$H = L \times strength, \tag{41.1}$$

where L is unit value of height, strength is the measure of classification accuracy of the classifier. Similarly, the length of each branch is

$$L_{length} = L \times s^{level}, \tag{41.2}$$

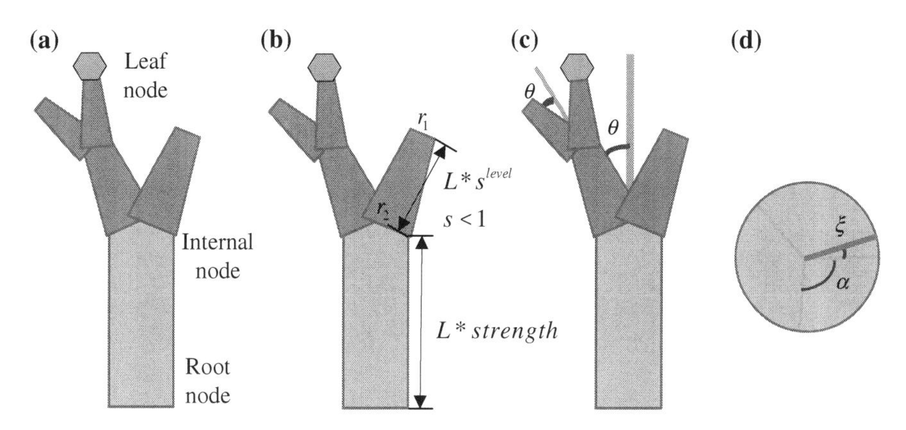

Fig. 41.2 The 3D virtual model of the decision tree: **a** structure of the decision tree, **b–d** the control parameters of the decision tree

where s is a float number satisfies $s < 1$, level denotes the branch level. Note that the level of trunk is 1 and we add 1 to the next level of branches. Each branch is denoted as a cylinder with two bottom radius r_1 and r_2. If current node is a leaf node, the radius is set to be a constant. Otherwise, if the node is an internal node, we set the radius of the cylinder at this position

$$r_2 = \frac{Numbers\ of\ cases}{Number\ of\ Total\ cases} \times strength, \tag{41.3}$$

where the statistical number of the cases is obtained from the randomly sampled records of the data set. We also define two angles θ and α to represent the direction of a branch. θ is the angle formed by child branch and main branch as shown in Fig. 41.2c and α is the angle formed by two child branches. Figure 41.2d shows a cross section view of an internal node. Here, α is the angle between different child branches. To make this structure more natural, we add a small random perturbation ξ.

Textures. Texture is often referred to a 2D image that used for adding visual characteristics to an on-screen object or area in computer graphics. Textures allow 3D models to look significantly more detailed and realistic than they would otherwise. The image texture can be generated procedurally or manually, or even from photographs. To improve the visual perception of the 3D decision tree model, we add textures to the tree model. Figure 41.3 shows different textures for branches and leaves. They are our texture resources and will be used for rendering the final decision trees. Note that the different colors of leaves denote different classification results.

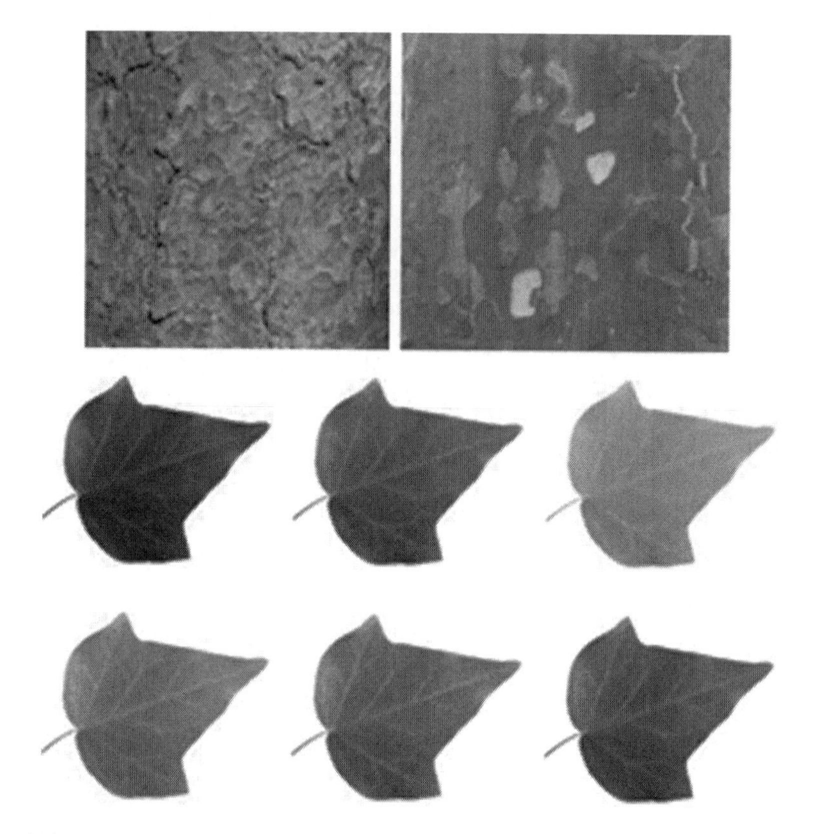

Fig. 41.3 Textures used in our paper. The *first row* shows the textures for branches and the *other rows* show the textures for leaves. *Different colors* denote different classification results

41.5 Visualization of the Forest

41.5.1 Random Forest

Random forest presented by Breiman [10] is composed by a number of decision trees or regression trees that generated from randomly selected samples from the same set of training data. By aggregating the classification or regression results of the decision trees, the random forest can be used for more accurate prediction. Specifically, in classification problems, majority vote is involved to get the final prediction results while in regression problems, an averaging technique is used.

The random selection from the training data allows us to get more robust decision results. If the size of the data sets is N and we are required to select N samples, the randomly selection method can get the same samples with different orders when training the decision tree. If we are required to select m samples that $m \ll N$, then m records are selected randomly. When growing the forest, m is constant. The above procedure makes the random forest be robust to noise.

41.5.2 Visualization Method

The visualization of the forest will focus on visualizing the positions of the decision trees. The positions of the tree denote their similarity. For example, if two trees are located very close to each other, they are of high similarity. To add more realistic factors in visualization, we also add a slope in the scene.

41.6 Results

We construct a system for visualizing decision trees and random forest in this paper. The system is built on a famous high performance 3D graphics toolkit OpenSceneGraph which is available from http://www.openscenegraph.org/. All the results in this paper are gathered on a PC with 2.6 GHz Intel Core 2 Duo CPU and 2 GB memory.

The left image of Fig. 41.4 shows the user interface of our system. In this system, we can browse the generated decision trees and random forest. Via 3D interactive tools, we can also select, delete and view detail information of each decision tree. For example, in the right image of Fig. 41.4, when we select a decision tree, we can see its detail information in the right bottom corner. Left image of Fig. 41.5 shows a 3D model of decision tree in this paper. Note that different leaves represent different classes. In our system, we can navigate the decision tree in arbitrary view point. The right image of Fig. 41.5 shows

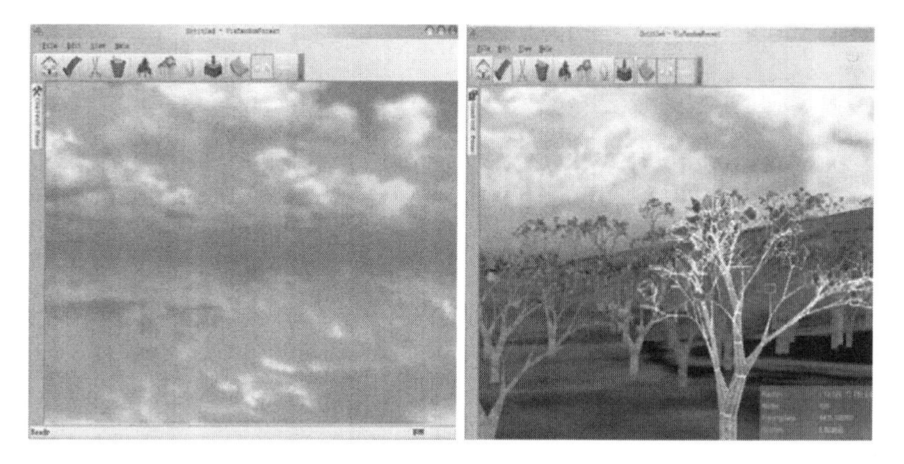

Fig. 41.4 Our visualization system. *Left* the user interface of our system. Besides visualization, the interface also provides us interaction tools that browse the forest, select a tree, delete a tree and even see the detail information of the decision tree. *Right* User can see the detail information of each decision tree by selection

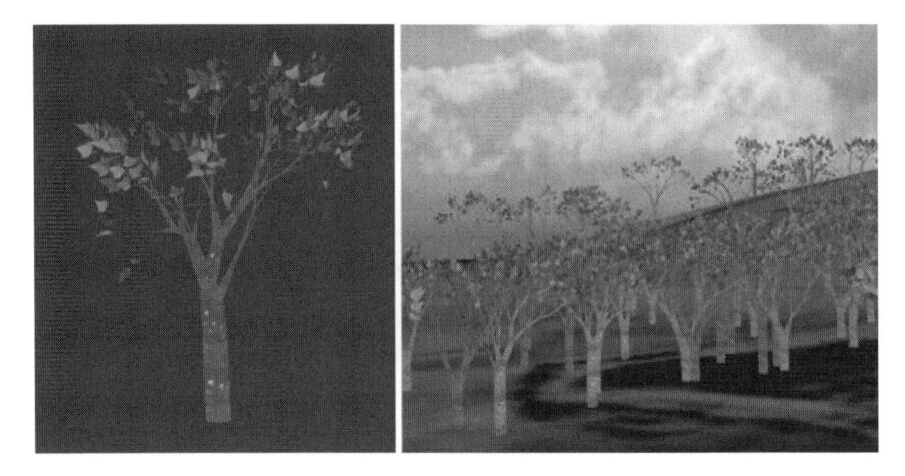

Fig. 41.5 The visualization results. *Left* The virtual 3D tree model of the decision tree. The textures are from Fig. 41.4. Branches denote the structure of the decision tree while leaves represent different classifications. *Right* The virtual forest model. Positions of the decision trees in the forest represent the similarities between decision trees

visualization result of a random forest. The positions of the trees represent their similarities. If two trees are located very close to each other, they are of high similarity in our system.

41.7 Conclusion

Visualization methods have been extensively studied and applied in the area of computer science. Inspired from the visualization method, we have presented a knowledge expression approach for virtual educational system. We take the decision tree and random forest algorithm as examples in this paper. We design a visualization system for decision trees and random forest. As for visualizing the decision tree, we focus on its structure and classification results. While for visualizing the random forest, we focus on the positions of the decision trees because the information represents the similarities of the decision trees.

Our visualization system also provides several interaction tools. They allow teachers and students to understand complex algorithms and procedures more intuitively and conveniently. The effective and understandable results from our system show that the visualization method is feasible in virtual education. We will extend the visualization method to other areas so as to improve the effectiveness of the knowledge expression in virtual educational system.

Acknowledgments This work is supported by National Natural Science Foundation of P.R.China under Grant Nos. 61202225, 61272094, 61104126, Project of Shandong Province Higher Educational Science and Technology Program under Grant No. J13LN13, and Shenzhen Basic Research Foundation under Grant No. JC201105190934A.

References

1. Serin O, Cyprus NN (2011) The effects of the computer-based instruction on the achievement and problem solving skills of the science and technology students. TOJET 10.1
2. Lowe JS, Holton III EF (2005) A theory of effective computer-based instruction for adults. Hum Resour Dev Rev 4(2):159–188
3. Weiss RE, Knowlton DS, Morrison GR (2002) Principles for using animation in computer-based instruction: theoretical heuristics for effective design. Comput Hum Behav 18(4):465–477
4. Xie C, Tinker R, Tinker B, Pallant A, Damelin D, Berenfeld B (2011) Computational experiments for science education. Science 332(6037):1516–1517
5. Guo H, Wang Z, Yu B et al (2011) TripVista: triple perspective visual trajectory analytics and its application on microscopic traffic data at a road intersection. In: Pacific visualization symposium (PacificVis) IEEE, pp 163–170
6. Herman I, Melançon G, Marshall MS (2000) Graph visualization and navigation in information visualization: a survey. IEEE Trans Visual Comput Graphics 6(1):24–43
7. Nagel HR (2006) Scientific visualization versus information visualization. In: Workshop on state-of-the-art in scientific and parallel computing, Sweden
8. Paton B (1999) Virtual laser laboratory. Retrieved 6 June 1999
9. Bin H (2008) Study for emotional interaction algorithm in virtual instruction based on facial expression computing. Master's thesis, Central China Normal University
10. Breiman L (2001) Random forests. Mach Learn 45(1):5–32

Chapter 42
Moral Education with the Background of Information Globalization

Liying Xiang

Abstract Information globalization brings the conflicts between different culture and customs. It also creates the diversity of values and personality. Nowadays, it is of significance to improve moral education in Chinese colleges, which is also regarded as an important approach to strengthen ethic education. This paper presents some principles and methods of moral education in practice. Hence, improving moral education is a good way to develop a perfect personality as well as ethic characteristics.

Keywords College student · Ethic · Develop education

42.1 Introduction

In the famous article "Youth China", Liang QiChao said, "The young Chinese to produce in the future, China youth of responsibility. Therefore, currently, the responsibility is not burdened on others, but on our youth." It is obviously that the quality of colleges student is heavily related with the development of themselves as well as the faith and future of the nation. A qualified student should therefore have a good training of ethic besides adequate knowledge of science, etc.

As indicated in the survey of state-of-the-art in one Chinese college which was carried out by the author, the importance ethic education has been heavily ignored. In question 3, 48 % students chose B which means the employment is solely depend on majority instead of ethic. A, both are important account for 32 %. C, ethic is more important account for 15 %, D-depend on real situation is 4 %.

L. Xiang (✉)
Department of Fundamental Education, Zhejiang Shuren University,
Hangzhou, People's Republic of China
e-mail: xly0001@sina.com

S. Li et al. (eds.), *Frontier and Future Development of Information Technology in Medicine and Education*, Lecture Notes in Electrical Engineering 269,
DOI: 10.1007/978-94-007-7618-0_42, © Springer Science+Business Media Dordrecht 2014

The survey also reveals that many students lack of sense of responsibility. Question 9, how about your sense of responsibility. Students who selected A, "I have strong sense of responsibility", account for 10 % of the total surveyed students. Students who selected B, "On common circumstances, I am very responsible, but just some occasionally whatever you please, no was very thoughtful", account for 10 % of the total surveyed students. Students selecting D, "although I have the responsibility, but generally are afraid of responsibility", count for 28 %. Students selecting E, "only responsible for myself" account for 29 %. Students selecting item E, "have no sense of responsibility", account for 15 %.

Another result of this survey is that students lack of rule consciousness. For example, as for the Question 6, the students who consider cheating in exam as normal phenomenon, but the students strongly disagree with this conduct only account for 22 %. As for Question 4, 45 % students believed that majority of college students would insinuate others and manage "guanxi" for fame and fortune. From this regard, strengthening of contemporary college students' moral education is urgently needed.

Develop education is based on the ideological and political education, but it focus on the moral quality of education and behavior habits. The cultivation of moral education is in the ideological and political education on the basis of people's morality, focus on quality and behavior of education. In daily life, work and study, through the behavior of the training, strict management and all kinds of education means, the colleges improve people's knowledge, feelings, and travel, and finally form the quality voluntarily comply with the social morals and the code of conduct and good moral character and behavior. At present, for the cultivation of university students' morals education, the society has a view that middle school students are worse than high school students, college students are worse than the primary school pupils. This shows the develop education university students in China is not optimistic. Therefore, it is important to strengthen and improve university students' ideological and moral education in an effective way.

Compared with the traditional social standard education, college students develop education in the pursuit and the value orientation, is a more distinct features of the Times, including education, education and standard deviations of mould education from the three aspects [1]. So the author thinks that the develop education can implement from several aspects.

42.2 Moral Cultivation Education

42.2.1 The Principle of Insisting on Moral System

In the survey questionnaire, Question 13 focuses on the students' self-evaluation of morals and ethics. The students whose self-evaluation is perfect only account for 11 %; and the students whose self-evaluation is general account for 33 %. From this respect, students' moral level has layers.

The traditional moral education emphasizes "sets up the lofty ideal, cultivate noble personality", encouraging each student to establish the highest ethical standards for themselves, which of course has its good on one hand, because under the strict request the whole moral standard of students have high starting point. However, it is undeniable that it has negative influence that cannot be ignored.

Students will soon find that it requires a great spirit of sacrifice in order to become this "perfect" moral model, and find people having this "perfect" moral are rare. Moreover, the phenomena that the majority of people in the society enjoy economic interests rather than spirit pursuit and highlight short-term interests instead of long-term interests have a negative impact on students so that many students find a big gap between education and reality, and have a view that becoming a "perfect" persons will surfer enormous sacrifices. Consequently, the result of moral teaching is that "you teaching your theories, but I go my way". Nowadays, moral education in colleges and universities in general commanding still does not go down from an ideal level to the moral status of the present reality, emphasizing the idealism and moral education is the focus of moral education.

The realm of moral personality has multiple levels. When cultivating college students' moral personality, not only the highest ethical requirements should be addressed, but also the actual level of their morality should be considered so that students could pursuit perfect moral realm step by step based on their actual situation [2]. Regarding the relationship between the personal interests and social interests, people's moral levels can be divided into four levels. The first also the highest level is selfless dedication; the second is the public interests priority; the third is looking after both public and personal interests; and the fourth level is the selfish. In the society, majority of people belong to the second and the third levels, and the situation of college students is the same. Therefore, the moral education should stand on the last line of moral requirements, which could ensure each member of the society obey the common rules and the social life run in an orderly manner. This last line of moral requirements include social common ethics and market rules, such fair competition, honesty and trust worthiness, respect, helpfulness, and so on [3]. Such last line is the basement of moral education. If the basement is unstable, the stricter requirements for morality cannot be achieved. Moreover, it is feasible to cultivate the students' personality referring to their own situation, and thereby achieve the objective of moral education.

42.2.2 Principle of Subjective Initiative

According to the teaching theory proposed by Markov and the theory of the whole development of students, it has been widely recognized that the school of education must be conceived in a social environment, and school education must be adapted to the needs of the community development. Teaching only touched the students' emotions and the will of the field, touch the spirit of the students need in order to play the efficient use. Education should be conceived in the society, and college education should adapt to the needs of social development. Teaching could be high effective and efficient on condition that it touches students' emotion and spiritual needs. As other social activities, teaching develops in the process of interactivities. The subjects of such interactivities are instructors and students. As for higher education, either educational theories or educational practices propose a requirement to study the objects of higher education at first, namely college students, which is the prerequisite of the implementation of teaching activities. It should be noticed that the psychological development of college students has been basically mature, cognitive ability is no longer just stay at the perceptual stage, but have strong rational thinking skills, and they are independent, autonomic and care for their personality development. Therefore, only if instructors fully respect the subjective status of students, care for students' the coordinated development of knowledge, intelligence, and behaviors, the objective of moral education, which aims to achieve the comprehensive development and the harmonious development of human, society and nature.

42.3 Cultivating Three Kinds of Awareness

42.3.1 Education of Rule Awareness

The modern society is a society of a "contract", in which social regulations and rules grant and safeguard the equal rights of each citizen and set requirements regarding citizen's obligations and responsibilities to other people and society. Obeying and respecting the rules in the society, and conscientiously fulfilling the responsibilities constitutes a basic obligation for modern citizens [4]. Obviously, rules are the basic elements of modern society. Harmonious society requires members of society have a higher awareness of the rules, and college students are the backbone of building a harmonious society. However, awareness of the rules of college students and is not optimistic. In 2007, the network on a hot post—"Top ten Chinese college students generally ugly phenomenon", citing China's college students cheating on exams, class late and leave early and not follow the rules of the vices to produce a sensational effect. Consequently, developing college students' good habits should begin from developing awareness of the rules.

Ethics and the law are to maintain social stability and development of the two most important social norms. The law than in the code of ethics in modern society under the rule of law, students still relatively admiration, while the code of ethics is often neglected, and even some students think this is a prejudice to their lives around rod. Teaching to make students do not look down that they called the shackles of their free moral constraints than hinder their lives around the pole, but to protect the barrier of their normal life. Appropriate desire to protect normal human life and joy, but the desire to Pandora's box open, they release a self-destructive life of the devil. If a person chooses to break through to those who they think is the moral constraints of the shackles of means to protect the safety disappear, no matter who he is. In this sense, whether the use of legal, code of ethics appropriate to divert a person's desires will become an important part in determining the success or failure of a person. There are numerous examples of failing to control the desire in a necessary extent and going beyond the moral constraints, which lead to tragedy.

42.3.2 Awareness of Responsibility

"People, a morally valuable person, must be responsible for something" [5]. Cultivation of the sense of moral responsibility will become moral subjects to do good tremendous impetus to become an important guarantee of conscious behavior to fulfill their social responsibilities.

In 1998, the first World Conference on Higher Education held in Paris makes it clear that the first task of higher education is to cultivate highly qualified graduates and responsible citizens. It shows that the responsibility concept of education has been widespread concerned and attached great importance to the international community. Due to various social factors, lack of sense of responsibility in a lot of college students in China is a general phenomenon. The lack of sense of responsibility of university students includes mainly the following aspects. First, lack the sense of self-responsibility, self-esteem, self-love, self-discipline, self-awareness of the game of life, wasted time. Second, lack moral responsibility. Moral sense, and ignore social ethics, comply with social ethics, as the performance of the pedantic. Dismissive of public opinion, ethics is not binding on them. Third, lack social responsibility. Everyone should be responsible to fulfill the social responsibility of each member of society can not be missing, especially in the contemporary college students to shoulder the great trust of the country, the hope of the nation. However, many students care their personal interests rather than social interests, and lack proper understanding and sense of responsibility when facing with the social responsibilities.

As for school education to develop students' sense of responsibility, it should enhance the students of the motherland, nation, society and the environment, family and others, their own sense of responsibility and spirit of responsibility, good sense of responsibility and responsibility character. Nowadays, the results of classroom teaching were pretty good. Second, it is to allow students to leave the campus to participate in social practice, to understand the community, understand the people's livelihood, to understand the country and, in practice, education, deepen understanding of responsibility in practice, in practice, know how everyone has their own responsibility, including on their own responsibility, family responsibility, social responsibility.

42.4 Moral Identity of Education

Moral identity of the individual or the social community, through interaction in the concept of a certain ethical and ethical recognition and sharing, or some kind of common ideals, beliefs, scale, the principle of the pursuit of goals to achieve in social life, and the value of positioning and orientation. Moral education of citizens a top priority is to educate the citizens' moral identity. From the theory of ethics, the formation of a harmonious society is the society's multi-stakeholder coordination of moral identity and behavior of selected and to meet human needs, and promote good moral of human development, social relations and spiritual atmosphere society [6]. The diversity of moral values is faced with an important subject of moral education. If not recognize and address can not be given to young people with the right guidance, it will lead to serious differentiation of their ideology, loss of common moral identity of the society as a whole, the spirit of a crisis of faith. For example, as for the item of No. 12 of the student questionnaire, the proportion of choosing the item A accounts 10 %, choosing the item B accounts 20 %, choosing C accounts 21 %, choosing D accounts 19 %, and choosing E accounts 30 %. Therefore, in the higher education sector should advocate the mainstream social values and the socialist concept of honor to create harmony, camaraderie and atmosphere. Adhere to the "three close" to a variety of ways and means to attract students, help students concerned about the domestic and international events, concerned about the life, objective and comprehensive understanding of the community. Thus, it is expected to provide spiritual support for the development of quality of students' concept of honor. The socialist concept of honor is the basic standards and ideas of glory and shame in the socialist society to maintain social stability, harmony and healthy development of all members of society. Teaching the socialist concept of honor education on college students aims to cultivate students' sense of national pride, self-confidence and patriotism, and to inspire them to work hard to learn, the rejuvenation of China and the consciousness of the struggle.

42.5 Focal Point

42.5.1 Honest Education

Max Weber addresses that in the modern economy, as long as the conduct is legal, earning money is the result of professional virtue and ability. The reason that honest is useful, because it can guarantee credit, punctual, industrious and thrifty [7]. The economist John Mueller also pointed out that without credit, benefits cannot be obtained from the capital [8]. Therefore, honest and trustworthy not only is the basic code of ethics, but also is a basic principle in Western civil law and known as the King terms.

As for Item 7, "how do you think about the personality of honesty of college students, the proportion of choosing A accounts 15 %, choosing B accounts 23 %, choosing C accounts 35 %, choosing D accounts 5 %, and choosing E accounts 22 %. All the ethic rules are established on the principle of honest and trustworthy. If loosing honesty, the whole moral system will be frangible. In other words, no honesty means no ethics. However, due to many reasons, there are a lot of phenomena of lacking honesty. Such phenomena also take place in college campus. For instance, some students like to plagiarism, cheating and other means to muddle through some weak sense of integrity, fraud to deceive teachers and classmates.

42.5.2 Consciously Abide by the Public Moral Education

The public morality in the society is the principle all citizens should follow in social interaction. With social progress and development of productive forces, the frequent interpersonal and people's social activities are increasing. In this regard, social morality and people's civil awareness in maintaining the normal order of society play an increasingly important role.

Consciously abiding the rules not only means the recognition of the value of morality, but also means emotional acceptance of the morality and honor experience. Only if students' awareness of consciously complying with the rule is increasing, the inconsistence of speech and conducts can be effectively reduced.

The author carries out the same questionnaire in classroom teaching in the last 3 year, requiring students to enumerate the top ten uncivilized phenomena. The result includes the following conducts: 1. loud noise in the library, and receive calls; 2. couples excessively intimacy at public places, especially in libraries, classrooms, academic lecture hall; 3. singing and doing something in the dormitory and boring others; 4. smoking and eating in classroom; 5. speaking, receiving calls and listening to music in class; 6. Being late, leaving early, being absent, and skipping classes; 7. do not line up; 8. Throwing away garbage disorderly; 9. trampling grass; 10. damaging public property. These indicate that students' awareness of consciously complying with the public rules is not strong. Therefore, it is necessary to instruct students to abide the moral norms through teaching.

42.5.3 Developing a Mental Health Attitude

In the modern society, it has been recognized that education of the mental healthy is a necessary approach of carrying out moral education. The World Health Organization (WHO) pointed out that the healthy means a person's physics and mental are completely in a good state of social adaptation rather than simply refers to diseases or sick. In other words, it is not only related to human psychology, and social and moral issues related to physical health, mental health, moral health, three aspects constitute the overall concept of health. Mental health and morality are closely related to good moral character and it is the prerequisite of ensuring mental health, good health, and psychological state. For this reason, college students a series of problem behavior, not only thinking of the quality of legal reasons, and often accompanied by psychological reasons. Obviously, ideological and moral is not only related with the level of knowledge and cultural literacy, but also related to the ability to self-awareness and evaluation capacity. If students self-awareness is not sufficient, it can not correctly understand and evaluation in the case of lack of proper guidance, they can not properly grasp of good and evil, and Africa, impartiality and favoritism, honesty and hypocrisy, noble and despicable boundaries, and thus moral a sense of misconduct. Consequently, we should regard the mental health education as the basis for moral education.

42.6 Conclusion

Developing moral education of college students has become an important task for the higher education in China. It is a good way to formalize a perfect humanity as well as ethic characteristic. As for such education, two principles should be obeyed: insisting on moral system, and subjective initiative. Colleges should help students develop the personality of honesty and mental health attitudes.

Acknowledgment This article is an achievement of the project "Establishing and Optimizing the Adaptation Mechanisms for Group Events Caused by Indirect Interest Conflicts", which is supported by "Education Scientific Planning Project" of Zhejiang Province, P.R.C. (SCG94).

Appendix

College Students Questionnaire of Moral Attitude

1. Are you ideal?

   A. Yes; B. No; C. I don't think about it; D. It does not matter.
2. Do you care for your parents?

   A. Yes; B. No; C. I don't think about it; D. It does not matter.
3. How do you think about professional knowledge and morals?

   A. Both of them are important;
   B. Only the former is important;
   C. Only the latter is important;
   D. The answer depends on the specific situation.
4. Are there a lot of college students favor other students for fame and fortune?

   A. A lot; B. No; C. Few; D. I have no idea about it.

5. How do you get along with people around?

   A. Normal; B. Very good; C. Good; D. Rarely get along with other people.
6. How do you think about cheating in the examination?

   A. It is a normal phenomenon;
   B. Hate it;
   C. It does not matter;
   D. The answer depends on the specific situation.
7. How do you think about the situation of the honesty personality of college students?

   A. Very good; B. Good; C. Normal; D. I have no idea about it; E. Not good.
8. What will you do when strangers ask for your help?

   A. I would like to favor others;
   B. Depend on my feeling;
   C. I will not provide help;
   D. The answer depends on the specific situation.
9. How do you think about your sense of responsibility?

   A. Very good; B. Good; C. Not good; D. Normal; E. My sense of responsibility is good only for my own matters.
10. What phenomena indicate that college students lack sense of morality?

    A. Trivial matters; B. Basic moral; C. Seriously fail to obey the social rules; D. I do not know.
11. How you do think the impacts of ethics on economic development?

    A. No impact; B. Positive impacts; C. Negative impacts.
12. Do you thing ethics effectively function on personal behaviors?

    A. Yes; B. Normal; C. No; D. No function at all; E. Function depends on the social environment.
13. How do you think your morality?

    A. Excellent; B. Very good; C. Normal; D. Not good.
14. What can we do in order to developing students' moral personality?

References

1. Xin GZ (2008) Taking moral education as an important approach of cultivating talents in higher education. Res Moral Polit Educ 3:29
2. Song K (2008) Discussing developing the moral personality of college students. Acad J Hunan Inst Metall Technol 8(2):46
3. Zhou Y, Lin Z (2008) Reconsideration of revolution of moral education. East South Dissem 6:133

4. Sun HX (2008) Study on developing moral responsibility of citizen. Acad J Liaoning Univ Technol (Soc Sci Ed) 10(3):9
5. Kant I (1986) Principles of metaphysics of morals. (Trans: Miao LT). Shanghai People's Publishing House, Shanghai, pp 6
6. Li XN Social identity and social harmony. http//:www.chinareform.org.cn/ad/2005_04/lunwen.asp
7. Max W (2002) The protestant ethic and the spirit of capitalism, vol 2. (Trans: Peng Q, Huang XJ). Shanxi Normal University Press, China, pp 24, 26
8. Mueller J Principles of economics. San Min Bookstore, Taipei, pp 447, 448

Chapter 43
A Bayes Network Model to Determine MiRNA Gene Silence Mechanism

Hao-yue Fu, Xiao-jun Lu and Xiang-de Zhang

Abstract MicroRNAs (miRNAs) are small noncoding RNAs that silence gene expression by base pairing to mRNAs. They play important gene regulatory roles via hybridization to target mRNAs. The functional characterization of miRNAs relies heavily on the identification of their target mRNAs. Determining whether mRNA genes are regulated by translational repression or by post-transcriptional degradation is the premise of accurately identifying miRNA target genes. Combining expression profiling method with computational sequence analysis method, we present a Bayes network model to identify miRNA target genes as well as to determine the gene silence mechanism. The result shows that the learning algorithm of the model has detected 49 % candidate miRNA target genes at 5 % false detection rate and has determined 80 % genes regulated by post-transcriptional degradation mechanism at 3 % false detection rate. Our model precisely predicts miRNA gene silence mechanism and presents an efficient method to find out miRNA targets.

Keywords MiRNA target identification · Gene silence mechanism · Bayes network · EM algorithm · Variational learning

H. Fu (✉) · X. Lu · X. Zhang
College of Sciences, Northeastern University, Shenyang, China
e-mail: fuhaoyue_neu@sina.com

X. Lu
e-mail: luxiaojun0625@sina.com

X. Zhang
e-mail: zhangxdneu@yahoo.com.cn

S. Li et al. (eds.), *Frontier and Future Development of Information Technology in Medicine and Education*, Lecture Notes in Electrical Engineering 269,
DOI: 10.1007/978-94-007-7618-0_43,

43.1 Introduction

At present, the two problems to be further solved in the miRNA study realm are to identify miRNA target genes and to determine miRNA regulation mechanism.

In order to identify miRNA target genes, a lot of sequence analysis computational algorithms have been developed [1–4]. These algorithms are on the basis of the nature of the pairing between miRNA and their targets gene. However, the accuracy and the effectivity of these computational algorithms have to be verified by biological methods. Combining computational method with gene expression method [5], GenMiR++ have more biological relevant evidence [6].

There is no exact answer as to how miRNA regulates gene networks. Nevertheless, researchers have confirmed miRNA regulates gene network by at the least two mechanism: post-transcriptional degradation and translational repression. It is uncertain that which genes are regulated by the former mechanism and which are done by the latter.

With these problems in mind, we present a switching model not only to identify miRNA target genes but also to determine the mechanism by which miRNA regulate gene network. First, we describe how genes are allowed to be regulated by anyone of the two mechanisms. The model is formulated in probabilistic graph model. Then, given miRNAs, mRNAs and protein expression data, the variational EM learning algorithm teases out the miRNA:target mRNA interaction pairs from the candidate set produced by computational algorithm TargetScanS and determines regulation mechanism. The result shows that our switching model can determine regulation mechanism effectively, at the same time, the accuracy with which the miRNA target genes are to be idendtified has been further improved.

43.2 Switching Model

The principle in which miRNA target genes can be identified by gene expression method is the phenomenon of high miRNA expression with low target gene expression because of the miRNA down-regulation action when miRNA and mRNA have interaction with each other.

Set point z, x, y respectively represents the expression data of miRNA, mRNA and protein. As shown in Fig. 43.1a, the directed edge from z to x represents the influence on mRNA owing to miRNA. The edge from x to y represents the influence on protein. The graph is in accordance with post-transcriptional degradation mechanism.

Translational repression mechanism is shown in the Fig. 43.1b. The mRNA expression is unaffected while the protein expression is decreased by this kind of mechanism. The switch random variable ω integrates the two mechanisms into one graph. As shown in Fig. 43.1a, when the switch is on, the graph equals to the first graph. Otherwise, it equals to the second graph.

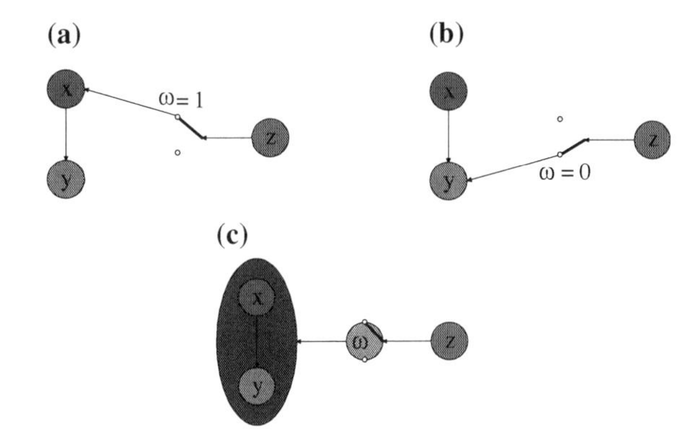

Fig. 43.1 Switching model of miRNA regulation

Including indicator random variable s, the graph can denote the situation whether miRNA and mRNA have interaction each other or not. The relationship among these variables can be expressed as such:

$$E\left[x_{it}\middle|s_{ij}=1,\omega_i=1,z_{jt},\Theta\right]=\mu_{xt}-\lambda_j z_{jt},\ \lambda_j>0 \tag{43.1}$$

$$E\left[x_{it}\middle|s_{ij}=0,\omega_i=1,z_{jt},\Theta\right]=\mu_{xt} \tag{43.2}$$

$$E\left[x_{it}\middle|s_{ij},\omega_i=0,z_{jt},\Theta\right]=\mu_{xt} \tag{43.3}$$

Co-regulation of multiple miRNAs to one target gene is an important characteristic of miRNA regulation. It has been embodied in the final graph model shown in Fig. 43.2. The final graph model is completed with multiple genes comprised of. The intention we construct the model is to obtain an accurate estimation about variable s and ω which respectively determine miRNA:target mRNA interaction pair and miRNA regulation mechanism. For the purpose of writing the model probability, it is necessary to define prior probability p(ω) and p(S|C), where C is a candidate miRNA:target mRNA interaction pair set predicted by computational algorithm TargetScanS.

$$P(X,Y,s,\omega|C,Z,\Theta)=\prod_i P(y_i|x_i,Z,s,\omega,\Theta)P(x_i|Z,s,\omega,\Theta)P(w_i|\Theta)\prod_j P\left(s_{ij}|C,\Theta\right) \tag{43.4}$$

If the parameter Θ denotes the prior probability of ω equals to 1 and parameter Π denotes the prior probability of s_{ij} equals to 1, the prior binomial distribution density expression are:

$$P(\omega|\Theta)=\prod_i P(\omega_i|\Theta)=\prod_i \delta^{\omega_i}(1-\delta)^{1-\omega_i} \tag{43.5}$$

$$P(s|C,\Theta)=\prod_{(i,j):C_{ij}=1} P\left(s_{ij}|C,\Theta\right)=\prod_{(i,j):C_{ij}=1} \pi^{s_{ij}}(1-\pi)^{1-s_{ij}} \tag{43.6}$$

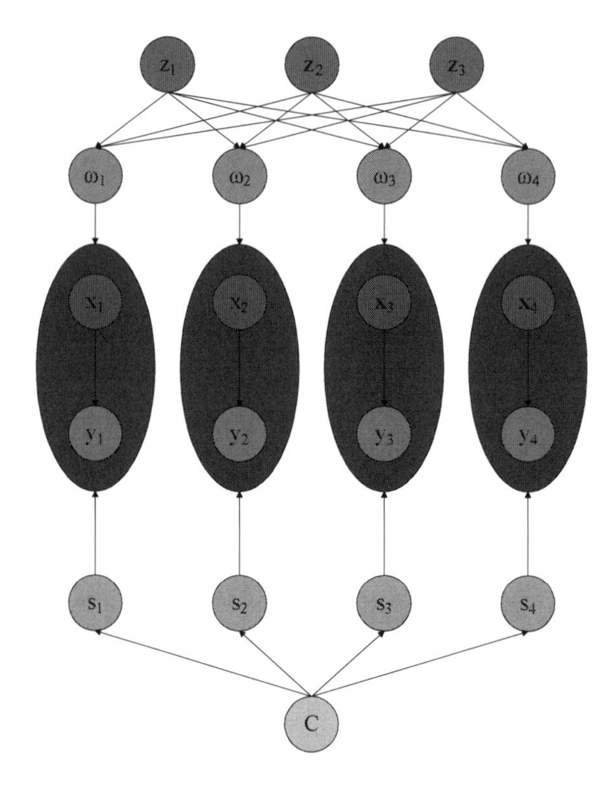

Fig. 43.2 Bayes network model of multiple miRNAs co-regulation

The model probability is written as:

$$P(y_i|x_i, Z, s, \omega, \Theta) = N\left(y_i; \mu_y - \xi \sum\nolimits_j \lambda_j s_{ij} z_j, \Sigma_y\right),\ \lambda_j \geq \varepsilon > 0 \tag{43.7}$$

$$P(x_i|Z, s, \omega, \Theta) = N\left(x_i; \mu_x - \omega_i \sum\nolimits_j \lambda_j s_{ij} z_j, \Sigma_x\right),\ \lambda_j \geq \varepsilon > 0 \tag{43.8}$$

Inference of our Bayes network modes is based on the posterior probability. Note that the complexity of computing the posterior probability is exponential in the number of miRNAs and the number of mRNAs. It is hardly to execute exact inference. Variational learning is a method to approximately infer probabilistic graph model [7, 8]. It turns the inference into a procedure of optimizing a set of variational parameter Φ. Therefore, the complexity has been greatly decreased and the inference can be executed practically.

43.3 The Variational Learning Algorithm of the Model

Consider the graph model with unobserved variables H and observed variables E. The posterior probability $P(H|E)$can be approximated by distribution $q(H;\Phi)$, where Φ is variational parameters. The variational learning is to find parameters Φ optimizing the fitness $P(H|E)$ with $q(H;\Phi)$.

The fitness is measured at kullback–Leibler divergence:

$$D(q\|p) = \int_H q(H;\Phi)\log\frac{q(H;\Phi)}{p(H,E)} = \sum\nolimits_{s,\omega} q(s,\omega|C)\log\frac{q(s,\omega|C)}{p(X,Y,s,\omega|C,Z,\Theta)} \tag{43.9}$$

The approximate distribution $q(s,\omega|C)$ is simplified as:

$$\begin{aligned} q(s,\omega|C) &= q(s|C)q(w) = \prod\nolimits_{(i,j):C_{ij}=1} q(s_{ij}|C)\prod\nolimits_i q(\omega_i) \\ &= \prod\nolimits_{(i,j):C_{ij}=1} \beta_{ij}^{s_{ij}}\left(1-\beta_{ij}\right)^{1-s_{ij}}\prod\nolimits_i \gamma_i^{\omega_i}(1-\gamma_i)^{1-\omega_i} \end{aligned}$$

If we write statistics $u_i, W_1, V_1, O_1, W_2, V_2$ as:

$$u_i = \sum\nolimits_{j:C_{ij}=1} \lambda_j\beta_{ij}z_j \tag{43.10}$$

$$W_1 = \frac{1}{N}\sum\nolimits_i (x_i - (\mu_x - \gamma_i u_i))(x_i - (\mu_x - \gamma_i u_i))^T \tag{43.11}$$

$$V_1 = \frac{1}{N}\sum\nolimits_i \gamma_i \sum\nolimits_{j:C_{ij}=1}\left(\beta_{ij} - \beta_{ij}^2\right)\lambda_j^2 z_j z_j^T \tag{43.12}$$

$$O_1 = \frac{1}{N}\sum\nolimits_i \left(\gamma_i - \gamma_i^2\right)u_i u_i^T \tag{43.13}$$

$$W_2 = \frac{1}{N}\sum\nolimits_i \left(y_i - \left(\mu_y - \xi u_i\right)\right)\left(y_i - \left(\mu_y - \xi u_i\right)\right)^T \tag{43.14}$$

$$V_2 = \frac{1}{N}\sum\nolimits_{(i,j):C_{ij}=1}\left(\beta_{ij} - \beta_{ij}^2\right)\lambda_j^2\xi z_j\left(\xi z_j\right)^T \tag{43.15}$$

The KL divergence can be simplified as:

$$\begin{aligned} D(q\|p) = &\sum\nolimits_{(i,j):C_{ij}=1}\left(\beta_{ij}\log\frac{\beta_{ij}}{\pi} + (1-\beta_{ij})\log\frac{(1-\beta_{ij})}{(1-\pi)}\right) + \sum\nolimits_i\left(\gamma_i\log\frac{\gamma_i}{\delta} + (1-\gamma_i)\log\frac{(1-\gamma_i)}{(1-\delta)}\right) \\ &+ \frac{N}{2}tr\left(\Sigma_x^{-1}(W_1 + V_1 + O_1)\right) + \frac{N}{2}tr\left(\Sigma_y^{-1}(W_2 + V_2)\right) + \frac{N}{2}\log|\Sigma_x| + \frac{N}{2}\log|\Sigma_y| \end{aligned} \tag{43.16}$$

Variational learning can be carried out by variational EM algorithm which will iteratively minimize $D(q\|p)$ with respect to variational parameters (E-step) and with respect to model parameters (M-step) until convergence. When taking derivatives of $D(q\|p)$ and setting to zeros, we get the following iterative equations.

43.3.1 E-Step

$$\frac{\beta_{ij}}{1-\beta_{ij}} = \frac{\pi}{1-\pi}\exp\Big(-\lambda_j\gamma_i z_j^T\Sigma_x^{-1}\Big(x_i - \Big(\mu_x - \gamma_i\sum\nolimits_{k\neq j:C_{ik}=1}\lambda_k\beta_{ik}z_k\Big) + \frac{\lambda_j}{2}z_j + (1-\gamma_i)\sum\nolimits_{k\neq j:C_{ik}=1}\lambda_k\beta_{ik}z_k\Big) - \lambda_j(\xi z_j)^T\Sigma_y^{-1}\Big(y_i - \Big(\mu_y - \xi\sum\nolimits_{k\neq j:C_{ik}=1}\lambda_k\beta_{ik}z_k\Big) + \frac{\lambda_j}{2}(\xi z_j)\Big)\Big) \tag{43.17}$$

$$\frac{\gamma_i}{1-\gamma_i} = \frac{\delta}{1-\delta}\exp\Big(-\Sigma_x^{-1}\Big(u_i^T\Big(x_i - \mu_x + \frac{1}{2}u_i\Big) + \frac{1}{2}\sum\nolimits_j\Big(\beta_{ij} - \beta_{ij}^2\Big)\lambda_j^2 z_j^T z_j\Big)\Big) \tag{43.18}$$

43.3.2 M-Step

$$\Sigma_x = diag(W_1 + V_1 + O_1) \tag{43.19}$$

$$\Sigma_y = diag(W_2 + V_2) \tag{43.20}$$

$$\mu_x = \frac{1}{N}\sum\nolimits_i(x_i + \gamma_i u_i) \tag{43.21}$$

$$\mu_y = \frac{1}{N}\sum\nolimits_i(y_i + \xi u_i) \tag{43.22}$$

$$\pi = \frac{\sum_{(i,j)\in C}\beta_{ij}}{card(C)} \tag{43.23}$$

$$\delta = \frac{\sum_i \gamma_i}{N} \tag{43.24}$$

$$\xi = \frac{diag\Big(\sum_i u_i(y_i - \mu_y)^T\Big)}{diag\Big(\sum_i u_i u_i^T + \sum_{(i,j):C_{ij}=1}\Big(\beta_{ij} - \beta_{ij}^2\Big)\lambda_j^2 z_j z_j^T\Big)} \tag{43.25}$$

$$\lambda_j = \max\left(-\frac{\sum_i\gamma_i\beta_{ij}z_j^T\Sigma_x^{-1}((x_i - (\mu_x - \gamma_i\sum_{k\neq j:C_{ik}=1}\lambda_k\beta_{ik}z_k)) + (1-\gamma_i)\sum_{k\neq j:C_{ik}=1}\lambda_k\beta_{ik}z_k) + \sum_i\beta_{ij}(\xi z_j)^T\Sigma_y^{-1}(y_i - (\mu_y - \xi\sum_{k\neq j:C_{ik}=1}\lambda_k\beta_{ik}z_k))}{\sum_i\gamma_i\beta_{ij}z_j^T\Sigma_x^{-1}z_j + \sum_i\beta_{ij}(\xi z_j)^T\Sigma_y^{-1}(\xi z_j)}, 0.01\right) \tag{43.26}$$

43.4 Results

Using data in literature [9–11], matrices $x_{155\times5}, y_{155\times5}, z_{22\times5}$ were build.

Each variable and parameter was initialized as: $\beta_{ij} = \pi = \delta = 0.5, \forall(i,j)$: $C_{ij} = 1$; $\lambda_j = 0.01, \forall j = 1, \ldots, M$; $\gamma_i = 0.5, \forall i = 1, \ldots, N$. μ_y, μ_x were initialized as the mean values of protein expression data and mRNA expression data respectively, and $\xi = \mu_y/\mu_x$. Σ_y, Σ_x were initialized as the covariance matrix of protein expression data and mRNA expression data respectively. The algorithm was iterated as most 200 times or the algorithm was converged with the error within 0.01.

The model performance evaluation is as follows. The candidate miRNA-mRNA pair (i,j) is evaluated by $score(i,j)$ defined as $score(i,j) = \beta_{ij}$. It is the $score(i) = \gamma_i$ that evaluates whether the gene i is regulated by post-transcriptional degradation. If the $score(i,j)$ is high, the miRNA-mRNA pair (i,j) would be more likely to become the real miRNA-mRNA interactional pair. Similarly, the high $score(i)$ shows the more possibility of the ith miRNA being regulated by post-transcriptional degradation. In order to determine an effective score threshold, it is necessary to calculate the average false detection rate of each score threshold. Therefore, a series of permutation tests must be executed. When the permutation test is done, the ordered number of miRNA expression data is randomly permutated and the algorithm is executed with the permutated order. A total of 100 permutation tests is executed. For a score threshold, the false detection number is the number of permutation tests whose score are higher than the threshold and the average false detection rate is the false detection number divided by 100. The ratio of the detected fraction (the number of detected candidate/the number of candidate) to the average false detection rate responses to the ration of the sensitivity to the specificity.

The results showed that, our algorithm predicted 49 % miRNA-mRNA pairs within 5 % false detection rate, while algorithm of literature [6] predicted 34 % miRNA-mRNA pairs within 5 % false detection rate. Furthermore, our algorithm

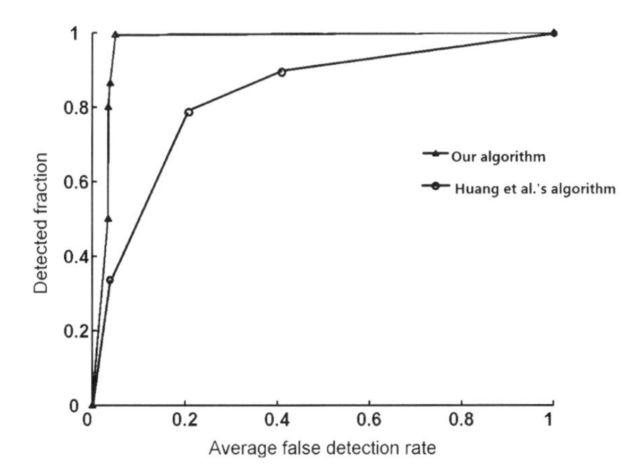

Fig. 43.3 Sensitivity and specificity curve to identify genes regulated by post-transcriptional degradation

also predicted the gene silence mechanism. It predicted 80 % genes were regulated by posttranscriptional degradation mechanism with 3 % false detection rate. The sensitivity and specificity curve to identify genes regulated by posttranscriptional degradation is showed in Fig. 43.3.

43.5 Conclusions

The Bayesian network methods of prediction miRNA targets based on expression profiling data have been included into the writings "Machine learning in bioinformatics" [12]. However, they assume that all the miRNAs are in accordance with the single gene silence mechanism. In our method, a new class of random variables is presented into the Bayesian network in order to predict the gene silence mechanism. The results show that our model precisely predicts miRNA gene silence mechanism and presents an efficient method to find out miRNA targets.

References

1. Stark A, Brennecke J, Russell RB et al (2003) Identification of drosophila MicroRNA targets. PLoS Biol 1:E60
2. Enright AJ, John B, Gaul U et al (2003) MicroRNA targets in drosophila. Genome Biol 5:R1
3. Lewis BP, Shih I, Jones-Rhoades MW et al (2003) Prediction of mammalian MicroRNA targets. Cell 115:787–798
4. Vejnar CE, Zdobnov EM (2012) miRmap: comprehensive prediction of microRNA target repression strength. Nucleic Acids Res 40(22):11673–11683
5. Lim LP et al (2005) Microarray analysis shows that some microRNAs downregulate large numbers of target mRNAs. Nature 433:769–773
6. Huang JC, Morris QD, Frey BJ (2006) Detecting microRNA targets by linking sequence, microRNA and gene expression data. In: Proceedings of the tenth annual conference on research in computational molecular biology
7. Jordan MI, Ghahramani Z, Jaakkola TS et al (1999) An introduction to variational methods for graphical models. Learning in graphical models. MIT Press, Cambridge
8. Neal RM, Hinton GE (1998) A view of the EM algorithm that justifies incremental, sparse, and other variants, learning in graphical models. Kluwer Academic Publishers, Boston
9. Babak T, Zhang W, Morris Q, Blencowe BJ et al (2004) Probing microRNAs with microarrays: tissue specificity and functional inference. RNA 10:1813–1819
10. Zhang W, Morris Q et al (2004) The functional landscape of mouse gene expression. J Biol 3:21–43
11. Kislinger T et al (2006) Global survey of organ and organelle protein expression in mouse: combined proteomic and transcriptomic profiling. Cell 125:173–186
12. Zhang Y, Rajapakse JC (2009) Machine learning in bioinformatics. Wiley, New Jersey

Chapter 44
The Novle Strategy for the Recognition and Classification of the Red Blood Cell in Low Quality Form Images

Qiyou Cao, Xueqing Li and Qi Zhang

Abstract In this paper, we describe a novle strategy for the recognition and classification of the red blood cell (RBC) in low quality form images. At present, the classification of red blood cells has become one of the routine inspection of hospital, the inspection result has the very vital significance for the clinical diagnosis. Under the microscope, however, the work is very time consuming, and the different person have different classification error. Therefore, people are trying to use computer technology to help people eye brain system to complete the work and in this area of research is still ongoing. This paper proposes a method can be better applied to the automatic identification of red blood cells, and the experimental results show that the research results can be applied to clinical diagnosis, reduce the labor intensity of professionals and is conducive to the doctor's diagnosis. The new cell recognition algorithm improves accuracy while the speed is suitable for practical applications. The Smear of this experiment is made by conventional method and use an Olympus camera magnified 800 times of cells on the film imaging, the grey scale 256.

Keywords RBC · Pattern recognition · Support vector machines (SVM) · Decision tree · Edge detection

Q. Cao (✉) · X. Li (✉) · Q. Zhang (✉)
School of Computer Science and Technology, Shandong University, Jinan 250101, China
e-mail: sducao@gmail.com

X. Li
e-mail: xqli@sdu.edu.cn

Q. Zhang
e-mail: cc_123662@163.com

S. Li et al. (eds.), *Frontier and Future Development of Information Technology in Medicine and Education*, Lecture Notes in Electrical Engineering 269,
DOI: 10.1007/978-94-007-7618-0_44,

44.1 Introduction

Image segmentation is the most important step and a key technology in image processing which directly affect the next processing. In human blood cell segmentation cases, it has appeared lots of particular segmentation methods and have achieved better results, but for the complex environment of cell image processing is still not ideal. This paper will propose an approach which is a part of study to perform automated recognition for RBC. The methods involve are wiener filtering, edge detection and SVM. The combination of wiener filtering and edge detection aim to remove noise and segment the image for all possible target (RBC). Then, in order to improve the accuracy of the classification, put forward an improved euclidean distance-based support vector machine decision tree construction method. A large number of experiments show that the ideal segmentation results, using our method. The Fig. 44.1 shows the flow of the segmentation.

44.2 The Preprocessing of Image

44.2.1 Restore The Montion-Blurred Images

Motion-blurring is caused by the relative motion between the camera and theobject. Photograph under flow state there will cause a transverse horizontal motion effect and blood cells move itself leads to motion-blurred image. We adopt the

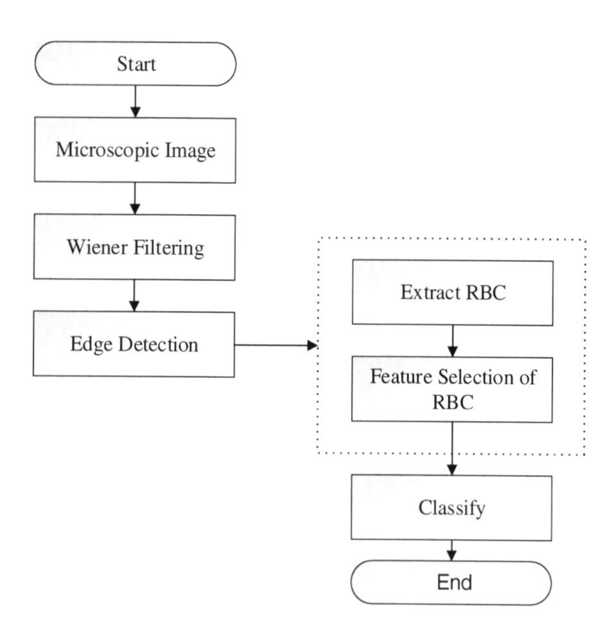

Fig. 44.1 The flow of RBC segmentation

wiener filter which is based on mathematical modeling method. The wiener filter minimizes the mean square error between the estimated random process and the desired process.

$$e^2 = E\left\{\left(f - \hat{f}\right)^2\right\} \tag{44.1}$$

E{·} is the value of expectation, f is the original image, $\hat{f}$ is the restored image.

$$\hat{F}(u,v) = \left[\frac{H*(u,v)S(u,v)}{S_f(u,v)|H(u,v)|^2 + S_\eta(u,v)}\right]G(u,v) \tag{44.2}$$

while the presence of white noise, $S\eta$ is a large constant and the power spectrum of the degradation of the image very little is known. Therefore this paper adopts the improved approximate expressions, as follows:

$$\hat{F}(u,v) = \left[\frac{1}{H(u,v)}\frac{|H(u,v)|^2}{|H(u,v)|^2 + K}\right]G(u,v) \tag{44.3}$$

K is a special constant.

During the processing of image restoration, the main problem is that the image information is incomplete, We divide the image into 4 × 4 and wiener filtering work on each piece. Experiments show that this method can effectively remove noise and reduce the edge error which the incomplete image information leads to. As a result, this achieve better results. As the Fig. 44.2 show.

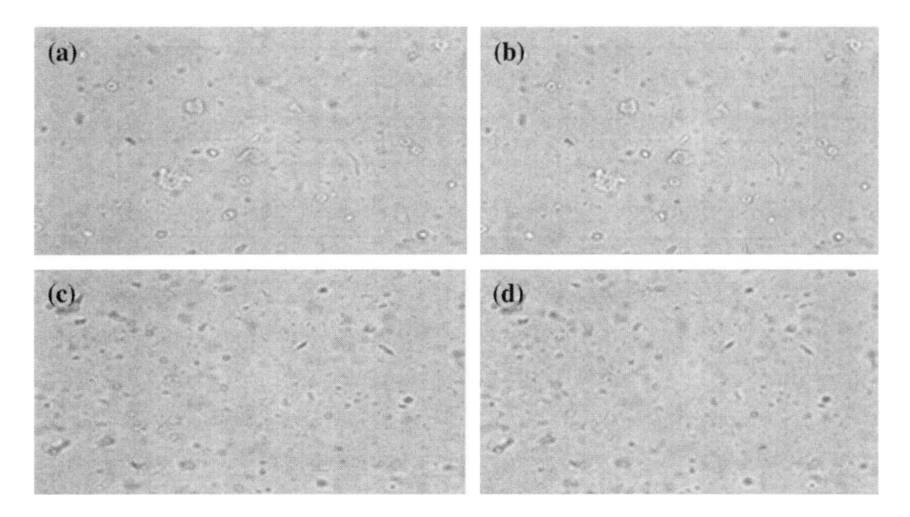

Fig. 44.2 The result of the wiener filter. **a** is the blurred image, **b** is the corresponding processed image, as well as the (**c**) and (**d**)

44.2.2 Edge Detection

Edge detection is the name for set of mathematical methods which aim at identifying points in a digital image at which the image brightness changes sharply or more formally, has discontinuities.

In this paper we adopt the image edge detection algorithm which is based on the improved canny operator by Wang xiaojun et al. It calculates the optimal high and low dual-threshold through iteration arithmetic, and uses mathematical morphology to detect image thinning. The threshold segmentation process is as follows:

1. Initialize the threshold T.

$$
\begin{aligned}
T_0 &= \{T_k | K = 0\} \\
T_0 &= \frac{Z_{\max} + Z_{\min}}{2}
\end{aligned}
\tag{44.4}
$$

K the iterations; Zmax, Zmin respectively the minimum and maximum grey value of image.

2. The image is divided into two parts the H1, H2.

$$
\begin{aligned}
H_1 &= \{f(x,y) | f(x,y) \geq T_k\} \\
H_2 &= \{f(x,y) | f(x,y) < T_k\}
\end{aligned}
\tag{44.5}
$$

3. Calculate M1, M2, the average grayscale of H1, H2.

$$
\begin{aligned}
M_1 &= \frac{\sum\limits_{f(i,j) \geq T_k} f(i,j)}{\sum\limits_{f(i,j) \geq T_k} N_H(i,j)} \\
M_2 &= \frac{\sum\limits_{f(i,j) < T_k} f(i,j)}{\sum\limits_{f(i,j) < T_k} N_L(i,j)}
\end{aligned}
\tag{44.6}
$$

4. Calculate the next threshold value Tk +1.

$$
T_{k+1} = \frac{M_1 + M_2}{2} \tag{44.7}
$$

5. If Tk = Tk + 1 or satisfy the constraint conditions end else K = K + 1 goto (2).
6. End the iteration, obtain M1, M2.

Experimental results prove that this algorithm can effectively reduce interference and noise edge, and make more prominent detection characteristics of medical cell image. The Fig. 44.3 show the processing results.

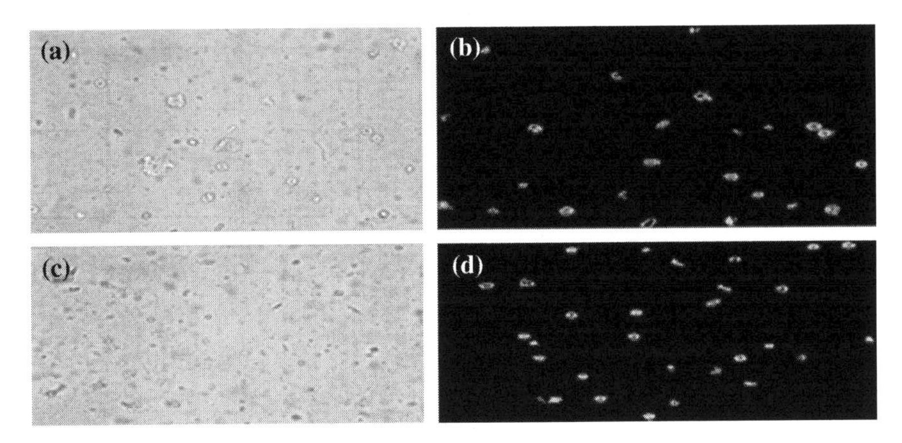

Fig. 44.3 The result of the edge detection. **a** is the original image, **b** is the corresponding processed image, as well as the (**c**) and (**d**)

44.3 Application of Support Vector Machine Red Blood Cell Recognition

44.3.1 Extract The Characteristics of RBC

Normal mature red blood cells are double concave disc, the area/volume ratio is larger which is suitable for gas exchange and its deformation, so we select the geometrical characteristics of RBC as the input of SVM. Involve: area S, circumference P, circularity C, rectangularity R, elongation E, maximum diameter Φ_{max}, minimum diameter Φ_{min}.

1. Area A. The area of the *i*th cell is Si $S_i = \sum_{x=1}^{N}\sum_{y=1}^{M} F(x,y)$, if foreground F(x, y) = 1 else 0.
2. Circumference P. $P = \sum_{(x,y)\in\Omega} P(x,y)$, if (x, y) belongs to the boundary p(x, y) = 1 else 0.
3. Circularity C. The circularity of the *i*th cell is $C_i = 4\pi S_i/P_i^2$.
4. Rectangularity R. The rectangularity of the ith cell is $R_i = {}^{S_i}/_{A_i}$, A_i the area of the external rectangle for the *i*th cell.
5. Maximum diameter Φ_{max}. The diameter of the circumscribed circle.
6. Minimum diameter Φ_{min}. The width of the external rectangular. This two geometrical characteristics can exclude the larger or smaller distruptors int the image.
7. Elongation E. $E = \min(w,l)/\max(w,l)$, This feature can separate the slender objects and square or circular object.

44.3.2 SVM Decision Tree Construction

In order to improve the efficiency and accuracy of classification, first of all, design an optimized SVM decision tree classifier. Collection u include all categories in a decision node, set of positive classes S1, set of negative classes S2, $U = S_1 \cup S_2$, N_{s1}, N_{s2} is the sizeof S1 and S2, X_i on behalf of the classes i samples set. The algorithm of obtaining the collection S1, S2 is as follows:

1. Obtain the center of each class.

$$c_i = \frac{1}{n_k} \sum_{x_i \in X_k} x_i \tag{44.8}$$

2. Calculate the center distance between the various of classes.

$$d_{ij} = \left\| c_i - c_j \right\| \tag{44.9}$$

3. Obtain the average distance D_{s1}, D_{s2} between any two class within the set of S1 and S2.

$$\begin{aligned} D_{s1} &= \frac{2}{N_{s1} * (N_{s1} - 1)} \sum_{i \in s_1, j \in s_1, i \neq j} d_{ij} \\ D_{s2} &= \frac{2}{N_{s2} * (N_{s2} - 1)} \sum_{i \in s_2, j \in s_2, i \neq j} d_{ij} \end{aligned} \tag{44.10}$$

assuming that $D_{s1} > D_{s2}$ and calculated the mean.

$$d_m = \frac{D_{s1} \times N_{s1} + D_{s2} \times N_{s2}}{N_{s1} + N_{s2}} \tag{44.11}$$

4. Cluster
   If $\|c_i - d_m\| \geq 0 \; i \cup S_1$ else $i \cup S_2$.
5. Circulate the process until all the categories are separate (Table 44.1).

Table 44.1 The mean of several types geometric features of RBC

Class name	$\overline{S}$	$\overline{P}$	$\overline{C}$	$\overline{R}$	$\overline{E}$
Spherocyte	1005.4423	131.9468	0.7257	0.9763	0.7652
Elliptocyte	1138.9687	156.9256	0.5812	0.5606	0.7937
Target-shaped cell	2615.5806	230.8527	0.6167	0.9450	0.7768
Somatocyte	476.5643	95.4681	0.6570	0.9021	0.7856
Sickle cell	1827.4562	226.4728	0.4477	0.3490	0.7523
Acanthocyte	1092.9631	230.0978	0.2594	0.6851	0.7265
Schistocytes	816.4538	142.6754	0.5040	0.5273	0.7031
Meniscocyte	760.8529	124.4572	0.6172	0.6549	0.8012
Teardrop-shaped cell	1970.7509	220.1196	0.5111	0.6739	0.6611

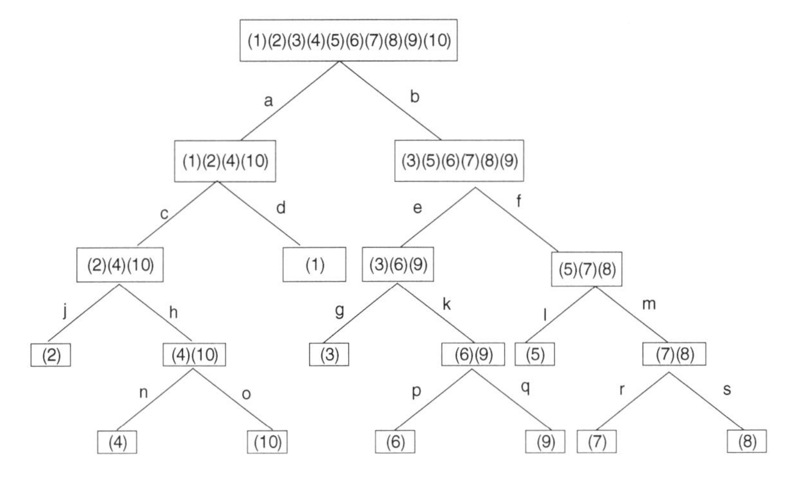

Fig. 44.4 Multi-class SVM classification structure

Due to the introduction of the SVM decision rules in this article, the complexity is not increased exponentially while the feature dimension increases, so using a priori knowledge of selecting characteristics which are favorable for classification using in each tree node to decision-making, so as to facilitate the classification. Experimental results show that the classification accuracy of acanthocyte is 70.7855 %, the target-shaped cell is 85 %, the meniscocyte, teardrop-shaped cell is 89.8732 %, the elliptocyte, sickle cell schistocytes 95.7523 %, the spherocyte, somatocyte is 100 % (Fig. 44.4).

44.4 Conclusions and Future Work

RBC is the dominant composition among the blood cells and the information extracted from its analysis can give a valuable data for a response index. This paper has presented the method for the recognition of blood cells under complex environment. The methods involve are wiener filtering, edge detection and SVM.The important point in this solution is the application of the SVM network classifier. We propose the improved decision tree construction and the experimental results very ideal in some way. The improvement need to be done for both segmentation and overlapped cell handling to obtain better result in the future.

References

1. Jerdnimo A-G, Femando P-C (2003) Multi-class support vector machines—a new approach. IEEE 781–784
2. Canny J (1986) A computational approach to edge detection. IEEE Trans Pattern Anal Mach Intell 8(6):679–698
3. Gonzalez RC, Woods RE (2004) Digital image processing, 2nd edn. Publishing House of Electronics Industry, Beijing, pp 243–276
4. Garrido A, Perez dela Blanca N (2000) Applying deformable templates for cell image segmentation. Pattern Recogn 33:821–832
5. Scotti F (2006) Robust segmentation and measurements techniques of white cells in blood microscope images. In: Proceedings of IEEE IMTC, Sorrento, pp 43–48
6. Hichem S, Donald G, Pietro P (2006) A hierarchy of support vector machines for pattern detection. J Mach Learn Res 7(10):2087–2123
7. Jiang K, Liao Q-M (2006) A novel white blood cell segmentation scheme based on feature space clustering. Soft Comput 10:12–19
8. Nasution AMT, Suryaningtyas EK (2008) Comparison of red blood cells counting using two algorithms: connected component labeling and backprojection of artificial neural network, PhotonicsGlobal@Singapore, IPGC 2008. IEEE, Singapore
9. Amari S, Wu S (1999) Improving support vector machine classifiers by modifying kernel functions. Neural Netw 12: 783–789
10. Haykin S (2002) Adaptive filter theory, 4th edn. Prentice-Hall, Upper Saddle River
11. Osowski S, Markiewicz T (2007) Support vector machine for recognition of white blood cells in leukemia. In: Camps-Valls G, Rojo-Alvarez JL, Martinez-Ramon M, (eds) Kernel methods in bioengineering, signal and image processing. Idea Group, London, pp 93–123
12. Takahashi F, Abe S (2002) Decision-tree-based multi-class support vector machines. IEEE Press, Singapore, pp 1419–1422
13. Vapnik VN (1998) Statistical learning theory. Wiley, New York
14. Hsu CW, Lin CJ (2002) A comparison of methods for multi-class support vector machines. IEEE Trans Neural Netw 13(2):415–425
15. Wang FS, Itose Y, Tsuji T et al (2003) Development and clinical application of nucleated red blood cell counting and staging on the automated hematology analyzer XE-2100. Clin Lab Haem 25:17–23
16. Wang X-J, Liu X-M, Guan Y (2012) Image edge detection algorithm based on improved canny operator. Comput Eng 38:196–198
17. Ma WY, Manjunath BS (1997) Edge flow: a framework of boundary detection and image segmentation. In: Proceedings of CVPR, pp 744–749

Chapter 45
Scalable and Explainable Friend Recommendation in Campus Social Network System

Zhao Du, Lantao Hu, Xiaolong Fu and Yongqi Liu

Abstract In the recent years, social networks have been growing in popularity and importance and to a certain degree contributing to a change in human life style. In a social network system, it's essential to offer well-designed and effective friend recommendation service for achieving high loyalty of users. Although Friend-Of-a-Friend (FOF) is widely used and proved to be effective, the straightforward implementation of FOF needs large amount of computation power which is a heavy burden for lightweight social network taking into account the restriction of resources. We propose a FOF-based friend recommendation algorithm in a campus social network system which is explainable and efficient. On one hand, we take multiple relationship factors into account for recommendation. On the other hand, we use incremental relationship data instead of the entire relationship data to generate latest recommendation list and detailed explanations. Ultimately, it achieves better performance in complexity and scalability.

Keywords Friend recommendation · Campus social network · FOF · Scalable and explainable

45.1 Introduction

In the recent years, social networks have been growing in popularity and importance and to a certain degree contributing to a change in human life style. Internet users tend to spend much more time on social networks than any other Internet

---

Z. Du (✉) · X. Fu
Information Technology Center, Tsinghua University, Beijing 100084, China
e-mail: dz@cic.tsinghua.edu.cn

L. Hu · Y. Liu
Department of Computer Science and Technology, Tsinghua University, 100084 Beijing, China

S. Li et al. (eds.), *Frontier and Future Development of Information Technology in Medicine and Education*, Lecture Notes in Electrical Engineering 269,
DOI: 10.1007/978-94-007-7618-0_45,

applications. Social networks become an indispensable part of people's lives. People exchange information, express ideas and make friends in social networks. Following this tendency, many organizations like enterprises and universities attempt to construct enterprise-level or campus-level social network services to their members. For instance, IBM started to provide its enterprise social network service from September 2007 [1].

It's valuable and essential to offer well-designed and effective friend recommendation service for achieving high loyalty of users in a social network. Friend recommendation proposes a limited, ordered and personalized list of potential friends to target users. Sometimes the recommendations are also accompanied with proper explanations which increase the probability of acceptance by users and ultimately help to enrich the connections in social network.

The recommender systems can be traced back to cognitive science, approximation theory, information retrieval, forecasting theories, management science and consumer choice modeling in marketing. It became an important research area since the introduction of collaborative filtering [1, 2] and has gained extensive attention more recently.

As an important part of social network, friend recommendation was studied by researchers in recent years for the tremendous success social network has achieved. There are dozens of algorithms that have been published for friend recommendation, including FOF [3], graph-based algorithms [4, 5], interaction-based algorithms [6] and content-based algorithms [3] etc. There into, FOF is the most widely used algorithm in social network, friend recommendation algorithms in Facebook, Twitter and LinkedIn are primary or partly based on FOF. The principle of FOF algorithm is the small world feature of social network as complex network that states "it's more probable that you know a friend of your friend than any other random person" [7]. In other words, the measured average distance in small world network is less than the measured average distance in a random graph [8]. On the other side, Graph-based algorithms and interaction-based algorithms also derive from FOF. Therefore, FOF is the most important algorithm for friend recommendation.

Although the principle of FOF is quiet clear and proved to be effective, its cost of computation power increases rapidly when it is applied in large-scale network. If we define the number of users and the average number of a user's friends as n and m respectively, the time complexity of FOF will be O (n^2m^2). It's perhaps not a problem for large enterprises like IBM which own abundant facilities and advanced technology but it's a heavy burden for lightweight social network taking into account the restriction of resources [9].

In this paper, we propose a FOF-based friend recommendation algorithm in a campus social network system which is explainable and efficient. The improvement is reflected in two aspects. On the one hand, we take more relationship factors into account. On the other hand, we use incremental relationship data instead of the entire relationship data to generate the latest recommendation list with detailed explanations for minimizing the cost of computation and achieving rapid reaction from the changes of users' relationships.

In the following sections, we first introduce the relationship model and dissemination of user information in our campus social network system. Then the details of friend recommendation algorithm will be represented. At last, we analyse the performance of friend recommendation from several aspects including time complexity, space complexity, scalability and interpretability.

45.2 Relationships in Campus Social Network System

The relationship model in campus social network system contains bi-directional confirmed friendship, one-directional follow relationship, and membership of groups. Users in campus social network system can designate the target users when they express opinions, share information, and exchange ideas.

45.2.1 Relationship Model

There are three categories of relationships in our campus social network, the two of them are relationships between two users called "Friend" and "Follower" respectively, and the last one is relationship between a user and a group called "Members". If two users want to become friends, the bi-directional confirmation is necessary. If user A wants to become a follower of user B, there is no need for bi-directional confirmation [10].

As shown in Fig. 45.1, user A has one friend and two followers; he is also the follower of the other two users. Besides, user A has also joined group P, as user F does. It's noteworthy that the relationship of two users cannot be both bi-directional and one-directional. In other words, when user A and user B become friends, they are removed from each other's followers list.

45.2.2 Dissemination of User Information

Although the majority of social network systems use either the bi-directional confirmed friend relationship model or one-directional follower relationship model, we decided to adopt a hybrid relationship model to give users larger flexibility in designating the target users of their opinions, information and ideas.

As shown in Fig. 45.2, user A has many friends that can be divided into three groups named university classmates, family members and colleges respectively. He also joins two groups called data mining group and young parents group. When user A wants to share information, he can designate the target users as one or more groups of his friends, or just let it be public. When he shares information to public, all his friends and followers will receive it. For the information user A shares in

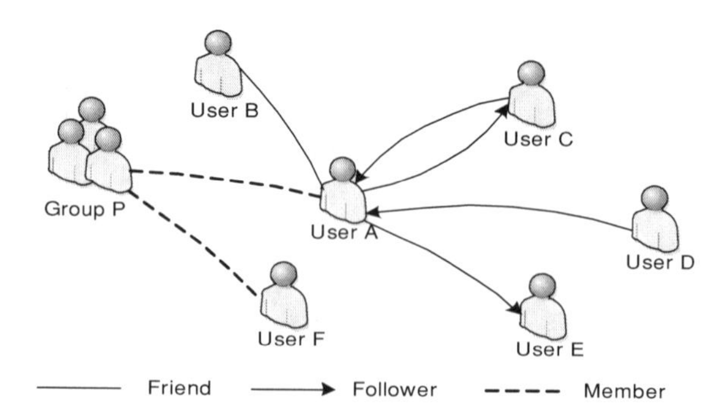

Fig. 45.1 Relationship model

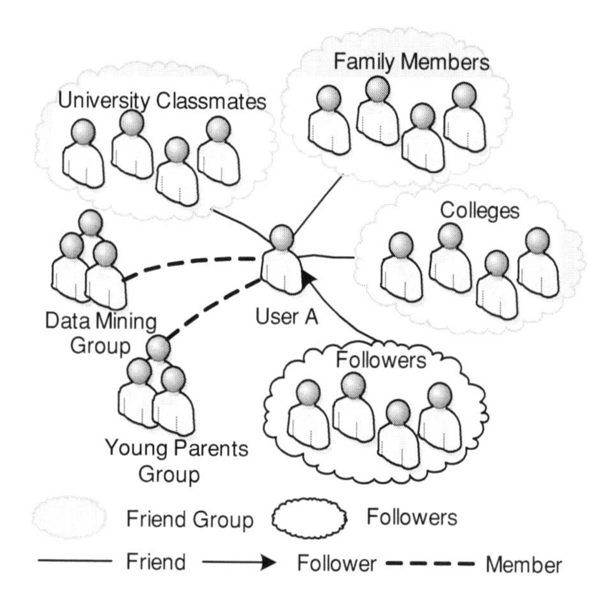

Fig. 45.2 Dissemination of user's information

any group that he has joined, all members in the same group will be the information receiver.

45.3 Friend Recommendation in Campus Social Network System

Our friend recommendation algorithm in campus social network system is primary based on FOF. In addition to the number of common friends of two users, we take into account the number of common followed users, common followers and common joined groups of them. In order to minimize the need for computational power and achieve rapid reaction from establishment of new connections or

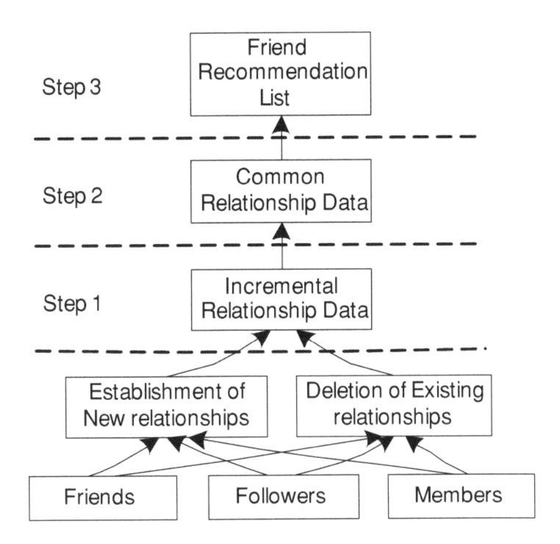

Fig. 45.3 Friend recommendation procedure

deletion of existing connections for friend recommendation, we use incremental relationship data instead of the entire relationship data to create the latest friend recommendation list with detailed explanations.

As shown in Fig. 45.3, friend recommendation consists of three steps. In step1, incremental relationship data are generated with the establishment of a new relationship or the deletion of an existing relationship simultaneously; in step2, incremental relationship data are merged into common relationship data to get the latest common relationships among users; in step3, friend recommendation list is updated according to common relationship data. It's noteworthy that the second step and the third step can be done independently; making it's more flexible to be scheduled when system is relatively idle.

45.3.1 Description of Incremental Relationship Data

We use five-tuples to keep record of the changes in users' relationship, that is, the incremental relationship data in the system:

Increment (User1, User2, User3, RType, CType)

In this five-tuple, "User1" and "User2" refer to the target user and the candidate for friend recommendation; "User3" refers to the user who has some the same type of relationship with "User1" and "User2"; "RType" refers to the type of relationship between "User3" and "User1" or "User2", it's value can be "Friend", "Follow" or "Member"; "CType" states the type of change in relationship between "User3" and "User1" or "User2", it's value can be either "Add" for establishment of new relationship or "Delete" for deletion of existing relationship.

45.3.2 Generation of Incremental Relationship Data

Incremental relationship data is generated when a new relationship is established or an existing relationship is deleted. Different incremental relationship data is generated for different scenarios of relationship changes.

There are three types of relationship change scenarios in our system. The first scenario type is change for "Friend" between two users; the second scenario type is change for "Follow" between two users; the third scenario type is change for "Member" between a user and a group. We will examine the creation of incremental relationship data in the three scenarios in detail.

As shown in Fig. 45.4a, when user A becomes a new friend of user B, user A becomes the new common friend of user B and user Ai ($1 \leq i \leq m$), and user B becomes the new common friend of user A and user Bj ($1 \leq j \leq n$). Here user Ai refers to existing friends of user A and user Bj refers to existing friends of user B. In this scenario, $m + n$ five-tuples will be generated to describe the new common friends. We use m five-tuples to describe user A as the new common friend of user B and user Ai:

Increment (B, Ai, A, "Friend", "Add")

We use other n five-tuples to describe user B as the new common friend of user A and user Bj:

Increment (A, Bj, B, "Friend", "Add")

When user A and user B are already friends, after one of them deletes the other from his/her friend list, user A will be deleted from the common friend list of user B and user Ai, and user B will be deleted from the common friend list of user A and user Bj. In this situation, $m + n$ five-tuples will also be generated to describe the deletion of common friend relationship:

Increment (B, Ai, A, "Friend", "Delete")
Increment (A, Bj, B, "Friend", "Delete")

When user A becomes a new follower of user B or deletes user B from his/her list of followed users. As shown in Fig. 45.4b, when user A becomes a new follower of user B, user A becomes the new common follower of user B and user Ai, and user B becomes the new common followed users of user A and user Bj.

We use m five-tuples to describe user A as the new common follower of user B and user Ai; use other n five-tuples to describe user B as the new common followed user of user A and user Bj:

Increment (B, Ai, A, "Follower", "Add")
Increment (A, Bj, B, "Followed", "Add")

Similar $m + n$ five-tuples will be created when user A deletes user B from his/her list of followed users. We should just change the value of "CType" from "Add" to "Delete" in the first m five-tuples and the next n five-tuples.

As shown in Fig. 45.4c, when user A joins group P, user A will have a new common group with all members of group P. We can use n five-tuples to describe group P as the new common group of user A and user Pi ($1 \leq i \leq n$):

Increment (A, Pi, P, "Member", "Add")

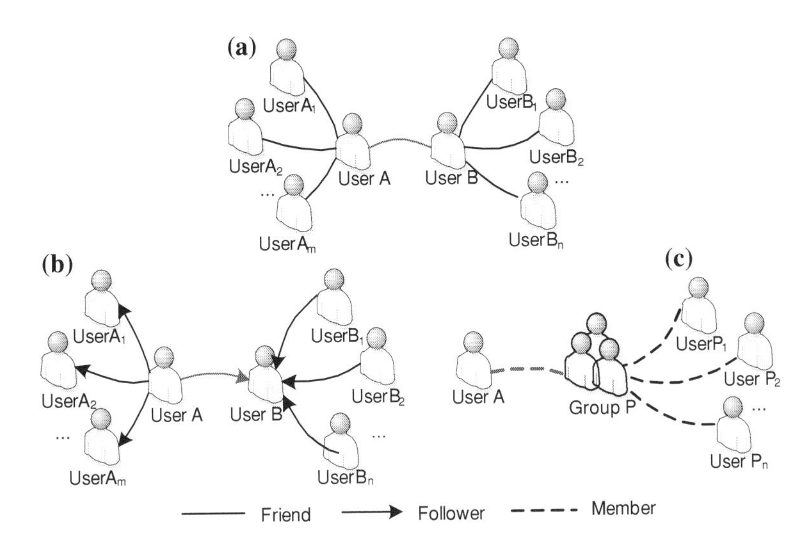

Fig. 45.4 Relationship change scenarios

When user A drop out from group P, we use other n five-tuples to describe group P as the deleted common group of user A and Pi:

Increment (A, Pi, P, "Member", "Delete")

Because all five-tuples are added to the database with the changes of users' relationships simultaneously, this task costs little computational power.

45.3.3 Merge of Incremental Relationship Data into Common Relationship Data

Common relationship data contains the two users who have one type of common relationship, the type of common relationship, the number of users with a certain type of relationship and the list of the common users between them. The frequency of data merge is primary determined by the application requirements and the distribution of low load states of servers. Generally speaking, increment relationship data will accumulate rapidly in system's start-up stage. As a result, it's necessary to merge incremental relationship data into common relationship more frequently during that period.

The key of merging is that once an item of increment relationship data is merged into common relationship data, it should be deleted from increment relationship data. In the end, all the increment relationship data will be deleted after one merge. By this way, we can minimize the time and computational power needed by the creation of incremental relationship data and merge procedure.

45.3.4 Update of Friend Recommendation List

Each item in the friend recommendation list consists of four elements: target user, potential friend, recommendation coefficient and explanations. Recommendation coefficient is the weighted sum of the number of common friends, common followed users, common followers and common joined groups between the target user and potential friend; explanations for recommendation contain the number and identifier list of common friends, common followed users, common followers and common joined groups between the target user and potential friend.

Update of friend recommendation list concerns three tasks. The first task is to calculate new recommend coefficients for the pairs of target user and potential friend whose common relationships have changed since the latest update of friend recommendation list. The second task is to update the potential friends of target users in friend recommendation list. In order to achieve good recommendation effect and high recommendation efficiency, the recommendation list only includes the top 20 potential friends according to their recommendation coefficient for each target user. The third task is to generate the latest explanations for the pairs of target user and potential friend whose common relationships have changed since the latest update of friend recommendation list.

45.4 Performance of Friend Recommendation

The performance of friend recommendation in campus social network system can be studied from the following aspects:

In the aspect of time complexity, if we define the number of users and the average number of a user's friends as n and m respectively in a social network, the time complexity of the straight-forward implementation of FOF will be $O(n^2m^2)$. It will be increasingly time-consuming with the growth of n and m. Because we use incremental relationship data to update the friend recommendation list, the time complexity is decided by the number of relationship changes since the last update and the average number of the friends or followers of a user or the average number of members of a group. If we use n' and m' to describe the two numbers, the time complexity of our incremental friend recommendation is $O(n'm')$, which will be much smaller than $O(n^2m^2)$ when the intervals of update are short.

In terms of space complexity, as the additional space which is used to keep incremental relationship data will be deleted immediately after it's merged into common relationship data, there is only limited increment for space. As a result, if we define the number of users who have at least one type of common connection as k, the space complexity of our incremental friend recommendation algorithm is O(k) which is the same as FOF.

Since the time complexity of our algorithm is decided by the number of relationship changes since the last update and the average number of the friends or followers of a user or the average number of members of a group, and there is only little requirement for additional space, we believe that it has good scalability. We also believe it has good interpretability because of the complete record of common relationships we keep during the process of data processing.

45.5 Conclusion and Future Work

In this paper, we propose a friend recommendation algorithm for campus social network based on FOF which to some extent solves the problem of FOF's high time complexity and the restriction of resources in campus social network system. Our study not only takes more relationship factors into account, but also achieves rapid reaction from changes in users' relationship by using incremental relationship data. The friend recommendation algorithm is proved to be scalable for its great improvement in time complexity compared to the original FOF. It's also explainable because we keep complete record of common relationships during the entire recommendation process.

Our future work concerns incorporation of users' social tags and other recommendation algorithms into campus social network to achieve better comprehensive effect and more efficient recommendation.

Acknowledgments This work is supported by the National Basic Research Program of China (No. 2012CB316000) and the Beijing Education and Science "Twelfth Five-Year Plan" (No. CJA12134).

References

1. Goldberg D, Nichols D, Oki BM, Terry D (1992) Using collaborative filtering to weave an information tapestry. Commun ACM 35(12):61–70. doi:10.1145/138859.138867
2. Adomavicius G, Tuzhilin A (2005) Toward the next generation of recommender systems: a survey of the state-of-the-art and possible extensions. IEEE Trans Knowl Data Eng 17(6):734–749. doi:10.1109/TKDE.2005.99
3. Chen J, Geyer W, Dugan C, Muller M, Guy I (2009) Make new friends, but keep the old—recommending people on social networking sites. In: Proceedings of ACM conference on human factors in computer systems (CHI 09). ACM Press, New York, pp 201–210. doi: 10.1145/1518701.1518735
4. Silva NB, Tsang I-R, Cavalcanti GDC, Tsang I-J (2010) A graph-based friend recommendation system using genetic algorithm. In: Proceedings of IEEE congress on evolutionary computation (CEC 10). IEEE Computer Society, pp 1–7. doi: 10.1109/CEC.2010.5586144
5. Lo S, Lin C (2006) WMR—a graph-based algorithm for friend recommendation. In: Proceedings IEEE/wic/acm international conference on web intelligence (WI 06). IEEE Computer Society, pp 121–128. doi: 10.1109/WI.2006.202
6. Zhang L, Fang H, Ng WK, Zhang J (2011) In trank: interaction ranking-based trustworthy friend recommendation. In: Proceedings IEEE international conference on trust, security and

privacy in computing and communications (Trust Com 11). IEEE Computer Society, pp 266–273. doi: 10.1109/TrustCom.2011.36
7. Mitchell M (2006) Complex systems: network thinking. Artif Intell 170(18):1194–1212. doi:10.1016/j.artint.2006.10.002
8. Kunegis J, Lommatzsch A, Bauckhage C (2009) The slashdot zoo: mining a social network with negative edges. In: Proceedings international word wide web conference (WWW 09). ACM Press, New York, pp 741–750. doi: 10.1145/1526709.1526809
9. Zhao D, Xiaolong F, Can Z, Ting L (2012) University campus social network system for knowledge sharing. In: Proceedings of international conference on systems and informatics (ICSAI 12), in press
10. Boyd DM, Ellison NB (2007) Social network sites: definition, history, and scholarship. J Comput Med Commun 13(1):210–230. doi:10.1111/j.1083-6101.2007.00393.x

Chapter 46
Application of Virtual Reality Technology in Medical Education

Yan-Li Shi

Abstract Medicine is a special discipline. The bottleneck of its teaching and learning lies in the difficulty of expressing many abstract teaching contents and obtaining many practical teaching contents and emotional experience in the course of teaching. The virtual reality technology is a new type of information technology. The VR technology have exerted increasingly important influence on the medical field due to its unique criticality, interactivity, imagination, and close combination with modern medicine. This article introduced the concept, characteristics, classification and the system of virtual reality (VR) technology, and discussed the application and significance of VR in medical education, as well as the trend and challenges for VR in medical education, to provide theoretical basis for the integration of VR teaching and traditional medical education.

Keywords Virtual reality technology · Medicine · Education · Progress

46.1 Introduction

With the rapid development of scientific technologies, new instructional media have been emerging. A new type of instructional media has become existent in the field of educational technology, namely, virtual reality technology. The virtual reality technology is a new type of information technology that came into existence in the 1990s. Like the birth of other emerging technologies or new media means, the development of virtual reality technologies will inject new vitality into the educational field, thus causing reforms of instructional means and teaching

Y.-L. Shi (✉)
College of Health Science and Nursing, Wuhan Polytechnic University,
Wuhan 430026 Hubei, China
e-mail: Shiyanli222@163.com

S. Li et al. (eds.), *Frontier and Future Development of Information Technology in Medicine and Education*, Lecture Notes in Electrical Engineering 269,
DOI: 10.1007/978-94-007-7618-0_46,

methods, which further will bring new opportunities and challenges to modern education.

Medicine is a special discipline. The bottleneck of its teaching and learning lies in the difficulty of expressing many abstract teaching contents and obtaining many practical teaching contents and emotional experience in the course of teaching. In recent ten years, virtual reality technologies have exerted increasingly important influence on the medical field due to its unique criticality, interactivity, imagination, and close combination with modern medicine. Therefore, the research on the application of virtual reality technologies in the medical education is especially important.

46.2 Introduction to VR technologies

46.2.1 Concept of VR Technologies

The VR technology is a computer-generated computer system that can create and experience the virtual world. It acts on the users by vision, hearing, and touching, etc. and brings the users immersive interactive scene simulation. It integrates computer graphics, image processing and pattern recognition, intellectual technology, sensing technology, language processing and audio technology, network technology and human behavioristic and many other disciplines. The VR technology is further development and application of modern simulation technology. Users interact naturally with objects in virtual environments with the help of necessary equipment, which will create immersive feeling and experience and make human–computer interaction more natural and harmonious.

46.2.2 Constitution of VR

General VR systems mainly consist of professional graphic processing computers, application software systems, input devices and demonstration devices, etc. In other words, people can feel the advanced user interfaces of designers' thinking through information channels such as vision, hearing, and touch.

Hardware platform: due to the complexity requirement of the virtual world and the requirement of computational efficiency, calculation needed to create virtual environments is immense, which raises high requirements for the configuration of central computers. Currently, foreign VR systems are generally configured with SGI or SUN workstation and large VR systems adopt computer parallel processing systems. Current research focuses on the desktop virtual reality system, which is cheap, easy to obtain and can meet some characteristic requirements of VR, and thus will be widely used.

Software systems: software systems are crucial to the realization of application of VR technologies. Application of VR technologies abroad is earlier than at home. Currently, typical desktop VR technologies include X3D, VRML, Java 3D, Cult3D Viewpoint, Atmosphere inWeb3D and Superscape VRT, EAI Sense 8 World ToolKit, MPI Vega applied to servers. They all provide tools for the application of VR technologies in virtual medical systems.

46.2.3 Classification of VR

According to the form and degree of immersion of users' involvement in virtual reality, virtual reality technologies can be classified into four classes.

(1) Desktop virtual reality system. The desktop virtual reality system carries out simulations via a personal computer and takes the screen of the computer as the window for users' to watch virtual environments. The participants can interact with the virtual reality world through various external devices and manipulate the objects in it. The biggest drawback of the desktop virtual reality system is lack of real experience, but it is easy to promote due to its simple structure and low price. Currently, the system is mainly used in the preparation of multimedia courseware.
(2) Immersive virtual reality system. It is also called "wearable" virtual reality system. This system provides completely immersive experience. It uses head-mounted displays or other devices to close participants' vision, hearing, and other feelings in order to provide a new and virtual feeling space. It also utilizes position trackers, data gloves, other manually operated input devices, sound, etc. to help participants create an immersive and totally involved feeling. "Sense of immersion" is mainly used in technical training.
(3) Distributed virtual reality system. The distributed virtual reality system makes full use of resources distributed in various areas and co-develops the application of different kinds of virtual reality in the Internet environment. It is generally development of immersive virtual reality systems and connects the immersive virtual reality systems distributed in different areas over the Internet to achieve a certain purpose jointly, taking distance education and remote medical consultation for example.
(4) Enhanced reality system. The enhanced reality system is also called the mixed reality system. It is a system combining real environments and virtual environments which cannot only reduce the expenses used to establish complex real environments (because some real environments are replaced by virtual environments), but also can perform operations on real objects (because some systems are real environments), which realizes a real and imaginary realm and marks the direction of future development.

46.2.4 Basic Characteristics of VR Technologies

As pointed out by Grigore and Philippe Coiffet in the book *Virtual Reality*, virtual reality has three outstanding characteristics, also the well-known three "I" characteristics of VR: interactivity, immersion, and imagination. Interactivity refers to the degree of inspection and operation of simulated environments realized by participants who use special devices and human natural skills. For example, users can directly grab the objects in simulated environments with their hands and they have the feeling about grabbing objects and can feel the weight of objects. The objects grabbed in the field of view should also move immediately as one's hands move. On the other hand, as VR is not simply a medium or a top end user interface, it can be used to solve some engineering, medical, and military problems. These applications are operated by both VR and designers and are designed for giving play to their creativity, which depends largely on human imagination. This is the second characteristic of VR: imagination.

The main technical characteristic of VR is "immersion". The goal of VR is to enable users to lie in a "totally immersive" status in the 3D virtual environments created by computers and have an immersive feeling, namely the so-called "immersion". It is also aimed to make users feel that they are part of the virtual environments rather than onlookers.

The "immersion" characteristic of VR distinguishes itself from general interactive 3D computer graphics greatly. Users can immerse themselves in data spaces and observe outward so that they are able to interact with data in a more natural and direct manner. They can also use immersion feature to isolate themselves from real environments and then immerse themselves in virtual environments, to be able to observe data truly.

46.3 VR Technology and Learning Theory

VR Technology provides a completely new platform for modern learning activities and an ideal stage for implementing various learning theories and ideas, especially for the combination of various kinds of learning theories. VR environment supports the "stimulus–response" and immediate reinforcement of behaviorism. Learning activities under the support of VR Technology can easily satisfy the learners' interior demand and motivations due to the emotional and impact force of its approaching real environment stimulus and feedback.

VR Technology can meet the requirements of the constructivism on scenario design perfectly. Moreover, Constructivism regards the learning as a procedure of learners' construction of their interior mental representations, and regards the interactions between the subjects and the environment as the determine factor of learning. Things created or simulated by VR Technology are produced with the realistic environments, and VR provides diversified natural interactive ways and conversational modes, allowing learners to move freely and explore the visual world in a controllable environment. Then the learners can acquire various perceptual or conceptual knowledge of objective things. This can motivate the imaginal thinking and research thinking of the learners, thereby deepen the concepts and construct new ideas and creations.

VR can fulfill the educators' idea of humanism. The creation of visual environment provides a new pattern for teaching and communicating. The open environment, abundant resources, realistic environment, engorged emotion, students-oriented environment, and supporting for cooperation of the new pattern enable students to get rid of the coldness of teaching by textbooks and machine screens and take part in active learning and practices. Moreover, all of this reflects the thought of humanism—"people-oriented", "emotional interaction" and "cultivating integrated people".

46.4 VR Technology and Medical Education

46.4.1 The Application of VR Technology in Medical Education

VR technology has changed the passive way of human–computer interaction, and had a profound impact on the traditional teaching mode, teaching methods and teaching approaches. It is developing smoothly as an effective teaching tool in the field of medical education, the main applications of which include theoretical teaching, practical training, virtual experiments, and so on.

46.4.1.1 Theory Teaching

The human body which is built with virtual reality technology is called the virtual human. Virtual human body is by means of computer technology to digitalize the human body structure, convert it into computer language, and reproduce realistic model of the human body. Through regulating, the virtual human can mimic various reactions of realistic human beings; combining with professional medical knowledge and needs, it can generate a variety of medical application models and provide powerful auxiliary tools for medical theoretical teaching.

The first and broadest application of virtual human in the medical theory teaching is its application on the human anatomy virtual three-dimensional expression. At present, the best human anatomy atlas database in the world is the visualization database. Initiated by the U.S. National Library of Medicine and built based on the visual human body plan, it is a digital human image library mouth consisting of three-dimensional human body tomography, nuclear magnetic resonance imaging, and anatomical section. Reconstructed human organs of virtual human can be rotated, of which the organizational structures such as blood vessels can be displayed individually. Learners can adjust the size, transparency, and direction of various organ models and deep structures to facilitate their comprehensive and intuitive understanding of the anatomical structures and relationships between the various organs. Digital anatomical atlas is with no need to be labeled complicatedly. As long as the computer mouse is moved to on a particular anatomical structure, a detailed description of the structure can be shown through the hyperlinks, making it easy to learn and use.

Dynamic visible human model is a more complex version. It can dynamically display the human physiological events and indicate the state of motion of various organs and systems under normal or disease states and how to respond to a variety of external forces. Such a model has a very broad prospect in medical education. Our research in this area is just entering the first stage, only built human parts data sets on the aspect of virtual visible human in Shanghai, Chongqing, Guangzhou and other provinces, which provides preliminary information for the follow-up study. In addition to the simulation of the completely human body, there also have emerged a large number of local organ VR models in medicine. Satava and others have developed an abdominal virtual reality model which allows the learner to observe the anatomical structure not only from the external of the organs but also from their interior, with the example of roaming in the alimentary canal to observe the gall bladder and pancreas as conducting an endoscopic examination. Lim group have developed a series of consecutive short local tissue anatomical models to demonstrate the local anesthesia related anatomic landmarks and needle control levels. Zito and his partners have generated high-resolution histopathology with VR technology based on a large number of microscopic digital photos of tissues. This sort of virtual slice can have multi-point analysis on key parts, and can be played in a variety of multimedia, which makes the pathological teaching get rid of the shackles of the microscope, and greatly reduces the number and cost of the biopsy.

46.4.1.2 Practice Training

Traditional medical practice training is more performed on the human body model, with part of operations also carried out on a real patient. Such practice-training mode, however, is not only with high cost but also may increase the patient's risk, so it is gradually being limited. The expanding of VR technology applications has promoted the practical training courses onto a higher level. A virtual practice training system usually consists of virtual operating environment, operating related hardware peripherals, back-end database. Utilizing high-resolution, high-contrast advanced image acquisition and other modern technologies, the system maximizes the simulation of real environment, feedbacks the learner's feels on different human organization textures with feel and forces of joystick and other devices, achieving the purpose of training through repeated simulation.

Currently, the most widely used system is the virtual endoscopic operation-training simulator. Collaborated with the School of Computer Science at National University of Defense Technology, the People's Liberation Army General Hospital has developed a virtual endoscopic sinus operation simulation system with a duration of two years. This system introduces feel into the multimedia teaching process and uses the 3D pen power to feedback the device Phantom; it carries out a three-dimensional reconstruction of the human nasal structure with human frozen section data, the result of which is consistent with the nasal structure of the yellow race. With optimized linear elastic model the system has built a virtual nasal tissue organ physiological—physical model; it has conducted research on the real-time elastic deformation algorithm of model; it has fulfilled a realistic demonstration of varying degrees of feedback force of the nasal soft tissues and organs under different pressure and tension of the training equipment; it has also utilized the virtual mechanical sensor and feedback system so that the beginners can experience the whole process of endoscopic operation. Furthermore, the system can provide different perspectives of the endoscope transformation in the entire process. Three degree-free tactile stimulations can even show different feels for minor operating equipment touching the mucosa and bone tissue and penetrating the lateral nasal wall. There are some other invasive operation simulation trainings, such as low colonoscopy training, bronchoscopy training, and venipuncture training under the condition of biological protection. Virtual training system for practical training has showed good results. The features of the virtual system being zero risk and repetitive facilitate the students to practice repeatedly according to the system given feedback until they master the whole skill. In addition, VR training system generally provides a plurality of evaluation parameters, and the database can record the entire operation process, enabling the evaluation function of the practical training. For example, the endoscopic simulation training system, using fuzzy logic methods, can record the time of surgery, vascular cutting length, knotting position and sturdiness procedures, the length of the cut line, the degree of smoothing of the instrument moving and efficiency, and other indicators to determine the operator's operative capacity.

46.4.1.3 Virtual Experiment

Virtual experiment is a visual 3D experimental environment that uses VR technology, computer multimedia technology, database technology, network technology and other virtual technologies and has similar functions with traditional laboratories. In this laboratory, students with full experiment autonomy are able to simulate various practical or even invisible, untouchable, inaccessible and high-risky experiments and imaginative experimental scenes, reducing the dependence of experimental teaching on objective material conditions, with students having chance to do experiments all day. The virtual laboratory makes some boring and difficult to operate experiments and trainings interesting and easy to understand and grasp, which is helpful to stimulate students 'creative thinking, tap their potentials, and cultivate their interest in learning, practical ability and research ability. For some expensive precision instruments and meters, it is necessary so that students can first use the virtual instrument and then have hands-on real practical operation of the equipment and instruments to rich their perceptual knowledge. Many experiments in medical education and clinical experiments can be conducted in a virtual lab. The hardware of the virtual experiment is only around smothering the input and output of the signal, while the software is the key. The software can easily change, increase or decrease, or improve the function and scale of the system. The software are generally written graphically based on LAB VIEW languages. Coleman experiment at University of California has developed the EXP software, which is a virtual reality-based, multi-function software for neurophysiology virtual experiment.

46.4.2 The Application Value of VR Technology in Medical Education

46.4.2.1 Beneficial Supplement for Theoretical Study

The emergence of VR technology helps to cultivate students' interest in learning, to broaden the students' scope of knowledge and to effectively support the theoretical study. If students can make comparison between a virtual environment and reality in virtual experiments, explored on the basis of cooperation, it can develop the concept in medical field, and help students to develop problem-solving skills, and the ability to migrate from the virtual real-life situation, which will have a great educational value.

46.4.2.2 Avoid the Danger of Real-life Situation

In the past, the teaching of some medical procedures and experiments were generally completed through TV video instead of students' direct involvement in order to obtain the perceptual. However, with VR technology, students can safely do a variety of human trials, such as the virtual heart bypass surgery, to avoid "patient" death medical malpractice injury caused by operational errors.

46.4.2.3 Break the Time and Space Constraints

With VR technology, the space limitations can be completely broken up in medical education. From the body structure to biomedical molecular structure, students can enter the interior of these structures to have observations. VR technology can also break the restrictions of time to present some change processes, which may take months or even decades to observe, through virtual reality technology in a very short time. Some of the laws of inheritance in biological genetics, for example, may take months to do the experiments with animals, but the virtual technology can achieve the same results within a class.

46.5 Development Trends and Challenges of VR Technology in Medical Education

The adoption of a new education strategy is performed in the diversity of learning styles, structured learning programs, and multidisciplinary teamwork. With the promotion of medical education reform and development of VR technology, how to make full use of the advantages of VR technology and use specific teaching strategies to improve the effectiveness of teaching has become the focus of attention of medical educators. Educators increasingly realize that adult learning programs need to reflect and encourage more active, more independent learning approaches. Therefore, the construction of VR study guide program pay more attention to promote the diversification of learning methods to better integrate theoretical knowledge into the medical skills and practical procedures.

In recent years, the medical profession has made provisions of the medical core curriculum contents and the corresponding communication skills, inspection skills, and practical program are increasingly integrated into the VR training program. In order to fulfill the teaching objectives and tasks better, designers try to design question-based program in VR teaching, and integrate a variety of teaching methods in the horizontal and vertical level in order to ensure that all students master the same content.

The development of the world's health-care system today calls for teamwork that is more multi-disciplinary. Medical VR teaching is paying more and more attention to the cooperative learning between the multidisciplinary. In the early stages of learning, students of various health care majors learn together and late in the learning, some content can be shared.

46.6 Conclusion

With the continuous increase of the hardware cost-effective as well as the continuous development and enhancement of VR technology, virtual technology will surely become more mature, and gradually popularization. In the future of education, virtual teaching and traditional teaching will run neck and neck and become further organic integration, produce new combination of the virtual and real teaching model, and with its powerful level of immersion, interactivity, multi-aware user-friendly features will have a profound impact on the practice-oriented field of medical education. Therefore, we have reason to believe that the virtual reality technology, which keeps pace with network technology and multimedia technology, will have even broader application and development prospects.

References

1. Andolsek DL (1995) Virtual Reality in Education and Training. Int J media 22(2):145–155
2. Chiou GF (1995) Learning rationales and virtual reality technology in education. J Educ Technol Syst 23(4):327–336
3. Burdea G, Coiffet P (2003) Virtual real technology. Wiley, John & Sons, USA
4. Wang P Becker AA Jones IA (2006) A virtual reality sugery simulation of cutting and retraction in neurosurgery with force feedback. Comput Methods Programs Biomed 84(1):11–18
5. Webster R, Sassani J, Shenk R (2004) A haptic surgical simulator for the continuous eurvilinear capsularhexis procedure during cataract satgery. Stud Health Technol Inform (98):404–406
6. Banks EH, Chudnoff S, Karmin I (2007) Does a surgical simulator improve resident operative performance of laparoseopic tubal ligation. Am J Obstet Gyneeol 197(5):541–545
7. Kockro RA, Stadie A, Schwandt E et al (2007) A collaborative virtual reality envimnment for neurosurgical planing and training. Neurosurgery,61(2 Supp 2):379–391
8. Walsh RM, Tymianski M, Wallace MC et al (2000) The transmastoid partial labyrinthectomy approach to mediaI skull base lesions. Rev Laryngol Orol Rhinol Bord 121:13–20

Chapter 47
An Improved Outlier Detection Algorithm Based on Reverse *K*-Nearest Neighbors of Adaptive Parameters

Xie Fangfang, Xu Liancheng, Chi Xuezhi and Zhu Zhenfang

Abstract The outlier detection algorithm based on reverse k-nearest neighbors can detect isolated points. The time complexity of finding the k-nearest neighbor is $O(kN^2)$, which is not suitable for large data set, and the selection of the parameters k have a great impact on getting the outliers in large data set. This paper used an adaptive method to determine the parameters k, and proposed an efficient pruning method by the triangle inequality, which reduced the computation in detecting outliers. The theoretical analysis and experimental results demonstrated the feasibility and efficiency of the algorithm.

Keywords Adaptive parameters · k-nearest neighbors · Outliers detection · Reverse k-nearest neighbors

47.1 Introduction

Outlier mining is an important field of data mining technology and the purpose is to find out data objects that do not get the general charateries in data base. They have different properties with other data, and may be the result of the error of measurement or perform or the data variation.

X. Fangfang · X. Liancheng (✉)
School of Information Science & Engineering, Shandong Normal University, Jinan 250014, China
e-mail: cisesdnu@163.com

X. Fangfang · X. Liancheng
Shandong Provincial Key Laboratory for Novel Distributed Computer Software Technology, Jinan 250014, China

C. Xuezhi
Shandong Poice College, Jinan 250014, China

Z. Zhenfang
School of Information Science and Electric Engineering, Shandong Jiaotong University, Jinan 250357, China

S. Li et al. (eds.), *Frontier and Future Development of Information Technology in Medicine and Education*, Lecture Notes in Electrical Engineering 269,
DOI: 10.1007/978-94-007-7618-0_47,

There are two strategies to treat the outliers in data mining: one is to clear them out from data set as the noise to improve the accuracy of the model; sometimes outlier is generated by a different mechanism that may contains special information, new knowledge is found often in identifying outliers, so another strategy is to treat outliers as research object to carry out outlier detection. Outlier detection is to identify the outliers in data set to analyze, this method can be used in different areas such as financial fraud, data management, forensics and site monitoring. At present the research on outliers has been more in depth abroad, which also attracted the attention of domestic group of professionals of outliers. There have been many articles on outliers published in the recent years, research on outlier especially the outlier analysis of anomalies will be an important research direction in the near future.

Currently, outlier detection algorithm is mainly depth-based, statistical-based, distance-based and so on, and the distance-based algorithm is valid for outlier definition, which uses of distance between each data point to its nearest to identify the isolated degree of each data point. This algorithm is easy to implement, and has been researched and applied extensively.

It's a valid outlier detection method of distance-based to calculate data k-nearest neighbor and reverse k-nearest neighbor. First calculate k-nearest neighbor of object *p*, then calculate the distance between point p and each point included detection datasets *D* and any positive integer *k*. Select adjacent to the *k* most recent (in addition to point *p*) point denoted as its *k*-nearest neighbor, and then calculate reverse *k*-nearest neighbor. The concept of reverse *k*-nearest neighbor (RkNN) is first proposed by Korn and Muthukrishnan and extended by improving the concept of reverse nearest neighbor to reverse k-nearest neighbor RkNN. The reverse *k* nearest neighbor of point *p* is a point set of those k-nearest neighbors containing *p*. reverse *k* nearest neighbor has been applied in decision support systems and other fields. Therefore, research on reverse *k*-nearest neighbor has an important practical significance as well.

There is an inefficient problem in existing K-nearest neighbor detection algorithm, which is improved in this paper based on reverse *k*-nearest neighbor method. The value of parameter k is determined by adaptive method first, and then the prune operation is carried out when calculating *k*-nearest neighbor of each data, which reduces the computational steps to improve efficiency.

47.2 Outlier Detection Algorithm Based on Reverse k-Nearest Neighbor

47.2.1 Related Definitions

Definition 1 The k-nearest neighbor of object p $KNN_k(p)$

For the test data set *D* and arbitrary positive integer *k*, calculate the distance between p and all the other points, and select adjacent recent *k* points (except *p*) as the *k*-nearest neighbor of object *p* which is denoted as $KNN_k(p)$.

Definition 2 The isolation degree of point p $D_k(p, D)$

The parameters k, $p \in D$ is given for the data set D. the sum of the distance between point p and k-nearest neighbors is the isolation degree of point p which is denoted as $D_k(p, D)$.

$$D_k(p, D) = \sum_{i=1}^{k} z_{i \in KNN(p)} \, dist(p, q_i) \quad (47.1)$$

Definition 2 uses the average distance between the point p and k-nearest neighbors as its isolation degree, although this method considers the isolation degree between p and its neighbor object, but does not take the point p of the scope of the whole neighborhood density into account, so the accuracy is not high, and when the outliers gathers together, some normal data may be treated as outliers, the error detection rate rises. In order to solve this problem, the distance between point p and its k-nearest neighbors and the internal distance between p and its k-nearest neighbors are used in this paper together to characterize the isolation degree of point p.

Definition 3 The internal distance between p and its k-nearest neighbors $W_k(p, D)$

For any data set D, which includes N data objects, the internal distance between p and its k-nearest neighbors in D defined is $W_k(p, D)$.

$$W_k(p, D) = \sum_{q \in KNN_k(p);\, r \in KNN_k(p);\, q \neq r} dist(q, r) \quad (47.2)$$

The smaller $W_k(p, D)$ of the object p, the smaller the degree of deviation from P and its neighbors, and the neighborhood of P will be more intensive; on the contrary, the greater the value of $W_k(p, D)$, the more sparse the neighborhood range of point p, the more likely the p will be an outlier.

Definition 4 Isolation factor of point p $D_k(p)$

Both $D_k(p, D)$ and $W_k(p, D)$ are affected by parameters k serious, so the ratio of the sum of $D_k(p, D)$ and $W_k(p, D)$ and k is used in this paper to represent the isolation degree of an object p and k-nearest neighbors,

$$D_k(p) = \frac{D_k(p, D) + W_k(p, D)}{K} \quad (47.3)$$

Definition 5 The reverse k-nearest neighbor of point p $RKNN_k(p)$

For the test data set D and arbitrary positive integer k, Object p reverse k-nearest neighbor is a collection of point p containing those k-nearest neighbors which is denoted as $RKNN_k(p)$.

$$RKNN_k(p) = \{p_i | p_i \in D \cap P \in KNN_k(p_i)\} \quad (47.4)$$

47.2.2 The Description of the Original Algorithm

47.2.2.1 ODRKNN Algorithm

Input: data set *D*, parameter *k*, *n*, (*k* is the number of nearest neighbors of point *p*, *n* is n the number of isolated point)
Output: the top n data selected from the data set with the smallest RKNN
The algorithm is described as follows: Firstly, calculate the *k*-nearest neighbors of every data according to the definition 1, obtain the distance between *p* and all other points, and then sore the distance values, store the top *k* data with the smallest values into the distance matrix *M*[*N*][*K*](*N* is the size of the data set *D*), the *k*-neighbor of one data is stored in each row of the matrix. Then calculate the number of each point of the reverse *k* neighbor by definition 3, namely, scanning the *k*-nearest neighbors of each point in the matrix sequentially. If the *k*-nearest neighbors of point p contain the point *p*, then the number of reverse *k*-neighbors of point *p* plus one. Finally, sort the data from small to large according to the size of the RKNN values, and select the top *n* data as the outliers.

47.2.3 The Problem of the Outliers Algorithm Based on Reverse k-Nearest Neighbor

Although the above-mentioned method can detect outliers well, but there are some larger human factors in determining the value of parameters *k*, affecting the accuracy when calculating the *k*-nearest neighbors of every data, it may have high time complexity, as follows:

you must make sure the value of parameter *k* When detecting the outliers first, the value of parameter *k* has an direct impact on the performance of the algorithm, so it is crucial to select appropriate parameters, the parameter *k* is artificial that does have some limitations; it is necessary to calculate the *k*-neighbors of every data in step 1, so the time complexity is $O(kN^2)$, it is not suitable for large data sets. It has to calculate the reverse *k*-neighbor of point p in step 2, and needs to traverse the entire matrix, this also needs a great deal of computation time. The number of isolated points is very few in a data set, so there is no need to calculate each point k-neighbor, to determine the data as the isolated point as early as possible could reduce the number of computing times, so as to reduce the amount of calculation and improve the operational efficiency of the algorithm.

47.3 Improved Methods and New Algorithmic Process

Aiming at the problems above, this paper presents the improved method:

47.3.1 The Pruning Operation on Data Sets

According to the efficiency problem of the algorithm, it accounts for the vast majority of the data set for normal data, if we can ensure the isolated point as early as possible in each data of k-nearest neighbor searching process, the nearest neighbor searching progress can be interrupted immediately to reduce the number of distance calculation, this process is known as the approximate nearest neighbor searching, identifying the isolated points in the process is also known as the pruning process.

The method of reducing the r distance calculation is to take the current minimum value of $D_k(p)$ outlier in the sample as the pruning threshold to remember as $O_{\min}$, the value increases with the increase of checked data set. And the value of $D_k(p)$ which is calculated by the current k-nearest neighbor of point p decreased gradually with the discovery of the new neighbor points. So if the current $D_k(p) < O_{\min}$, you can judge that p is not an isolated point, so it does not have to calculate the distance between point p and the remaining points in the data set.

For $D_k(p)$ of point q calculated in the sample, to prune the rest data based on this and pruning rules is shown below:

When searching the k-nearest neighbor of point P, check whether the q and p is the neighbors or not through calculating distance, and assume that $D_k(q)$ of point q has been calculated, so the $D_k(q)$ and the triangle inequality can be used to calculate the upper bound of $D_k(p)$, if the upper bound is less than the $O_{\min}$, then object p is trimmed and there is no need to re-evaluate its k-nearest neighbor.

Certification process: point q is an outlier as known in the sample, and the outlier factor is $D_k(q)$, when searching the k-nearest neighbor of p, take q and p to calculate the distance to check whether they are close neighbor or not. Point q, p and the k-nearest neighbors of point q can form K triangles according to the triangular inequality:

$$\begin{aligned} k \times dist(p,q) + \sum_{i=1}^{k} z_{i \in KNN(p)}\, dist(p,q_i) + w_k(q,D) \\ > \sum_{i=1}^{k} z_{i \in KNN(p)}\, dist(p,z_i) + w_k(q,D) \end{aligned} \quad (47.5)$$

Both sides of the formula (47.5) are divided by k to obtain:

$$dist(p,q) + D_k(p) > \frac{1}{k}\left(\sum_{i=1}^{k} z_{i\in KNN(p)}\, dist(p,z_i) + w_k(q,D)\right) \tag{47.6}$$

The k-neighbor of q is not necessarily the k-neighbor of p, so there is:

$$\frac{1}{k}\left(\sum_{i=1}^{k} z_{i\in KNN(p)}\, dist(p,z_i)\right) > \frac{1}{k} D_k(q,D) \tag{47.7}$$

$$\frac{1}{k}\left(\sum_{i=1}^{k} z_{i\in KNN(p)}\, dist(p,z_i) + W_k(q,D)\right) > D_k(q,D) \tag{47.8}$$

By formula (47.6), (47.7) and (47.8):

$$dist(p,q) + D_k(q) > D_k(p) \tag{47.9}$$

So we can get the upper bound of $D_k(p)$. If the upper bound is smaller than the pruning threshold, that is to say, the Formula (47.10) is right, so p is not an isolated point, there is no need to calculate the k neighbor of p any more.

$$dist(p,q) + D_k(q) < O_{\min} \tag{47.10}$$

47.3.2 Adaptive Selection of k Value by Calculating the Sample

When selecting the parameter k, adopt the method based on sample bẏ the calculation and analysis of the isolated points and normal data in the sample to select the appropriate value of k adaptively. Select the value of k as following method according to normal data and outlier data in sample. In the k neighborhood of point p, the isolated factor $D_k(p)$ can show the difference between normal data and isolated points, so use the figure of $D_k(p)$-k to observe the effects of k on the $D_k(p)$. Figure 47.1 is the $D_k(p)$-k between an isolated point and a normal data.

As is shown in Fig. 47.1: when the value of k is small, outlier data is far from its neighbor, the value of $D_k(p)$ rises very quickly; when the value of k increases to a certain value influenced by the normal data, $D_k(p)$ changes gently with the value of k increases, but the normal data value changes relatively flat; when the value of k continues to increase to a certain value, it rises very quickly for a period of time affected by the isolated point, the position of the maximum gap between the two lines is labeled as pk points so as to maximize the differences between isolated points and normal data and ensure the accuracy of the subsequent outlier detection algorithm.

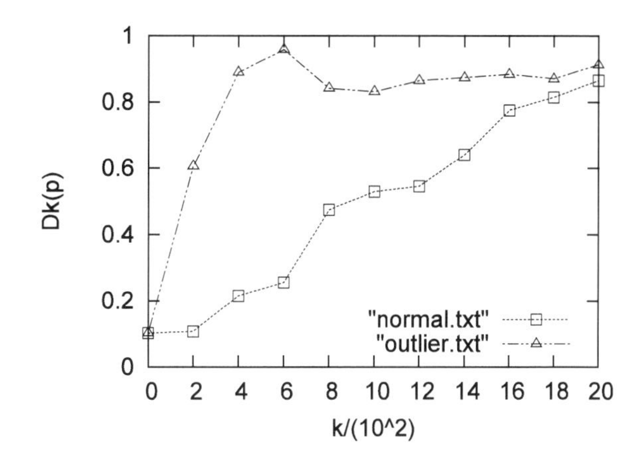

Fig. 47.1 The $D_k(p)$-k between an isolated point and a normal data

47.3.3 New Algorithmic Process

Input: sample data sets M (outlier data and normal data is shown) and the test data set N;

Output: outlier set.

Step 1 Take a normal data n and an outlier m from the sample data according to the formulae (47.2) and (47.3) to calculate the k of corresponding value $D_k(p)$ from 1 to $|M|$, which are denoted as $D_k(m)$, $D_k(n)$. so $y = D_k(m) - D_k(n)$, use the k corresponding to maximum of y as required in present method.

Step 2 Calculate the isolated factor for the outlier data in sample data and choose the minimum value as the pruning threshold.

Step 3 the pruning process If $D_k(p) < O_{\min}$, so p is not an outlier If $dist(p, q) + D_k(q) < O_{\min}$, so p is not an outlier Otherwise point p may be an outlier, add it to distance matrix.

Step 4 Find the k-nearest neighbor distance for the data in the matrix.

Step 5 Find the reverse k-nearest neighbor, and sort them in ascending order, the top n data are outliers.

47.4 Algorithm Analysis and Experimental Analysis

47.4.1 Algorithm Analysis

Although the time complexity of k determined in Step 1 is $O(kN^2)$, the sample data remains small relative to the data for the entire data set, and asks for less on the memory. The pruning process in step 2 is: when the isolated factor has been calculated in the sample data. it only needs to calculate the distance between q and p (point q is an outlier that had been known) for the calculation of the isolated factor of the test data to compare, so it reduces the distance computational between point p and each data point, the approximate time complexity is linear $O(N)$, the normal data can be excluded out from the data set in step 2 because the most data are not the isolated point. For steps 3 and 4, it only makes the small portion possible isolated points for data validation, and therefore will not take up too much memory.

47.4.2 The Accuracy and Efficiency in the Implementation of the Algorithm Analysis

The accuracy and implementation efficiency analysis of the algorithm

The performance of algorithm LOF, ODRKNN, IODRKNN is compared in this paper to test the accuracy and implementation efficiency. The above-mentioned dataset and simulated dataset-test dataset is used in this experiment. It is mainly to see the isolated point detected proportion by algorithm in true isolated points in data set to evaluate a detection algorithm. The higher the proportion, the higher accuracy of the algorithm, at the same time the shorter running time, the higher efficiency of the implementation. Accuracy is expressed as the ratio of number of isolated points measured by algorithm and the total number isolated points.

The experimental results are shown in Figs. 47.2 and 47.3. As shown in Figs. 47.2 and 47.3, the implementation efficiency of algorithm IODRKNN is much higher than LOF and ODRKNN. The dataset is pruned in Algorithm IODRKNN, reducing the distance between each data and the amount of computation. The accuracy of algorithm IODRKNN is close to LOF while much higher than ODRKNN, it is the value of K determined by adaptive method that played an important role in the accuracy of the algorithm.

47.4.3 Efficiency Analysis

This experiment adopts KDDCUP99 data set to validate the effectiveness of the improved algorithm, which is a network environment from the Lincoln Laboratory simulation of the U.S. Air Force LAN data kDDCUP99 data set contains five million connection records. Each record consists of 42 properties, of which the last attribute value describes whether the connection is normal or some sort of intrusion behavior. This paper considers intrusion behavior data as abnormal data which are called isolated points. Test environment is: CPU for the Intel (R) Core (TM); For 2G memory; The OS is Windows XP; Experimental platform for Matlab 7.0.

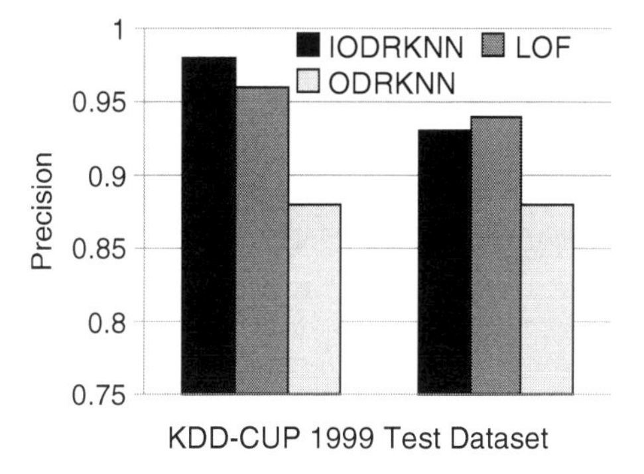

Fig. 47.2 The accuracy comparing of 3 kinds of algorithms

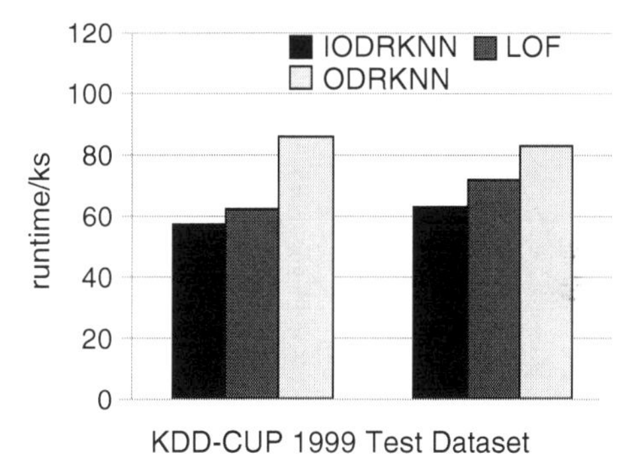

Fig. 47.3 The performance comparison of 3 algorithms

The data set used in experiment is a two-dimension data sets in the literature [8], a total of 494,021 records in the data set, in which the normal number of records is 97278, and the rest are abnormal data. 8397 records are selected in this paper from the data as the experimental data, of which 142(1.7 %) are abnormal data, and the abnormal proportion in line with the assumptions in anomaly detection abnormal data are far less than the normal data.

The purpose of the test is to verify the improved algorithm consistent with LSC and LOF algorithm for outlier. First randomly select 2026 normal data and five attacks data from experimental data as test data, the sample data number of k obtained after training is 200, then prune the operation, the Table 47.1 is experimental comparison, taking a large degree of isolation of the top 10 points, it can be seen that the IDRKNN algorithm can also obtain the isolated point that obtained by the LOF algorithm.

The reason why the record number of 832 data is the strongest point that we can see is that it is a DOS attack that produces a large number of connection records, and thus be more different from normal data. Secondly, looking down, the corresponding 10 attacks are different from normal data records.

Table 47.1 LOF algorithm and IDRKNN algorithm comparison on real data sets

Order	LOF		IDRKNN	
	ID	LOF	ID	RKNN
1	8	12.854	832	8
2	4	11.371	412	15
3	2	9.913	23	24
4	3	9.156	358	29
5	1	8.543	151	34
6	9	5.871	9	38
7	2	4.962	251	45
8	8	4.568	856	53
9	1	3.797	105	57
10	8	3.215	86	64

47.5 Conclusion

This paper proposes an improved outlier detection algorithm based on reverse k-nearest neighbors of adaptive parameters, it based on the reverse k-neighbor outlier detection algorithm, and proposes an improved algorithm, the algorithm not only keeps the advantages of original algorithm, but also can detect outliers well, and the efficiency of the algorithm is improved since the pruning process is joined in, it reduces the number of calculation of the distance between the data points, Tests show that the improved algorithm is an effective and efficient detecting outlier algorithms.

Acknowledgments This work is supported partly by National Nature Science Foundation of China (60873247), Science and Technology Plan in Colleges and Universities of Shandong Province (J12LN21).

References

1. Han J, Kamber M. (2011) Data mining concepts and techniques. Morgan kaufmann Machinery industry press, p 295
2. Wu M, Jermaine C (2006) Outlier detection by sampling with accuracy guarantees. In: Proceedings of the 12th ACM SIGkDD international conference on knowledge discovery and data mining. ACM, Philadelphia, pp 767–772
3. Gu H, Rastogi R, SHIM K (1998) Cure: an efficient clustering algorithm for large databases In: Proceedings of the 1998 ACN SIGMOD international conference on management of data montreal. ACM, pp 73–84
4. Herman CA (1952) Measure of asymptotic efficiency for tests of a hypothesis based on the sum of observations. Ann Math Stat 23(4):493–507
5. Saha BN (2009) Ray N, Zhang H. snake validation: a PCA-based outlier detection method. IEEE Signal Process Lett 16(6):549–552
6. Jie H, Gongde G (2009) Distributed intrusion detection architecture based on incremental kNN model. Microcomput Appl 30(11):29–32

7. Korn F, Muthukrishna S (2000) Influence sets based on reverse nearest neighbors queries. In: Proceedings of ACM, SIGMOD, pp 201–212
8. Chenyi X, Hsu W, Lee ML, et al. (2006) BODER: efficient computation of boundary points. IEEE Trans knowl Data Eng, 18
9. Sheng L, Shimin L. (2004) Distance-based outlier detection research. Computer Eng Appl 40 (33):73–75
10. Yue F, Baozhi Q (2007) The outlier detection algorithm based on reverse *k* neighbor. Comput Eng Appl, lancet (7):182–184
11. ShengZong L, XiaoPing F (2012) Applies to connection properties outlier test samples of the adaptive parameters. Appl res Comput 29(9):3259–3262
12. Bhaduri K, Matthews BL, Giannella CR (2011) Algorithms for speeding up distance-based outlier detection In: Proceedings of the 17th ACM SIGKDD international conference on knowledge discovery and data mining.[S.I SCM Press, London
13. Sambasivam S, Theodsopoulos N (2006) Advanced data clustering methods of mining Web documents. Issues Informing Sci Infor Technol 3:563–579

Chapter 48
A Practical Study on the Construction of Diversified Network Monitoring System for Teaching Quality

Jia Bing, Jiang Fengyan and Li Di

Abstract Teaching quality monitoring is core content of management of teaching quality in medical colleges. Based on modern network technology, diversified network monitoring system for teaching quality is built up, which is inevitably the best solution to the current problems in teaching quality management. This paper was written on the basis of an empirical study,for the purpose of constructing the teaching quality network monitoring system by means of the theory about teaching total quality management (TTQM), the building of teaching quality monitoring system and its operating mechanism, as well as the researches and designs of teaching quality network monitoring system, in which both sides of the interest parities, whether on-campus or off-campus, could participate. The result of our practice shows that the application of the system, with the participation of whole faculties, has met the needs of implementing teaching quality monitoring thoroughly and systematically, and greatly improved work efficiency.

Keywords Diversified · Network · Teaching quality · Network monitoring system · Study

Teaching quality is always the lifeline for the survival and development of colleges and universities. With rapid development and in-depth application of modern network technology, especially perfection of internet and campus network software and hardware construction, an effective approach can be carried out by the whole faculties to realize teaching quality management thoroughly and

---

J. Bing
Guangxi Medical University, Nanning 530021 Guangxi, China

J. Fengyan (✉)
Room 801, Teaching Complex Guangxi Medical University No. 22 Shuangyong Road, Nanning City 530021 Guangxi, China
e-mail: fyjianggx@163.com

L. Di
Nanning Daqin Network Corporation Ltd, Nanning 530021 Guangxi, China

S. Li et al. (eds.), *Frontier and Future Development of Information Technology in Medicine and Education*, Lecture Notes in Electrical Engineering 269,
DOI: 10.1007/978-94-007-7618-0_48,

systematically, especially by means of the theory of total quality management and launching the study on application of teaching quality network monitoring system via modern network technology.

48.1 Necessity of Network Construction for Teaching Quality Monitoring in Medical Colleges

48.1.1 Disadvantage of Traditional Teaching Quality Management Mode

Owing to the small management span and multiple management levels, the traditional teaching quality management mode used to base on paper media, which is hard for the teaching management personnel to carry out timely and effective management for important teaching events. It is even more difficult to improve and manage elements and links that affect teaching quality from an overall height.

Information collection and feedback channel is blocked, and severe hysteretic nature exists in teaching quality evaluation and feedback, so instantaneity and effectiveness of teaching quality monitoring work are bad [1]. Stopgap measures are often taken when the practical problems in teaching quality need to be solved via trans-department cooperation. Therefore, problems that affect teaching quality have been mentioned for several times, but there are still no effective solutions. As time passes, the so-called quality management becomes a mere formality.

Besides, in order to cope with insufficiency of clinical teaching materials like teachers and practical teaching base, not a few medical colleges have cooperated with local hospitals throughout the country, to establish non-directly affiliated hospital and undertake the task of full-course teaching. However, owing to the limitation in cross-school and cross-region aspects as well as human, financial and material resources, traditional teaching quality management tool cannot improve the full-course teaching quality.

48.1.2 Adaptation to the Requirements of Medical Education Reform

The core content of modern teaching quality management is to emphasize the essence of management activity which is to promote development of students, and satisfy the relevant interest group demands of colleges and universities timely and effectively [2]. Development of medical education reform and implementation of education reform theory is dependent on acknowledgement, participation and support from relevant interest groups. Meanwhile, we should guarantee the central position of students; try to satisfy demands of diversified interest groups including all students, teachers and teaching management personnel; carry out tracking, evaluation, feedback, analysis, decision and improvement in time. The traditional teaching quality management mode will not only consume a mass of administration cost and time cost, but is also difficult to satisfy the requirements of interaction and communication among diversified interest groups.

48.2 The Thought of Constructing Teaching Quality Network Monitoring System in Medical Colleges

48.2.1 Establishment of Teaching Total Quality Management (TTQM) Theory [3]

Correct quality thought and quality culture is the premise, core and guidance of constructing teaching quality network monitoring system in medical colleges. TTQM theory is application and reflection of system theory and all-round development of human being theory. It emphasizes the concept of system integrity, and advocates that elements and links that affect teaching quality should be improved and managed continuously. In this point, it is in consistence with the basic requirements of medical education standard. Its core idea is "comprehensiveness, full course and all personnel".

By combining with teaching quality management process of medical colleges, comprehensive quality management emphasizes the central position of students. It starts from the training objective of medical knowledge, practical skill, ideology and morality, and professional quality. Comprehensive quality management is carried out for all factors and links that affect academic quality, teaching quality, management quality and service quality. All-personnel quality management is accepted by all school members and off-campus interest part representatives. School members include teachers, students, supporting staff, teaching management personnel and all people serving the education; off-campus interest part representatives cover higher authorities, employers, parents of students and graduates. Full-course quality management covers recruiting process, formulating process of teaching plan, teaching operation process, operation process of aided teaching, study process, test-taking process, training process for clinical skill, and graduate quality management.

48.2.2 Formation of Teaching Quality Monitoring System and its Operating Mechanism on the Basis of TTQM

Scientific and perfect teaching quality monitoring system is the premise and base of constructing teaching quality network monitoring system. Through a series of measures like perfecting institutional framework and duty, expanding supervision contents, strengthening system guarantee, developing multi-evaluation, setting up information feedback platform, supervising implementation of reform, and perfecting incentive mechanism, the teaching quality monitoring system (as shown in Fig. 48.1) based on TTQM that suits medical education characteristics was designed by starting from the requirements of medical education standard and "comprehensiveness, full course and all personnel" of TTQM theory. This system consists of seven interrelated parts; it has good operation mechanism of both incentive function and restriction function, and carries out full-course monitoring for teaching input, teaching process and teaching output.

The teaching quality management mode is dominated by self-management "from bottom to top" and assisted by superior supervision and guidance. By combining with six major links which are "formulation of teaching plan", "evaluation of teaching quality", "teaching operation process", "teaching effect and graduate quality", "teaching management service level", and "performance appraisal and incentive for teachers' job", it has highlighted the dominant position of quality management in secondary colleges as well as its teaching and research section; besides, it has also clarified tasks and duties of secondary management institutes, its administrative staff, teachers, and students in teaching quality monitoring and evaluation. It will be beneficial to effective operation of teaching quality monitoring network system to streamline administration and delegate power to the lower levels.

48.2.3 Research and Development of Diversified Teaching Quality Network Monitoring System

48.2.3.1 Development Environment and Technology of Teaching Quality Network Monitoring System

By combining with the operation mode and function requirements of teaching quality monitoring system, and through comprehensive consideration about

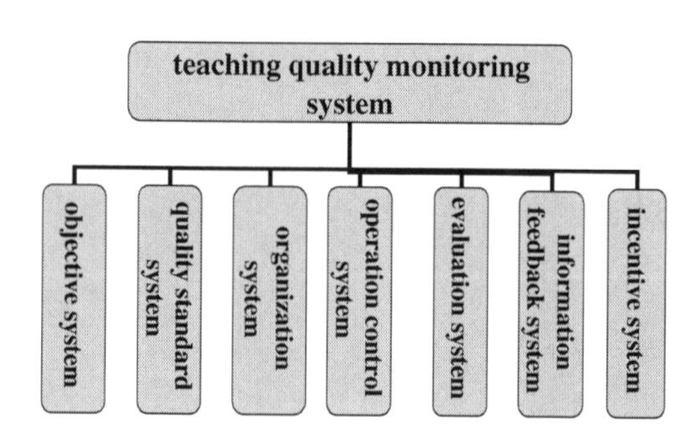

Fig. 48.1 Constitution of teaching quality monitoring system of Guangxi Medical University

software and hardware performance requirement, acquisition cost, operation and maintenance cost, as well as openness, expandability and timeliness of the system, finally Tomcat6.0 was selected to constitute the application server; dynamic and interactive teaching quality monitoring system based on Web data base was researched and developed by adopting open-source java language. Open-source framework technology of SSH (Struts +Spring +Hibernate) was used; myeclipse6.0 was set as the development platform; MySql5.0 was adopted as the backend database. On the basis of data security and stability, teaching quality network monitoring system is composed by depending on the campus network. It includes two platforms which are intranet and extranet. Users of extranet platform have to get data authorization and distribution of intranet platform, to visit data on intranet platform.

48.2.3.2 Major Functional Design of Teaching Quality Network Monitoring System

Teaching quality network monitoring system is composed of six functional modules which are system management module, information feedback module, decision analysis module, online communication module and job reminding module, as shown in Fig. 48.2.

By establishing basic status data base, system management module brings data related to teaching, on-campus institutions (including affiliated hospitals), and all members into real-time on-line management of network monitoring system.

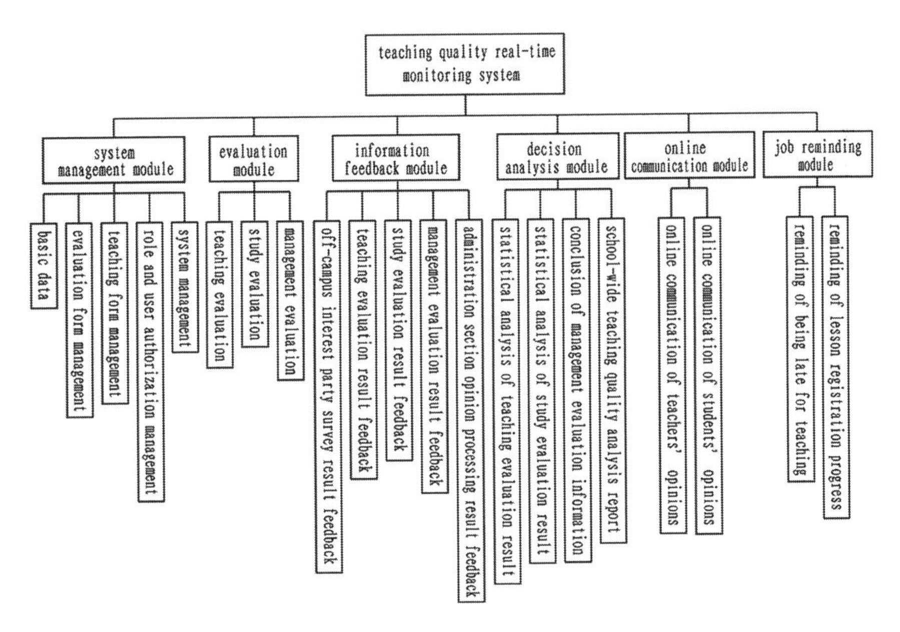

Fig. 48.2 Functional module chart of teaching quality network monitoring system

"Evaluation—information feedback—decision analysis" is the core plate of the system. Different roles and users can log in the system at any time to record information, evaluate (supervise) teaching, evaluate (supervise) study, evaluate (supervise) management, look up the evaluation result or opinions, make statistical analysis, and dispose and reply opinions according to their permissions. "Job reminding module" can feed back severe teaching problems like being late for teaching and missing classes, and help the administrative department investigate and handle these problems in time. Online communication module faces all teachers and students, 24 h in service. Teachers and students can log in and leave a message at any time.

48.2.4 Characteristics of Diversified Teaching Quality Network Monitoring System

48.2.4.1 Diversification of Monitoring Subject and Monitoring Object

Monitoring subject covers all on-campus members (including students covering overseas student, teachers, supervision experts, and administrative staff at different levels) and off-campus interest part representatives (including higher authorities, employers and graduates); monitoring object involves all teachers, students and on-campus administrative departments at different levels.

48.2.4.2 Diversified Permission Setting Function to the Aspect Oriented Technology

Real-time monitoring system sets different permissions for each user who enters this system to guarantee the privacy rights of information about monitoring subject and monitoring object. In this way, different roles or users can coordinate their jobs in the safest mode.

48.2.4.3 Diversification of Evaluation Contents

According to different evaluation purposes, flexible and diverse evaluation index was set by centering on course and practical teaching quality (including theory course, experimental course, clinical practice skill and operation, etc.), teaching content and method reform (such as integrated curriculum, Problem-based Learning teaching, bilingual teaching, etc.), medical quality ability (including lifelong learning ability, empathy, entrepreneurial ability, etc.), teaching management quality and service level, etc. Unilateral teaching has transferred to interactive "teaching evaluation ← → study evaluation" and "management evaluation".

48.2.4.4 Diversification of Evaluation Method

Qualitative and quantitative evaluation methods were combined together, to provide corresponding functions of others' evaluation, mutual evaluation, and self-evaluation for different roles and users, such as teaching evaluation and study evaluation of supervisors, teachers and administrative staff at different levels, stage peer evaluation for study effect of integrated curriculum, study evaluation of teachers, self-evaluation of students, self-evaluation or mutual evaluation of students for PBL teaching, etc.

48.2.4.5 Function of Comprehensive and Timely Information Feedback and Disposal

Teaching administrative department and relevant administration sections can dispose recordings according to various evaluation results and feedback opinions. They will work out teaching quality report or implementation report of rectification measures in each term, and thus form school-wide teaching quality analysis report.

48.3 Practice Effect of Teaching Quality Network Monitoring System

For almost 6 years of research and exploration, by centering on core links of teaching quality management, Guangxi Medical University has successfully developed "real-time monitoring system of teaching quality of Guangxi Medical University" in which all on-campus and off-campus interest parties can participate. The system still requires ceaseless improvement, but compared with traditional supervision model in the teaching quality management process, it has already shown irreplaceable superiority (Figs. 48.3, 48.4 and 48.5).

48.3.1 The Improvement of Teaching Quality Management with the Application of Teaching Quality Network Monitoring System

Through construction and practice of teaching quality network monitoring system, off-campus interest party representatives and all teachers and students can fully perform their knowledge rights, participation rights, expression rights and supervision rights. Quality awareness and self-management awareness have been increased obviously among teachers, students and staff of this school.

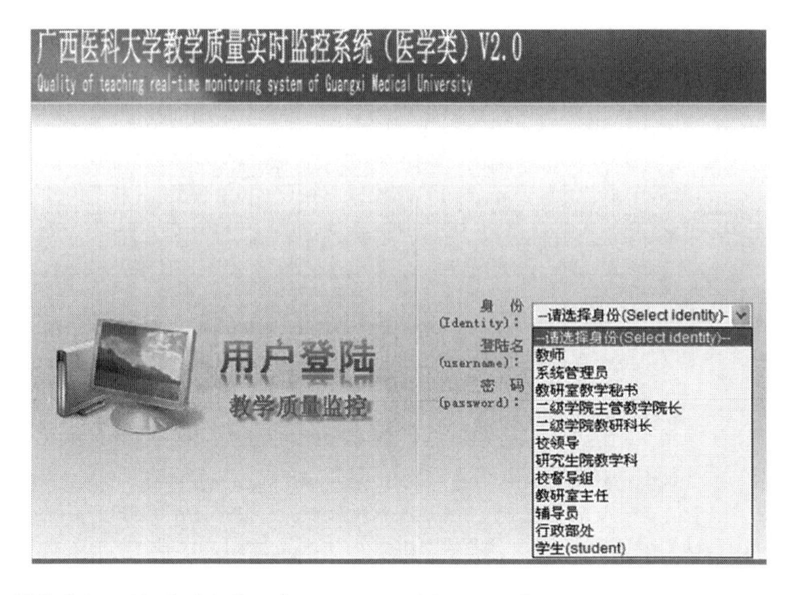

Fig. 48.3 Intranet login interface for on-campus interest parties

Fig. 48.4 Extranet login interface for off-campus interest parties

The awareness of centering on students and serving education has been enhanced greatly among administrative departments at different levels. In the process of applying network system, teaching quality monitoring has changed from

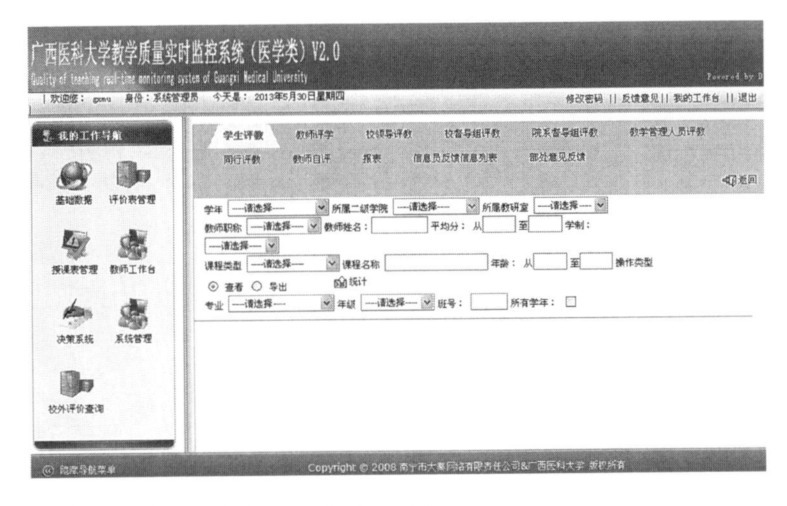

Fig. 48.5 Surface chart of decision analysis module

post-action control to real-time control. This has broken the management barrier among different departments of the school, stepped over the restriction of time and space, effectively overcome the hysteretic nature of information feedback and disposal in traditional teaching monitoring, guaranteed timeliness and effectiveness of evaluation information feedback, and realized integration of "evaluation—feedback—decision".

Since "real-time monitoring system of teaching quality of Guangxi Medical University" was formally put into use in 2007, it has been an important channel and communication platform of information collection and feedback [4]. Off-campus interest party extranet evaluation function of this system has reduced time cost and administration cost to some degree since its application at the end of 2011. It can satisfy demands of different social interest groups, and plays the role of promotion well.

48.3.2 Constant Improvement of Satisfaction Degree of On-campus Teachers and Students for Teaching Quality Network Monitoring System

Teaching quality network monitoring system has undergone four times of function re-development. In comparison of the sampling questionnaire survey result among on-campus teachers and students in 2011 with that in 2009 (as shown in Table 48.1), it presents that satisfaction degree of on-campus teachers and students for its application effect has been increased constantly. Nearly 1,000 teachers and 5,000 students of this school participate in online teaching evaluation in each term.

Table 48.1 Satisfaction survey for teaching quality monitoring system among teachers and students

Survey item	Survey object	Satisfaction degree (%)	
		2009	2011
The demand of teaching quality management can be satisfied through functions of our present teaching quality real-time monitoring system	Teacher	80	90
"Students' evaluation for teachers has positive influence on teachers' lecturing"	Student	Above 74	Above 85
Effect of online evaluation is equal to or better than effect of paper evaluation	Teacher, student	Above 80	Above 95
"Result of adopting quantitative and qualitative evaluation method is more objective and just". We have the ability to correctly use evaluation information provided by teaching quality real-time monitoring system of our school	Teacher	80	90
Check the evaluation information one by one, and treat every opinion or suggestion seriously and objectively	Teacher	Above 70	Above 88
Implementation of teaching quality real-time monitoring system will increase our teaching quality to some extent; the evaluation result and feedback opinion can also improve teachers' lecturing level to some degree	Teacher, student	Above 80	Above 90

Data source obtained by organizing questionnaire data of teachers' version and students' version in 2009 and 2011

Rate of voluntarily participation in online evaluation among students has increased from 25 % for traditional paper evaluation to about 90 %, and it is still rising stably.

48.4 Conclusion

Given the complicated influencing factors and long-term sustainability of teaching quality, we need to resort to the diversified teaching quality network monitoring system and motivate the participation of different parties both on-campus and off-campus to be parts of teaching quality management via so that the idea of implementing TTQM could affect the quality of teaching,and thus a virtuous cycle—the evaluation of teaching quality, feedback, analysis of the results, decision making, improvement and evaluation again—could be formed. The practice is helpful for the independent management and regulation of improvement and continuous promotion of teaching quality in medical education. This study shows that with the participation of the whole faculties, the construction of a diversified network teaching quality monitoring system could be one of the effective ways to achieve a comprehensive and integrate teaching quality management.

Fund Program

1. Unit Funding Planning Task of Ministry of Education in 2010 at the "11th Five-Year Plan" of Nationwide Science of Education: (FFB108163);
2. Guangxi New Century Education Reform Engineering Project in 2011 (2011JGB025).

Achievement and Rewards

The second award of teaching results at autonomous level of Guangxi higher education in 2012, one of the series achievements of "Construction and Practice of Teaching Quality Monitoring System and Its Networking Platform in Medical Colleges".

References

1. Jia B, Jiang F, Cao Y (2010) The discussion of teaching quality monitoring operating mechanism of medical college under the new situation. Res Med Educ 4:436–438
2. Compiled by Expert Group of Higher Education Evaluation Center (2009) Evaluation for internal quality assurance system and classified curriculum of colleges and universities. Higher Education Press, Beijing, pp 430, 431
3. Zhang D (2006) An Exploratory Thinking on Management of Teaching Quality in Colleges and Universities. Continue Educ Res 3:58–60
4. Jiang F, Jia B, Jing L et al. (2010) The practice and exploration of diversified teaching quality evaluation systems. Chinese J Med Educ 5:788–790

Chapter 49
Reformation and Application of "Project-Tutor System" in Experimental Course Teaching of Fundamental Medicine

Li-fa Xu and Jian Wang

Abstract This paper firstly makes an analysis of the necessity in reforming the teaching and proposes that the preparations such as textbook compiling, teaching staff training and the improvement of experimental conditions should be made. Meanwhile, in this paper, efficient evaluation of the teaching effect and timely summarization of the steps in teaching are also mentioned as the keys to "Project-Tutor System". We can conclude from the teaching practices that "Project-Tutor" system has seen its obvious effect in experimental course teaching.

Keywords Fundamental medicine syllabus · Project-Tutor system · Reformation of experimental course teaching

49.1 Introduction

By "Project-Tutor System" experimental course teaching, we mean the new-type teaching methods applied in the experimental course in which the teaching contents, based on the requirements of syllabus, are compiled into complete and relatively independent experimental projects similar to research subjects and the students are required to finish the experiments with the guide of project teachers [1]. Since the Anhui Provincial Project "Research on 'Project-Tutor' System in Medical Fundamental Course" was approved, the project team has always been doing the research in experimental course teaching of medical fundamental course, with plenteous achievement reported as follows.

L. Xu · J. Wang (✉)
Department of Aetiology and Immunology, Medical College, Anhui University of Science and Technology, Huainan 232001 Anhui, China
e-mail: wangjian8237@sina.com

L. Xu
e-mail: ahhnlfxu@126.com

S. Li et al. (eds.), *Frontier and Future Development of Information Technology in Medicine and Education*, Lecture Notes in Electrical Engineering 269,
DOI: 10.1007/978-94-007-7618-0_49,

49.2 The Necessity of Launching Study on "Project-Tutor System" Experimental Course Teaching

49.2.1 The Demand of Cultivating Innovative Talents

The twenty first century-oriented action plan for invigorating education proposed by The Ministry of Education points out: That we are lacking in the innovative talents of international leading level has become one of the major factors restricting the innovation and competence in our country. However, in the current syllabus, the experimental course teaching in medicine fundamental courses is mostly affiliated to the corresponding theoretical courses and is overlooked in its significance. Judging from the educational objectives, there exist many problems in the current experimental syllabus: the class hours of experimental course are not sufficient, which is not beneficial to improving students' practical skills; the experimental contents are old-fashioned and mostly are replication experiment, which will do harm to the development of students' comprehensive experimental skills because the pioneering knowledge in medicine can not be reflected and applied in their experiments; the common overlaps in experiments among different subjects result in the waste of limited resources and inadequacy of class hours; the lack of being systematic, scientific and complete and hierarchy in experimental syllabus, especially the failure to train students' ability to do scientific research would be no good for the development of their individuality and innovative ability; the lack of integration of related subjects causes inflexibility in experimental contents; the low efficiency and replacement rate of experimental equipment would hinder the process of getting laboratories modernized, scientific and regularized; the teachers would not be motivated for what they are allocated by the educational administration department; the experimental equipment is old and thus leads to incompletion of experiments for the students for the lack of experiment funds [2]. All these mentioned problems have seriously hindered the experimental course teaching quality and calls for urgent measures from the authority to overcome the weak points of the traditional experimental course teaching. It is therefore essential to establish a teaching model which could be beneficial to develop the students' intelligence, to cultivate the awareness of invention and to improve the professional skills.

"Project-Tutor" System experimental course teaching transforms replication experiment from researching and conventional experiment into comprehensive experiment, in-class experiment report into conclusively comprehensive report, which could enhance completeness, science, practicality and sustainability of the experiments and thus be beneficial to training the students' experiment skills, improving experimental practicality, developing students' awareness of science research and initiative to do research. In order to improve students' ability to do the experiment, the experiment groups, in this system, are scaled down from 36 per group to 10–12 per group, providing more chances for the students to practice; the schedule of experiment is also more flexible, compared with the traditional fixed lab-opening time, in order to make the best of the teaching resources and relieve the conflict between the enlarged number of students after the enrollment expansion and the insufficiency of experimental equipment. The experimental project consists of two parts, namely, appointed part and optional part, from which the students could make their own choice according to their learning conditions, ability and interests [3, 4]. Tutors and students could make two-way selection each other. In this way, more and more competent teachers with higher professional titles would be willing to be the tutors, which would enhance their awareness of competition. During the whole process, the students would become more active in learning and broaden their horizon, motivating their awareness of innovation. Therefore, it is of great necessity that the research of "Project-Tutor System" experimental course teaching should be done in no time [5].

49.2.2 The Emphasis on the Necessity and Significance of Teaching Reformation

In the seminar of education reformation held in our school, our project team offered a series of discussions with different subjects such as "to reform the experimental course teaching model and improve the quality of the students", "to deepen the reformation of experimental course teaching and establish new experimental course teaching system", "to improve practical teaching and cultivate high-quality medical professionals", "to construct new experimental course teaching model to adapt to new requirements of talents in twenty first century", "to reform practical teaching model to develop the students' capability of innovation and practice", "to enhance the reformation of experimental course teaching to ensure the training quality", "to take the project system in experimental course teaching to improve the training of medical professionals" and "to transform the traditional teaching conception and compile the guidance for experimental course teaching".

Among the students, the discussions at different levels from classes to grades to majors were launched and then the representatives of the students would get together to present their viewpoints and suggestions concerning "Project-Tutor" System experimental course teaching reformation; the teachers would also firstly be organized to have the discussion in terms of teaching and research sections and majors and then they would get together to express their opinion and suggestions on "Project-Tutor" System experimental course teaching reformation. Through those various discussions at different levels, the teachers as well as the students have therefore been aware of the necessity and the significance of "Project-Tutor" System experimental course teaching reformation, and they have also been clear of the practical requirements of this system, which is the guarantee of the implementation of the experimental course teaching reformation.

49.3 The Preparation for "Project-Tutor" System Experimental Course Teaching Reformation

49.3.1 To Compile the Guide of "Project-Tutor" System Experimental Course Teaching

All the teaching and research sections in our medical school firstly collected the existing experimental textbooks published by different medical colleges and universities, and then recomposed them into an experimental textbook in which relatively independent experimental projects are similar to research projects. The contents in the textbook are constructed based on the status quo of experimental conditions of the teaching and research section and staff. Those experiments are practical, innovative, representative and operational. In terms of the complexity of experimental contents and the usage of funds, "Project-Tutor" System experiments are classified to be appointed and optional. There were in all 110 experimental guides made by all the teaching and research sections, appointed experimental guide 63 and optional experimental guide 47. The compiled experimental guide Book I was used by the students and the teachers in the school.

49.3.2 To Train the Experimental Course Teaching Staff

"Project-Tutor" System experimental course teaching places higher demands for the teachers. In order to meet the demands, the medical school authority made an arrangement to train the teachers. Firstly, teachers with higher professional titles were appointed to deliver lectures to the staff; then the teachers with higher professional titles or experienced teacher would take responsibility for young teachers' experimental course teaching preparation and coaching. Especially, the tutorial system was carried out to set the training program and to arrange demonstration teaching for the young teachers [6]. The young teachers were required to look up a large amount of relative literature, and consult the experienced teachers when they come across some difficulties. Before class, they should rehearse the experiment on their own, from the preparatory work such as reagent to the obtainment of experimental results, and should be very familiar with the operation and adjustment of the experimental equipment. Moreover, the young teachers should predict the questions which would be asked by the students during the experiments and provide answers to them.

49.3.3 To Purchase Experimental Equipment and to Improve Experimental Conditions

In order to improve the experimental conditions, the medical school tried to raise funds as much as possible. Based on the requirements of the syllabus and "Project-Tutor" System experimental course teaching, the plan to purchase equipment and instrument was made according to the appointed "Project-Tutor" System experiment projects in all the teaching and research sections.

49.4 The Organization of "Project-Tutor" System Experimental Course Teaching

49.4.1 Mobilization

In order to publicize the necessity and significance of "Project-Tutor" System experimental course teaching among the students, a conference involving deans, teaching secretaries, heads of the teaching and research sections, students instructors was held to clarify how to take the course of experimental projects. The procedure was: the appointed experiments course were what the students must take, in which the students were divided into three groups, with each group consisting of 10–12 students; the experimental project tutors or tutor groups were selected according to these groups. Every tutor or tutor group would have to guide students no more than 50 % of the students of the same major, otherwise, the teaching and research section would make some adjustment. While the optional experiments were what could be selected by the more competent students according to their own conditions. The procedure is shown in Fig. 49.1.

49.4.2 Selection of Courses

The courses to be selected were arranged according to majors, grades and classes beforehand, and then the students were asked to make the selection with the assistance of the instructors. The results of the students' selection then were reported to the educational administration department. The medical school accordingly distributed the experiment guide book and experiment report book. All the teaching and research sections then appointed the tutors or tutor groups to make preparation for the experimental course teaching according to the students' selection.

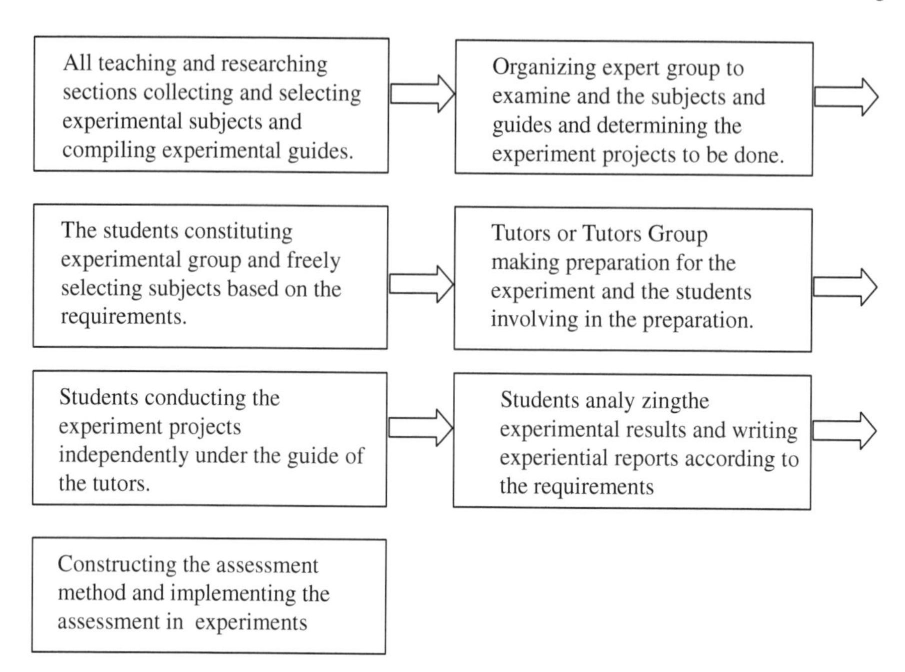

Fig. 49.1 Basic procedures of "Project-Tutor System" experimental course teaching method

49.4.3 To Set the Teaching Plan and Make Preparation for Experiment

The tutors or the tutor groups of all the experiment projects, together with the students, checked out the teaching plan, including the time and place of the experiment projects, and proposed for the students the specific requirements concerning the teaching contents and the data retrieval.

49.4.4 Implementation of the Project

The tutors or the tutors groups of the experiment projects delivered systematic lectures concerning the research significance, the application of the related experiment projects at home and abroad, research contents and technical route. Under the guidance of the tutors, the students conducted the experiments independently, which was beneficial not only to developing the students' ability to practice and innovate but also to familiarizing them with the experiment contents as well as its design.

49.4.5 The Establishment of Objective and Scientific Assessment Method

The assessment method involved many parts, such as inviting the experts to inspect the students' conducting the experiment, to attend the in-class lectures at random, assessing the experiment report and making questionnaires to know the students' assessment on teaching effect of "Project-Tutor System" teaching method.

49.5 Summarization and Improvement of "Project-Tutor System" Teaching Method

49.5.1 Advantages of "Project-Tutor System" Teaching Method

"Project-Tutor System" teaching method, judging from the teaching practice, fully motivated both the teachers and the students involved and fostered the responsibility of teaching in the teachers which urged the teacher to be more responsible and to alter their teaching method—from teaching them what to learn to teaching them how to learn. "Project-Tutor System" teaching method, aiming at students-centeredness, developed initiative and enthusiasm in students and allowed the students to select the tutors and experimental contents to some extent [7].

The teaching method of "Project-Tutor System" is the essential measure to improve the teaching quality in under-graduation education. It could foster the concepts of valuing teaching in the teachers and transforming their passive teaching into active teaching by means of competing-from "I teach because I am made to teach" to "I teach because I am ready to teach". In "Project-Tutor System" teaching method, the specific experimental contents would be allocated to the tutor and then the tutor would, under the pressure or, say, the trust, deliberate his teaching method, consult related literature, conduct the preparatory experiment by himself and explore and make clear of every detail or the possible error in the experiment. Through the experiment course teaching, the tutor could accumulate and enrich his academic knowledge and thus the quality of experimental course teaching would be improved as a whole by tutors' systematic teaching.

"Project-Tutor System" teaching method could enhance the skill-training on a comprehensive basis. Every experiment consists of many procedures from preparation, operation, and result analysis to conclusion. During the experiment course teaching, the tutor would first ask the students to look up the theoretical knowledge and consult the new technology and methods related to the given experiment, from which the students would learn the ways for reference such as surfing the internet, searching in the library and have a general idea of the experiment; and then the students, under the guide of the tutor, design the technique route of the experiment, make up all the needed reagents independently and finish doing the experiment by themselves. As to the problems emerging from the experimental process, the students would be first encouraged to discuss by themselves and then have them analyzed by the tutors, which would make the students fully understand the experimental procedures and enhance their ability and their comprehensive quality in experiment. Moreover, "Project-Tutor System" teaching method could help develop innovative ability in students and foster their perseverance in doing the scientific research as medical experiment itself is a science in which some related experimental knowledge and rare experimental phenomen remain to be further illustrated though many of the experimental results have been testified. In the experiments, there would be some disagreements between what the students have done and what is indicated in theory, which demands students' careful observation, serious analysis and painstaking exploration in order to find out the reasons. As a result, the students would get more practice in both mind and will.

49.5.2 Teaching Effect of "Project-Tutor System" Teaching Method

Two seminars on "Project-Tutor System" teaching method have been held in our medical school, in which all the teaching and research sections and the tutors of all experimental projects have gathered to discuss and exchange their experiences from their teaching practice. Many achievements have been made, such as teaching and researching papers, 89 in all, which were compiled into two papers collections, and 15 of which were published in journals at different levels in our country; four published in experiment textbooks.

The successful implementation of "Project-Tutor System" teaching method in medical fundamental courses was acclaimed by the students as well as the tutors due to the proper procedures, forceful measures, strong pertinence and assured effect in its design. Now the method has been popularized in all the experiment courses in our school. The students benefit much from this method, and up to now they have published 20 papers concerning experiment researching in different journals and were awarded by our college authority. "Project-Tutor System" teaching method has been one of the featured projects, with a full appreciation by the experts.

The experimental practice demonstrated that "Project-Tutor System" teaching method could fully motivate both the teachers and the students due to its impeccable mechanism of management, competition and restriction. On the one hand, this method could help the tutors foster strong sense of responsibility and dedication in profession and the strong awareness of competition supposing they want to have a successful experimental class. On the other hand, this method would not only provide more chances for the students to practice and improve their interest in academic study and their ability to do experiment, but help foster in them the realistic and scientific working style and help them acquire more theoretical knowledge and equip them with more experimental skills. Therefore, it is worthy of being further popularized.

Acknowledgments This research was supported by the grants from Educational Science Foundation of Anhui Province (2012jyxm209), China, and also supported by the key grants from Educational Science Foundation of Anhui University of Science & Technology (No: 2010jyxm025 and No:2012-27).

References

1. X L, Li C (2004) Initial exploration on application of Project-Tutor system teaching method to medical fundamental experimental courses teaching. J Ah Univ Sci Technol (Social Sci) 6(2):672–674
2. Sun J, Liu J, Sun Y (2012) Study on application of project-tutor system teaching method in experimental courses teaching in human parasitology. J Int Med Hum Parasitol 39(1):127–128
3. Xu L, Wang J, Zhang R (2006) Study on application of project-tutor system teaching method to experimental courses teaching in medical immunology. Pract Gen Med 4(3):314–315
4. He J, Zhu Y, Wang J (2006) Application of project-tutor system teaching method to experimental courses teaching in human parasitology. Pract Gen Med 4(1):62–63
5. Li C, Wu Q (2004) To develop "project-tutor system" experimental course teaching method to foster high-quality medical talents. Med Educ 48(3):482–484
6. Yu Y, Zhu W (2006) Basic requirements of excellent medical fundamental course teachers. Chin Med Educ 26(5):29–31
7. Li L (2008) Study of tutor system in Oxford university from the perspective of sociology. Higher Educ Explor 5:34–37

Chapter 50
A Knowledge-Based Teaching Resources Recommend Model for Primary and Secondary School Oriented Distance-Education Teaching Platform

Meijing Zhao, Wancheng Ni, Haidong Zhang, Ziqi Lin and Yiping Yang

Abstract In distance education systems, the ranked list of resources is very important for learners and teachers to find useful resources effectively. Apart from user's interest, the knowledge point of subject is a crucial factor for education system, especially for primary and secondary school oriented distance education. Much of the previous work are models based on recommender systems, however, these models considered only user's interest, ignoring the crucial impact of subject knowledge. In order to improve the performance of recommender systems, we considered both the subject knowledge and user's interest. To get this target, Latent Knowledge Model (LKM) is adopted. LKM is a knowledge-based and teaching task-oriented model. It enables subject knowledge resources through knowledge tree extended search strategy, and gets personalized resources through user feature mining strategy. LKM is realized on real data sets which are obtained from a popular distance education teaching platform. Recall and precision rate are used to evaluate the performance of our proposed method for resources recommendation tasks. Experimental results show that the LKM captures subject knowledge and personal preferences for resources selection, which yields significant improvement in recommendation accuracy.

M. Zhao · W. Ni (✉) · H. Zhang · Z. Lin · Y. Yang
Department of CASIA-HHT Joint Laboratory of Smart Education, Institute of Automation Chinese Academy of Science, Beijing 100190, China
e-mail: wancheng.ni@ia.ac.cn

M. Zhao
e-mail: meijing.zhao@ia.ac.cn

H. Zhang
e-mail: haidong.zhang@ia.ac.cn

Z. Lin
e-mail: ziqi.lin@ia.ac.cn

Y. Yang
e-mail: yiping.yang@ia.ac.cn

S. Li et al. (eds.), *Frontier and Future Development of Information Technology in Medicine and Education*, Lecture Notes in Electrical Engineering 269,
DOI: 10.1007/978-94-007-7618-0_50,

Keywords Distance education • Knowledge tree • Extended search • User feature • Recommender system

50.1 Introduction

The concept of distance education has been getting more and more popular during the last half decade. As a result, network educational resources and the number of various network educational platforms have drastically increased. However, the lack of effective organization of the overloaded educational resources brought difficulty to users, especially to teachers in teaching task (such as teaching design, courseware or homework assignment) to get effective resources quickly and accurately. Effective recommender algorithms can separate useful resources from mass of information. Thus, recommender system becomes a very good idea to solve this problem.

Personalized recommendation approaches are firstly proposed and applied in ecommerce area for product purchase. It helps customers find products which they would like to purchase by producing a list of recommended products [1–3]. There are some well-known recommendation techniques [4]: the items are recommended to users based on user's past activities (interest) in content-based recommender system; the items are recommended to users based on people with similar interests liked in the past in collaborative filtering recommender system; the items are recommended to users based on rules that enable precisely the recommended items to those that limiting particular conditions in rule-based recommender system. To improve performance, sometimes these techniques combine together as a hybrid recommendation [5, 6]. The system justifications can be obtained from preferences directly expressed by users, or from the customer experience represented by data [7].

However, education resource, especially resource in primary and secondary school oriented distance education, has its own unique characteristics. These unique characteristics can be used in resources management systems or recommendation systems. We summarized these unique characteristics as follows:

1. Education resources are closely related with subject knowledge.
2. Education resources have hidden semantic relations, so resources can contact with each other through teaching knowledge nodes.
3. Subject knowledge formed a complex and orderly network.
4. Knowledge points of certain subject play more important role than teacher's preferences and interests in subject learning, especially in China's primary and secondary school.

In order to help teachers find adequate and useful resources from mass of online teaching resources, we make use of these unique characteristics. In our proposed approach, we considered both the user's interest and subject knowledge. To realize this idea, a knowledge-based teaching task-oriented recommendation model called Latent Knowledge Model (LKM) is proposed. It enables subject knowledge resources through knowledge tree extended search strategy, and gets personalized resources through user feature mining. The LKM achieves significant improvement in recommendation accuracy.

The rest of this paper is organized as follows: a brief literature review in topics related to this paper is given in Sect. 50.2. Section 50.3 is a core section explaining the composition of LKM which contains the concept of extended search strategy and user feature mining strategy. In Sect. 50.4 the proposed LKM based recommendation system is introduced, with a discussion on how to get parameters and how to recommend resources. Section 50.5 gives the recommendation evaluation results. Finally Sect. 50.6 gives an overall discussion and conclusion, together with directions for future research.

50.2 Related Works

In recent years, the mainly knowledge-based approach employed in resources recommender system is ontology-based resource management method. In [7], it introduced an ontology-based framework for semantic search of education content in E-learning, and its main idea is that the domain ontology is used to represent the learning materials. The ontology here is composed by a hierarchy of concepts and sub-concepts. However, this method still cannot meet the extended search requirement because of the absence of relationship between resources. In another work [8], the education resources are recommended using the semantic relationship between learning materials and the learner's need. But this recommender model makes the learner's need as the recommend center rather than the teaching goal. As a result, there will have a deviation in the final resources recommendation list. The research purpose in [9] is to study the personalized service of basic data resources integration platform based on ontology, to combine the traditional personalized service technology with ontology, to analyze user's preferences and demands, and then to design a user model based on ontology direct to the features of basic data resources integration platform which includes multiple fields of specialty, multiple information resources and multiple subsystems. This work also focus in user's preferences and demands, ignored the knowledge points hidden in subjects.

Our proposed method, LKM, is different from the aforementioned methods because the relations among resources are organized through knowledge tree. There are three innovation points: extended search, extending depth controllable and large potential of knowledge mining. Apart from enjoying good performance, LKM, also maintains personalized teaching style reflected by user features.

50.3 Latent Knowledge Model

In this section, we provide the core theories on the problem of education resources recommendation, LKM, which include knowledge-based extended search strategy and user feature mining strategy. We first describe the organization of knowledge tree, and then introduce our knowledge-based extended search work briefly. The user feature mining strategy will be explained later for the integrity of LKM.

50.3.1 Knowledge Tree Structure

In order to implement knowledge mining among resources, we need to construct knowledge trees which contact education resources with each other. The principle of constructing knowledge tree can be summarized as follows:

1. Knowledge tree is composed of a hierarchy of knowledge nodes and sub knowledge nodes.
2. The hyponymy relation and synonymy relation between knowledge nodes contain parent-child relation and leader-membership relation. The parent-child relation has inherited attribute and the leader-membership relation has reverse inherited attributes.
3. Every knowledge node is composed of several attributes, and each attribute is represented by attribute name and attribute value. These attributes reflect the knowledge points of the current knowledge node.

After the comprehensive and careful investigation of teaching material of Chinese primary and secondary schools, we build our domain knowledge tree for distance education resources. We determined the basic resource knowledge tree organization model—"1 + n" knowledge tree structure, which include one basic tree (textbook transverse knowledge tree) and n extended trees (such as subject longitudinal knowledge tree, people tree, events tree, place tree and etc.).

The textbook transverse knowledge tree is organized by national textbook classification criteria, takes the "section" as each branch's terminated note, and makes several attributes to represent the knowledge of this "section". In a similar way, we obtain our subject longitudinal knowledge tree through summarizing the longitudinal knowledge of certain subject in a period of time. The people tree, events tree and place tree contain the important persons, events and place that referred in textbooks. Figure 50.1 is a textbook transverse knowledge tree schematic diagram of the text "Qilv·Changzheng", the attributes of this section are author, background, genre and place.

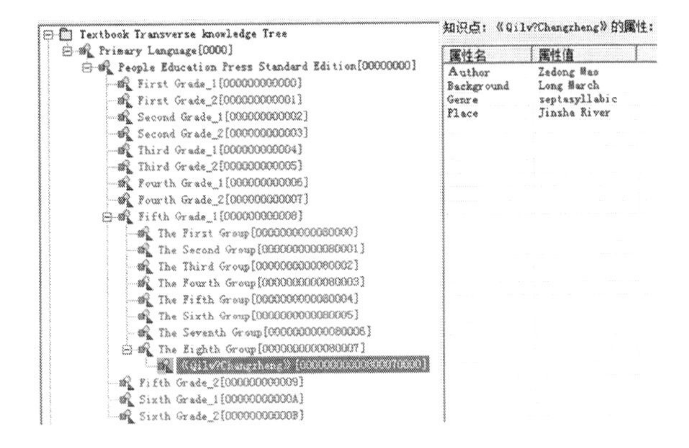

Fig. 50.1 The textbook transverse knowledge tree schematic diagram of text "Qilv·Changzheng"

50.3.2 Knowledge-Based Extended Search Strategy

Knowledge-based extended search strategy searched the semantic related attributes of a given teaching task through several knowledge trees. And then the most important resources of this given teaching task can be founded. With the constructed knowledge tree structure, we implement our extended search strategy according to the following steps:

1. Teaching object locate: locate the current teaching object to a certain section of the basic knowledge tree (textbook transverse knowledge tree).
2. Attributes search: search other related attributes of knowledge nodes from several extended knowledge trees through attribute values of the basic knowledge tree.
3. Attributes extended search: repeat the above step using the current attribute values until the extending depth meet requirement. It should be pointed out that the depth of extended search can be defined by users, and usually 1–3 times attributes query will offer enough information.
4. Recommended resources list construct: take the searched attribute values as keywords to search the related resources. Different extended depths of researching sources have different weights. Usually, the deeper the search extended, the smaller the weights are.

Assuming the teaching task is courseware design, we implement the strategy on a special object "Qilv·Changzheng": through the attribute of textbook transverse knowledge tree, we get the author of the text "Qilv·Changzheng" is Zedong Mao, and then we can extend to the knowledge node of "Zedong Mao" of the people tree, through which we can obtain more information and resources about "Zedong Mao", such as the attribute about his literary works or the attribute about his achievements. In a similar way, through other attributes of textbook transverse knowledge tree, we can extend to the rest of the five trees and get enough

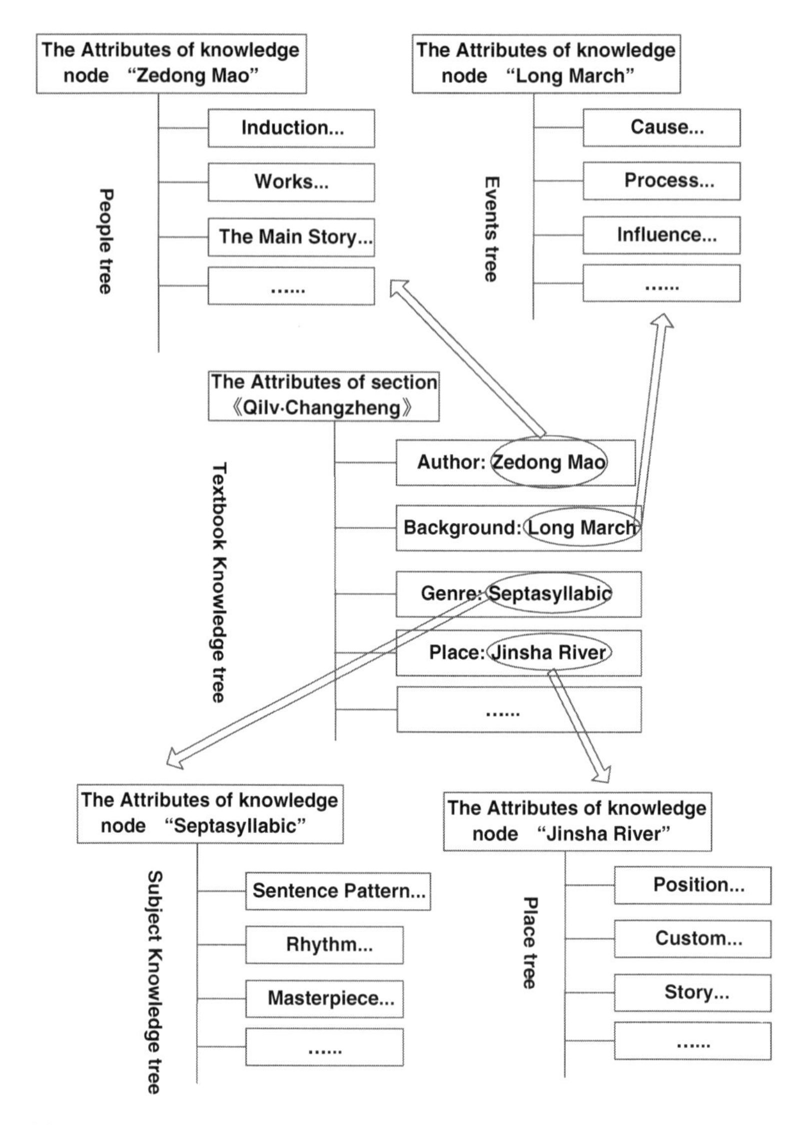

Fig. 50.2 The extended search process schematic diagram of text "Qilv·Changzheng"

information of this section. Then we take those semantic related attribute values as keywords to search for resources. Figure 50.2 is the extended search process schematic diagram of section "Qilv·Changzheng".

50.3.3 User Feature Mining Strategy

In teaching platform, each teacher user has individual differences, such as age, gender, address, cognitive level, educational background, hobbies, etc. The teachers in the teaching platform tend to reflect personalized style. User feature mining strategy can help teachers get personalized recommendation to meet each teacher's unique requirement. For this purpose, the user features are represented by a vector space $U_N(\cdot)$ representing N features. Take the features age, gender and address for example, the user features can be described as follows:

$$U_N(\cdot) = U_N(1, 1, 010) \tag{50.1}$$

On the above equation, age = 1 denotes the user's age below a certain number, gender = 1 denotes the user is male and address = 010 denotes the user living city is Beijing. Different feature has different affect in the process of recommending, therefore, our user feature mining task is to find the weight of each feature.

The feature weights can be acquired by calculating the distribution of downloading resources. In our strategy, we take the overall variance of resources in each feature as the initial weights firstly. And then the accurate weights are obtained by dataset training using recall and precision rate for resources recommendation tasks. The weights of user features are represented by another vector space $W_N(\cdot) = W_N(a, b, c\ldots)$ which will be calculated in the final recommend rank algorithm.

50.4 Resources Recommendation Using Latent Knowledge Model

In the knowledge-based recommender system, LKM attempt to obtain the top-K resources which reflect both the knowledge points of the current teaching object and teacher's personalized teaching style. In this section, the way to achieve this goal through the proposed recommender system architecture is explained.

50.4.1 Recommender System Architecture

The inputs of recommender system are depth of extended search and teaching task tag, while the output is recommended resources list. The idea of system can be summarized as follows:

1. Construct the "1 + n" knowledge tree structure.
2. Implement extended search strategy to obtain related teaching semantic object keywords.

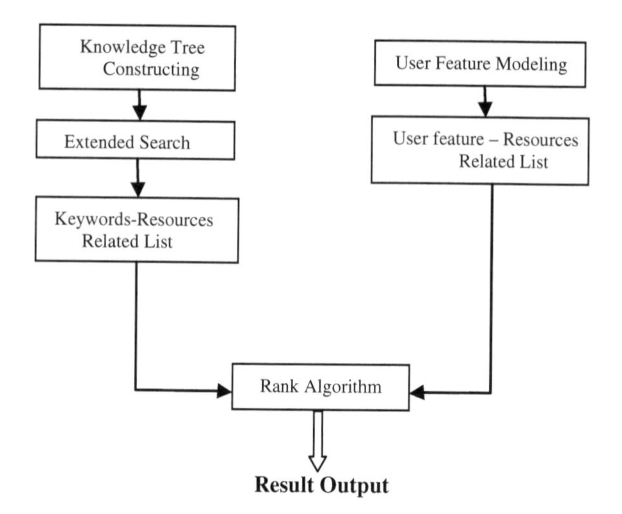

Fig. 50.3 Graphical recommendation system architecture

3. Generate knowledge-based recommended resources list.
4. Implement user feature mining strategy to obtain the user features which reflect teacher's personalized teaching style.
5. Generate knowledge-based recommended resources list.
6. Generate the final recommended resources list through resources rank algorithm.

The Graphical system architecture is presented in Fig. 50.3.

50.4.2 Rank Algorithm

We use the following formula to compute the final recommendation result:

$$L = \sum w_{ki} L_k(i) + \sum w_{uj} L_u(j) \tag{50.2}$$

On the above equation, L is the final ranked resources recommendation list, $L_k(i)$ and $L_u(j)$ denotes the ranked resources recommendation list obtained from extended search and user feature mining respectively. The index i denotes the notes recommendation results decided by jth user feature. Variables w_{ki} and w_{uj} express the weights of each recommendation results. We obtained the final ranked recommendation result by finding the optimal weights.

50.5 Experiment Results

In this section, the experiment results are reported on two different teaching object data sets collected from the CASIA-HHT Joint Laboratory of Smart Education.[1] The first (small) data set consists of 42 users, 684 resources and 931 tags. The second (big) data set consists of 106 users, 911 resources and 3885 tags. 90 % of data for training and 10 % for testing, and experiment with ten times repeat. We choose the user features of age, gender and address for personalized training, and set the extended search depth as two.

Recommendation performances in resources recommendation task are evaluated by precision/recall. Assuming R(u) denotes resources recommended to user u, and T(u) denotes resources tagged by user u, the precision/recall functions are defined as follows:

$$\text{Precision} = \frac{\sum_{u}|R(u) \cap T(u)|}{\sum_{u}|R(u)|} \tag{50.3}$$

$$\text{Recall} = \frac{\sum_{u}|R(u) \cap T(u)|}{\sum_{u}|T(u)|} \tag{50.4}$$

The parameters optimized through training based on recall from small dataset are $w_{k1} = 0.92$, $w_{k2} = 0.33$, $w_{u1} = 0.67$, $w_{u2} = 0.81$, $w_{u3} = 0.12$, while the parameters optimized through training based on recall from big dataset are $w_{k1} = 0.39$, $w_{k2} = 0.11$, $w_{u1} = 0.18$, $w_{u2} = 0.28$, $w_{u3} = 0.04$. We compare the recommendation results between our LKM and DM (which based on simply recommend the top-N resources according to download rate). Table 50.1 reports the recall values at top-20 and top-100 resources. The results in Table 50.1 clearly show the superiority of LKM approach. Resources recommendation recall values of LKM are consistently higher than those of the DM-based method, up to about 33 % in accuracy. Note that except the precision/recall accuracy, LKM approach can also recommend some amazing and unexpected resources which may be very useful to teachers due to the subject knowledge organized in knowledge trees.

Table 50.1 Recall @ 20 and Recall @ 100 values of LKM and DM for resources recommendation in the two datasets

Method	Dataset	Recall @20	Recall @ 100
LKM	Small	0.429	0.857
DM	Small	0.286	0.714
LKM	Big	0.667	0.916
DM	Big	0.583	0.833

[1] The education resources datasets can be collected from: http://www.910edu.com/reslibsrv/web/index/index.do.

50.6 Conclusions and Future Work

In this paper, we introduce our work of a novel knowledge-based personalized teaching resources recommendation method called LKM. The advantage of this approach is the ability to joint subject knowledge and personalized feature. Experiments on real datasets show the effectiveness performance of LKM in both small and big dataset. Note that besides the precision/recall accuracy, LKM approach can also recommend some amazing and unexpected resources which may be very useful to teachers due to the subject knowledge organized in knowledge trees. The recommender model has three innovation points:

1. Extended search: we implement extended search through attributes of these five knowledge trees.
2. Extending depth controllable: the depth of extended search can be defined by users.
3. Large potential of knowledge mining: besides the attributes of knowledge nodes, other features of knowledge tree can also be considered for semantic mining, such as the hyponymy of knowledge nodes.

In the proposed method, a core problem is the organization of knowledge tree. A strong knowledge tree structure may help user find enough and satisfied teaching resources. On the other hand, effective user features play important impact on personalized recommendation. Those two issues are the subjects of our further work.

Acknowledgments We thank Dayong Wen and the subject experts for their helpful comments and suggestions about extracting subject knowledge nodes from the special subject.

References

1. Yunus Y, Salim J (2008) Framework for the evaluation of e-learning in Malaysian Public Sector from the pedagogical perspective. In: International symposium in information technology, pp 1–8
2. Basu C, Hirsh H, Cohen W (1998) Recommendation as classification: using social and content-based information in recommendation. In: Proceedings of the fifteenth national conference on artificial intelligence, pp 714–720
3. Pan P, Wang C, Horng G, Cheng S (2010) The development of an ontology-based adaptive personalized recommender system. In: 2010 international conference on electronics and information engineering, pp V176–V180
4. Adomavicius G, Tuzhilin A (2005) Toward the next generation of recommender systems: a survey of the state-of-the-art and possible extensions. IEEE Trans Knowl Data Eng 17(6):734–749
5. Drachsler H, Hummel H, Koper R (2007) Recommendations for learners are different: applying memory-based recommender system techniques to lifelong learning. SIRTEL workshop at the EC-TEL 2007 Conference

6. Burke R (2002) Hybrid recommender systems: survey and experiments. User Model User-Adapt Interact 12:331–370
7. Saman S, Seyed Yashar B et al (2011) Review of personalized recommendation techniques for learners in e-learning systems. In: 2011 international conference on semantic technology and information retrieval, pp 277–281
8. Isabela G, Daniel L et al (2009) Quality ontology for recommendation in an adaptive educational system. In: 2009 international conference on intelligent networking and collaborative systems, pp 329–335
10. Liu X, Liu N, Du H (2011) Research on personalized service of basic data resources integration platform based on ontology. In: 2011 international symposium on it in medicine and education (ITME), pp 299–304

Chapter 51
A Fast and Simple HPLC–UV Method for Simultaneous Determination of Emodin and Quinalizarin from Fermentation Broth of *Aspergillus. ochraceus* lp_0429

ShaoMei Yu and Ping Lv

Abstract A rapid, sensitive and reproducible high performance liquid chromatographic (HPLC) method was developed and validated for simultaneous quantification of Emodin and Quinalizarin from Fermentation Broth of *Aspergillus. ochraceus* lp_0429. Isocratic RP-HPLC system with C18 column (4.6 mm × 250 mm i.d., 5 μ particle size) and a detector UV-VWD was employed. The mobile phase of 0.05 M disodium hydrogen phosphate and acetonitrile (25:75, v/v) containing 0.5 mL/L triethylamine at pH 5.8 was delivered at flow rate of 0.1 mL/min at ambient temperature. The UV detection of emodin and quinalizarin was set at 254 nm. Total run time was 10 min and retention times for Emodin and Quinalizarin were 2.08 and 6.12 min, respectively.

Keywords HPLC–UV · Emodin · Quinalizarin Aspergillus Ochraceus

51.1 Introduction

Emodin (1,3,8-trihydroxy-6-methyl-anthraquinone) is a naturally occurring pigment found in many plants [1], molds and lichens, exhibiting diverse biological activities including anticancer functions [2–4] and anti-inflammatory functions [5]. Early studies on its therapeutic benefits were mainly focused on its laxative functions as it is abundant in traditional Chinese medicinal herbs used for laxative formulation, such as rhubarb, the root and rhizome of Rheum palmatum [6].

S. Yu · P. Lv (✉)
Department of Biotechnological and Environmental Engineering, Tianjin Professional College, Tianjin 300410, China
e-mail: bestman_0429@163.com

S. Yu
e-mail: ysm913@163.com

S. Li et al. (eds.), *Frontier and Future Development of Information Technology in Medicine and Education*, Lecture Notes in Electrical Engineering 269,
DOI: 10.1007/978-94-007-7618-0_51,

Recently, the health benefit of emodin has been linked to its involvement in many cellular processes, such as the suppression of tumor-associated angiogenesis through the inhibition of extracellular signal-regulated kinases [7]. There was also a report that emodin can sensitize certain types of breast cancer cells to the treatment of paclitaxel [8]. Its inhibitory effect on tumorogenesis-associated cell signaling pathways has made emodin an interesting molecular entity for anti-neoplastic studies and formulations.

The traditional function of Quinalizarin (1,2,5,8-tetrahydroxyanthraquinone) is determination of beryllium, magnesium, calcium, aluminum and boron reagents. Karami [9] reported that Quinalizarin (QA) was loaded on an octadecyl silica-polyethylene mini-column for the retention of Hf and Zr ions in complex form in order to determinate Hf and Zr by ICP-atomic emission spectroscopy. Zanjanchi [10] used quinalizarin as coloring reagents in Rapid determination of aluminum by UV–vis diffuse reflectance spectroscopy. Kumar [11] manufactured a new polymer matrix of Amberlite XAD-2 coupling to quinalizarin for solid-phase extraction of metal ions for flame atomic absorption spectrometric determination. However, the research on physiological functions of Quinalizarin was developed at present. Cozza [12] identified quinalizarin as ail inhibitor of CK2 that is more potent and selective than emodin and proved quinalizarin able to inhibit endogenous CK2 and to induce apoptosis more efficiently than the commonly used CK2 inhibitors TBB (4.5,6,7-tetrabromo-1H-benzolriazole) and DMAT (2-dimethylamino-4,5,6,7-Tetra-bromo-1H-benzimidazole).

We report our studies on a strain of *Aspergillus ochraceus* isolated from Chinese potato, which constantly and efficiently produced an red pigment mixture (including Emodin and quinalizarin) [13]. So it was important to find a fast and simple HPLC–UV method for simultaneous determination of emodin and quinalizarin from fermentation broth of *Aspergillus. ochraceus lp_0429.*

51.2 Experimental

51.2.1 Chemicals and Reagents

HPLC-grade Acetonitrile and methanol were from Sigma Chemicals Co. (St. Louis, MO, USA). Emodin and quinalizarin were from Merck (Darmstadt, Germany). All other reagents were of analytical grade. NaNO3, MgSO4·7H20, KCl, KH2PO4, FeSO4·7H20 and ZnSO4·7H2O were purchased from Tianjin Chemical Reagent Co. Ltd (Tianjin, China) and Shanghai Chemical Reagent Co. Ltd (Shanghai, China). Glucose, chloroform and methanol were supplied by Sinopharm Chemical Reagent Co. Ltd. (Shanghai, China) and distilled water, prepared from deionized water, was used throughout the study.

51.2.2 Medium and Culture Grown

Aspergillus. ochraceus strain lp_0429 was grown in Czapek-Dox (CD) medium. This contained (in g/L): glucose 40, NaNO3 2, MgSO4·7H2O 0.5, KCl 0.5, KH2PO4 1.0, FeSO4·7H2O 0.01, ZnSO4·7H2O 0.01. The pH of the medium was adjusted to 6.8 before autoclaving. Flasks containing 100 mL of Czapeck Dox medium were inoculated with conidial suspension from a 5-day-old culture and were incubated at 29–300 C on a rotary shaker (220 rpm) for 120 h and the pigment mixture occurred.

51.2.3 Sample Preparation

An accurately weighed mycelium sample of 30 g centrifuged, filtered and dried from 400 mL fermentation liquid and 100 mL chloroform were added to a flask, and extraction was conducted in anultrasonic bath for 15 min. The extraction process was repeated three times. The primary extracts were combined, filtered, evaporated under vacuum.

51.2.4 Silica Gel Column Chromatography

The silica gel column chromatograph was applied to separate the red pigment (including of emodin and quinalizarin) from primary extracts. The solid phase was activated silica gel (100–200 mu), mobile phases was chloroform and methanol which changed from v:v = 9:1 to v:v = 2:8. The red eluting fraction were collected by their ABS254 and color, and then evaporated under vacuum.

51.2.5 Instrumentation and Chromatographic Conditions

An isocratic HPLC system of Agilent technologies 1200 series consisted of a pump with a column of Thermo Electron Corporation USA (ODS hypersil C18 4.6 mm × 250 mm), a UV-detector (VWD) with data processing Chem station software employed to assay the prepared plasma samples. The UV detection of emodin and quinalizarin was set at 254 nm, respectively. The mobile phase of 0.05 M disodium hydrogen phosphate and acetonitrile (25:75, v/v) containing 0.5 mL/L triethylamine at pH 5.8 was delivered at flow rate of 0.1 mL/min at ambient temperature.

51.2.6 Statistical Analysis

Statistical analysis was performed to determine variability level between the samples. The data was analyzed statistically using SPSS11 at 95 % confidence level.

51.3 Results

51.3.1 Assay Development

To examine the contents of emodin in the dry cell mass after Silica gel column chromatography, a mobile phase was optimized with various combinations of buffer solutions and organic solvents. Acetonitrile, methanol and buffer (acetate, phosphate buffers) in different percentages were investigated and finally a mobile phase of disodium hydrogen phosphate-acetonitrile in the ratio of 25:75 % (v/v) containing triethylamine 0.5 mL/L showed higher elution and resolution with sharp peaks for emodin and quinalizarin. The pH and molarity of mobile phase was also selected after various trials. The pH of 5.8 was found suitable for the desired objectives of no interference at low wavelength and was sufficient in concentration to avoid peak tailing because silica-based particles are unstable at low pH. An optimal flow rate of 0.1 mL/min was found appropriate for peak resolution with short run time of only 10 min. The retention times for emodin and quinalizarin were 2.08–6.12 min, respectively. A representative chromatogram has been shown in Fig. 51.1.

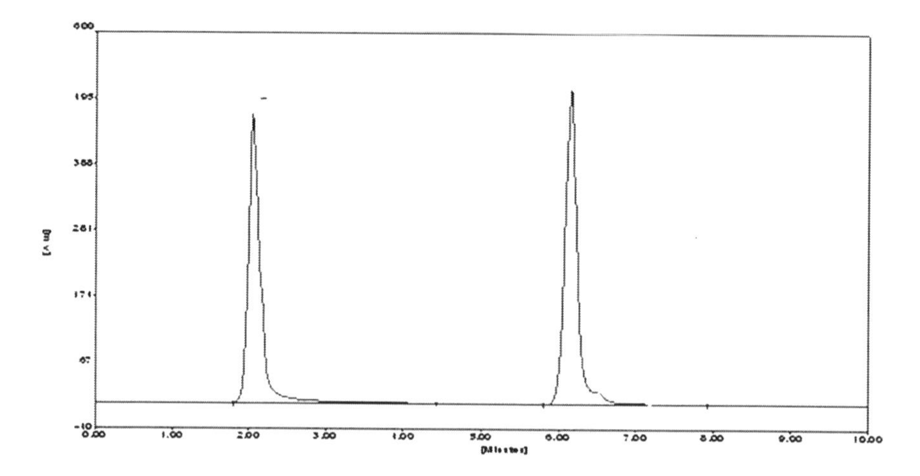

Fig. 51.1 Representative chromatogram of emodin and quinalizarin

51.3.2 *Method Validation*

51.3.2.1 Linearity

The standard curves of emodin and quinalizarin were produced using known sample concentrations within ranges of 0.01–50 μg/mL (emodin) and 0.01–50 μg/mL (quinalizarin). Linear regression was applied to fit straight line. Mean R2 values for emodin and quinalizarin were determined as 0.9991 and 0.9978, respectively and values of slope, intercept and R2 are shown in Table 51.1

51.3.2.2 Precision and Accuracy

Percent coefficient of variation (% CV) was calculated to find out intra-day precision, inter-day precision and accuracy of the present method for emodin and quinalizarin. The findings are shown in Table 51.2. The validation run consists of

Table 51.1 Standard curve parameters (mean ± SD) for emodin and quinalizarin

Sample	Slope	Intercept	R2
Emodin	16.818 ± 0.6	4.867 ± 0.32	0.9991 ± 0.003
Quinalizarin	21.726 ± 0.5	11.842 ± 0.58	0.9978 ± 0.004

Table 51.2 Intra-day and Inter-day precision and accuracy of emodin and quinalizarin

Parameter	Emodin			Quinalizarin		
	LQC (μg/mL)	MQC (μg/mL)	HQC (μg/mL)	LQC (μg/mL)	MQC (μg/mL)	HQC (μg/mL)
Intra-day						
Nominal Conc.	0.1	10	50	0.1	10	50
Mean	0.0987	9.821	49.995	0.0988	9.961	49.687
S.D.	0.0004	0.008	0.32	0.00084	0.012	0.38
Precision CV (%)	0.004053	0.000815	0.006401	0.008502	0.001205	0.007648
Accuracy (%)	0.987	0.9821	0.9999	0.988	0.9961	0.99374
Inter-day						
Nominal Conc.	0.1	10	50	0.1	10	50
Mean	0.996	9.921	49.895	0.993	9.951	49.782
S.D.	0.00101	0.003	2.587	0.00087	0.003	0.234
Precision CV (%)	0.001014	0.000302	0.051849	0.000876	0.000301	0.0047
Accuracy (%)	9.96	0.9921	0.9979	9.93	0.9951	0.99564

Table 51.3 Percent extraction yield of emodin and quinalizarin

	Conc. found in samples	Conc. found in standard solutions	Conc. found in samples	Conc. found in standard solutions
Emodin parameters	*Conc. Added (0.1 μg/ml)*		*Conc. Added (50 μg/ml)*	
Mean ± S.D.	0.0961 ± 0.00042	0.0984 ± 0.00036	49.751 ± 0.476	49.802 ± 0.664
CV (%)	0.437	0.3659	0.9568	1.333
PEY (%)	97.66		99.91	
Quinalizarin parameters	*Conc. Added (0.1 μg/ml)*		*Conc. Added (50 μg/ml)*	
Mean ± S.D.	0.0951 ± 0.00041	0.0972 ± 0.00030	49.684 ± 0.493	49.729 ± 0.654
CV (%)	0.441	3.086	0.992	1.3151
PEY (%)	97.83		99.90	

calibration curve and three replicates of each; low, medium and high quantification concentrations. For inter-day, analysis of three batches of each of samples was performed on three different days.

51.3.2.3 Quantification Limits

Limit of detection (LOD) and Limit of quantitation (LOQ) of emodin and quinalizarin as mean ± SD were 0.068 ± 0.0004 μg/mL and 0.187 ± 0.0006 μg/mL (emodin), 0.093 ± 0.0005 μg/mL and 0.158 ± 0.006 μg/mL (quinalizarin). Lower quantification limits showed the higher sensitivity of present method for two samples in single run.

51.3.2.4 Extraction Yields

Percent extraction yield was calculated by comparing mean drug concentration from samples (extracted) with mean concentration from standard solutions (true solutions of emodin and quinalizarin), determined from response (peak areas). Mean extraction recoveries were determined by analyzing four replicates of samples at three concentration levels of each drug of emodin and quinalizarin combination. The values of extraction yields are presented in Table 51.3 for emodin and quinalizarin.

51.4 Conclusion

The present chromatographic method provides a reproducible, accurate, selective and simultaneous quantification of emodin and quinalizarin. The method was applied successfully for analysis of emodin and quinalizarin from fermentation broth of Aspergillus. ochraceus lp_0429 and was propitious to the research and application of emodin and quinalizarin.

Acknowledgments The financial support of Tianjin Natural Science Foundation (A Study of Biosynthesis Pathway and Induced Mechanism from Reactive Oxygen Species of Emodin by Fermentation from Aspergillus ochraceus, No: 12JCYBJC19000), is gratefully Acknowledged.

References

1. Izhaki I(2002) Emodin - a secondary metablosite with multiple ecological functions in higher plants. New Phytol 55:205–217
2. Lin SY, Lai WW, Ho CC et al (2009) Emodin induces apoptosis of human tongue squamous cancer SCC-4 cells through reactive oxygen species and mitochondria-dependent pathways. Anticancer Res 29:327–335
3. Muto A, Hori M, Sasaki Y et al (2007) Emodin has a cytotoxic activity against human multiple myeloma as a Janus-activated kinase 2 inhibitor. Mol Cancer Ther 6:987–994
4. Srinivas G, Babykutty S, Sathiadevan PP et al(2007)Molecular mechanism of emodin action: transition from laxative ingredient to an antitumor agent. Med Res Rev 27:591–608
5. Ding Y, Zhao L, Mei H et al(2008)Exploration of Emodin to treat alpha-naphthylisothiocyanate-induced cholestatic hepatitis via anti-inflammatory pathway. Eur J Pharmacol 590:377–386
6. Wang L, Li D, Bao C et al(2008)Ultrasonic extraction and separation of anthraquinones from Rheum palmatum L. Ultrason Sonochem 15:738–746
7. Kaneshiro T, Morioka T, Inamine M et al (2006) Anthraquinone derivative emodin inhibits tumor-associated angiogenesis through inhibition of extracellular signal-regulated kinase 1/2 phosphorylation. Eur J Pharmacols 553:46–53
8. Zhang L, Lau YK, Xia W et al (1999) Tyrosine kinase inhibitor emodin suppresses growth of HER-2/neu-overexpressing breast cancer cells in athymic mice and sensitizes these cells to the inhibitory effect of paclitaxel. Clin Cancer Res 5:343–353
9. Karami H, Mousavi MF, Yamini Y (2006) On-line solid phase extraction and simultaneous determination of hafnium and zirconium by ICP-atomic emission spectroscopy. Microchim Acta 154(3–4):221–228
10. Zanjanchi MA, Noei H, Moghimi M (2006) Rapid determination of aluminum by UV-vis diffuse reflectance spectroscopy with application of suitable adsorbents. Talanta 70(5):933–939
11. Kumar M, Rathore DPS, Singh AK (2001) Quinalizarin anchored on Amberlite XAD-2. A new matrix for solid-phase extraction of metal ions for flame atomic absorption spectrometric determination. Fresen J Anal Chem 370(4):377–382
12. Cozza G, Mazzorana M, Papinutto E (2009) Quinalizarin as a potent, selective and cell-permeable inhibitor of protein kinase CK2. Biochem J 421(3):387–395
13. Lu P, Zhao XM, Cui T (2010) Production of emodin from Aspergillus ochraceus at preparative scale. Afr J Biotechnol 9(4):512–517

Chapter 52
Alteration of Liver MMP-9/TIMP-1 and Plasma Type IV Collagen in the Development of Rat Insulin Resistance

Jun-feng Hou, Xiao-di Zhang, Xiao-guang Wang, Jing Wei and Kai Jiao

Abstract Insulin resistance (IR) is a risk factor of many diseases and present in various metabolic abnormalities including obesity, type 2 diabetes. Although several factors are believed to contribute to the initiating course of IR, fatty liver, hepatic injury or hepatic fibrosis is a prominent feature during IR development. Although a correlation between IR and hepatic injury has long been suspected, it remains unclear whether accumulation of fat in the liver is causally related to hepatic injury which in turn induces systemic IR. Using rat IR model with high-fat diet (HFD), the present study shows a time courses of expression of matrix metalloproteinases (MMP-9)/tissue inhibitors of metalloproteinases (TIMP-1) mRNA and protein in the liver as well as plasma type IV collagen (collagen-IV), and liver histology. The results showed that expression of MMP-9 mRNA and protein significantly increased in rat liver after 15 days in HFD group but decreased thereafter. In contrast, liver TIMP-1 and plasma collagen-IV levels gradually increased and reached to a peak at the end of 60 days in HFD group. Histological analysis revealed that livers from HFD group exhibited steatosis, and more collagen fibers were formed in the interspace among disse cavea and intruded into the tight junctions among hepatocytes detected by transmission electron microscope. The results indicated that the IR induced alteration of MMP-9 to TIMP-1 ratio may play a role in elevation of collagen-IV, which may participate in development of inchoate hepatic fibrosis in the later course of IR.

Jun-feng Hou, Xiao-di Zhang contributed equally to this work.

J. Hou · X. Zhang · X. Wang · J. Wei
Department of Toxicology, Fourth Military Medical University, Xi'an 710032, China

K. Jiao (✉)
Department of Endocrinology, Tangdu Hospital, Fourth Military Medical University, Xi'an 710038, China
e-mail: tdjkaijk@fmmu.edu.cn

S. Li et al. (eds.), *Frontier and Future Development of Information Technology in Medicine and Education*, Lecture Notes in Electrical Engineering 269,
DOI: 10.1007/978-94-007-7618-0_52,

Keywords Insulin resistance · Hepatic steatosis · Hepatic fibrosis · Type IV collagen · MMP-9/TIMP-1

52.1 Introduction

Insulin resistance (IR) is a condition of tissues to be resistant to insulin, and often present in various metabolic abnormalities, predominantly in the type 2 diabetes mellitus, dyslipidemia, and hypertension [1, 2]. IR is also associated with nonalcoholic fatty liver disease (NAFLD) [3–7], which is a common hepatic disorder characterized by fat accumulation in the liver and can range from a simple fatty liver to nonalcoholic steatohepatitis (NASH) [8, 9]. Ultimately, and of major clinical significance, NASH can progress to fibrosis, cirrhosis and even hepatocellular carcinoma [10, 11]. The prevalence of NAFLD may affect up to 75 % of subjects in obese population, whereas the prevalence of NAFLD and NASH in a general population is only approximately 20 and 3 %, respectively [12–14]. In the morbidly obese, steatosis has been found in almost all subjects, with NASH being present in 25–70 % of these individuals [15, 16]. Metabolic syndrome and NAFLD are commonly associated and the presence of metabolic syndrome frequently predicts development of NAFLD [17]. Forty-eight percent of subjects diagnosed with metabolic syndrome in one clinical study were found to have fatty liver by ultrasound [18].

Since NAFLD patients frequently display hepatic as well as whole-body IR, weight loss and low fat diet are often recommended as treatment for NAFLD or NASH. Most importantly, the liver functions and histology can be significantly improved by weight loss and clinic interventions of fibrates, metformin and thiazolidinediones for reducing triglycerides and increasing insulin sensitivity [19]. It is not clear whether IR is a cause or a consequence of hepatic steatosis in the pathogenesis of NAFLD. To test whether systemic IR causes liver steatosis and/or hepatic fibrosis, we induced rat IR model by high-fat diet (HFD), detected the expression of matrix metalloproteinase-9 (MMP-9)/tissue inhibitors of metalloproteinase-1 (TIMP-1) mRNA and protein in liver tissue and plasma content of type IV collagen (collagen-IV), surveyed morphological change of rat liver. The results of the present study may provide some cue for inchoate hepatic fibrosis of IR subjects.

52.2 Materials and Methods

52.2.1 Animals and Treatments

Two-month-old male Sprague–Dawley albino rats (Laboratory Animal Center of the Fourth Military Medical University, Xi'an, China), weighed 180–200 g, were randomly divided into two groups: 24 rats were received a normal chow diet as control group, and 24 rats were fed with a high-fat diet (HFD) for 60 days as the HFD group. HFD was composed of 51 % (mass percentage) normal diet, 20 % lard, 20 % sucrose and 9 % egg yolk powder [20]. Body weights, plasma triglycerides (TG), plasma free fatty acids (FFA), fasting blood glucose and fasting plasma insulin levels were measured. Liver tissues were dissected and frozen in liquid nitrogen for 24 h and kept at −80 °C until RNA and protein extraction. All experiments were carried out in accordance with the Institute Guideline for the Care and Use of Laboratory Animals.

52.2.2 *Blood Sampling and Chemistry Assays*

Blood samples were collected by shearing tail tip between 8:00 and 9:00 from animals after overnight fasting. Fasting blood glucose levels were measured with One Touch II blood glucose meter (Lifescan Inc., California, USA). Plasma samples were collected by centrifuge at 12,000 g for 15 min, and stored at −80 °C until assays. Plasma TG was detected with TG kit (Jiancheng Bioengineering Institute, Nanjing, China) and plasma FFA was detected with FFA kit (Applygen Technologies Inc., Beijing, China). The fasting plasma insulin levels were measured with ^{125}I-Insulin Radioimmunoassay Kit (Chemclin Biotech Co. Ltd., Beijing, China) following the manufacturer's protocol.

52.2.3 *Homeostasis Model Assessment of Insulin Resistance (HOMA-IR)*

For evaluation of insulin sensitivity, HOMA-IR was calculated using the formula, HOMA-IR = [fasting plasma insulin (mIU/l) × fasting blood glucose (mmol/l)]/ 22.5 as described [21, 22].

52.2.4 *Liver Histology*

Rats were anesthetized with sodium pentobarbital (80 mg/kg; Sigma) and then infused with 2.5 % glutaraldehyde and 4 % paraformaldehyde in 0.1 M phosphate buffer (pH = 7.4) Liver tissues were dissected and fixed by immersion in 3 % glutaraldehyde in 0.1 M phosphate buffer (pH = 7.4), at 4 °C overnight. Liver morphology was analyzed with hematoxylin & eosin (HE) or van Gieson (VG) staining. For VG staining, image analysis was performed with Image-pro-plus 6.0 on five fields in each section and three slides per rat liver tissue. Percentage of red collagen fibers area to the total visual field area was calculated as collagen content [23]. The other fixed specimens for transmission electron microscope (TEM) followed by osmication in 1 % osmium tetroxide in 0.1 M sodium cacodylate buffer for 2 h at room temperature were dehydrated in a graded acetone series: 50, 75, 90, and 100 % acetone for 10 min each. After having soaked and embedded in epoxy resin for 2 h, the specimens were heated at 60 °C for 48 h. The sections dyed with acetic acid uranium and acetic acid lead were surveyed and taken photos under TEM (JEM-2000EX, JEOL Ltd., Japan) [24].

52.2.5 RNA Analysis

Lives tissue (50–100 mg) was isolated using Trizol reagent (Invitrogen Carlsbad, USA), according to the manufacturer's protocol. Total liver RNA (1 μg) was used to synthesize first-strand cDNA with AMV reverse transcriptase (TOYOBO, Japan) and oligo (dT) primers (Invitrogen Carlsbad, USA) to a final volume of 20 μl. PCR was conducted with primers specific for MMP-9 (rat MMP-9; GenBank NM_174744, forward primer: 5′-GGCACCACCACAACATCA-3′, reverse primer: 5′-GCGGTCGGC GTCGTAGTC-3′, expected PCR fragment: 452 bp), TIMP-1 (rat TIMP-1; GenBank NM_213857; forward primer: 5′-GCAACTCCGACCTTGTCA TC-3′, reverse primer: 5′-AGCGTAGGTCTTGGTGAAGC-3′, expected PCR fragment: 326 bp). The cDNA in each tube was denatured at 94 °C for 5 min for the first cycle and then stepped into 30 PCR cycles containing denaturation at 94 °C for 30 s, extension at 72 °C for 45 s with 30 s of annealing at various temperatures: 53 °C for MMP-9, 58 °C for TIMP-1, and 1 cycle of 5 min at 72 °C. An 8 μl portion of the amplified product was resolved on 2 % agarose gels containing 0.5 μg/ml ethidium bromide and DNA was visualized by Molecular Imager ChemiDoc XRS System (Bio-Rad). The gel images were captured by a scanner, and PCR products were quantified by using Quantity One 1-D Analysis Software (BIO-RAD). Each RT-PCR product was normalized by β-actin from the same cDNA template. Experiments were repeated three times [25].

52.2.6 Western Blot Analysis

Rat liver tissues were homogenized on ice in a buffer (50 mM Tris–HCl, pH 7.4, 1 % NP-40, 1 mM EDTA, 1 mM Na_3VO_3, 1 mM NaF, protease inhibitor cocktail 5 μl/ml), and centrifuged at 12,000 g for 30 min and the supernatant was stored at −70 °C until further analysis. Total protein (10 μg) was denatured and separated on 10 % sodium dodecyl sulphate polyacrylamide mini gels, and transferred electrophoretically to nitrocellulose membranes using a Semi-Dry transfer system (Bio-Rad). The nitrocellulose membranes were incubated 1 h in 8 % non-fat milk/TBST blocking buffer (20 mM Tris Base, 137 mM NaCl, 2 M HCl, 0.1 % Tween 20, pH 7.6), and then incubated with primary antibody of either rat anti-MMP-9

(1:500) or rat anti-TIMP-1 (1:500) (Santa Cruz Biotechnology) in blocking buffer at room temperature for 30 min, then 37 °C for 20 min. Membranes were washed in blocking buffer for 10 min, four times and then incubated with secondary antibody of HRP-conjugated anti-rat (1:1000) at 37 °C for 20 min. Membranes were developed using enhanced chemiluminescence (ECL+, Amersham, Piscataway, NJ) and analyzed using Scion Image (Bio-Rad). All data were normalized to saline control values that are matched to the treated animals from the same experiments.

52.2.7 Measurement of Plasma Collagen-IV Levels

Plasma collagen-IV levels were measured using an ELISA kit following the manufacturer's protocol (Uscnlife, Wuhan, China), and the intensity of the color was read spectrophotometrically at 450 nm using a ZS-2 microplate reader (HRD Co. Ltd., Beijing, China).

52.2.8 Statistical Analysis

All data were expressed as mean ± SEM. The data between control group and HFD group were compared by using one way ANOVA post hoc analysis (Least significant difference, LSD). P value < 0.05 was considered to be statistically significant.

52.3 Results

52.3.1 Generation of Rat IR Model

Body weights of rats treated with HFD for 60 days were similar to that of rats with normal chow diet (Fig. 52.1a), but plasma TG and FFA levels increased markedly in HFD treated rats starting on day 20 compared to control group (Fig. 52.1b, c). Fasting blood glucose levels in HFD treated rats tended to be higher than control rats after 25 days on HFD but did not reach statistically significant, and they were maintained within normal range throughout the course in both groups (Fig. 52.1d). In contrast, compared to control rats, fasting plasma insulin levels in HFD treated rats increased significantly after 20 days on HFD (Fig. 52.1e). Insulin sensitivity evaluated by HOMA-IR in control group was not changed during the experimental course, but it was significantly increased in HFD group since day 20 after HFD treatment (Fig. 52.1f), indicating the HFD treated rats developed IR.

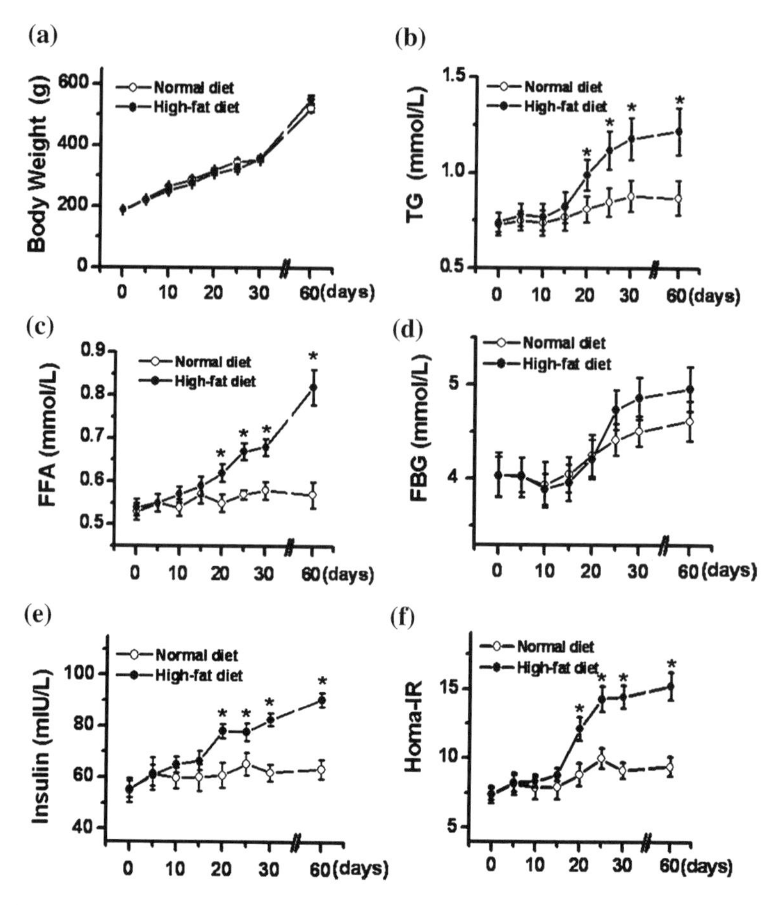

Fig. 52.1 Establishment of IR rat model. **a** Change of body weight within two experimental groups. **b** Change of plasma TG values within two groups. **c** Change of FFA values within two groups. **d** Change of FBG values within two groups. **e** Change of fasting plasma insulin concentration within two groups. **f** Change of Homa-IR within two groups. Values are mean ± SEM (n = 6). $*P < 0.05$ compared with control group

52.3.2 Liver Morphology

At the end of 60-day treatment of chow or HFD, the liver tissues from control rats showed normal structures observed with HE staining (Fig. 52.2a) and VG staining (Fig. 52.2c). In contrast, the liver tissues from HFD treated rats showed steatosis with multiple lipid droplets (Fig. 52.2b), and extensive collagen fibers shown on dark brown color by VG staining (Fig. 52.2d). Percentage of area with the dark brown collagen fibers to total visual field area in HFD group was significantly higher than that of control group (Fig. 52.2e). Under TEM, plasmocytes tightly touched hepatic stellate cells in the control livers (Fig. 52.3a), but in the liver of

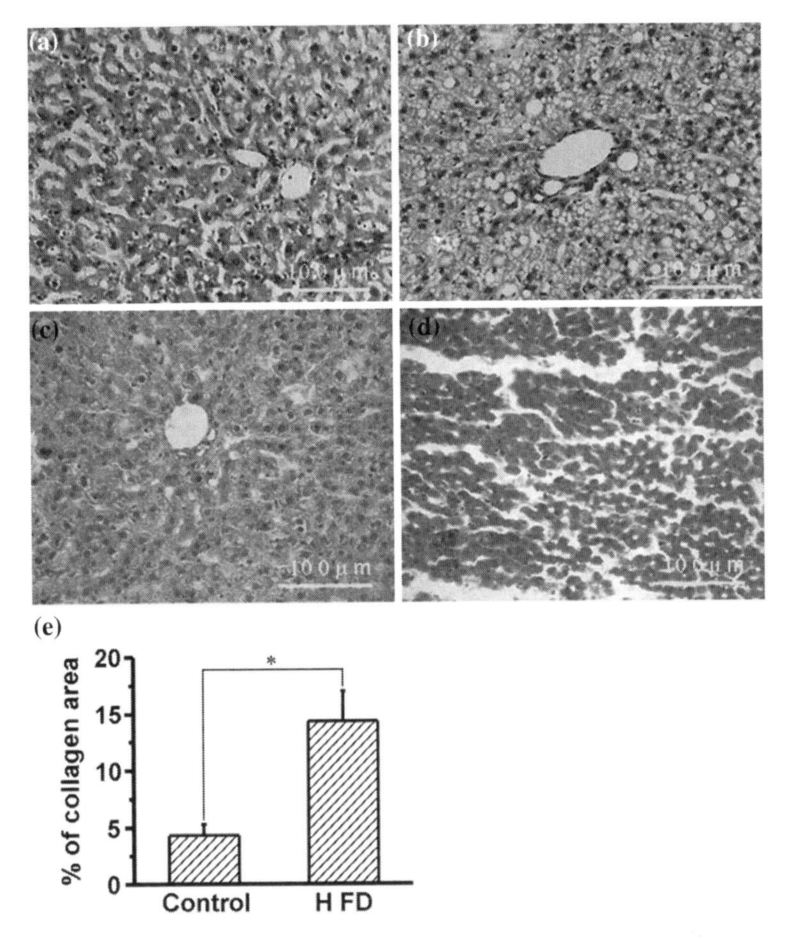

Fig. 52.2 HE staining of liver from control group (**a**) and HFD group (**b**) on 60th day of HFD. VG staining of liver from control group (**c**) and HFD group (**d**) on 60th day respectively. Percentage of red collagen fibers area was calculated as fractions of total visual field area for VG staining (**e**). $*P < 0.01$ compared with control group

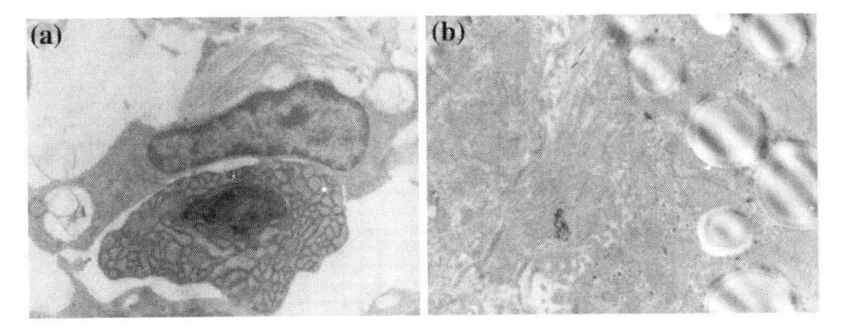

Fig. 52.3 TEM of hepatic stellate cell (**a**) and collagen (**b**). (Original magnification: $\times$ 7500)

HFD group inequality of sizes of lysosomes and lipid droplets emerged in cytoplasm, and more collagen fibers were formed in the interspace among disse cavea and intruded into the tight junctions among hepatocytes (Fig. 52.3b).

52.3.3 Expression of MMP-9 and TIMP-1 mRNA and Protein in Rat Liver Tissue

In HFD group, liver MMP-9 mRNA was significantly increased on day 15 after HFD treatment compared to that of basal condition (day 0), but reduced to basal level on day 30 and lower than basal level on day 60 after HFD treatment (Fig. 52.4a, upper panel), whereas TIMP-1 mRNA from HFD group showed a

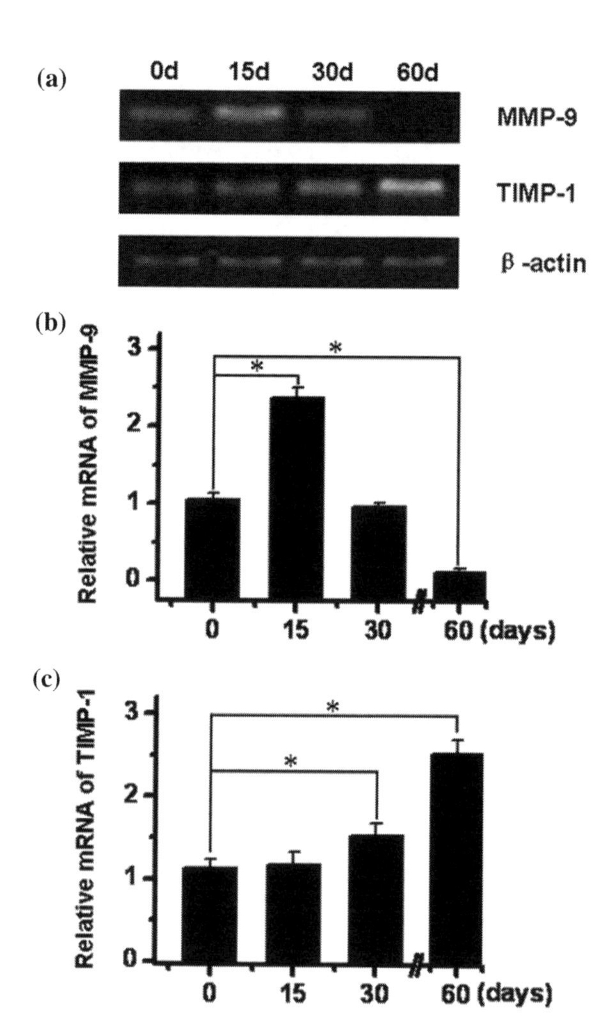

Fig. 52.4 Different expressions of MMP-9 and TIMP-1 mRNA in rat live tissue detected by RT–PCR. **a** The expressed MMP-9 and TIMP-1 mRNA. The cDNA products of the housekeeping gene β-actin were constantly expressed in all experimental groups. Gene expression of MMP-9 and TIMP-1 were normalized with that of β-actin from the same template and shown as a ratio. **b** The relative abundance of MMP-9 mRNA in liver tissue. **c** The relative abundance of TIMP-1 mRNA in liver tissue. Experiments were repeated three times with similar results each time. Values are mean ± SEM (n = 3). $^{*}P < 0.01$

significant increase on day 30 and reached to the highest level on day 60 after HFD treatment (Fig. 52.4a, middle panel). Amount of MMP-9 and TIMP-1 mRNA was normalized by shown on Fig. 52.4b and c respectively. Changes in protein levels of MMP-9 and TIMP-1 from HFD livers exhibited similar patterns with increased MMP-9 protein on day 15 and TIMP-1 protein on day 60 after HFD treatment (Fig. 52.5).

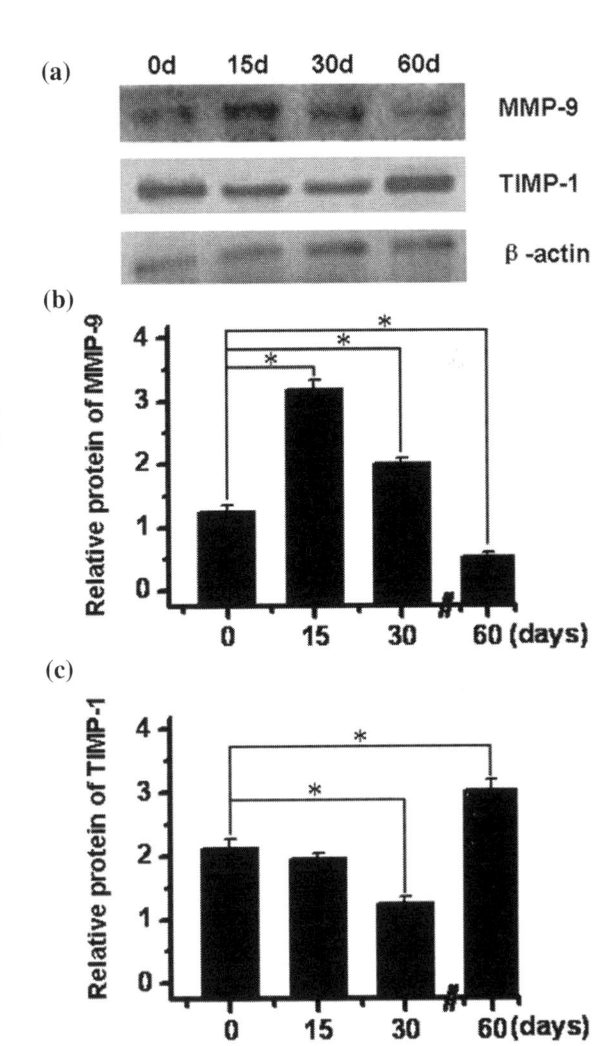

Fig. 52.5 Protein levels of MMP-9 and TIMP-1 in rat live tissue detected by Western blot. **a** Proteins of MMP-9 and TIMP-1 were loaded onto SDS-PAGE gels and followed by Western blot analysis. *Lowest panel* is the loading control staining with anti-β-actin antibody. **b** Data were normalized to the level of β-actin and expressed relative to MMP-9 protein. **c** Data were normalized to the level of β-actin and expressed relative to TIMP-1 protein. Experiments were repeated three times with similar results each time. Values are mean $\pm$ SEM (n = 3). $*P < 0.01$ compared with control group

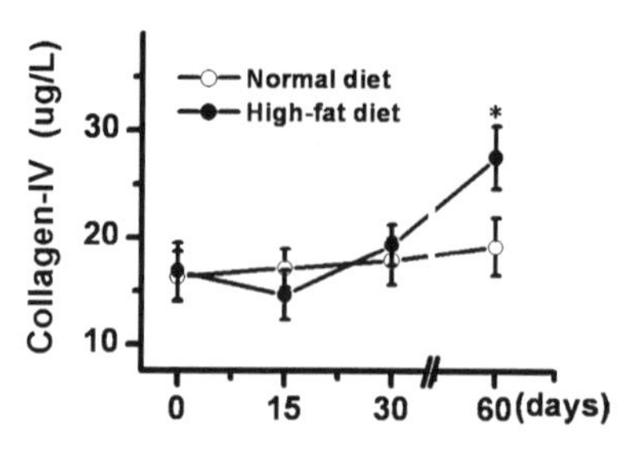

Fig. 52.6 Dynamic changes of plasma collagen-IV content within two groups. $*P < 0.01$ compared with control group

52.3.4 Change in Plasma Collagen-IV Content

Plasma collagen-IV levels in HFD group were comparable to control group before day 30 after HFD treatment, and was significantly elevated on day 60 compared to that of control group (Fig. 52.6).

52.4 Discussion

The high fat lard diet has been shown to induce IR effectively in rodent models [26]. Our previous study showed a similar effect of high lard diet on IR in rats [20]. Using the same high fat lard diet in the present study, we generated the IR rat model with elevated plasma TG and FFA. Fasting blood glucose levels were maintained in normal range in both control and HFD treated groups, whereas fasting plasma insulin of HFD group elevated significantly compared with that of control group, and Homa-IR results further confirmed that high fat diet induced IR on rat successfully.

Although numbers of studies have shown the cross-sectional associations between IR and nonalcoholic fatty liver disease (NAFLD) [27–29], it is not clear whether the accumulation of fat in the liver is a primary event leading to hepatic and then later peripheral IR [30, 31]. In our previous study [20], we found that lipid deposition in the liver and IR emerged at the same time, so that a causal relation between IR and fatty liver could not been confirmed. In the present study, we prolonged HFD treatment to 60 days, and found that hepatic steatosis occurred as well as hepatic collagen increased significantly at the end of experiment even though no confirmed hepatic fibrosis and IR was induced in the middle of the experimental course. We also observed that plasmocytes tightly touched hepatic stellate cells under TEM, suggesting that HFD induces hepatic inflammation. The inflammatory reactions have been shown to contribute to IR [32, 33]. In our previous study [20], we also found an elevated inflammatory mediator of rat fed with high-fat diet. Whether the HFD-induced NAFLD process is responsible for systemic IR via hepatic inflammatory reaction needs to be further clarified.

The fact of elevated plasma collagen levels in HFD group indicates an imbalance between matrix production and degradation processes, although hepatic fibrosis was not confirmed in these animals. One pathological character of hepatic fibrosis is accumulation of extracellular matrix (ECM), which involves excessive production and diminished degradation of ECM. The latter plays a predominant effect during the later course of hepatic fibrosis progress. When type I, III, IV collagen and other ECM increase excessively, they destruct hepatic tissue and damage hepatic functions. Early disruption of the normal hepatic matrix by matrix-degrading proteases hastens its replacement by scar matrix, which has deleterious effects on cell functions.

A critical element in matrix remodeling is a family of MMPs. They are calcium-dependent enzymes that specifically degrade collagens and non-collagenous substrates [34–36]. MMPs activity is regulated at three levels, i.e., gene transcription, proteolytic activation of the proform, and inhibition of the active form. The latter is ensured by a variety of proteinase inhibitors, among which specific TIMPs are of importance [34, 37]. MMPs and TIMPs both involve in hepatic fibrosis progress and recovery. MMPs can degrade excessive ECM, at same time TIMPs inhibit MMPs activity appropriately to avoid MMPs damage normal hepatic tissue. Thus both sides maintain homeostasis of hepatocellular microenvironment [38]. Once causative agent disturbs the balance, hepatic injury or hepatic disease will occur and develop ceaselessly. In addition, hepatic stellate cells play an important role on hepatic fibrosis occurrence [36]. Stellate cells may secrete MMP-9 [39, 40], collectively known as gelatinases, which degrades collagen-IV. Stellate cells can also produce functional TIMP-1 and TIMP-2 [41], and ongoing production of these proteins during liver injury could inhibit the activity of MMPs, leading to reduced degradation of the accumulating ECM during liver injury. Our results indicated that the balance between MMP-9 and TIMP-1 is impaired by HFD treatment. Increased collagen-IV indicates the abnormal change of MMP-9/ TIMP-1 ratio, which ultimately causes hepatic fibrosis. Assessment of plasma collagen-IV could be used as a biomarker of imbalance of MMPs/ TIMPs in order to conduct clinic interventions for prevention from inchoate hepatic fibrosis.

Acknowledgments The work was supported by grants from the Scientific Technological Research Planning of Shaanxi Province (2010K15-05-04). We also acknowledged the assistance from the Electronic Microscope Center of the Fourth Military Medical University.

References

1. Reaven GM (1988) Role of insulin resistance in human disease. Diabetes 37:1595–1607
2. DeFronzo RA, Ferrannini E (1991) Insulin resistance: a multifaceted syndrome responsible for NIDDM, obesity, hypertension, dyslipidemia, and atherosclerotic cardiovascular disease. Diabetes Care 14:173–194

3. Marceau P, Biron S, Hould FS et al (1999) Liver pathology and the metabolic syndrome X in severe obesity. J Clin Endocrinol Metab 84:1513–1517
4. Schwimmer JB, Deutsch R, Rauch JB et al (2003) Obesity, insulin resistance, and other clinicopathological correlates of pediatric nonalcoholic fatty liver disease. J Pediatr 143:500–505
5. Marchesini G, Brizi M, Morselli-Labate AM et al (1999) Association of nonalcoholic fatty liver disease with insulin resistance. Am J Med 107:450–455
6. Marchesini G, Brizi M, Bianchi G et al (2001) Nonalcoholic fatty liver disease: a feature of the metabolic syndrome. Diabetes 50:1844–1850
7. Chitturi S, Abeygunasekera S, Farrell GC et al (2002) NASH and insulin resistance: insulin hypersecretion and specific association with the insulin resistance syndrome. Hepatology 35:373–379
8. Ludwig J, McGill DB, Lindor KD (1997) Review: nonalcoholic steatohepatitis. J Gastroenterol Hepatol 12:398–403
9. Brunt EM, Janney CG, DiBisceglie AM et al (1999) Nonalcoholic steatohepatitis: a proposal for grading and staging the histological lesions. Am J Gastroenterol 94:2467–2474
10. Powell EE, Cooksley WG, Hanson R et al (1990) The natural history of nonalcoholic steatohepatitis: a follow up study of forty-two patients for up to 21 years. Hepatology 11:74–80
11. Angulo P (2002) Nonalcoholic fatty liver disease. N Engl J Med 346:1221–1231
12. Ground KE (1982) Liver pathology in aircrew. Aviat Space Environ Med 53:14–18
13. Hilden M, Christoffersen P, Juhl E et al (1977) Liver histology in a 'normal' population: examinations of 503 consecutive fatal traffic casualties. Scand J Gastroenterol 12:593–597
14. Bellentani S, Saccoccio G, Masutti F et al (2000) Prevalence of and risk factors for hepatic steatosis in Northern Italy. Ann Intern Med 132:112–117
15. Dixon JB, Bhathal PS, O'Brien PE (2001) Nonalcoholic fatty liver disease: predictors of nonalcoholic steatohepatitis and liver fibrosis in the severely obese. Gastroenterology 121:91–100
16. García-Monzón C, Martín-Pérez E, Iacono OL et al (2000) Characterization of pathogenic and prognostic factors of nonalcoholic steatohepatitis associated with obesity. J Hepatol 33:716–724
17. Hamaguchi M, Kojima T, Takeda N et al (2005) The metabolic syndrome as a predictor of nonalcoholic fatty liver disease. Ann Intern Med 143:722–728
18. Fan JG, Zhu J, Li XJ et al (2005) Fatty liver and the metabolic syndrome among Shanghai adults. J Gastroenterol Hepatol 20:1825–1832
19. Neuschwander-Tetri BA, Caldwell SH (2003) Nonalcoholic steatohepatitis: summary of an AASLD single topic conference. Hepatology 37:1202–1219
20. Jiao K, Liu HL, Chen JK et al (2008) Roles of plasma interleukin-6 and tumor necrosis factor-α and FFA and TG in the development of insulin resistance induced by high-fat diet. Cytokine 42:161–169
21. Matthews DR, Hosker JP, Rudenski AS et al (1985) Homeostasis model assessment: insulin resistance and beta-cell function from fasting plasma glucose and insulin concentrations in man. Diabetologia 28:412–419
22. Matthews DR, Hosker JP, Rudenski AS et al (2002) Homeostasis model assessment: insulin resistance and beta-cell function from fasting plasma glucose and insulin concentrations in man. Diabetes Care 25:1891–1892
23. Ishak K, Baptista A, Bianchi L et al (1995) Histological grading and staging of chronic hepatitis. J Hepatol 22:696–699
24. Doggenweiler CF, Frenk S (1965) Staining properties of lanthanumon cell membranes. Proc Natl Acad Sci 53:425–430
25. Chen CL, Huang SK, Lin JL et al (2008) Upregulation of matrix metalloproteinase-9 and tissue inhibitors of metalloproteinases in rapid atrial pacing-induced atrial fibrillation. J Mol Cell Cardiol 45:742–753

26. Buettner R, Parhofer KG, Woenckhaus M et al (2006) Defining high-fat-diet rat models: metabolic and molecular effects of different fat types. J Mol Endocrinol 36:485–501
27. Gupte P, Amarapurkar D, Agal S et al (2004) Non-alcoholic steatohepatitis in type 2 diabetes mellitus. J Gastroenterol Hepatol 19:854–858
28. Assy N, Kaita K, Mymin D et al (2000) Fatty infiltration of liver in hyperlipidemic patients. Dig Dis Sci 45:1929–1934
29. Donati G, Stagni B, Piscaglia F et al (2004) Increased prevalence of fatty liver in arterial hypertensive patients with normal liver enzymes: role of insulin resistance. Gut 53:1020–1023
30. Biddinger SB, Kahn CR (2006) From mice to men: insights into the insulin resistance syndromes. Annu Rev Physiol 68:123–158
31. Samuel VT, Liu ZX, Qu X et al (2004) Mechanism of hepatic insulin resistance in non-alcoholic fatty liver disease. J Biol Chem 279:32345–32353
32. Martinez Ortega, de Victoria E, Xu X, Koska J et al (2009) Macrophage content in subcutaneous adipose tissue: associations with adiposity, age, inflammatory markers, and whole-body insulin action in healthy Pima Indians. Diabetes 58:385–393
33. Haus JM, Kashyap SR, Kasumov T et al (2009) Plasma ceramides are elevated in obese subjects with type 2 diabetes and correlate with the severity of insulin resistance. Diabetes 58:337–343
34. Iredale JP (2001) Hepatic stellate cell behavior during resolution of liver injury. Semin Liver Dis 21:427–436
35. Arthur MJ (1995) Collagenases and liver fibrosis. J Hepatol 22:43–48
36. Benyon RC, Arthur MJ (2001) Extracellular of matrix degradation and the role of hepatic stellate cells. Semin Liver Dis 21:373–384
37. Van Pham TD, Couchie N, Martin-Garcia Y et al (2008) Expression of matrix metalloproteinase-2 and -9 and of tissue inhibitor of matrix metalloproteinase-1 in liver regeneration from oval cells in rat. Matrix Biol 27:674–681
38. Nagase H (1996) Zinc metalloproteinases in health and disease. Taylor & Franics, London, pp 153–204
39. Han YP (2006) Matrix metalloproteinases, the pros and cons, in liver fibrosis. J Gastroenterol Hepatol 21(Suppl.3):S88–S91
40. Han YP, Yan C, Zhou L et al (2007) A matrix metalloproteinase-9 activation cascade by hepatic stellate cells in trans-differentiation in the three dimensional extracellular matrix. J Biol Chem 282:12928–12939
41. Arthur MJ (2000) Fibrogenesis II. Metalloproteinases and their inhibitors in liver fibrosis. Am J Physiol Gastrointest Liver Physiol 279:G245–G249

Chapter 53
Evaluation Method for Software System Reliability

Han Lu, Shufen Liu, Zhao Jin and Xue Fan

Abstract Evaluation method for software system reliability is the foundation of studying software system reliability. In this paper, we propose an evaluation method for software system reliability, and flight simulation system is used as an example to illustrate in detail how this method is used to construct evaluation model for system reliability. The method has certain reference value for reliability evaluation work of large and complex software systems.

Keywords Software system · Reliability evaluation · Model · Weight coefficient grading method · Module

53.1 Introduction

With the development of computer technology, software systems become more and more complex. If the reliability can't meet the requirement of higher standard, the possibility of system failure will be larger and the loss will be larger too. Hence, the reliability of software system catches more and more attention.

The model of software system reliability is the foundation of system reliability analysis and evaluation, the more complex the system is, the more complex the model will be. The study of reliability evaluation method has very important guiding significance to the improvement of system reliability and enhancement of system quality.

In this paper, we first give a brief introduction to weight coefficient grading method. Then we propose a weight coefficient grading method based on reliability evaluations of various function modules by using G–O (Goel–Okumoto) software

H. Lu (✉) · S. Liu · Z. Jin · X. Fan
College of Computer Science and Technology, Jilin University, Changchun, 130012, People's Republic of China
e-mail: hanlu@jlu.edu.cn

S. Li et al. (eds.), *Frontier and Future Development of Information Technology in Medicine and Education*, Lecture Notes in Electrical Engineering 269,
DOI: 10.1007/978-94-007-7618-0_53,

reliability model [1, 2]. Using flight simulation system as an example, we point out the advantage of this method compared to conventional methods, and illustrate how the method is used to do reliability analysis. Finally, we give conclusions and prospects to the application of the method.

53.2 Weight Coefficient Grading Method

In a software system, some modules will be executed only when called, they will not participate in execution when not called. To evaluate the software reliability of the whole system more efficiently, we assume all function modules in the system will be called during every execution of the whole system. As each module in the software system has different importance and different execution time, and the complexity and working time are also different, one can use a grading method to determine the occupation percentage of each module in the reliability model of whole system. The grading coefficients include:

(1) Complexity of the module

The software reliability of a system often is determined by the complexity of the software system. The more complex the system is, the less its reliability will be, and vice versa. So system complexity is inverse proportional to system software reliability. In a simulation system, each module can be treated as independent sub-system, the complexity can be measured by using the number of code lines. Complexity factor $\gamma j1$ can be used as grading coefficient of complexity. The grading coefficient is given as the ratio of number of code lines of sub-system to that of whole software system. The formula is:

$$\gamma_{j1} = B_{j1} / \sum B_{j1} \tag{53.1}$$

B_{j1} is the number of code lines of the j sub-system, i.e. the higher the percentage of code lines occupied by this sub-system in the whole system code lines, the more complex the sub-system will be.

(2) The importance of module in a system

As not all modules participate in all works during software system running, from the software reliability point of view, the more essential a module is to the running of whole software system, the more important it will be in the software system. So the core modules and the modules supporting the system to complete information running are more important. And non-core modules are of less importance. A importance factor γ_{j2} can be used as grading coefficient to evaluate the importance. The factor can be given by specialist according to their experience, or can be given by the ratio of tasks each module participated in. The formula is:

$$\gamma_{j2} = B_{j2} / \sum B_{j2} \tag{53.2}$$

B_{j2} is the number of functions the j sub-system participated in, i.e. the higher percentage of function numbers a sub-system participated into the whole function numbers of the system, the more important the sub-system will be [3].

(3) Maturity of module

The maturity of each module in a software system also has strong influence to the software reliability of the system. The maturer the development technique and module structure of the module and the more it is reused, the higher the stability and quality it will be of, the higher the corresponding software reliability will be. For a simulation system, because of existing development experiences, each module will have different maturity. Reused modules or modules with similar development experiences will have higher maturity. But new demand-oriented function modules will have lower maturity. Because the concept of how to distinguish existed or to be developed module is rather obscure, in this paper, we adopt the method of grading by specialists according to their experiences [4, 5]. Maturity factor γ_{j3} is used as grading coefficient to measure system maturity. The maturity of each module will be graded by specialists according to their experiences. Then the ratio of maturity of each module to that of the whole system will be calculated according to the grades. The formula is:

$$\gamma_{j3} = B_{j3} / \sum B_{j3} \tag{53.3}$$

B_{j3} is the grade for the j sub-system, i.e. the higher percentage of a certain sub-system's maturity occupied in the whole system's maturity, the higher maturity the sub-system will be. In the development of simulation software, high maturity modules need to be reused or similarly developed to construct key modules, so as to ensure the software reliability of whole system meets standard.

(4) Running time of module

When the software system is running, the running time of different module is different. Hence the influence of different module to the reliability of whole system will be different. Running time thus becomes a weight coefficient of measuring the influence to software system reliability [6]. As a real time system, the influence of time to reliability of the whole flight simulation system is especially obvious. When measuring, software execution time (i.e. the time the software is run by CPU) should be used as the time measuring unit. Time factor γ_{j4} is used as grading coefficient for measuring influence of module running time to software reliability of the whole system. Real running time of each module and that of the whole system need to be obtained, and the ratio of each module's running time occupied in the running time of whole system is calculated. The formula is:

$$\gamma_{j4} = B_{j4} / \sum B_{j4} \tag{53.4}$$

B_{j4} is the real running time of j sub-system, i.e. the higher percentage a sub-system's running time to that of the whole system's running time, the higher weight of the influence to system's software reliability will be.

After determining the grades of the above four aspects which influence software reliability occupied in the whole system, we need to determine the influence of each module to the software reliability of whole system, i.e. the weight coefficient of each module in the system [7]. The weight coefficient is denoted by K_j. And the formula is:

$$K_j = W_j / \sum W_j \quad (53.5)$$

in which, W_j is the product of all grading coefficients, i.e.

$$W_j = \prod_{i=1}^{n} \gamma_{ji} \quad (53.6)$$

in which n is the number of grading coefficients. In flight simulation system, $n = 4$. γ_{ji} is the value of i grading coefficient for j module.

If a module has higher influence to the whole software system, its coefficient K_j will be larger, and higher reliability of the module will need to be ensured.

53.3 Reliability Evaluation of Each Function Module Based on G–O Software Reliability Model

Because every module developer has similar experiences, and every error in each module will cause invalid run of the module, the requirement of similar tested possibility and seriousness is fulfilled.

During test and running of the flight simulation system, system developer, tester and user will record the phenomena of errors as failure reports, when they detect a system error. Software engineers thus can trace the problem and find the reason according to these reports, hence can make corresponding changes to the system. Data needed for analysis of reliability are also collected, to evaluate software reliability.

For each module in the system, G–O software reliability model is used in reliability evaluation. In this model, accumulated failure number N(t) of each module is used as a function of time, and described using non-homogeneous Poisson Process Model [8, 9]. Assumed preconditions satisfy:

(1) Running environment should be similar to anticipated operating environment

In the design and development of command and guide system, the executing operating environment is considered. Running environment is similar to anticipated operating environment.

(2) Detected error numbers in different period should be independent

During test period, each module is tested, modules can communicate only through communication ports, the test and failure detection are independently performed.

(3) The seriousness of every error and the possibility of detecting it should be similar

Because every module developer has similar experiences, and every error in each module will cause invalid run of the module, the requirement of similar tested possibility and seriousness is fulfilled.

Let N(t) be accumulated invalid number at time t, m(t) be the expected value of N(t). According to the reliability model of G–O software, we have the following equation:

$$m_i(t) = a_i\left(1 - e^{-b_i t}\right) \tag{53.7}$$

$$\lambda_i(t) = a_i b_i e^{-b_i t} \tag{53.8}$$

in which, a_i, b_i, are the expected value of total possible detected error number and remaining failure incidence, they are special parameters of the model and are approximated by maximum likelihood of the parameters. They can be determined by the following equation [10]:

$$a_i\left(1 - e^{-b_i t_m}\right) = n_m \tag{53.9}$$

$$a_i t_m e^{-b_i t_m} = \sum_{j=1}^{m} \frac{\left(n_j - n_{j-1}\right)\left(t_j e^{-b_i t_j} - t_{j-1} e^{-b_i t_{j-1}}\right)}{e^{-b_i t_{j-1}} - e^{-b_i t_j}} \tag{53.10}$$

Assuming $a_i = a$, $b_i = b$, from G–O software reliability model, we get:

$$MTBF = \frac{1}{\lambda(t)} = \frac{1}{ab} e^{-bt} \tag{53.11}$$

$$n(t) = ae^{-bt} \quad (n(t) \text{is the residue error number}) \tag{53.12}$$

Hence, according to the above model, after collecting measured error number and running time of each module, the software reliability of each module can be approximated, described by MTBF (Mean Time Between Failures) and n (residue failure number).

53.4 Integrated Software Reliability Model of Flight Simulation System

After evaluation of each module in system by using G–O software reliability model, combining structure characteristics of the whole system and function

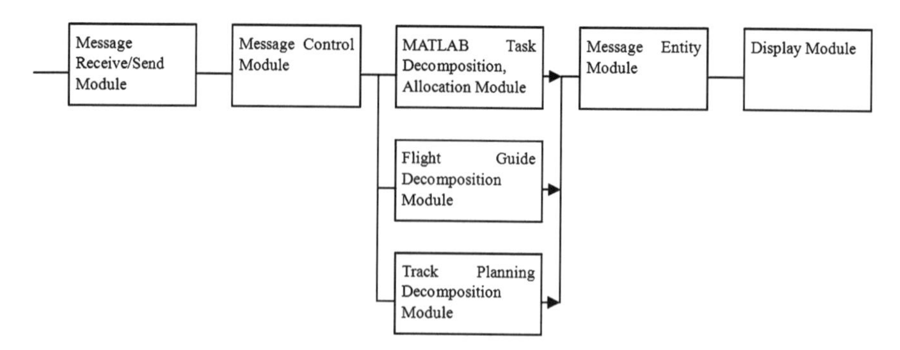

Fig. 53.1 Reliability block diagram of flight simulation system software

calling relations, reliability modeling is performed on simulation system. The reliability block diagram is shown in Fig. 53.1.

In the system, message receive/send module, message control module, message entity module and message display module are essential modules for system running, they participate in every task of the system. MATLAB task decomposition and allocation module, track planning module and flight guide module form a combination connection model, and fulfill system core tasks together. In such combination connection model, the participation rate of each module is similar; hence the proportionality factor of the combination connection model is 1/3.

Since the weight coefficient of each module in the system is different, according to the grading method introduced in the second section of this paper the grading weight coefficient of each module can be obtained, let it be K_i, and substitute grading weight coefficient of each module in the system. Assuming the measured reliability of each module is R_i, in which the reliability of message receive/send module is R_1, weight coefficient is K_1; reliability of message control module is R_2, weight coefficient is K_2; reliability of MATLAB task decomposition and allocation module is R_3, weight coefficient is K_3; reliability of flight guide module is R_4, weight coefficient is K_4; reliability of track planning and decomposition module is R_5, weight coefficient is K_5; reliability of message entity is R_6, weight coefficient is K_6; reliability of message display module is R_7, weight coefficient is K_7. The following system software reliability evaluation model can be obtained:

$$R = R_1K_1R_2K_2\left(\frac{1}{3}R_3K_3 + \frac{1}{3}R_4K_4 + \frac{1}{3}R_5K_5\right)R_6K_6R_7K_7 \tag{53.13}$$

In this model, R_i is the reliability of each module which can be measured by using basic G–O model, K_i is the weight proportion of each module in the system which can be calculated by using formulas (53.5) and (53.6) in the second section, measuring the complexity, running time, importance and maturity of each module in the system. The test data of each module of command and guide simulation system during debugging period are shown in Table 53.1.

Tab. 53.1 Some reliability data of certain debugging period of flight simulation system

Module	Code lines	Measured Failure number	Test time (h)
Message receive/send module	2378	13	12
Message control module	2171	16	12
Message entity module	1326	17	12
Message display module	1824	23	12
Matlab task decomposition and allocation module	2731	31	4
Track planning module	1742	22	4
Flight guide module	1087	19	4

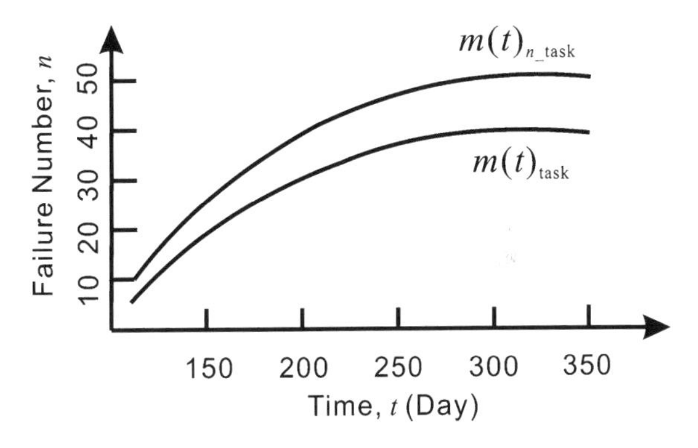

Fig. 53.2 Comparison of module weight coefficient reliability model curve with G–O software reliability model curve

The failure numbers in the table are the failure numbers detected during entire test period. The test data can be substituted into software reliability model of flight simulation system based on module weight coefficient, the software reliability evaluation functions and future reliability expected values can be obtained [11].

Figure 53.2 shows simulated comparison in MATLAB environment of software reliability model curve of system adopting modularized weight coefficient method with software reliability model curve of system adopting normal G–O software reliability model.

From the graph, we can see that software reliability model failure number average value curve based on modularized weight coefficient $m(t)_{\text{task}}$ is lower than the failure number average value curve $m(t)_{\text{n\_task}}$ of normal G–O software reliability model.

53.5 Conclusions and Prospects

With the development of science and technology, the complexity of software system is increasing. The problem of how to perform proper and effective evaluation of the reliability of large complex software system is catching more people's attention. In this paper, through the investigation of system reliability evaluation methods, based on existing reliability evaluation model, we proposed a new weight coefficient grading method. When applying the new method to the evaluation of large complex system's reliability, it can reduce the problem of function and unit loss effectively, it can increase the accuracy of system reliable modeling. It also gives suggestions to lowering the complexity of software system reliable modeling and to multi-people cooperation.

References

1. Huang XZ (2002) Software reliability security and quality. Publishing House of Electronics Industry, Beijing
2. Shi Z, He XG, Wu Z (2000) Software reliability and its estimation. J Comput Appl 11:2–5
3. Cai KY (2000) Towards a conceptual framework of software runreliability modeling. Inform Sci 126:137–163
4. Far B (2007) Software reliability engineering for agile software development. In: Canadian conference on electrical and computer engineering, pp 694–697
5. Sun SJ, Chu RZ, Liu YR (2010) The analasis and evaluation of a new software reliability model. In: Proceedings of the international conference on computer application and system modeling, vol 8, V8425–V8429
6. Li HF, Lu MY, Li QY (2006) Software reliability metrics selecting method based on analytic hierarchy process. In: Proceedings of the international conference on quality software, pp 337–344
7. Cai X, Lyu MR (2007) Software reliability modeling with test coverage: experimentation and measurement with A fault-tolerant software project. In: Proceedings of the international symposium on software reliability engineering, pp 17–26
8. Condon E, Cukier M, He T (2007) Applying software reliability models on security incidents. In: Proceedings of the international symposium on software reliability engineering, pp 159–168
9. Cao Y, Zhu QX, Yang B (2009) The prediction model of software reliability based on fractals. Commun Comput Inf Sci 30:124–136
10. Huang CY, Lyu MR (2011) Estimation and analysis of some generalized multiple change-point software reliability models. IEEE T Reliab 60:498–514
11. Wu Y, Lu M, Ruan L (2006) Software reliability qualitative evaluation method based on unascertained mathematics. In: Proceedings of the European safety and reliability conference 2:1451–1458

Chapter 54
P System Based Particle Swarm Optimization Algorithm

Qiang Du, Laisheng Xiang and Xiyu Liu

Abstract Particle Swarm Optimization algorithm is a kind of excellent optimization algorithm, and has been widely used in many fields. In order to overcome the premature convergence and improve the accuracy of the PSO, we combine some related theories of membrane computing with PSO. The new algorithm can effectively balance the global search and partial optimization. Simulation results based on three bench functions show that the new algorithm can effectively solve the problem of premature, and effectively improve the convergence precision. At the same time, the algorithm in solving TSP problem also shows good optimization ability.

Keywords Membrane · Computing · Particle swarm optimization · Global search · Partial optimization

54.1 Introduction

Particle swarm optimization algorithm, simply called PSO, originated in the research of feeding behavior of birds and fish. Because of its versatility and simple algorithm formula, and have strong ability of global optimization, the PSO quickly become a powerful tool to solve difficult problems [1]. PSO algorithm has been widely used in electric power system optimization, clustering analysis, neural network training, and many other fields.

Q. Du · L. Xiang (✉) · X. Liu
School of Management Science and Engineering, Shandong Normal University, Jinan, China
e-mail: creazydu@163.com

Q. Du
e-mail: 807630393@qq.com

S. Li et al. (eds.), *Frontier and Future Development of Information Technology in Medicine and Education*, Lecture Notes in Electrical Engineering 269,
DOI: 10.1007/978-94-007-7618-0_54,

Although the particle swarm optimization has so many advantages, in the late iteration algorithm, the algorithm is easy to fall into local optimum because of the reduction of species diversity; we also call this phenomenon of premature convergence [2]. Many researchers have done a lot of work to improve the basic algorithm. Besides inertia weight improvement strategy, many scholars introduced other algorithms into the particle swarm optimization: Wu Dinghai introduces the chaotic mutation into PSO algorithm, and presents a model of double particle swarm optimization based on chaotic mutation [3]. Ren Zihui put forward a kind of particle swarm optimization algorithm based on improved entropy [4]. Yao Kun introduces the genetic algorithm into the particle swarm optimization algorithm [5]. Besides, there are adaptive PSO [6] and a series of improved PSO algorithm. Various algorithms above have different characteristics but also exist some defects.

Membrane computing is a new branch of natural computation, which abstracts the computing model from cell structure and function, and from the group collaboration of tissues and organs [7]. Membrane computing is put forward by Paun, academician of European academy of sciences and academy of sciences of Romania, in research report of the computer center in Turku, Finland, and formal papers saw the publication in 2000 [8]. Therefore membrane computing system is also called P, P system is mainly composed of three parts: hierarchical structure of the membrane, multisets and evolution rule. P system is a computation model of great parallel, distributed and non-deterministic. Research shows that simple P system calculation model is equal to Turing machine's computation ability [9].

Inspired by membrane computing, this paper proposes a new particle swarm optimization method based on P system. We simply call it P-PSO. It put particles in different membranes of P system, and according to the different function, we divide the membranes into main membrane and auxiliary membrane. Particles in the main membrane are primarily responsible for local optimization; particles in auxiliary membrane are mainly for the global search, in order to find the target area, which contains the optimal solution. Auxiliary membrane will be effective to avoid algorithm falls into local optimum, which prevent the problem of premature convergence. Different membrane (different particle swarms) exchange information through the membrane calculation rules.

54.2 PSO and P System

This section will present PSO and P systems briefly.

54.2.1 Particle Swarm Optimization

PSO is a kind of optimization algorithm based on swarm intelligence, and originated in studies on bird of prey. According to the experience of the group and their experiences, birds, in search of food in the flight, will be constantly to adjust the flight status. If the bird is seen as a particle in the space, and the location of the food is seen as the optimal solution of optimization algorithm, then the birds foraging process becomes a solving process of particle swarm. In the PSO algorithm, each particle adjust its speed and position, according to its most optimal location recorded by its own experiences (individual optimal) and the group optimal position (global optimal).

Each particle updates its speed and position, according to the following iterative formula, and produces a new particle of the next generation.

$$v_{id}^{t+1} = wv_{id}^{t} + c_1 r_1 \left(p_{id}^{t} - x_{id}^{t}\right) + c_2 r_2 (p_{gd}^{t} - x_{id}^{t}) \tag{54.1}$$

$$x_{id}^{t+1} = x_{id}^{t} + v_{id}^{t+1} \tag{54.2}$$

v_{id}^{t+1} is the speed of dimension d of particle i in the $(t + 1)$th generation. v_{id}^{t} is the speed of dimension d of particle i in the tth generation. x_{id}^{t+1} is the position of dimension d of particle i in the $(t + 1)$th generation. x_{id}^{t} is the position of dimension d of particle i in the tth generation. p_{id}^{t} is individual history optimization position of particle i in the tth generation. p_{gd}^{t} is optimization position of particles in the tth generation. r_1 and r_2 are elements from uniform random sequence in range (0, 1), c_1 and c_2 are the acceleration coefficients, usually $c_1 = c_2 = 2$. w is the weight coefficient.

54.2.2 P System

Inspired by biological cells, Paun, European academy of sciences, put forward P system. In this article we only study the Cell-like P system, Tissue-like and Neural-like P systems are beyond the scope of this article. Basic Cell-like P system can be expressed as the following multiple groups [10]:

$$\prod = (V, T, \mu, w_1, \cdots w_m, (R_1, \rho_1), \cdots, (R_m, \rho_m)) \tag{54.3}$$

(1) V is the alphabet of objects;
(2) T is the output alphabet;
(3) μ is a membrane structure of degree m; The structure with m membranes and the regions labeled by H; $H = \{1, 2, \ldots, m\}$;
(4) $wi \in V^*(1 \le i \le m)$ are the multisets of objects associated with the m regions of μ;
(5) $R_i, 1 \le i \le m$,are the finite sets of multiset rewriting rules associated with the m regions ofμ;

Figure 54.1 is a simple diagram of membrane structure

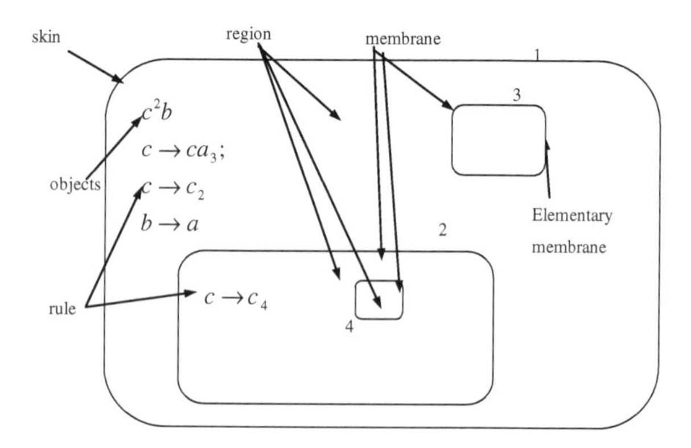

Fig. 54.1 Example of membrane structure

54.3 P System Based Particle Swarm Optimization Algorithm

Inspired by P system and the limitations of PSO algorithm, this paper proposes particle swarm optimization based on P system (P-PSO). It put particles in different membranes of P system. According to the function different, we divide the membranes into main membrane and auxiliary membrane. There is a main membrane, several auxiliary membranes. Particles in auxiliary membranes are responsible for the exploration (global search); Particles in main membranes are responsible for the development (partial optimization). According to these principles, particles in different membrane need to update their position and velocity through different ways: for the purpose of exploring, particles in Auxiliary membranes will be as far as possible to keep the population diversity, and to search the whole space; for the purpose of development, particles in main membrane will search optimal solution carefully, after receiving the message from the auxiliary membranes. Exchange of information between different membranes is through communication rules which between different membranes.

54.3.1 Design of P-PSO

In the P-PSO, each particle's position (the corresponding solution of optimization problem) is seen as an object in the membrane. Membrane structure is shown in Fig. 54.2, the P system can be expressed as the following multiple groups:

$$\prod = (V, T, \mu, w_1, \cdots w_6, n_1, \cdots n_6(R_1, \rho_1), \cdots, (R_6, \rho_6)) \qquad (54.4)$$

Among them, V is the alphabet, T is output alphabet, μ is a membrane structure, $w_1, \cdots, w_6$ are multisets within the membranes, $n_1, \cdots, n_6$ are numbers of particles in membrane, $R_i (1 \leq i \leq 6)$ is the rule corresponding to membrane i, $\rho_i (1 \leq i \leq 6)$ is the priority of rules in membrane i.

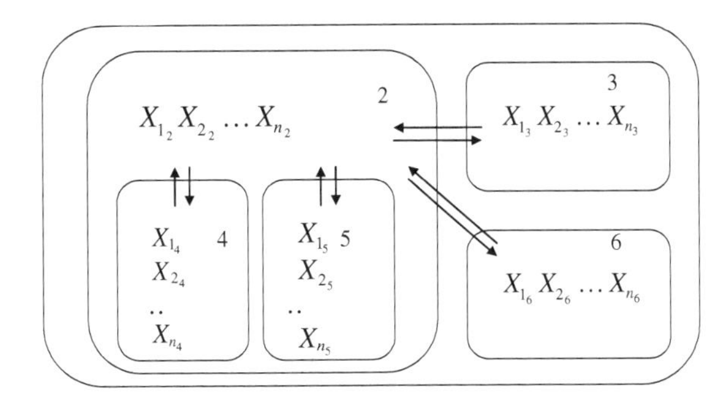

Fig. 54.2 Membrane structure of P-PSO

54.3.2 Encoding Rule

In traditional membrane computing, letters are seen as objects. In order to meet the needs of the new algorithm, in the new algorithm we will adopt a new kind of coding way, we use the real number to encode directly. $X_i^t = (x_{i1}^t, x_{i2}^1, \cdots, x_{id}^t)$ is seen as an object. multi-sets of objects in the ith region can be expressed as $w_i = (X_{1_i} X_{2_i} \cdots X_{n_i})$, i = 1, 2, 3, 4, 5, 6. n is the number of particles in membrane i. $X_{1_i}^t, X_{2_i}^t, \cdots, X_{n_i}^t$ are positions of particles of tth generation in region i, besides $X_{n_i}^t = (x_{n_i1}^t, x_{n_i2}^t, \cdots, x_{n_id}^t)$, and d is the dimension of search space. The total number of objects of each generation in the membrane system is $\sum_{i=1}^{6} n_i$.

54.3.3 Evolutionary Rules

Membrane 2 is the main membrane, and 3, 4, 5 and 6 are auxiliary membranes. Membrane 1 is responsible to recycle particles that are abandoned by the main membrane, there is no specific operation in 1. Particles in auxiliary membranes are responsible for the exploration (to find the general area of optimal solution). Particles in the auxiliary must have strong global search ability, thus this need the particles to keep population diversity in the iterations of algorithm, so as to guarantee the population to search every area. Particles in main membranes are responsible for the development (to find the concrete position of the optimal solution), thus this need the particles to have strong local optimization ability. So main membrane receive good particles to guide the optimization of the algorithm.

In order to ensure that particles in membrane 3 have strong global search ability in the iteration process, we will introduce the population diversity [11] into the P-PSO algorithm.

$$diversity(S) = \frac{1}{|S| \cdot |L|} \cdot \sum_{i=1}^{|S|} \sqrt{\sum_{j=1}^{N} (p_{ij} - \bar{p}_j)^2} \qquad (54.5)$$

$$V_{id}^{t+1} = v_{id}^{t} - c_1 r_1 (p_{id}^{t} - x_{id}^{t}) - c_2 r_2 (p_{gd}^{t} - x_{id}^{t}) \tag{54.6}$$

Population diversity are given in the range of (*dir_low, dir_hig*). During the iterations of the algorithm, we will l measure population diversity in each generation. If the value of diversity within the scope, the particle's velocity and position will update according to the formula (54.1) and (54.2). If the value is less than lower limit *dir_low*, particle velocity and position will update according to the formula (54.6) and (54.2). Thus these measures increase the population diversity, and ensure the global search ability of the particles. In each generation, we will sort the particles according to the fitness from small to large. The first 20 particles will be sent into the membrane 2. Membrane exchange rule is shown as below:

$$r_3 : X'_{1_3} \cdots X'_{20_3} \cdots X'_{n_3} \rightarrow X'_{1_3} \cdots X'_{20_3} \cdots X'_{n_3} (X'_{1_3} \cdots X'_{20_3})_{in2} \tag{54.7}$$

Thus, $X'_{1_3} \cdots X'_{20_3} \cdots X'_{n_3}$ is the sequence after sorted.

Particles in the membrane 4 update speed and position according to the formula (54.1) and (54.2). Firstly, We will sort the particles according to the fitness from large to small; secondly, initialize the worst s (set number for s) particles; lastly, reorder the particles. After that, sent the first 20 particles into membrane 2. The corresponding rules are as follows:

$$r_4 : X'_{1_4} \cdots X'_{(n-s)_4} X'_{(n-s+1)_4} \cdots X'_{n_4} \rightarrow X'_{1_4} \cdots X'_{(n-s)_4} X^{init}_{(n-s+1)_4} \cdots X^{init}_{n_4} \tag{54.8}$$

$$X'_{1_4} \cdots X'_{20_4} \cdots X'_{n_4} \rightarrow X'_{41} \cdots X'_{20_4} \cdots X'_{n_4} (X'_{1_4} \cdots X'_{20_4})_{in2}$$

To abandon the worst part of particles, and re-initialize them, may find better fitness value. More important of this operation is that it increases the diversity of the population, and will ensure the global search ability of the algorithm.

Particles in membrane 5 iterate according to the standard particle swarm algorithm. The particle velocity and position updating formula according to (54.1) and (54.2), particles will be sorted after every iteration. The first 20 particles will be sent into membrane 2. The corresponding rules are as follows:

$$r_5 : X'_{1_5} \cdots X'_{20_5} \cdots X'_{n_5} \rightarrow X'_{1_5} \cdots X'_{20_5} \cdots X'_{n_5} (X'_{1_5} \cdots X'_{20_5})_{in2} \tag{54.9}$$

Particles in the membrane 6 update speed and position according to the formula (54.1) and (54.2). Among them, the inertia weight w will adopt strategies based on tangent function [12]. w updates according to the formula (54.10).

$$w(t) = (w_{start} - w_{end}) \times \tan(0.875 \times (1 - (t/t_{\max})^k)) + w_{end} \tag{54.10}$$

The first 20 particles will be sent into membrane 2. The corresponding rules are as follows:

$$r_6 : X'_{1_6} \cdots X'_{20_6} \cdots X'_{n_6} \rightarrow X'_{1_6} \cdots X'_{2_6} \cdots X'_{n_6} (X'_{1_6} \cdots X'_{20_6})_{in2} \tag{54.11}$$

Particles in the main membrane 2 update speed and position according to the formula (54.1) and (54.2). After receive 80 particles from auxiliary membranes, particles will be sorted according to the fitness. The worst 80 particles will be discarded into membrane 1. In order to guide particles in auxiliary membrane to search more effectively, the main membrane send the best particle into every auxiliary membrane. The corresponding rules are as follows:

$$r_2 : X'_{1_2} \cdots X'_{n_2} \cdots X'_{n+60} \rightarrow X'_{1_2} \cdots X'_{n_2} (X'_{n+1} \cdots X'_{n+60})_{in1} \tag{54.12}$$

$$X'_{1_2} \rightarrow (X'_{1_2})_{in3} (X'_{1_2})_{in4} (X'_{1_2})_{in5} (X'_{1_2})_{in6} \tag{54.13}$$

To sum up, the P-PSO model can be expressed as the following multiple groups:

$$\prod = (V, T, C, \mu, w_1, \cdots w_6, n_1 \cdots n_6 (R_1, \rho_1), \cdots, (R_6, \rho_6))$$

$$\begin{cases} \mu = [_1 [_2 [_4]_4 [_5]_5]_2 [_3]_3 [_6]_6]_1 \\ w_i = X_{1_i}, \cdots, X_{n_i} (1 \leq i \leq 6) \\ R_i = \{ r_i; r_{i,\ update} \} (1 \leq i \leq 6) \\ r_2 : X'_{1_2} \cdots X'_{n_2} \cdots X'_{n+80} \rightarrow X'_{1_2} \cdots X'_{n_2} \left(X'_{n+1} \cdots X'_{n+80} \right)_{in1} \\ r'_2 : X'_{1_2} \rightarrow \left(X'_{1_2} \right)_{in3} \left(X'_{1_2} \right)_{in4} \left(X'_{1_2} \right)_{in5} \left(X'_{1_2} \right)_{in6} \\ r_3 : X'_{1_3} \cdots X'_{20_3} \cdots X'_{n_3} \rightarrow X'_{1_3} \cdots X'_{20_3} \cdots X'_{n_3} \left(X'_{1_3} \cdots X'_{20_3} \right)_{in2} \\ r_4 : X'_{1_4} \cdots X'_{(n-s)_4} X'_{(n-s+1)_4} \cdots X'_{n_4} \rightarrow X'_{1_4} \cdots X'_{(n-s)_4} X^{init}_{(n-s+1)_4} \cdots X^{init}_{n_4} \\ r'_4 : X'_{1_4} \cdots X'_{20_4} \cdots X'_{n_4} \rightarrow X'_{1_4} \cdots X'_{20_4} \cdots X'_{n_4} \left(X'_{1_4} \cdots X'_{20_4} \right)_{in2} \\ r_5 : X'_{1_5} \cdots X'_{20_5} \cdots X'_{n_5} \rightarrow X'_{1_5} \cdots X'_{20_5} \cdots X'_{n_5} \left(X'_{1_5} \cdots X'_{20_5} \right)_{in2} \\ r_6 : X'_{1_6} \cdots X'_{20_6} \cdots X'_{n_6} \rightarrow X'_{1_6} \cdots X'_{2_6} \cdots X'_{n_6} \left(X'_{1_6} \cdots X'_{20_6} \right)_{in2} \\ \rho_i = \{ r_{i,\ update} > r_i \} (1 \leq i \leq 6) \end{cases} \tag{2.8}$$

54.3.4 The Procedure of P-PSO Algorithm

Step 1 initialization: build the P system structure, initialize the position and velocity of the particle in membranes, and find individual optimal value (Pi) and the global optimal value (Pg) in every membrane.

Step 2 particles in auxiliary membranes update position and velocity respectively according to their corresponding formula.
Step 3 particles in auxiliary membranes will be sorted respectively, and good particles will be sent into the main membrane according to the rules (54.7) (54.8) (54.9) (54.11).
Step 4 after receive 80 particles from auxiliary membranes, particles will be sorted according to the fitness. The worst 80 particles will be discarded into membrane 1. Send the best particle into every auxiliary membrane.
Step 5 the residual particles in main membrane update their speed and position according to the formula (54.1) and (54.2).
Step 6 if the current number of iterations to achieve preset maximum number of iterations, or the result is less than convergence accuracy, stop the iteration and output optimal solution. Otherwise, back to Step2

54.4 Experiments and Result Analysis

54.4.1 Benchmark Functions

Experiments use the commonly used three benchmark functions to test the performance of the algorithm. The three bench functions are respectively: Griewank function Rosenbrock function and Rastrigin function.

$$f_1(x) = \frac{1}{4000}\sum_{i=1}^{n} x_i^2 - \prod_{i=1}^{n}\cos\left(\frac{x_i}{\sqrt{i}}\right) + 1$$

$$f_2(x) = \sum_{i=1}^{n-1}\left(100(x_{i+1} - x_i^2)^2 + (x_i - 1)^2\right)$$

$$f_3(x) = \sum_{i=1}^{n}\left(x_i^2 - 10\cos(2\pi x_i) + 10\right)$$

54.4.2 Experimental Methods

Using MATLAB2010, we use the standard PSO algorithm and the proposed P-PSO to solve the above three test functions respectively, and compared the simulation results. In the test we set the evolution generations t = 500 times, learning factor c1 = c2 = 1.429, standard PSO inertia weight w = 0.729, particle number n = 100, function dimension d = 10.

Table 54.1 Fitness of both methods

Function	P-PSO-fitness-average	PSO-fit-average	P-PSO-fit-best	PSO-fit- best
Griewank	0.39	163.01	0.01	25.25
Rosenbrock	6.28	21.94	1.20	7.63
Rastrigin	5.02	9.49	0.79	2.67

54.4.3 Experiment Analysis

In order to reduce the effect of random factors on experimental results, we conducted 10 consecutive repeating experiments, the experimental results take 10 times test average.

We can see from the image curve trend that P-PSO algorithm has faster convergence speed. In 50 generations, the P-PSO algorithm has basically found out the optimal value of bench functions.

We can see from Table 54.1: Fitness, Corresponding to P-PSO, on Griewank, Rosenbrock and Rastrigin are: 0.01, 1.20 and 0.79. Fitness, Corresponding to PSO, on Griewank, Rosenbrock and Rastrigin are: 25.25, 7.63 and 2.67. This shows that the new algorithm has played a very positive role in the development phase, and improved the convergence precision of the algorithm. Therefore, P-PSO algorithm has higher optimizing efficiency than the standard PSO algorithm.

54.5 An Application of P-PSO

In order to test the ability of P-PSO algorithm to solve practical problems, we will use the new algorithm to solve the problem of standard 14 points TSP problem. The TSP problem is the NP-hard problem in operations research, graph theory and combinatorial optimization. The description of the problem is as follows: Given n cities and the distance between two cities, sales man needs to find the shortest route, which passes by every city only one time, and the staring point is the same as the destination. Assume that d_{ij} is the distance between *i* and *j*. x_{ij} is decision variable.

$$x_{ij} = \begin{cases} 1, \text{ if the salesman visit j after he have visited i} \\ 0, \text{ otherwise} \end{cases}$$

The objective functions for the TSP:$\min Z = \sum_{i,j=1}^{n} x_{ij} d_{ij}$

The description of 14 points TSP problem is shown in Table 54.2 By now, the best solution for 14 points TSP problem is 30.878 5, the route is 1-10-9-11-8-13-7-12-6-5-4-3-14-2-1.

Table 54.2 14 points of TSP

Number	1	2	3	4	5	6	7
X	16.47	16.47	20.09	22.39	25.23	22.00	20.47
Y	96.10	94.44	92.54	93.37	97.24	96.05	97.02
	8	9	10	11	12	13	14
X	17.20	16.30	14.05	16.53	21.52	19.41	20.09
Y	96.29	97.38	98.12	97.38	95.59	97.13	94.55

Table 54.3 Experimental results

Method	Optimal value	Averalge	Average number of iterations	Rate of convergence (%)
PSO	30.8785	32.3573	251.3	35
GA	30.8785	31.0057	64.2	85
P-PSO	30.8785	30.9973	20.8	97

For comparison, we will use the P-PSO algorithm, genetic algorithm and basic PSO algorithm to experiment respectively for 30 times. The population of particles are 50, maximum number of iteration is 2,000. Experimental results are shown in Table 54.3, touring path is consistent with the known best solution.

From the data in Table 54.3, we can see that compared with basic PSO, convergence rate and convergence speed of the P-PSO algorithm are improved obviously. Compared with the genetic algorithm, convergence speed of P-PSO algorithm is higher than the genetic algorithm. Thus, P-PSO algorithm has better ability to solve practical problems.

54.6 Conclusions

This paper proposed an improved PSO algorithm P-PSO, the algorithm introduced membrane computing knowledge into PSO algorithm. Experiments show that P-PSO algorithm has stronger optimization ability than PSO algorithm. The optimal solution is more accurate, and bench functions have fast convergence speed. Also notes that the PSO algorithm combining with the membrane computing is still in its infancy, the algorithm need to be more perfect, this also is later research.

Acknowledgments This work is supported partially by National Science Fund of China (No. 61170038), Science Fund of Shandong province (No. ZR2011FM001), Social Science Fund of Shandong province (No. 11CGLJ22).

References

1. Kennedy J, Eberhart R (1995) In: Particle swarm optimization: proceedings of IEEE international conference on neural networks, 1995[C]. Perth, Australia, IEEE, 1942–1948
2. Duan XD, Gao HX, Zhang XD (2007) Relations between population structure and population diversity of particle swarm optimization algorithm. Comput Sci 34(11):164–167
3. Wu DH, Zhang PL, Li S (2011) Adaptive double particle swarms optimization algorithm based on chaotic mutation. Control Decis 26(7):1083–1086
4. Ren ZH, Wang S (2009) Improved particle swarm optimization algorithm based on entropy. Syst Eng 27(8):106–113
5. Yao K, Li FF, Liu XY (2007) Multi-particle swarm co-evolution algorithm. Comput Eng Appl 43(6):62–64
6. Luan LJ, Tan LJ, Niu B (2007) A novel hybrid global optimization algorithm based on particle swarm optimization and differential evolution. Inf Control 36(6):708–714
7. Paun G, Rozenberg G, Salomaa A (2009) Handbook of membrane computing. Oxford University Press, Oxford, pp 35–40
8. Paun G (2000) Computing with membranes. Comput Syst Sci 61(1):108–143
9. Krishna SN (2007) Universality results for P systems based on brane calculi operations. Theoret Comput Sci 371(1–2):83–105
10. Paun G, Rozenberg G (2002) A guide to membrane computing. Theoret Comput Sci 287(1):73–100
11. Riget J, Vesterstrom JS (2002) A diversity-guided particle swarm optimizer-the ARPSO. J RIGET, Aarhus
12. Li L, Niu B (2009) Particle swarm optimization algorithm, Metallurgical Industry Press, Beijing, pp 44–51

Chapter 55
Specifying Usage of Social Media as a Formative Construct: Theory and Implications for Higher Education

Tao Hu, Ping Zhang, Gongbu Gao, Shengli Jiao, Jun Ke and Yuanqiang Lian

Abstract Theoretical advances the in the conceptualization and operationalization of usage of social media (SM) are lacking in Information Systems (IS) research area. This study extends the conceptualization of IS usage and specifications of formative constructs into the SM context, and proposes a formative model of SM usage. The model conceptualizes and operationalizes SM usage as a multidimensional formative construct. For estimating and validating the proposed model, the research of next steps is reported pertaining to data collection, instrument development, and data analysis. Contributions of this study for IS research and practical implications for SM companies and high education are discussed; limitations and avenues for future research are also addressed.

Keywords Information systems · Social media · Social networking · Usage · Formative · Construct

T. Hu (✉) · G. Gao · S. Jiao · J. Ke · Y. Lian
College of Business Administration, Yangzhou University, Jiangsu 225009, China
e-mail: thu@king.edu

G. Gao
e-mail: gbgao@yzu.edu.cn

S. Jiao
e-mail: sljiao@yzu.edu.cn

J. Ke
e-mail: kejun@yahoo.cn

Y. Lian
e-mail: yqlian@yzu.edu.cn

T. Hu
School of Graduate & Professional Studies, King University, Bristol, TN 37620, USA

P. Zhang
Department of Mathematical Sciences, Middle Tennessee State University, Murfreesboro, TN 37132, USA
e-mail: pzhang@mtsu.edu

S. Li et al. (eds.), *Frontier and Future Development of Information Technology in Medicine and Education*, Lecture Notes in Electrical Engineering 269,
DOI: 10.1007/978-94-007-7618-0_55,

55.1 Introduction

Social media (SM) refer to an integrative collection of telecommunication and computing technologies that builds on the creation and exchange of user generated content to deliver a wide variety of online applications and services to meet people's social needs for fun, self-expressing, information sharing, and relationship developing. SM as an application/service platform in blogging, wikis, and social networking has been viewed as the most exciting interactive interface on the Internet. People are using SM en masse (Edison 2011). In today's higher education, SM play an increasing role in creating, storing, and disseminating information and knowledge. Leading colleges are now reengineering curricula with the Internet-based backbone and moving to the e-education age [22].

The wide use of SM has pushed the research in the burgeoning phenomenon a "hot topic" in the Information Systems (IS) area [38]. A few studies (e.g. [24, 23]) have examined SM usage as a key component of theoretical frameworks. Despite the studies aiming at explaining SM usage behaviors, the dependent variable, SM usage, is conventionally modeled as a unidimensional construct. The conceptualization and operationalization of SM usage in this manner has ignored the rich context-specific nature of the construct, and lacks sound theoretical basis for choice of usage measures or sufficient empirical validation of the construct [1, 4].

Yet, IS research has realized that establishing theory-driven multidimensional conceptualization and verification of IS usage is important (e.g., [1, 4, 16, 41, 44]). This has theoretical and practical implications especially for the exploration of the ever pervasive phenomenon, SM usage [38]. Built on the conceptualization of IS usage, specifications of formative constructs, and extensive literature review of SM usage, this present study takes into account the overall interactions of SM usage, and develops a typology of SM usage behaviors. We further proposed modeling SM usage as a formative construct to describe multi-dimensions of SM usage behaviors of relationship developing, information searching, self-expressing, entertaining, and usage levels.

The proposed formative model reinforces the need for IS research to justify, both theoretically and empirically, the choice of usage measures, and suggests a rich set of dimensions that collectively and uniquely define the nature of SM usage. For SM usage practice, measuring usage behaviors appropriately is essential to examine the antecedents of SM usage, and evaluate the overall success of SM companies [10, 11], and therefore bears practical implications. Specifically for educators and administrators of higher education, the conceptualization and operatoinalization of SM usage offers a meaningful metrics in understanding individual and organizational performance of SM usage in a setting of higher education.

The reminder of the paper is organized as follows. The next section provides a literature review of the conceptualization of IS usage and specifications of formative constructs, upon which the overall interactions of key components of SM usage are described, and a typology of major dimensions of SM usage behaviors is developed. A formative model is then proposed to specify SM usage construct as a multidimensional formative construct. The subsequent section presents research of next steps in data collection, instrument development, and data analysis for estimating and validating the proposed model. The last section discusses contributions and implications of this study, as well as limitations and avenues for future research.

55.2 Theoretical Background

55.2.1 Conceptualization of IS Usage

IS research defines IT artifacts as "those bundles of material and cultural properties packaged in some socially recognizable form such as hardware and/or software" [37, p. 121]. By definition, IT artifacts are not only a concrete objective entity with engineered features and technical characteristics, but also socially recognizable in that they are constructed and used by human individuals and agencies. IT artifacts are therefore imprinted with behaviors, interests, perceptions, and value of a wide variety of human stakeholders. As IT artifacts are ingrained in a system of time, space, discourse, and relationships, their technicality and conditions are essentially interrelated with the historical and cultural aspects of social entities. The emergence, configuration, and advance of IT artifacts is interconnected with human social-economic practices; its nature is dynamic and flexible [37]. Along with advances of technologies and human activities, new features and designs of IT artifacts are invented, existing functions are updated, and new standards and protocols are established. Human beings at the same time keep testing and implementing IT artifacts for new different practices and purposes.

Premised upon "the centrality of IT in everyday socio-economic life" ([37], p. 121), IS research defines IS usage as the use of features, functions, and outputs of IT artifacts to perform tasks [1, 4]. By definition, IS usage is a set of interactive behaviors including what entities do using what features and functions of IT artifacts at what usage levels for what ends in what kind of contexts [1, 28]. Within the interactions, the user may be a person or an organization who adapts, modifies, and uses any element of IT artifacts to accomplish tasks, whereas a task "is a goal-directed activity" undertaken by the social actor/user [4, 28]. In this sense, IS usage is conceptualized as a collection of "structurational" interactions of interrelated components—IT artifacts, social actors (individual and/or organizational entities), personal/organizational tasks, and organizational properties and practice [28, 36].

The interactive process encompasses the overarching characteristics of IT artifacts. Firstly, IS is "a product of human agents"; its usage is an organizational practice that is characterized by social and technical properties of "antecedent conditions, encounters, episodes, and outcomes" [35]. IS usage in this sense reflects integral organizational properties, and usage patterns and effects may be varying across organizational settings. Secondly, at the individual level, depending on usage requirements, and personal identifies, preferences, and cognitions, social actors use multiple features of IT artifacts to undertake different activities often in varying roles cross multiple social contexts [1]. Their usage responses vary in terms of usage satisfaction, participation, and involvement [10], and exert different impact on IS choice and selection [28]. The dual nature of IT artifacts as "an objective reality and socially constructed product" along with the complex interactions of key components make IS usage a comprehensive flexible construct, which calls for a holistic multidimensional conceptualization and operationalization across rich social contexts. This help IS research capture a composite set of usage behaviors to address interdependent nature, effects, and capabilities of IT artifacts [1, 5, 28].

IS Research attempts have been made towards this direction. For example, [5] showed that IS usage can be modeled multidimensionally in terms of usage behavior, usage cognition, and usage affect. [41] suggested that IS use be factored into multiple dimensions. [16] developed a set of multidimensional measures of IS usage in terms of decision support, work integration, and customer service functions. [4] clarified the richness of IS usage measures, and demonstrated different aspects of IS usage can be integrated to derive a contextualized construct. [1] categorized IS use-related activities into three sets of behavior categories—technology interaction, task-technology adoption, and individual adaptation. While the IS usage behaviors have multiple dimensions, the breadth and structures of usage behaviors can be manifested with multiple levels, for which context-specific dimensions have been conceptualized and measured [4, 16].

55.2.2 Specifications of Formative Constructs

A formative construct (or composite variable) is composed of multiple observable quantifiable indicators that define and determine the nature of the construct. That is, the combination of the variant measures describes the underlying properties of the formative construct. For formative constructs, the disturbance error term is usually taken into account at the construct level [14, 25]. A measurement model with at least one formative construct is considered to be a formative model.

One major difference between reflective and formative models is that, with a formative model, all the measures as a group jointly impact the formative construct. A measure is thus required in order to fully represent the content domain of the construct; dropping any measure may affect the extent to which the construct is completely captured [30]. Putting in the context of [2] regression equation, this means each measure has a nonzero beta weight associated with the formative construct. Omitting any of the measures is to eliminate the contribution the measure makes to the entire domain of the construct, and adversely affect the variance explained by the composite set of the measures [39].

Diamantopoulos and Winklhofer [14, 25] established a set of criteria to distinguish between formative and reflective constructs. The first relates to the direction of causality between the construct and measures. For formative constructs, it flows from the measures to the construct. That is, because the measures are considered to define the characteristics of the construct, the changes in the composite set of measures are expected to cause changes in the construct. The second relates to the interchangeability of the measures, which is not expected for formative constructs. The third relates to the extent to which measures covary with each other. For a formative model, covariation among measures is not necessarily assumed, and changes in the value of one of measures do not necessarily cause changes in other measures. The fourth relates to the extent to which measures have the same antecedents and consequences. For a formative model, "there is no reason to expect the measures to have the same antecedents and consequences." (p. 203). In IS research, there has been emerging interest in formative constructs (e.g., [1, 6, 7, 39]). One of the purposes of our study is to draw upon the specifications of formative constructs to address the methodological issues of SM usage.

55.3 Specifying SM Usage as a Formative Construct

55.3.1 Conceptualization of SM Usage

The conceptualization of IS Usage provides a theoretical background that informs the specific conceptualization of SM usage tapping multidimensional SM usage behaviors. Following this line of reasoning, the core IT artifact of SM usage involves an integrative collection of telecommunication and computing technologies that deliver a wide variety of services and applications allowing people to create and exchange user generated content. The interactive behaviors of SM usage include activities that a social actor uses the bundle of applications and services at varying levels to meet social needs for fun, self-expressing, information sharing, and relationship developing in a non-organizational voluntary setting. The conceptualization of SM usage in this sense reflects the dual nature of IT artifacts as "an objective reality and socially constructed product", and takes into account the overall interactions of SM artifacts, goal-directed tasks, individual users, and organizational properties and practice. Built upon the conceptualization and an extensive literature review of SM research and practice, this study next proposes a typology of usage behaviors that make up the dimensions of SM usage. These dimensions are conceptually symbiotic and interrelated, and, as a group, jointly define the underlying nature of SU usage.

Relationship Developing. In the use of SM, people are engaged in various activities such as blogging and social networking to maintain and develop relationships with families, friends, colleagues, strangers, and even virtual avatars. SM applications and services offer people the benefits of managing and building wider and deeper social networks by making them stay in touch with others [3]. As such, SM build virtual communities of tightly interconnected and emotionally close groups, and develop "mutual acquaintance and recognition" for individual users – a life sense of social interdependence, identities, and belongingness [33]. We thus propose relationship developing as the first dimension of SM usage.

Information Sharing. SM usage constructs a rich source of information channels for exchanging common contexts, interests, hobbies, and experience among a large pool of contacts and contents. People can use SM for the sharing of information anytime anywhere. Thanks to the high communicative connectivity and flexibility, information flow in SM portals has been expanded into "friends of friends and their friends" for people to share events, news, gossip, and ideas within the communities. As such, SM usage links weak informational ties beyond existing social reaches. We thus propose information sharing as the second dimension of SM usage.

Self-Expressing. In the use of SM, people not only showcase their factual interests, but also craft sets of fantasies, personas, and avatars to express their social status and egocentric networks [17]. In the virtual environment, people weave different situations, portraits, perspectives, and traits of self-beings, and eagerly present themselves to the audience. People even take great pains and construct faked personas to disclose egotism and topical preferences and fancies about themselves [40]. With these online shows, SM provides people the opportunity to articulate various cultural roles and social norms and contexts to re-characterize themselves into active virtual beings. We thus propose self-expressing as the third dimension of SM usage.

Entertaining. In the use of SM, people can get access to a lot of online games to gain exciting entertaining experience. Furthermore, the informational, relational, and self-expressing interactions can be embellished so well as to carry hedonic entertaining fantasies. The online environment is not a simple extension of real social lives, but rather a "My space", where appeals of ceaseless novelty in the flow of people and information come and go [17]. Casually sneaking into online gaming, video/audio postings, blogging, and private pages, and interacting with friends or any accessorized digital bodies, people satisfy intrinsic curiosity into active virtual lives symbolizing a surreal playground for shared mindsets and interactions. Because these virtual shows and dramas are often hilarious and offer various fun after-school activities, people can be very cognitively spontaneous, playful, and excited in the use of SM. The entertaining activities can be so enjoyable and pleasure-focused that people are easily self-fulfilled in the use of SM. We thus propose entertaining as the fourth dimension of SM usage.

Usage Levels. People use SM features at different levels to meet social needs. Specifically, people's assessments of and behavioral responses to SM usage vary, and exert different impact on their usage choices and levels. As such, within a specific period of time, usage intensity, frequency, duration, and usage types vary across demographics, contexts, and SM applications [29]. To conceptually capture this variation, we specify usage levels as the fifth dimension of SM usage. Adopting the well-established attributes of IS usage levels from prior research

Table 55.1 Typology of SM usage dimensions

Construct	Dimension	Description
SM usage	Relationship developing	People use SM to develop relationship and stay connected with others
	Information sharing	People use SM to search and share information, events, and ideas
	Self-expressing	People use SM to self-express interest, status, and events
	Entertaining	People use SM to pursue entertaining enjoyable experience in its own right
	Usage levels	People use SM at different levels in terms of usage duration, frequency, and intensity

(e.g., [43]), we argue that the levels of SM usage are mainly reflected in such attributes as usage duration (how long people use SM), intensity (the extent to which people use SM), and frequency (how often people use SM). We present the typology and dimensional descriptions of SM usage in Table 55.1.

Meanwhile, each of the five dimensions is conceptually distinct from others, and defines a unique prominent aspect of SM usage behaviors. Firstly, people use SM to perform specific activities. These activities are most relevant to task performance per se, whereas the dimension of usage levels is different from these usage activities in that it taps the extent, duration, and frequency that a usage activity occurs within a period of time. Secondly, the dimensions of relationship developing, information sharing, and self-expressing represent the utilitarian instrumental nature of SM usage in that people employ SM to enhance task performance [31, 42]; whereas the dimension of entertaining reflects people's enjoyable exciting experience with SM use, which represents "a distanced appreciation" of usage activities [21]. Thirdly, among the three utilitarian dimensions of SM usage, self-expressing captures people's internal desire that they wish to convey through the use of SM in controlling the virtual impressions their online connections and contacts form of them [26]; whereas the dimensions of SM usage in relationship developing and information sharing reflect people's external social interactions within a virtual community. And fourthly, the dimension of relationship developing reflects people's use of SM in building interpersonal relations that are interdependent upon each other over time "through a history of interactions"; whereas the dimension of information sharing represents searching and exchanging activities for information and opportunities within various heterogeneous groups of different practices [33].

55.3.2 Modelling SM Usage as a Formative Construct

The conceptualization of SM usage with the five dimensions suggests a promising theoretical basis for modelling SM usage as a formative construct. For the construct, the disturbance term (ξ) is taken into account at the construct level.

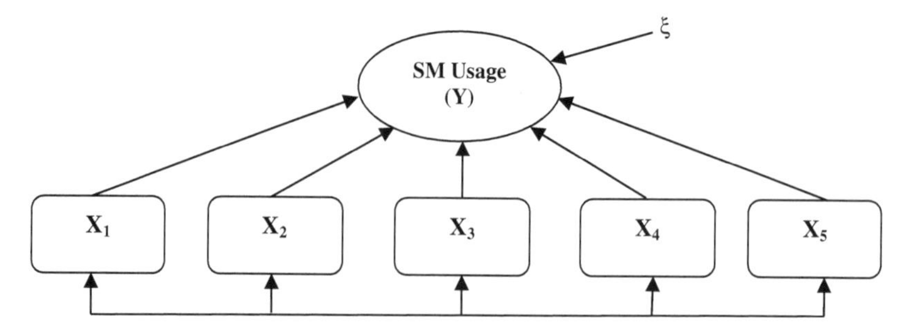

$$Y = \beta_1 X_1 + \beta_2 X_2 + \beta_3 X_3 + \beta_4 X_4 + \beta_5 X_5 + \xi$$

Where,
Y: The formative construct being estimated, SM usage.
$\mathbf{X_i}$: The scores/observations for the measurement indicators – relationship developing (X_1), information sharing (X_2), self-expressing (X_3), entertaining (X_4), and usage levels (X_5).
• : The beta weights for measurement indicators.
• : The disturbance term.

Fig. 55.1 Formative Model of SM Usage

The five dimensions constitute the measurable indicators; each of them has a nonzero beta weight, and captures a unique non-interchangeable aspect of SM behaviors. The combination of the five dimensions represents the full content domain of SM usage behaviors, and determines underlying context-specific nature of the construct.

Through the lens of [14, 25], SM usage as a formative construct displays the measurement characteristics as follows. Firstly, the direction of causality between the construct and the five observable indicators—relationship developing, information sharing, self-expressing, entertaining, and usage levels—occurs from the indicators to the latent construct, implying that changes in the indicators lead to changes in the construct. Secondly, because the five dimensions are conceptually distinct from each other, the interchangeability of the measurement indicators is not expected, and covariation among them not assumed. This implies that the five indicators do not share a common theme, or have the same antecedents and consequences. As such, changes in any of the indicators are not expected to cause changes in others. The formative model of SM usage is presented in Fig. 55.1.

55.4 Next Step Research: Validating the Formative Model of SM Usage

Researchers have suggested that the estimation and validation items for formative models focus on multicollinearity among measures, and content, construct, and nomological validity [13, 25, 39]. Content validity assesses whether the domain of a formative construct is fully represented by the composite set of measures. Construct validity can be assessed through examining the item weightings for measures. Finally, to validate the nomological validity of formative constructs, it is suggested that the formative construct be associated to other constructs in a nomological network [14]. For operationalizing and assessing the proposed formative model of SM usage, we next report the research of next steps pertaining to data collection, instrument development, and data analysis

Data Collection. While usage nuances and contexts of SM vary, online social networking services (OSNS) have been viewed as the most popular application of SM (Kaplan and Haenlein 2011) serving as an excellent research context in studying SM usage behaviors. Because the target population for this study is SM users, we will conduct a cross-sectional field survey of undergraduate and graduate students enrolled in several large universities in North America as college students are considered to be a major OSNS user group [29]. The survey consists of questions with multi-item scales to capture the constructs encompassed in the proposed formative model. The survey will provide rich contextual information to ensure respondents complete it while thinking about the one OSNS they have used most often during the last 3 months. Demographic data including age, gender, and ethnicity will be gathered along with other OSNS usage data including work status, OSNS sites used, and usage experience. Variables associated with these data will be treated as control variables controlling effect on SM usage.

Instrument Development. In this study, we model SM usage as a second-order formative construct, for which the five dimensions of SM usage behaviors serve as the subconstruct indicators. We will draw upon the measurement guidelines outlined in [14, 25] to operationalize the construct from a formative perspective. Furthermore, we model the five sets of subconstruct indicators as the first-order reflective constructs. Measurement scales of entertaining and usage levels will be directly adapted from previously validated scales in IS usage literature; and the measures of relationship developing, information sharing, and self-expressing will be newly developed following the standard procedures of instrument construction.

Data Analysis. The SEM-based approach with SmartPLS 2.0 will be used to analyze the data for the estimation and validation of the formative model. The SEM-based partial least squares (PLS) analysis provides a powerful procedure in addressing key IS research questions [7]. The technique uses a component based approach to estimation, and places minimal restrictions on measurement scales, sample size, and residual distributions [8]. The results of data analysis will be interpreted following the guidelines outlined in [6, 14, 25].

55.5 Discussions

55.5.1 Contributions to IS Research

IS research has long called for deeper examination of IS usage construct to address the complex interactions of key usage components – users, IT artifacts, performance tasks, and organizational properties and practice. This current study responds to the call by conceptualizing and operationalizing the construct, SM usage. This study contributes to IS theory in several aspects.

Overarching Conceptualization of SM Usage. This study conceptualizes SM usage as a composite set of behaviors that a social actor uses the bundle of SM applications and services at varying levels to meet social needs for fun, self-expressing, information sharing, and relationship developing in a non-organizational voluntary setting. The conceptualization recognizes the complex interactive nature of SM artifacts, and captures multidimensional SM usage behaviors. The conceptualization describes SM usage from an individual's point of view, and portrays SM usage as a function of a wide variety of online activities that social users undertake at various levels to accomplish relational, informational, entertaining, and self-expressing tasks in varying usage contexts. The proposed dimensions of usage-related behaviors clarify the content of SM usage, and help IS researchers to develop a full domain and context-specific measures of SM usage while minimizing measurement errors and model misspecification. This should in turn assist IS studies to obtain meaningful accumulative findings about the relationships between SM usage and its antecedents and consequences at multiple levels and contexts [5].

Theory-Driven Operationalization of SM Usage Construct. The objective of this study is to describe the nature and attributes of SM usage. For this purpose, a formative model assumes greater explanatory power over a reflective one [14, 19]. Basing on the conceptualization of SM usage and specifications of formative constructs, we proposed a formative model of SM usage and operationalize SM usage as a second-order formative construct. The formative construct comprises five subconstruct indicators, which are modelled as the first-order reflective constructs capturing key dimensions of SM usage behaviors The operationalization offers a promising research direction towards empirical investigations to reach insights about SM usage in an aggregate manner regarding what behaviors are involved, and the degree and extent to which the behaviors are undertaken. In this sense, the proposed model presents an organizing theory-driven framework for designing and testing formative models on content, parsimony and criteria validity of derived measures. IS research in this direction should enable empirical indicative understanding of SM artifacts and its usage through identifying how SM companies design and deliver applications and services, and how the individual and organizational impact of SM usage can be leveraged for long term performance [41].

55.5.2 Implications for Practice and High Education

The conceptualization and operationalization of SM usage advanced in this study provides practical guidelines for SM companies and managers to measure people's usage behaviors and evaluate overall organizational performance. The multidimensional formative measures can facilitate SM managers and designers to understand key antecedent factors that drive users to use SM applications and services, how to use them at what levels for what purposes, and what usage behaviors matter most for them. Such understandings assist to build SM applications and services effectively to retain users. Meanwhile, IS usage has downstream impact on individual and organizational performance [10, 11]. People's effective use of SM has been considered the major determinant for the success of SM companies [27, 32]. Thus, the proposed formative model enables SM companies to investigate the patterns and extent of SM usage along relevant dimensions for developing long-term strategies for business survival and marketing extension.

Specifically for educators and administrators of higher education, where SM are widely used for knowledge creation and delimitation, this study bears important implications. Because the estimation and validation of the proposed model will be conducted upon data sampled from college students, the findings will provide meaningful insights into how college students use SM to develop relationships with peers, faculty members, and administrators, how they use SM for information searching and sharing in a typical educational platform, how they use SM as a tool for entertaining and self-expressing, and how different usage behaviors may affect their value assessments of SM. These findings help higher education institutions assess educational outcomes properly and create effective SM applications and services to retain students and meet various educational purposes.

55.5.3 Limitations and Future Research

This study represents a first attempt in conceptualizating and operationalizing SM usage from a formative perspective. It has limitations in several respects, which should be addressed in future research.

Firstly, we draw upon the general conceptualization of IS usage and extensive literature review of SM research and practice to develop the typology of SM usage behaviors. Although this is consistent with the guidelines for developing formative constructs (e.g., [14, 25, 39], a deeper understanding of the multidimensional nature of SM usage may benefit from further theoretical and literature refinement. This will ensure that the full formative domain of the construct is covered. For example, the salience and meaningfulness of incorporating usage costs into SM usage behaviors needs to be considered in future research. We urge researchers to consult a wider variety of theories and literature to determine whether it is possible to reach a more integrated understanding of SM usage.

Secondly, this study conceptualizes SM usage as a behavioral construct. The mental aspects of SM usage as indicated in activity theory (e.g., [15, 34]) have not been covered in the conceptualization. Thus, one future research for the improvement of SM usage construct could be to integrate in the domain of the construct additional dimensions and usage elements implied in activity theory such as psychological states and feelings. We believe great opportunities exist to extend the formative model of SM usage in this direction.

Thirdly, this study operationalizes SM usage as a formative construct. We believe it provides a greater explanatory power over a reflective model in describing the nature and dimensions of SM usage behaviors. However, because operationalizing a construct from a literature with a strong reflective or formative tradition may introduce measurement biases [9], this suggests one direction for improving the operationalization of SM usage construct. For further research, improved procedures for operatoinalizing formative indicators should be considered.

55.6 Conclusion

In this study, we extend the general conceptualization of IS usage and specifications of formative constructs into the context of the ever pervasive phenomenon, SM usage. We conceptualize and operationalize SM usage as an aggregate higher-order formative construct with multi-dimensions of usage behaviors in relationship developing, information searching, self-expressing, entertaining, and usage levels. In response to the research call for improving and enhancing IS usage construct, the proposed formative model of SM usage takes into account the complex interactions of key usage components, and contributes to IS theory in several aspects. For SM usage practice and higher education, the model enables organizations to investigate the patterns and extent of SM usage for developing long-term strategies for business survival and marketing extension. We hope that this study will encourage future research that will examine SM usage within different theoretical models and usage contexts, helping provide a better understanding of SM usage behaviors.

References

1. Barki H, Titah R, Boffo C (2007) Information system use-related activity: an expanded behavioral conceptualization of individual-level information system use. Inf Syst Res 18(2):173–192
2. Bollen K, Lennox R (1991) Conventional wisdom on measurement: a structural equation perspective. Psychol Bull 110(2):305–314

3. Boyd D, Ellison N (2007) Social network sites: definition, history, and scholarship. J Comput-Med Commun 13(1):210–230, http://jcmc.indiana.edu/vol13/issue1/boyd.ellison.html
4. Burton-Jones A, Straub DW (2006) Reconceptualizing system usage: an approach and empirical test. Inf Syst Res 17(3):228–246
5. Burton-Jones A, Gallivan MJ (2007) Toward a deep understanding of system usage in organizations: a multilevel perspective. MIS Q 31(4):657–679
6. Cenfetelli RT, Bassellier G (2009) Interpretation of formative measurement in information systems research. MIS Q 33(4):689–707
7. Chin WW (1998) The partial least squares approach to structural equation modeling. In: Marcoulides GA (ed) Modern business research methods. Lawrence Erlbaum Associates, Mahwah
8. Chin WW, Marcolin BL, Newsted PR (2003) A partial least squares latent variable modeling approach for measuring interaction effects: results from a monte carlo simulation study and an electronic-mail emotion/adoption study. Inf Syst Res 14(2):189–217
9. Colman T, Devinney TM, Midgley DF, Venaik S (2008) Formative versus reflective measurement models: two applications of formative measurement. J Bus Res 61:1250–1262
10. DeLone WH, McLean ER (1992) Information system success: the quest for the dependent variable. Inf Syst Res 3(1):60–95
11. DeLone WH, McLean ER (2003) The delone and mclean model of information systems success: a ten-year update. J Manage Inf Syst 19(4):9–30
12. Diamantopoulos A (2006) The error term in formative measurement models: interpretation and modeling implications. J Model Manage 1(1):7–17
13. Diamantopoulos A, Siguaw JA (2006) Formative versus reflective indicators in organizational measure development: a comparison and empirical illustration. Br J Manag 17(4):263–282
14. Diamantopoulos A, Winklhofer HM (2001) Index construction with formative indicators: an alternative to scale development. J Mark Res 38(2):269–277
15. Ditsa G (2003) Activity theory as a theoretical foundation for information systems research. Inf Manage pp. 192–231
16. Doll WJ, Torkzadeh G (1998) Developing a multidimensional measure of system-use in an organizational context. Inf Manage 33(4):171–185
17. Donath J (2007) Signals in Social Supernets. J Comput-Med Commun 13(1):231-251, http://jcmc.indiana.edu/vol13/issue1/donath.html
18. Enders A, Hungenberg H, Denker H, Mauch S (2008) The long tail of social networking: revenue models of social networking sites. Eur Manage J 26(3):199–211
19. Formnell C, Bookstein FL (1982) A comparative analysis of two structural equation models: lisrel and pls applied to market data, In: Fornell (ed) A second generation of multivariate analysis, Vol 1, Praeger, New York, pp. 289–324
20. Goffman E (1959) The presentation of self in everyday life. Doubleday Anchor Books, New York
21. Holbrook MB (1994) The nature of customer value: an axiology of services in the consumption experience. In: Roland TR, Richard LO (eds) Service quality: new directions in theory and practice. Sage, Newbury Park, pp 21–71
22. Hu T, Zhang X, Dai H, Zhang P (2012) An examination of gender differences among college students in their usage perceptions of the internet. Edu Inf Technolo 17:315–330
23. Hu T, Poston R, Kettinger W (2011) Non-adopters of online social network services: is it easy to have fun yet! Commun Assoc Inf Syst 29(1):441–458
24. Hu T Kettinger W (2008) Why people continue to use online social networking services: developing a comprehensive model. In: Proceedings of 2008 ICIS, Paris, France, 14–17 Dec 2008
25. Jarvis CB, MacKenzie SB, Podsakoff PM (2003) A critical review of construct indicators and measurement model misspecification in marketing and consumer research. J Consum Res 30(2):199–218

26. Kaplan AM, Haenlein M (2010) Users of the world, unite! the challenges and opportunities of social media. Bus Horiz 53:59–68
27. Kim SS, Son JY (2009) Out of dedication or constraint? a dual model of post-adoption phenomena and its empirical test in the context of online services. MIS Q 33(1):49–70
28. Lamb R, Kling R (2003) Reconceptualizing users as social actors in information systems. MIS Q 27(2):197–236
29. Lenhart A, Purcell K, Smith A, Zickuhu S (2010) Social media & mobile internet use among teens and young adults http://web.pewinternet.org/~/media/Files/Reports/2010/PIP_Social_Media_and_Young_Adults_Report_Final_with_toplines.pdf. Accessed 31 March 2013
30. MacKenzie SB, Podsakoff PM, Jarvis CB (2005) The problem of measurement model misspecification in behavioral and organizational research and some recommended solutions. J Appl Psychol 90(4):710–730
31. Mathwick C, Malhortra N, Rigdon E (2001) Experiential value: conceptualization, measurement and application in the catalog and internet shopping environment. J Retail 77(1):39–56
32. Mithas S, Ramasubbu N, Krishnan MS, Fornell C (2007) Designing web sites for customer loyalty across business domains: a multilevel analysis. J Manage Inf Syst 23(3):97–127
33. Nahapiet J, Ghoshal S (1998) Social capital, intellectual capital, and the organizational advantage. Acad Manag Rev 23(2):242–266
34. Nardi BA (1996) Activity theory and human computer interaction. In: Nardi BA (ed) Context and consciousness: activity theory and human-computer interaction. The MIT Press, Cambridge, pp 1–8
35. Newman M, Robey D (1992) A social process model of user-analyst relationships. MIS Q 16(2):249–266
36. Orlikowski W (1992) The duality of technology: rethinking the concept of technology in organizations. Organ Sci 3(3):398–427
37. Orlikowski WJ, Iacono SC (2001) Research commentary: desperately seeking the "it" in it research – a call to theorizing the it artifact. Inf Syst Res 12(2):121–134
38. Parameswaran M, Whinston AB (2007) Research issues in social computing. J Assoc Inf Syst 8(6):336–350
39. Petter S, Straub D, Rai A (2007) Specifying formative constructs in information systems research. MIS Q 31(4):623–656
40. Rosen C (2007) Virtual friendship and the new narcissism, New Atlantis 17:15–31
41. Straub D, Limayem M, Karahanna E (1995) Measuring system usage: implications for is theory testing. Manage Sci 41(8):1328–1342
42. Sweeney JC, Soutar GN (2001) Consumer perceived value: the development of a multiple item scale. J Retail 77(2):203–220
43. Venkatesh V, Brown SA, Maruping LM, Bala H (2008) Predicting different conceptualizations of system use: the competing roles of behavioural intention, facilitating conditions, and behavioural expectation. MIS Q 32(3):483–502
44. Venkatesh V, Thong JYL, Xu X (2012) Consumer acceptance and use of information technology: extending the unified theory of acceptance and use of technology. MIS Q 36(1):157–178

Chapter 56
Unsupervised Brain Tissue Segmentation by Using Bias Correction Fuzzy C-Means and Class-Adaptive Hidden Markov Random Field Modelling

Ziming Zeng, Chunlei Han, Liping Wang and Reyer Zwiggelaar

Abstract Unsupervised brain tissue segmentation in magnetic resonance imaging (MRI) is a key step in brain analysis, such as computer-aided surgery, clinical diagnosis, pathological analysis, surgical planning. Due to the noise and bias field in MRI, it is difficult to automatically segment brain tissue. In order to improve the segmentation accuracy, we propose an unsupervised method which combines an improved bias correction Fuzzy C-means (BCFCM) and class-adaptive hidden markov random field Modelling (HMRF). The BCFCM segmentation result is used as the initial labelling for class-adaptive HMRF, which is utilized to refine the segmentation results. Experiments are evaluated on simulated MR images. Comparing with the ground truth, the results show that the proposed method can perform well on MR brain images with noisy MRI and bias field.

Keywords MRI · Brain · Segmentation · Noise · Bias field

56.1 Introduction

Segmentation of magnetic resonance imaging (MRI) is a challenging problem due to the complexity of the images. The brain has a particularly complex structure, and its segmentation is an important step for many problems. Manual

Z. Zeng (✉)
Information and Control Engineering Faculty, Shenyang Jianzhu University, Shenyang 110168 Liaoning, China
e-mail: zengziming1983@gmail.com

Z. Zeng · L. Wang · R. Zwiggelaar
Department of Computer Science, Aberystwyth University, Aberystwyth SY23 3AL, UK

C. Han
Turku PET Center, Turku University Hospital, 20520 Turku, Finland

S. Li et al. (eds.), *Frontier and Future Development of Information Technology in Medicine and Education*, Lecture Notes in Electrical Engineering 269,
DOI: 10.1007/978-94-007-7618-0_56,

segmentation is time consuming and highly variable [1]. Some unsupervised segmentation method are proposed, the fuzzy c-means (FCM) algorithm [2] has been successfully applied for brain tissue segmentation. Several developments have been proposed to the standard FCM algorithm to deal with noise and intensity inhomogenity. Ahmed et al. [3] modified the objective function of the standard FCM algorithm to compensate for inhomogeneities. Chen et al. [4] developed the FCM object function with spatial constraints based on a kernel distance measure. Sasikala et al. [5] used a Genetic Algorithm to optimize a modified FCM function. However, the segmentation results are not accurate enough when significant noise exists in MR image. The HMRF-EM framework [6] was proposed to segment brain MRI which can be effectively performed on noisy images. However, it does not perform well on images with bias field. In this work, we use the class-adaptive HMRF [7] which is initialized by using BCFCM method to segment brain tissues. Firstly, we modified the weighting of the objective function and the iteration criteria from Ahmed [3] to estimate the bias field, then the calculated cluster centers for each group are used as the initial labelling for class-adaptive HMRF [7] with a class adaptive weighting function to compensate the immediate neighborhood influence.

56.2 The Proposed Method

The proposed segmentation method contains three steps. In the first step, the brain skull is removed. In the second step, an improved BCFCM is used to remove the bias field, and initialize the group labelling. In the third step, an anisotropic diffusion model is used to reduce the noise, then the noiseless image is segmented by using class-adaptive HMRF.

56.2.1 Brain Skull Removing

As a pre-processing step, the noise and bone (and closely associated tissue) need to be removed, because the density of the non-brain tissues are similar as the density of brain. Firstly, the fuzzy c-means method with two clusters is used to distinguish between the background and brain tissue. Then erosion with a circular structuring element is used to disconnect the brain from the other regions. Subsequently, a labelling method is used to identify the brain region (assuming the brain to be the largest region present). After that, the eroded area is regained by a matched dilation [8]. Finally, the binary mask is used to extract the corresponding pixels from the brain MR image.

56.2.2 Bias Field Removing by Using an Improved Bias-Corrected Fuzzy C-Means

In this step, an improved bias correction Fuzzy C-means method is used for bias field estimation and initial segmentation. In [3], the objective function with a spatial neighborhood regularization term is defined as:

$$J_m = \sum_{i=1}^{c}\sum_{k=1}^{N} u_{ik}^{p}\|y_k - \beta_k - \upsilon_i\|^2 + \sum_{i=1}^{c}\sum_{k=1}^{N} u_{ik}^{p} \sum_{y_r \in \mathcal{N}_K} \omega(yk, yr)\|y_r - \beta_r - \upsilon_i\|^2 \tag{56.1}$$

where $\|\cdot\|$ is the Euclidean norm, $\{\upsilon_i\}_{i=1}^{c}$ are the prototypes of the clusters and the array $[u_{ik}] = U$ represents a partition matrix, y_k and β_k are the observed log-transformed intensity and the bias field at the k_{th} voxel, respectively. In this term $y_k - \beta_k$ is the true log-transformed intensity at the k_{th} voxel. $\mathcal{N}_k$ is the set of neighbors that exist in a window around y_k. $\omega(y_k, y_r)$ is a weighting function which is defined as:

$$\omega(y_k, y_r) = \frac{\alpha}{N_R},\ 0 \le \alpha \le 1 \tag{56.2}$$

where N_R is the cardinality of $\mathcal{N}_k$, the parameter α, which is chosen experimentally, is used to control the weight of the neighboring term (the second term in Eq. 56.1). In this work, we considered the local spatial distance and the local intensity difference between the neighbouring pixel r and the central pixel k and modified Eq. 56.2 as

$$\omega(y_k, y_r) = \frac{1}{\sqrt{2\pi\sigma^2}} e^{-\frac{\|y_k - \mu\|^2}{\sigma^2}} \frac{\sqrt{\sum_{y_r \in \mathcal{N}_k} \|y_k - y_r\|^2}}{N_R} \tag{56.3}$$

where μ and σ can be automatically estimated by calculating the mean and standard deviation of all the grey level values in a small window around y_k.

Formally, the optimization problem can be estimated in the form $\min_{u_{ik}, \upsilon_i, \beta_k} J_m$. The objective function can be calculated by taking the first derivatives of J_m with respect to $u_{ik}, \upsilon_i, \beta_k$ and setting them as zero gradient conditions. The parameters can be estimated as:

$$u_{ik}^{*} = \frac{\left(A + \sum_{y_r \in N_k} \omega(y_k, y_r) B\right)^{1/(1-p)}}{\sum_{j=1}^{c}\left(A + \sum_{y_r \in N_k} \omega(y_k, y_r) B\right)^{1/(1-p)}} \tag{56.4}$$

$$\upsilon_i^{*} = \frac{\sum_{k=1}^{N} u_{ik}^{P}\left((y_k - \beta_k) + \omega(y_k, y_r)\sum_{y_r \in \mathcal{N}_k}(y_r - \beta_r)\right)}{1 + \sum_{k=1}^{N} \omega(y_k, y_r) u_{ik}^{p}} \tag{56.5}$$

$$\beta_k^* = y_k - \frac{\sum_{i=1}^{c} u_{ik}^p \upsilon_i}{\sum_{i=1}^{c} u_{ik}^p} \tag{56.6}$$

where u_{ik}^* is the membership function, υ_i^* is the cluster prototype function, and β_k^* is the bias-field estimation function. $A = \|y_k - \beta_k - \upsilon_i\|^2, B = \|y_r - \beta_r - \upsilon_i\|^2$. The traditional termination criterion in [3] is defined as $\|V_p - V_{p-1}\| \leq \varepsilon$, where $V = [\upsilon_1, \upsilon_2, \cdots, \upsilon_c]$ are the vectors of group centers, and p is the iteration number. This only considers the difference of group center values between iterations which ignores the spatial difference and potentially converges to local minima rather than global extremum. Here a new iteration termination criteria is defined as

$$\left(MI\left(S_p, S_{p-1}\right) - MI\left(S_{p-1}, S_{p-2}\right)\right)^2 \leq \varepsilon, \tag{56.7}$$

where S is the segmentation labelling, $MI(\cdot,\cdot)$ is the mutual information [9] of two images which is defined as $MI(A,B) = H(A) + H(B) - H(A,B)$, where $H(A)$ and $H(B)$ are the entropy of image A and B, respectively. $H(A,B)$ is the joint entropy of image A and B. Finally, the bias field removed image can be generated by subtracting the estimated bias field β from the original image.

56.2.3 Segmentation by Using HMRF-EM

When significant noise exists in MRI, the segmentation result generated by using BCFCM only is usually not accurate enough and the bias field removed image can still contains significant noise. We introduce a class-adaptive Hidden Markov random field modelling approach to refine the previous segmentation result. Firstly, the noise in the bias field removed image is reduced by using an anisotropic diffusion model [10]. Then we can achieve accurate and robust segmentation results by incorporating both a class-adaptive Hidden Markov random field model [7, 11] and expectation–maximization into a HMRF-EM framework.

For the class-adaptive HMRF modeling, a set of observation field is given as $Y = \{y_1, \ldots, y_i, \ldots, y_N\}$. Given a set of group labels as $L = \{1, 2, \ldots, c\}$ which are initialized by using the results from the previous step. The label assignment which is defined as $X = \{x_1, \ldots, x_i, \ldots, x_N\}$ is initialized by using the segmentation result in the previous step. An optimal labeling should satisfy the maximum posteriori probability (MAP) criterion:

$$x^* = arg\,max_x(P(x|y)) = arg\,max_x(P(y|x)P(x)) \tag{56.8}$$

According to the Hammersley-Clifford theorem [12], the prior probability $P(x)$ satisfies a Gibbs distribution: $P(x) = Z^{-1}exp(-U(x))$, where Z is a normalisation factor. Then the posterior energy can be calculated as $U(x|y) = U(y|x) + U(x)$, where $U(y|x)$ is computed by the sum of the likelihood potentials at all sites which are approximated by using Gaussian distribution function with parameters $G(y_i, \theta_c)$. Assuming that the distribution of intensities of brain tissue follows a

Gaussian distribution $G(y_i, \theta_c)$ with parameters $\theta_c = (\mu, \sigma_c) = (\upsilon_c, \sigma_c)$, which can be initialized by using the BCFCM method. $U(x)$ is computed by the sum of binary clique energies. Subsequently, we formulate the MAP-MRF by using expectation maximization (EM) algorithm to calculate the maximum posterior probability. The processing of the EM algorithm can be summarized as the following steps:

(1) E part: It tries to calculate maximum likelihood of posterior probability.
(2) M part: Updating the penalty factor as well as the mean μ_c and variance σ_c of each Gaussian component by using the maximum likelihood obtained in E-step.
(3) Repeat E and M parts until $\left|\left(U^{*(t+1)} - U^{*(t)}\right)/U^{*(t)}\right| \leq \psi$, where U^* is the energy for pixel labels, t denotes the iteration number, ψ is a constant value.

56.3 Evaluation and Discussion

Experiments are evaluated on synthetic images and simulated brain images. Figure 56.1 shows a comparison with the BCFCM [3] and HMRF [13] methods. We generated two synthetic images (256 $\times$ 256) with bias field by adding different bias fields as shown in Fig. 56.1b to two noisy images shown in Fig. 56.1a from the IBSR dataset [14]. The bias field is estimated by using the improved BCFCM shown in Fig. 56.1d. Compared with the ground truth, we can see the HMRF method can effectively deal with noise, and can deal with the small scale bias field, such as the first test image in Fig. 56.1f. However, it fails to perform equally on the second example due to large scale bias field changes. For the BCFCM method, we can see that it can deal well with the bias field, but is affected by noise. Visually, our method provides the best results on these synthetic images.

The proposed method is used to segment nine simulated T1-weighted brain MR images which were randomly selected from Brainweb [15]. Figure 56.2 shows some segmentation results compared with BCFCM [3] and HMRF [13]. All the images have 9 % noise and 40 % bias field. We use the simple FCM and morphology method introduced in the preprocessing step to remove non-brain tissues. Then the skull removed images are used as the test images to evaluate the proposed and alternative methods. Figure 56.3 shows zoom in areas of some selected segmentation results. Compared with our results in Fig. 56.3d, the HMRF could not give appropriate results as shown in Fig. 56.3b. We can clearly see that the results of HMRF have over segmentation of GM (see the purple arrows in Fig. 56.3b) and CSF (see the green arrows in Fig. 56.3b). Especially for the white matter (WM) at the bottom of some images, which is misclassified as grey matter (GM) and cerebrospinal fluid (CSF). It can be explained that the phenomenon of misclassification is caused by the bias field. In Fig. 56.3c, the segmentation results of BCFCM are not smooth and the result still contain noise. The results of BCFCM

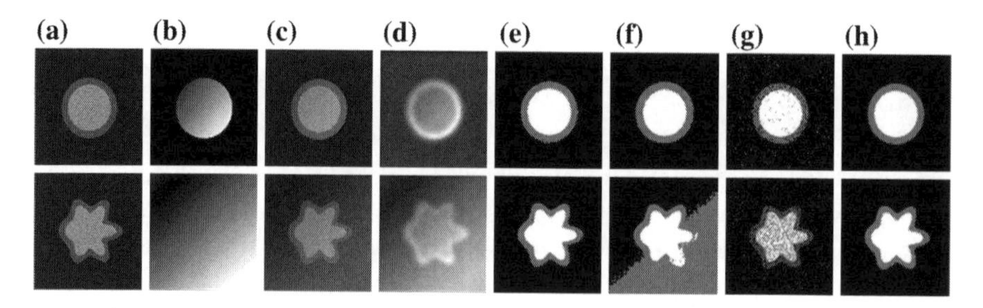

Fig. 56.1 Examples of segmentation results on synthetic images: **a** Original image with noise from the IBSR database [14], **b** Bias field, **c** Synthetic image with additional bias field, **d** Estimated bias field, **e** Our result, **f** HMRF, **g** BCFCM, **h** Ground truth

have more scatter noise points in the WM (see the red arrows in Fig. 56.3c) and the boundary of GM is not smooth (see the blue arrows in Fig. 56.3c). Since the anisotropic diffusion method and class-adaptive HMRF are used to smooth the results in the proposed method, our results can effectively segment brain tissue (especially the WM) and are more robust with regard to noise and bias field compared with the alternative approaches.

To further evaluate the accuracy of the segmentation method, two measurements are used for the simulated brain images. The first two measurement are the

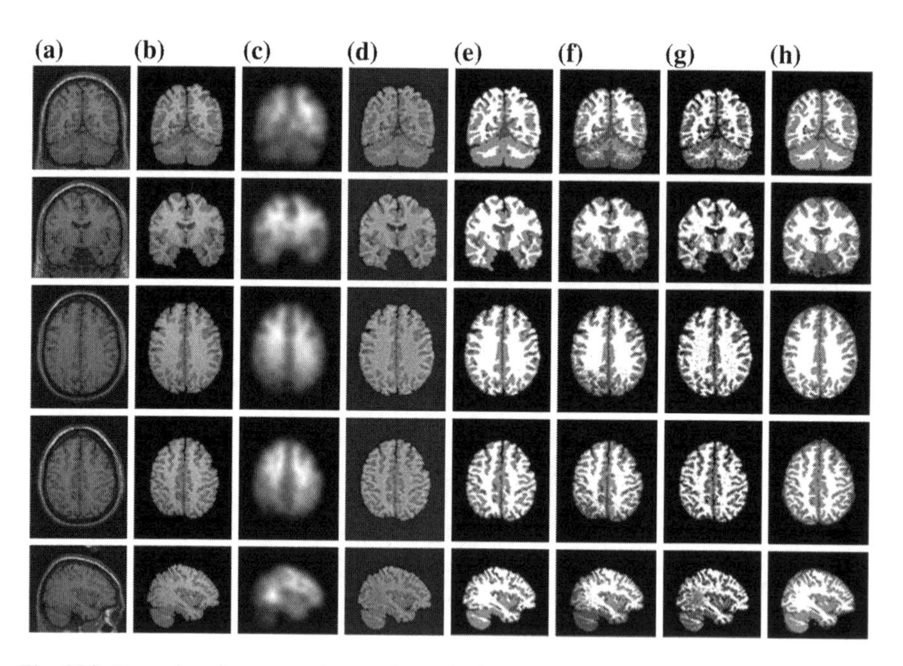

Fig. 56.2 Examples of segmentation results on brainweb data: **a** Original MR images with 9 % noise 40 % density inhomogenity, **b** MR images after brain skull removal, **c** Estimated bias field, **d** MR images after bias field removal, **e** Our result, **f** HMRF, **g** BCFCM, **h** Ground truth

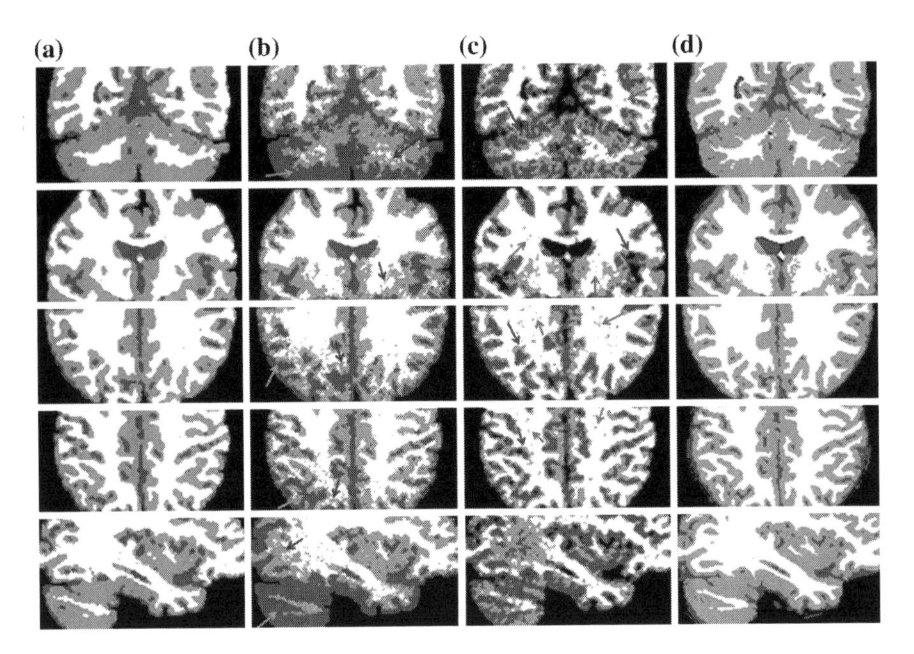

Fig. 56.3 Zoom in of the segmentation results on brainweb data: **a** Our result, **b** HMRF, **c** BCFCM, **d** Ground truth

Table 56.1 Dice index for tissues segmentation on brainweb data for 9 % noise and 40 % bias field

Algorithm	MAP-MRF-EM			BCFCM			Our method		
Brain tissue	CSF	WM	GM	CSF	WM	GM	CSF	WM	GM
Dice	0.413	0.861	0.696	0.149	0.858	0.590	0.483	0.893	0.842
SD (dice)	0.129	0.038	0.096	0.043	0.049	0.078	0.139	0.036	0.028
PPV	0.364	0.933	0.783	0.131	0.899	0.767	0.717	0.853	0.889
SD (PPV)	0.144	0.034	0.099	0.042	0.033	0.116	0.184	0.058	0.066

Dice similarity coefficient (DICE) and positive predictive value (PPV). Their results are shown in Table 56.1. In all cases except the WM PPV, our method performs better than the other methods, although some standard deviations (SD) for CSF and WM are slightly higher than the alternative methods. The third measurement for segmentation results is confusion matrices which are shown in Table 56.2. The overall segmentation accuracy of the proposed method, BCFCM and HMRF are 77.86, 62.02 and 73.16 %, respectively. The segmentation results for WM and GM are improved on alternative methods with WM and GM achieving 93.81 and 80.39 % accuracy, respectively. The CSF are largely misclassified as the background, because some CSF outside of the GM shown in Fig. 56.3a are segmented as the background by using FCM and morphology when extracting the brain tissues.

Table 56.2 Confusion matrices of results represented as percentages on all the simulated brainweb images [15]

	Tissues	Ground truth			
		BG	CSF	WM	GM
(a) (Overall accuracy = 77.86 %)					
Out	BG	99.38	49.34	0.03	0.98
	CSF	0.29	37.87	0.02	5.55
	WM	0.02	0.01	93.81	13.08
	GM	0.31	12.78	6.14	80.39
(b) (Overall accuracy = 62.02 %)					
BCFCM	BG	99.59	81.99	0.03	1.89
	CSF	0.31	17.77	0.57	42.43
	WM	0.01	0	82.39	7.36
	GM	0.09	0.24	17.01	48.32
(c) (Overall accuracy = 73.16 %)					
HMRF	BG	99.42	50.08	0.03	0.98
	CSF	0.42	49.22	0.20	30.80
	WM	0.04	0	80.33	4.55
	GM	0.12	0.70	19.44	63.57

56.4 Conclusion

This paper proposed an unsupervised segmentation method for brain MRI based on an improved BCFCM and class-adaptive HMRF. Evaluations were carried out by using synthetic data, simulated brain MR images with significant noise and bias field. Comparing with the alternative methods, the segmentation results showed that the proposed method improves the accuracy of segmenting on the different type of brain tissue. In the future, further clinical evaluation could be completed and robust skull removing could be developed. In addition, there is a need to cover partial volume effects and the unsupervised determination of the optimal number of segmentation groups.

References

1. Breen SL, Publicover J, De Silva S, Pond G, Brock K, Osullivan B, Cummings B, Dawson L, Keller A, Kim J, Ringash J, Yu E, Hendler A, Waldron J, Waldron J (2007) Intraobserver and interobserver variability in gtv delineation on fdg-pet-ct images of head and neck cancers. Int J Radiat Oncol Biol Phys 68(3):763–770
2. Pohle R, Toennies KD (2001) Segmentation of medical images using adaptive region growing. In: Proceedings of SPIE medical imaging, pp 1337–1346
3. Ahmed MN, Yamany SM (2002) A modified fuzzy c-means algorithm for bias field estimation and segmentation of MRI data. IEEE Trans Med Imaging 21(3):193–199

4. Chen S, Zhang D (2004) Robust image segmentation using fcm with spatial constraints based on new kernel induced distance measure. IEEE Trans Syst, Man, Cybernetics 34(4): 1907–1915
5. Sasikala M, Kumaravel N, Ravikumar S (2006) Segmentation of brain MR images using genetically guided clusting. In: The proceedings of IEEE EMBS annual international conference, pp 3620–3623
6. Zhang YY, Brady M, Smith S (2001) Segmentation of brain MR images through a hidden Markov random field model and the expectation-maximization algorithm. IEEE Trans Med Imaging 20:45–57
7. Wang W, Feng Q, Liu L, Chen W (2008) Segmentation of brain MR images through class-adaptive Gauss-Markov random field model and the EM algorithm. J Image Graphics 13(3):488–493
8. Yu D, Tuan D, Zhou X (2009) Analysis and recognition of touching cell images based on morphological structures. Comput Biol Med 39:27–39
9. Kraskov A, Stogbauer H, Grassberger P (2004) Estimating mutual information: physical review. E, Statistical, Nonlinear, Soft Matter Phys 69(6):1–16
10. Perona P, Malik J (1990) Scale-space and edge detection using anisotropic diffusion. IEEE Trans Pattern Anal Mach Intell 12(7):529–539
11. Zeng Z, Wang W, Yang L, Zwiggelaar R (2011) Automatic estimation of the number of segmentation groups based on MI. Lect Notes Comput Sci 6999:532–539
12. Hammersley JM, Clifford P (1971) Markov fields on finite graphs and lattices. IEEE Trans Med Imaging 9(1):84–93
13. Wang Q, (2012) HMRF-EM-image: implementation of the hidden markov random field model and its expectation-maximization algorithm, arXiv:1207.3510 [cs.CV]
14. Massachusetts general hospital (2006) Internet brain segmentation repository (IBSR). http://www.cma.mgh.harvard.edu/ibsr/
15. McGill universit montreal neurological Institute (2006) Brain web. http://www.bic.mni.mcgill.ca/brainweb/

Chapter 57
An Adaptive Cultural Algorithm Based on Dynamic Particle Swarm Optimization

Liu Peiyu, Ren Yuanyuan, Xue Suzhi and Zhu Zhenfang

Abstract To avoid the local optimum problems and to improve convergent speed when particle swarm optimization algorithm in solving complex problems, an adaptive cultural algorithm based on dynamic particle swarm optimization algorithm was proposed. Particle swarm algorithm introduced evaluation premature convergence degree of index to judge the population space condition to determine the role of the influence function time. The inertia weight of the particle was adjusted adaptively based on the premature convergence degree of the swarm. The diversity of inertia weight makes a compromise between the global convergence and the speed of convergence. The proposed algorithm was tested with four well-known benchmark functions. The experimental results show that the new algorithm has great global search ability convergence accuracy and convergence velocity is also increased and avoid the premature convergence problem effectively.

Keywords Adaptive · Particle swarm · Cultural algorithm · Inertia weight · Influence function

L. Peiyu (✉) · R. Yuanyuan · X. Suzhi
School of Information Science and Engineering, Shandong Normal University, Jinan 250014, China
e-mail: liupy@sdnu.edu.cn

L. Peiyu · R. Yuanyuan · X. Suzhi
Shandong Provincial Key Laboratory for Novel Distributed Computer Software Technology, Shandong Normal University, Jinan 250014, China

Z. Zhenfang
School of Information Science and Electric Engineering, Shandong Jiao Tong University, Jinan 250357, China

S. Li et al. (eds.), *Frontier and Future Development of Information Technology in Medicine and Education*, Lecture Notes in Electrical Engineering 269,
DOI: 10.1007/978-94-007-7618-0_57,

57.1 Introduction

Particle swarm optimization (PSO) [1, 2] is a kind of evolutionary algorithm based on swarm intelligence which was proposed by Kennedy and Eberhart in 1995. Particle swarm optimization algorithm move to the global optimal position of the individual and the individual optimal realization of individual evolution. Cultural algorithm (CA) was firstly purposed by Reynolds [3] in 1994.

In order to overcome the defects of PSO algorithm, improve the ability of local optimization. Many improved methods have been proposed for the particle inertia weight by domestic and foreign scholars. Previous studies have typically used, linear decreasing inertia weight strategy was proposed Shi [4], however, the strategy couldn't adapt to the complex nonlinear optimization problems. Related scholars have made some research and experimentation to optimize the inertia weight, such as adaptive changes [5], changes exponentially [6], fuzzy adaptive inertia weight [7] etc. Compared with the standard PSO algorithm, these methods can improve the convergence speed and optimization precision. But just inertia weight optimization, the improved algorithm is still being trapped in a local optimum possibly.

In response to these issues, an adaptive cultural algorithm based on dynamic particle swarm optimization algorithm was proposed. PSO is embedded into the framework of standard CA, combined with the PSO algorithm for global optimization ability and the double evolutionary mechanism of cultural algorithm. A cultural particle swarm optimization was constructed.

Usually in the literature about cultural particle swarm algorithm [8–10], influence function always acts on the population space. Uninterrupted mutation implementation of the variation of the parent particle position, not only be able to maintain the diversity of the population space, but also to prevent the population space particles from falling into the local optimum. But this mutation operation of the guidance population space with a certain degree of blindness, so that the whole culture particle swarm algorithm is difficult to converge. To solve this problem, the evaluation of particle swarm premature convergence indicators introduced into population space is proposed in this paper. Convergence speed and precision optimization PSO algorithm is far superior to a single when solving complex multi-extreme problem.

57.2 Adaptive Cultural Algorithm Based on Dynamic Particle Swarm Optimization

57.2.1 Dynamic Particle Swarm Optimization

57.2.1.1 Particle Swarm Optimization (PSO)

PSO is a population-based stochastic algorithm that starts with an initial population of randomly generated particles. PSO algorithm to evaluate the pros and cons of the individual based on the individual fitness value in the search space size, and the optimization of potential solutions of the problem as the search space not only the speed and position of the mass and volume of particles. For a search problem in a D-dimensional space, a particle represents a potential solution presented by their velocity and position. There is a population size of N particle swarm, where each particle $i(i = 1, 2, \ldots, N)$, the position of the *i*th particle is $x_i(x_{i1}, x_{i2}, \ldots, x_{iD})$, the velocity of the *i*th particle is $v_i(v_{i1}, v_{i2}, \ldots, v_{iD})$.During a search process, each particle is attracted by its previous best particle (p_i) and the global best particle (p_g) as follows.

$$v_{id}^{t+1} = wv_{id}^{t} + c_1r_1(p_{id}^{t} - x_{id}^{t}) + c_2r_2(p_{gd}^{t} - x_{id}^{t}) \quad (57.1)$$

$$x_{id}^{t+1} = x_{id}^{t} + v_{id}^{t+1} \quad (57.2)$$

where r_1, r_2 are generated within the interval of [0, 1] randomly. The parameter w, called inertia factor, which is used to balance the global and local search abilities of particles, c_1 and c_2 are two learning factors which control the influence of the social and cognitive components, and t indicates the iteration number. In order to prevent particles out of the search space in the iterative process, need to be limited to the range of particle velocity and position. If limited $|x_i| \leq x_{\max}$, then the speed is $v_{\max} = \alpha x_{\max}$, where $0.1 \leq \alpha \leq 1.0$.

57.2.1.2 Premature Convergence Judgment

Evolutionary population has always been to maintain diversity is a prerequisite for algorithm effectively running, and the greater the diversity of particle swarm, the population is more likely to produce excellent individuals. The course of particle swarm algorithm will lead to the gradual loss of the diversity of particle swarm, once the diversity is lost, the individuals in population will be of mutual convergence, and thus the convergence phenomenon is easy to happen. So to judge the state of the particle swarm can help to research the changes of particle fitness value, to determine whether the algorithm converges.

The indicator of evaluation particle swarm premature convergence is proposed. Set the size of the particle swarm is n, fitness value of the particle *i* in the *k*th iteration is f_i^k, optimal particles adaptation value is f_m^k, the average fitness value of the particle swarm is f_{avg}^k, fitness value obtained by averaging the fitness value is better than f_{avg}^k is $\overline{f_{avg}^k}$. Defined as follows:

$$\rho = \left| \frac{f_m^k - \overline{f_{avg}^k}}{f_m^{k-1} - \overline{f_{avg}^{k-1}}} \right| \tag{57.3}$$

where ρ can be used to evaluate the degree of convergence of the particle swarm algorithm, the smaller the ρ shows that particle swarm is more tend to converge.

57.2.1.3 Dynamic Inertia Weight Adjustment

It claimed that a large inertia weight facilitates a global search while a small inertia weight facilitates a local search. By changing the inertia weight dynamically, the search capability is dynamically adjusted. This is a general statement about the impact of w on PSO's search behavior shared by many other researchers.

Standard particle swarm algorithm have used a linear decreasing change inertia weight, there are two flaws, one is that cannot react the complex nonlinear behavior effectively in the actual search process of particle swarm, so the convergence rate and precision is still not ideal; the other one is that the slope of the inertia weight value decreases linearly depend on the specific problem, there is no slope that suitable for all optimization problems [11]. Because linearly decreasing inertia weight changes single, and the search process of particle swarm algorithm is very complex and non-linear, so its ability to adapt and adjust the complex problems is very limited. To solve the above problems, a strategy of adjusting the inertia weight dynamically is proposed in this paper, and the change of inertia weight and the indicators of evaluating particle swarm premature convergence will link together. Inertia weight adjustment formula is as follows:

$$w_i(t) = 1 - (1 + e^{-\rho})^{-1} \tag{57.4}$$

As can be seen by the above formula, the value of inertia weight changes in (0, 1). Where $w_i(t)$ describes the inertial of particle ith in generation t impact on velocity. The ability of global optimization and local optimization capability can be adjusted according to the value of the inertia weight. The higher the value of $w_i(t)$, the stronger the ability of global optimization. On the contrary, the ability of global optimization was reduced and the ability of local search was strengthened. Appropriate inertia weight value can improve the performance of the algorithm, to improve the optimization capability, while reducing the number of iterations. When the state of PSO is convergence, it requires a large inertia weight increase search step length, thereby enhancing the ability of global optimization of PSO. When the PSO in the global search, it requires a small inertia weight reduce search step length, thereby enhancing local search ability of the PSO.

57.2.2 Adaptive Cultural Particle Swarm Optimization Algorithm

57.2.2.1 Algorithm Framework

Cultural algorithm is an evolutionary algorithm which best represents a social system and consists of two levels of evolution: the microevolution in a population space and the macroevolution in a belief space. Through an acceptance function, the experiences of individuals in the population space are used to generate problem solving knowledge that is to be stored in the belief space. The belief space manipulates the knowledge, which in turn guides the evolution of the population space by means of an influence function.

Fixed proportion elites are selected from population space to construct the swarm of belief space through acceptance function. Then, the belief space updates its normative knowledge and situational knowledge according to the elite particles, and the elite-swarm in the belief space performs PSO operation according to the update knowledge and generates new particles. A framework for Cultural Particle Swarm Optimization Algorithm can be depicted in Fig. 57.1.

57.2.2.2 Design of the Belief Space

The belief space is made up with the knowledge and experience of the individuals. Iacoban et al. [12] defines five kinds of decision-making is very useful knowledge.

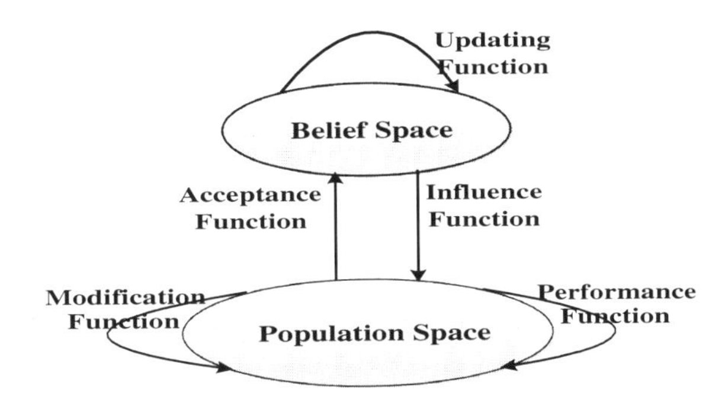

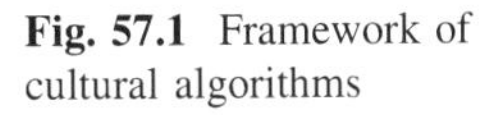
Fig. 57.1 Framework of cultural algorithms

There are five basic knowledge types: normative knowledge, situational knowledge, domain knowledge, history knowledge, and topographical knowledge. One of the most commonly used is the normative knowledge (NK) and situational knowledge (SK) that $BLF = <NK, SK>$.

The normative knowledge source is used to store the maximum and minimum values for numeric attributes. For nominal or discrete attributes a list of possible values that the attribute can take are stored. The normative knowledge contains the intervals for each domain variable in order to move the new individuals towards to the good solutions. For each parameter$j$, $NK = < I_j, L_j, U_j, >$. where I_j denotes the internal layout of the parameter$j$, which is defined as follows:

$$I_j = [l_j, u_j] = \{x | l_j \le x \le u_j, x \in R\} \tag{57.5}$$

where l_j and u_j are the lower and upper bounds of the belief space$B_i.U_j$ and L_j are the values of the fitness function corresponding to the bound l_j and u_j. Then the normative knowledge is renewed according to the Eqs. (57.6) and (57.7) under the assumption that the lower bound of jth particle is affected by ith particle and upper bound is affected by kth particle. The normative knowledge update rules as follows:

$$l_j^{t+1} = \begin{cases} x_{i,j}^t & x_{i,j}^t \le l_j^t \, or \, f\left(x_{i,j}^t\right) < L_j^t \\ l_j^t & otherwise \end{cases} \quad u_j^{t+1} = \begin{cases} x_{k,j}^t & x_{k,j}^t \le u_j^t \, or \, f\left(x_{k,j}^t\right) < U_j^t \\ u_j^t & otherwise \end{cases} \tag{57.6}$$

$$L_j^{t+1} = \begin{cases} f\left(x_{i,j}^t\right) & x_{i,j}^t \le l_j^t \, or \, f\left(x_{i,j}^t\right) < L_j^t \\ L_j^t & otherwise \end{cases} \quad U_j^{t+1} = \begin{cases} f\left(x_{k,j}^t\right) & x_{k,j}^t \le l_j^t \, or \, f\left(x_{k,j}^t\right) < L_j^t \\ U_j^t & otherwise \end{cases} \tag{57.7}$$

Situation knowledge consists of the best exemplar found along the evolutionary process. It represents a leader for the other individuals to follow. Situational knowledge to be adjusted according to the update function update (), the expression as follows:

$$P_g^{t+1} = \begin{cases} x_{best}^t & f\left(x_{best}^t\right) < f\left(P_g^t\right) \\ P_g^t & otherwise \end{cases} \tag{57.8}$$

where x_{best}^t represents the best individual of the tth generation. If the optimal particle x_{best} in current population is better than p_g, and available x_{best} instead of p_g to complete update the situational knowledge.

57.2.2.3 Design of Communication Protocol

Communication protocol, a bridge for transferring information between the two spaces, plays an important role in the whole evolution process. One is acceptance function, the other is influence function. The acceptance function selects individuals which can directly impact the information of current belief space. The number of the accepted particle can be represented as follows:

$$\eta_{accept} = (p\,\% + p\,\%/t) * N \tag{57.9}$$

where p is the probability, given according to the needs and is normally set to 20 %; t is current iteration; N is the size of population.

In algorithm design, how to take advantage of the knowledge of the belief space affect the generation of the next generation population is very important. After the belief space to complete its own update by affecting the function of the population space particles exert influence. This requires that by the following equation to adjust the position of the particle in the population space.

$$x_{id}^{t+1} = \begin{cases} x_{id}^{t} + |size(I_d) * N(0,1)| & (x_{id}^{t} < p_{gd}) \\ x_{id}^{t} - |size(I_d) * N(0,1)| & (x_{id}^{t} > p_{gd}) \\ x_{id}^{t} + \eta * size(I_d) * N(0,1) & (x_{id}^{t} = p_{gd}) \end{cases} \tag{57.10}$$

where N (0, 1) is the standard normal distribution random number, $size(I_d)$ is the belief space variable d adjustable interval length, η is the step length contraction factor.

57.2.2.4 Influence Function of Adaptive Guidance

In the past, many literatures which based on cultural particle swarm optimization algorithm, the influence function always acted on the population space. When the population space is still in the state of the global search, influence function mutation operation makes the particles lose the current position and forced to re-optimization, thus the original particle swarm structure is disturbed, lead to the population space can't conduct on a precise local search, slow down the speed of convergence of cultural particle swarm algorithm and its efficiency decline.

In fact, in the cultural particle swarm optimization, when PSO algorithm during the stage of global random search, it is unnecessary to take advantage of influence function conduct the mutation operation for fathers individuals in the population space, so it can maximize use the PSO algorithm approach the global solution subspace, to accelerate the speed of convergence of the algorithm. When the population space into the state of convergence, the mutation operation by influence function can improve the local search capability, and accelerate the speed of convergence of the algorithm. Therefore, a mechanism which can determine the time of the influence function acts on population space particles must be provided.

The key to this problem is to determine when the PSO algorithm in the population space in the state of premature convergence.

To judge the state of the particle swarm, a study on changing the value of the particle fitness in population space was conducted, thereby determine whether the algorithm convergence. To this end, evaluation of particle swarm premature convergence indicator ρ mentioned above was employed to judge the degree of convergence of the population space algorithm. The indicator ρ is smaller; the population space more tends to convergence. On the contrary, the particles more tend to randomly search. In this paper, the value of ρ is less than a certain threshold value is set C to determine convergence, where C is the population evolutionary capacity threshold. When $\rho > C$, indicating the state of the PSO algorithm in global search, the influence function doesn't operate at this time. When $\rho < C$, the PSO algorithm tend to convergence, the influence function conducts on the mutation operation and update operation, thereby gain new descendents, the individuals re-iterate in the population space. So the cycle until the algorithm find the global optimum solution. Not only ensure both groups space structure of the PSO algorithm optimization, but also the influence function plays a role in guiding effectively, improve the convergence speed and the efficiency of the optimization of culture particle swarm algorithm.

57.2.3 The Main Procedure of CA-DPSO

Step1 Initialization

Randomly initialize the positions of all particles $X = (X_1, X_2, \ldots, X_N)$ of size N
Initialize the Velocity $(V_1, V_2, \ldots, V_N)$
Set generation counter t = 1
Build population space and belief space, and initialize all the individuals in the two spaces randomly
Set the population evolutionary capacity threshold C
Determine the search space $[-x_{\max}, x_{\max}]$ and maximum speed $v_{\max}$
Evaluate the fitness values $F = (fit_1, fit_2 \ldots, fit_N)$ of X
Set X to be $p_{id} = (p_{1d}, p_{2d} \ldots, p_{Nd})$ of each particle
Set the particle with best fitness to be p_g

Step 2 Reproduction and loop

For i = 1: N
  Update the inertia weight Eq. (57.4)
  Update the velocity v_i and position x_i Eqs. (57.1) and (57.2)
  Evaluate the fitness value fit_i of the new particle X_i
  If X_i is the better than p_{id}
    Set X_i to be p_{id}
End if

If X_i is the better than p_g
Set X_i to be p_g
End if
End for
Evaluate the number of replaces the worst particle in belief space $\eta_{accept} = (p\% + p\%/t) * N$

$$\text{if } \rho = \left| \frac{f_m^k - \overline{f_{avg}^k}}{f_m^{k-1} - \overline{f_{avg}^{k-1}}} \right| < C$$

The location of each particle was updated in population space by the influence function Eq. (57.10).
End if
Set t = t+1

Step 3 If termination condition is not met, go to Step 2, otherwise end.

57.3 Experiment Results and Analysis

To evaluate the performance and effectiveness of CA-DPSO, four benchmark test functions are chosen to simulate and compare the accuracy and convergence speed. Where D is the dimension of the functions, $X \in R^D$ is the definition domain, and $f(x^D)$ is the global optimum of the function see (Table 57.1).

$$f_1(x) = \sum_{i=1}^{n} \left(\sum_{j=1}^{i} x_j \right)^2 \tag{57.11}$$

$$f_2(x) = \sum_{i=1}^{n} \left[100(x_{i+1} - x_i^2)^2 + (x_i - 1)^2 \right] \tag{57.12}$$

$$f_3(x) = \sum_{i=1}^{n} \left[x_i^2 - 10\cos(2\pi x_i) + 10 \right] \tag{57.13}$$

Table 57.1 Dimensions, search spaces, and optimum values of functions used in Sect. 57.3

Test function	Function	Dimension	Search space	Global minimum
Uni-modal	f_1: Quadric	30/100	$[-100, 100]^D$	0
	f_2: Rosenbrock	30/100	$[-30, 30]^D$	0
Multimodal	f_3: Rastrigrin	30/100	$[-30, 30]^D$	0
	f_4: Griewank	30/100	$[-30, 30]^D$	0

Table 57.2 Comparison of AC-DPSO with PSO, CPSO and AG-CPSO on test function f_1–f_4

	PSO		CPSO		AG-CPSO		AC-DPSO	
	Average optimum	Standard deviations	Average optimum	Standard deviations	Average optimum	Standard deviations	Average optimum	Standard deviations
f1	3.5805e − 03	2.6490e + 03	5.7214e − 03	2.9523e + 03	4.7318e − 03	4.3218e + 03	2.1499e − 03	3.1206e + 03
f2	7.6756e + 03	3.7868e + 05	7.4032e + 03	5.7441e + 05	6.9156e + 03	3.1543e + 05	2.1554e + 03	3.0154e + 05
f3	4.7056e + 01	6.2729e + 01	5.4333e + 01	4.9354e + 01	4.1521e + 00	2.5596e + 01	2.7054e + 00	1.2501e + 01
f4	2.2621e − 02	5.5953e − 02	4.7710e − 02	6.4316e − 02	3.6509e − 02	3.7683e − 02	3.2548e − 02	2.4315e − 02

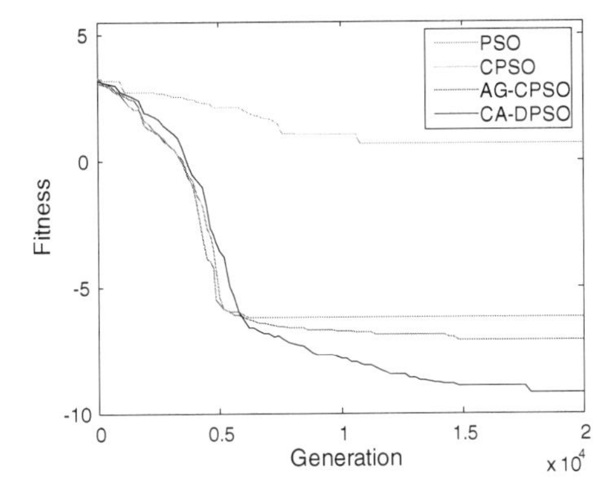

Fig. 57.2 The comparison of convergence property on Quadric Function

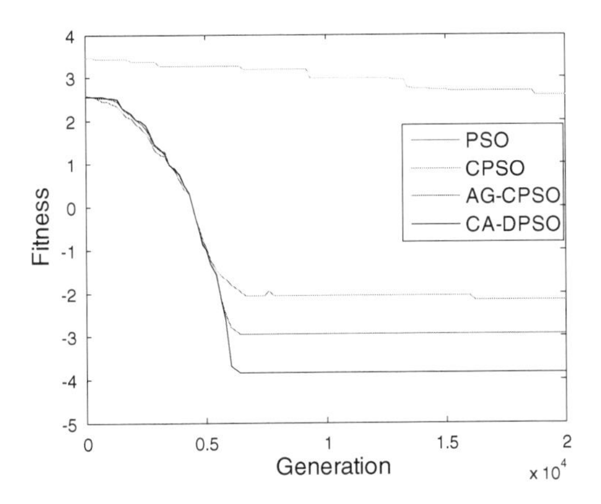

Fig. 57.3 The comparison of convergence property on Rosenbrock Function

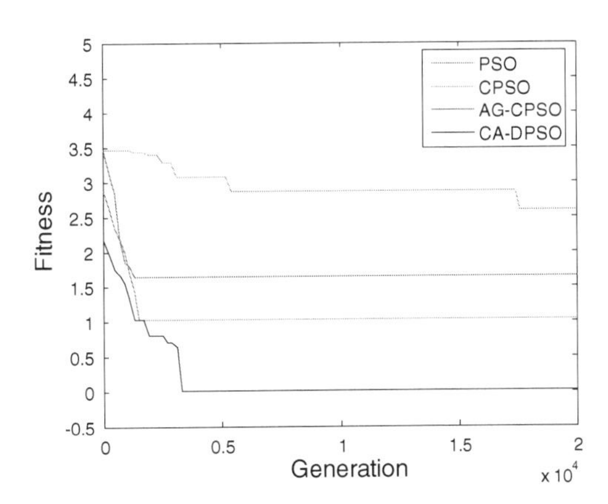

Fig. 57.4 The comparison of convergence property on Ratrigrin Function

$$f_4(x) = \frac{1}{4000}\sum_{i=1}^{n} x_i^2 - \prod_{i=1}^{n} cos\left(\frac{x_i}{\sqrt{i}}\right) + 1 \tag{57.14}$$

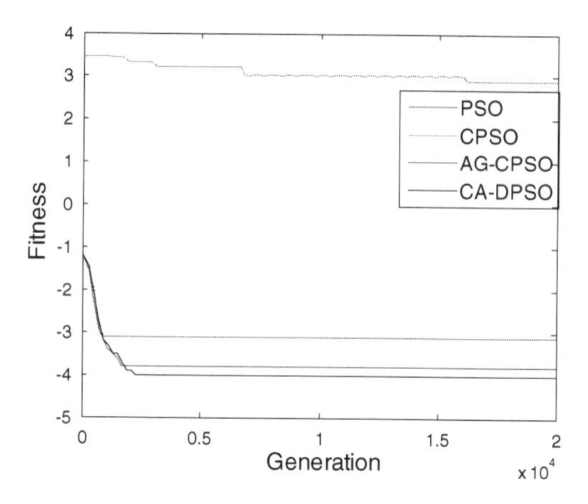

Fig. 57.5 The comparison of convergence property on Griewank Function

In order to show the effectiveness of the proposed method, the results have been compared with several previously published approaches, such as basic PSO, CPSO [13] and only used influence function of adaptive guidance cultural particle swarm optimization AG-CPSO. According to the experiences of a lot of experiments and literature, the main parameter settings of the methods are given as follows: acceleration constants c1 = c2 = 2; inertial weight w decreases from 0.9 to 0.4 linearly for PSO, CPSO and AG-CPSO; population size is 100; maximum number of iteration is 20000; set population evolutionary capacity threshold C = 0.05. Every test function using three algorithms is repeated for 30 times independently. The simulation results are summarized in Table 57.2 and shown in Figs. 57. 2, 57. 3, 57. 4 and 57.5.

Comparing the standard deviations of the four functions, we can find that the accuracy of the algorithm in this paper is better than the other three algorithms overall by analyzing the simulation results shown in Table 57.2. As can be seen from Figs. 57. 2, 57. 3, 57. 4 and 57.5, the improve algorithm in this paper has better global optimal solution search ability and faster convergence rate. This is due to using the influence function adaptive guidance the particle swarm algorithm in population space. The diversity of particle was enhanced. The inertia weight of the particle was adjusted adaptively based on the premature convergence degree of the swarm. The diversity of inertia weight regulates the global search and local search ability effectively and makes each search step changes with the convergence state of the particles.

As can be seen from Figs. 57. 2, 57. 3, 57. 4 and 57.5, the convergence effect of CPSO algorithm is worse than AG-CPSO algorithm. Due to not judging the status of particles in population space before the influence function guides the population space, thus the guidance of the influence function for population space has a lot of blindness and disturbs the structure of PSO algorithm in population space.

Ratrigrin function and Griewank function are multimodal functions which are used to test the performance of the global search. Figure 57.3 shows PSO, CPSO and AG-CPSO are easy to fall into local optimal late in search, while the influence function of the algorithm in this paper guides particles swarm in population space effectively escape from local optima.

Comprehensive above figures, they clearly illustrates that PSO is easy to fall into local minimum. In CPSO algorithm, due to mutation operation of influence function for population space the whole process, result in the convergence concussion becomes larger and convergence speed becomes slower. In AG-CPSO algorithm, due to linearly decreasing inertia weight changes single, so its ability to adapt and adjust the complex problems is very limited. The convergence speed of CA-DPSO is remarkably higher than that of the other algorithms.

57.4 Conclusions

An adaptive cultural algorithm based on dynamic particle swarm optimization algorithm was proposed in this paper. In CPSO algorithm, the mutation operator adopted by influence function may disturb the structure and convergence of PSO algorithm in population space. A new CPSO algorithm with adaptive guidance which the degree of evaluation premature convergence introduced into population space is proposed in this paper. The population space is prone to get into local best position in the last period of evolution. By calculating the degree of evaluation premature convergence, decisions are made whether to have mutated operation on population space. The improved algorithm can enhance the diversity of particle and improve the efficiency of the CPSO algorithm. Comparison of the performance of the proposed approach with PSO algorithm, CPSO algorithm and AG-CPSO algorithm was experimented. The simulation results of typical complex function optimization problems show that the improved algorithm can not only effectively solve the premature convergence problem, but also significantly speed up the convergence and improve the stability.

Acknowledgments This research was supported by the National Natural Science Foundation of China (No.60873247), the Natural Science Foundation of Shandong Province of China (No. ZR2009GZ007, ZR2011FM030), and National Social Science foundation of China (12BXW040).

References

1. Eberhart RC, Kennedy J (1995) A new optimizer using particle swarm theory. In: Proceedings of the sixth international symposium on Micro Machine and Human Science, Nagoya, pp 39–43
2. Kennedy J, Eberhart V (1995) Particle swarm optimization. In: Proceedings of the IEEE international conference on neural networks—conference proceedings, vol 4, Perth, pp 1942–1948
3. Reynolds V (1994) An introduction to culture algorithms. In: Proceedings of the third annual conference on evolutionary programming, San Diego, pp 131–139

4. Shi Y, Eberhart RC (1999) Empirical study of particle swarm optimization. In: Proceedings of the IEEE Congress on Evolutionary Computation, IEEE Computer Society, Washington, pp 1945–1950
5. Chen D, Wang GF, Chen ZY (2008) The inertia weight self- adapting in PSO. In: Proceedings of the 7th World Congress on Intelligent Control and Automation, Chongqing, pp 5313–5316
6. Chen GM, Huang XB, Jia JY et al (2006) Natural exponential inertia weight strategy in particle swarm optimization. In: Proceedings of the 6th World Congress on Intelligent Control and Automation, Dalian, pp 3672–3675
7. Shi Y, Eberhart RC (2001) Fuzzy adaptive particle swarm optimization. In: Proceedings of the 2001 Congress on Evolutionary Computation, vol 1, pp 101–106
8. Hou YL, Hu JW, Zhao CH et al (2007) Test set optimization using cultural particle swarm optimization. J Harbin Eng Univ 27(7):151–154
9. Sheng L, Wang X, You X (2007) Cultured differential particle swarm optimization for numerical optimization problems. In: Proceedings of the third international conference on natural computation, pp 642–646
10. Wang L, Cao C (2012) An Improved particle swarm algorithm based on cultural algorithm for constrained optimization. Adv Intell Soft Comput 135:453–460
11. Jaco FS, Albert AG (2005) A study of global optimization using particle swarms. J Global Optim 31:93–108
12. Iacoban R, Reynolds RG (2003) Cultural swarms: modeling the impact of culture on social interaction and problem solving. In: Proceeding of IEEE swarm intelligence symposium, Indianapolis, Indiana, pp 205–211
13. Wang Y, Ai J, Shi Y et al (2007) Cultural-based particle swarm optimization algorithm. J Dalian Univ Technol 47(4):539–544

Chapter 58
A Modified Approach of Hot Topics Found on Micro-blog

Lu Ran, Xue Suzhi, Ren Yuanyuan and Zhu Zhenfang

Abstract Due to the simplicity, immediacy and convenience, micro-blog is gaining more and more attention from all kinds of people, especially the researchers. Recently, topic detection on micro-blog has attracted more interests due largely to the rapid development of micro-blog. However, retrieving information from micro-blog is challenging, as the texts of the micro-blog are short, ungrammatical, and unstructured, and they are full of noise. Therefore, the traditional hot topic detection method performed less. In order to solve this problem, this paper proposed a method of hot topics found based on speed growth. In this method, the pretreated micro-blogs were divided into different windows, and the time information was extracted in each window; then, for each word, it was expressed as feature trajectory of binary group sequence; then, calculated the growth speed of the word and the users relevant to the word in every adjacent two windows, selected the words whose growth speed is greater than a certain threshold as hot keywords; then, hot topics were found through the hot keywords clustering. The experiment was done based on SINA micro-blog dataset, the miss rate and false detection rate were done to prove the feasibility of the algorithm, results showed that the method improved the efficiency of the detection to a certain extent.

Keywords Time information · Growth speed · Feature trajectory of binary group sequence

L. Ran (✉) · X. Suzhi · R. Yuanyuan
School of Information Science and Engineering, Shandong Normal University, Jinan 250014, China
e-mail: luran@sdnu.edu.cn

X. Suzhi · R. Yuanyuan
Shandong Provincial Key Laboratory for Novel Distributed Computer Software Technology, Jinan 250014, China

Z. Zhenfang
School of Information Science and Electric Engineering, Shandong Jiaotong University, Jinan 250357, China

S. Li et al. (eds.), *Frontier and Future Development of Information Technology in Medicine and Education*, Lecture Notes in Electrical Engineering 269,
DOI: 10.1007/978-94-007-7618-0_58,

58.1 Introduction

With the rapid development of social media, people are tend to gain and share information from social medias, such as blog, news website, forum and micro-blog, especially the micro-blog, due to its simplicity, immediacy and convenience, has gain increasing popularity from all kind of people. Because micro-blog is different from traditional media, it's highly interactive, and the user is not only a passive information receiver, but a originator of information, so the people's interests are highly aroused which lead to the rapid spread of information on the Internet, meanwhile some emergency are showed gradually. But due to the forms of micro-blog information are complicated and various, including text, music, pictures, video and other forms, combined with the large amount of information, which makes a challenge to get emergency from micro-blog [1]. Therefore, how to make full use of the advantages of sensitivity and the real-time to get hot topic timely from the vast amounts of data is more and more important.

Micro-blog is different from traditional forms of news, as the texts of the micro-blog are short, ungrammatical, and unstructured, so using the traditional clustering and classification method to extract hot topics is particularly difficult nowadays. A method based on the speed growth is proposed in this paper to detect hot topics on micro-blog. Firstly, the micro-blog is processed using the labels the micro-blog provided such as "@", "#", much information published by the zombie account and interactive dialogues are filtered out effectively. The reason for the above processing is as follows: Although micro-blog with the defects of shortness, non-standard language and so large amount of information, it has advantages of bursty, fissionability and immediacy, so we should make full use of the advantages the micro-blog provided combined with overcoming the shortcomings to process micro-blog text effectively. The Concrete processing methods are as follows: first, a assumptions in this paper is that information published by the users whose fans number is less than a certain threshold, and information with the format of "@", "#" influence largely on word frequency statistics but a small role, so this information is filtered out [2]. Second, instead of the traditional clustering algorithm, a method based on speed growth is used. In this paper, We calculates not only the growth speed of a certain word, but also the growth speed of the user numbers related to the certain word, the speed of two respects determine a hot keyword. The main content of this paper has two aspects as follows:

In topic detection, time information is attached more attention and it often plays a major role, the shorter the time interval of two posts, the greater the similarity. For every word, it is expressed as feature trajectory of binary group sequence, and then calculates the growth slope of every adjacent two windows in the all sequence to discover the hot keywords. By this means, we can predict and extract the hot keywords according to the trend curve.

After extracting hot keywords, hot keywords are clustered to extract hot topics, so measuring similarity of the words is needful. In this paper, the similarity of words is measured from two aspects: the similarity based on Chinese Thesaurus and probability co-occurrence of two words in the same micro-blog text. We can deduce the hot topics by hot keyword clusters which generated through clustering. The effectiveness of the proposed method has been verified.

58.2 Related Work

Topic detection and tracking (TDT) was put forward by Defense Advanced Research Projects Agency (DARPA) in 1996, and topic detection was a subtask in TDT evaluation workshops. Since the TDT was proposed, it has attracted intensive and persistent interests from many researchers and scholars. Meanwhile, topic detection appeared as a subtask in TDT also received great attention. In the beginning, researchers and scholars focused the research on news corpus, but recently, with the rapid rise of micro-blog and the superiority it performed, micro-blog has attracted the attention of the researchers. However, the micro-blog text is rather different from the news articles, it is short, ungrammatical, and unstructured, so the traditional method used on news articles performed badly on micro-blog [3]. However, micro-blog has a unique characteristic—immediacy, the number of related micro-blog is often greater than related news at the same time period, it is very sensitive to the emergency on the network. Therefore, nowadays, many researchers are trying to get hot topics on micro-blog. So far, extracting hot topics on micro-blog mainly from the following two aspects: from the angle of the users and from the angle of the micro-blog content. The related works are as follows:

A master's graduation thesis of Zhejiang University made full use of the user relationship to form a user network or the user tree, and then used the user tree for hot topic detection [4]. Shi et al. [1] introduced active index on micro-blog users to rank users with activeness.

The two researches were on the angle of the users.

A master's graduation thesis of Tongji University using the method of keyword detection and cluster discovered hot topics [5]. At present the analysis on the micro-blog content mostly focused on clustering algorithm, but the clustering algorithm performed badly because of the amount of noise.

Although as a new thing, study on it is not mature both at home and abroad, micro-blog as the favorite of the Web2.0, its booming trend has attracted the attention of many researchers and scholars at home and abroad as well as the famous international conference.

ACL conference in the year 2011, 2012 and academic conference of the eighth national information retrieval in the year 2012 both involved the searching and mining of social media (such as BBS, blog, micro-blog).

Mario Cataldi [6] proposed the method of Twitter hot topics found based on time Sequence and social relationship evaluation. He thought that over a period of time, if a topic was detected for many times, but rarely detected in before, by now, the topic was likely to become a hot topic.

Swip Phuvipadawa [7] proposed an approach to detect the burst on Twitter by using the methods of collecting, grouping and sorting.

Recently, many scholars' study on micro-blog was from two aspects of the perspective of the users and content. In this paper, a method based on time sequence was proposed to discover hot topics. In this approach, the growth speed was determined from the angle of the users and the angle of the micro-blog content, then calculated the similarity of the keywords into a cluster, and then the hot topics were detected.

58.3 Keywords Detection Based on Growth Speed

58.3.1 Related Concepts: Time Sequence

Time sequence is a concept proposed in this paper, it was obtained by the pre-treated micro-blog, and the pretreatment included filtering and sorting on micro-blog. The information on micro-blog platforms are not all useful, it contains much noise and advertising information, which affect the word frequency statistics seriously. Three kinds of filtering are as follows:

(1) Remove the information with "@username" format. The information with this format is similar to the chat dialogue in our daily life, the reason remove it is that less words, the words at random and not standard, and the context relationship is not obvious, besides, the possibility it directly describe the event is smaller. All of the reasons would seriously impact the clustering effect, so removing the information with this format.
(2) Remove the information with "# topic name" format. This topic is usually released by micro-blog platform themselves, such as "# national civil service exam", the number of participants is larger but the artificial factor is strong, it would affect the total number of users.
(3) Remove the information released by the users whose fans number is less than a certain threshold. Many advertisement users whose fans number is less and concern number is larger often release information that related to their interests, so removing the information released by them.

After filtering the micro-blog, sorting them as follows:

(1) Extract time information of micro-blog, and sort them in chronological order.
(2) Divide these micro-blog texts into several groups by a certain interval, each group is called a window (for example, 300 texts as a group).

In this paper, form a time sequence for every word, for example, for a word w, the time sequence denoted as

$$C_w = (C_w(1), C_w(2), C_w(3), \ldots, C_w(k))$$

Among them, $C_w(i) = TF_w(i)$ is the frequency of word w in the ith window.

After extracting time information of every micro-blog text, statistics the earliest time and the latest time of each window, and calculates the half of the difference between the two, denoted as td, by now, every word is expressed as feature trajectory of binary group sequence, denoted as

$$V_w = [(C_w(1), td_1), (C_w(2), td_2), (C_w(3), td_3), \ldots, (C_w(k), td_k)]$$

Namely, every binary group sequence consists of two parts: the frequency of word w in a certain window, and the middle time of the window.

58.3.2 Calculate Growth Rate

Currently there are many ways to judge whether a time sequence contains potential hot keywords [8], the typical is automata model proposed by Mr. Kleinberg and the model are tested and verified from many applications [9]. However, the micro-blog platform which is time sensitivity and immediacy, these typical methods achieved less. In this paper, we use slope to analyze the feature trajectory of binary group sequence, it is effective to discover evolution tendency of suspected hot keywords, so as to detect the hot topic timely.

Given a certain time sequence

$$V_w = [(C_w(1), td_1), (C_w(2), td_2), (C_w(3), td_3), \ldots, (C_w(k), td_k)]$$

The slope is used to calculate words w growth trend

$$SLO_w = \frac{C_w(i) - C_w(i-1)}{td_i - td_{i-1}}, \text{ the unit of } td_i \text{ is hour}$$

That is to say, for a certain word, calculates the slope of every two adjacent windows, if the slope increases gradually or the slope appears as growth trends roughly, it would be as hot keyword in all probability. At the moment, we just predict the growth trend of the word, the development trend also depends on the number of users who spread the word. Therefore, the growth rate of a certain word includes two parts: the growth rate of the word itself and the growth rate of different users related to the word, respectively denoted as GR_w and GR_{user}

$$GR_w = \frac{C_w(i)}{\sum_{i=1}^{i-1} C_w(i)/(i-1)}$$

$$GR_{user} = \frac{C_{wuser}(i)}{\sum_{i=1}^{i-1} C_{wuser}(i)/(i-1)}$$

That is to say, the frequency of the current window divided by the average frequency of the previous window. Among them, $C_{wuser}(i)$ is the number of users related to the word w in window of i, namely the number of different users whose micro-blog contains the words w.

$$GR = a * GR_w + b * GR_{user}$$

Among them, a, b are two parameters, they were set to be 0.5 in the experiment.

58.4 Topic Extraction

58.4.1 Keywords Extraction

What we have done in this paper aims at extracting hot topics, so the previous work is prepared for the topic extraction. Therefore, topic extraction includes the following five procedures: micro-blog pretreatment, expressed as feature trajectory of binary group sequence for every word, calculating the growth rate, extracting hot keywords, clustering keywords into clusters, and discovering hot topics.

Through the calculation of the third chapter we can find that some words increase rapidly and some increase slowly, even the growth slope is close to zero. The growth rate is sorted in order, and the word as hot keyword whose growth rate is greater than a certain threshold T.

58.4.2 Hot Keyword Clustering

After extracting the hot keywords, keyword clustering is an important step for hot topic extraction. In this section, we focus on the keywords clustering. In order to cluster better, the method of the similarity based on Chinese Thesaurus combined with probability co-occurrence of two words in the same micro-blog text is adopted to calculate the similarity. The reasons adopt the method is that the similarity of words not only depends on the similarity of words meaning, but also the similarity in the real context. For example, in Chinese Thesaurus, the similarity of two words based on a assumption: the more similar meaning words the greater the similarity, and if two words meaning is not close, it is generally thought as independence. But factually, this assumption does not conform to the actual situation. For example, "grain output improved generally this year, the wheat output increase largest, ten percent more than last year", if we only use similarity calculation method based on Chinese Thesaurus, we would get {grain, wheat}, rather than {grain, wheat, yield, improve}we want to get. Therefore, we also use the similarity calculation method based on the real context.

For the similarity calculation based on the real context, it is measured through the computation of conditional probability. The following method is adopted to calculate similarity, for keywords t1 and t2, statistics the conditional probability of t1, t2 that appeared at the same time in each window, namely

$$P(t_1/t_2) = \frac{P(t_1, t_2)}{P(t_2)} = \frac{C(t_1, t_2)}{C(t_2)}$$

Namely, the number of micro-blog appeared t1, t2 at the same time divided by the number of micro-blog appeared t2.

$$Sim(t_1, t_2) = \max P(t_1/t_2)$$

Namely, the similarity values of t1, t2 are expressed as the maximum in all Windows.

For the two similarity calculation methods, the former one only considered the inherent similarity of words, it takes a assumption that if two words meaning is closer and the similarity is larger, the chances they belong to the same topic is greater. It has a defect that it ignored the real context of two words, the latter makes up for the defect. Therefore, as a result, a keyword cluster method based on Chinese Thesaurus combined with probability co-occurrence of two words in the same micro-blog text is adopted in this paper. The specific clustering procedure is as follows:

First, the similarity is calculated based on Chinese Thesaurus. For keywords t1, t2, looking up Chinese Thesaurus get the two words similarity, if the similarity value is judged to be similar, then proceeds to the next step. Second, for keywords t1, t2, if $sim(t_1, t_2)$ is greater than a certain threshold T1, the t1, t2 are thought to belong to the same cluster. At this moment, several clusters are got, and each cluster contains one or more keywords, we could deduce hot topics from these clusters. For example, as a cluster {china, Diaoyu Islands, Japan}, we could get a topic of "China and Japan compete for Diaoyu Islands".

58.5 Test Results and Analysis

In order to verify the accuracy and efficiency of the proposed method in this paper, the experiment was done as follows.

58.5.1 Data Preparation

The dataset for the evaluation is extracted from SINA micro-blog for ten days. The dataset consists of 2 million micro-blog texts collected during 2012-5-15 to 2012-5-24. The texts are pretreated including micro-blog filtering and sorting. And then, the noise and stop words are removed on micro-blog. We annotate the hot topics manually during the time, including "north Korea arrest Chinese fishing boat", "China and Philippines confront in the south sea", "An old man in Daqin resist others pull down his house", and "Civil servants force the boss kneel down to him" and so on.

58.5.2 Results and Discussions

In this section, we will discuss the evaluation from both the results using our method in this work and the baseline results—without using our method. Namely, the experiment results using our method compares to the baseline system on the performance.

We adopt miss rate and false detection rate proposed by National Institute of Standards and Technology (NIST) to evaluate the efficiency. They are respectively denoted as P_{miss} and P_{FA},

$$P_{miss} = \frac{c}{a+c} \quad P_{FA} = \frac{b}{b+d}$$

Among them,

a the number of related micro-blog text that have been detected;
b the number of unrelated micro-blog text that have been detected;
c the number of related micro-blog text that have not been detected;
d the number of unrelated micro-blog text that have not been detected.

The miss rate is defined as the system has not detected the new topic while the topic should be a new hot topic; the false detection rate is defined as the system judges the follow-up reports of the original topic to be a new topic mistakenly.

In the experiment, the intention is to evaluate the influence of the size of window, T, T1 on topic detection respectively. In order to assess the influence of these parameters effectively, we divide the dataset into 8 groups. The values of these parameters are determined by the average calculated by the 8 group data. The specific settings of these parameters are described in the following paragraphs.

Firstly, in order to verify the effectiveness of the proposed approach, the experiment was done to calculate the miss rate and false detection rate, and the accuracy (comprehensive assessment of miss rate and false detection rate) was used to prove the efficiency of the proposed method in this paper. Besides, we take a comparison on the accuracy between the approach using the method proposed in this paper and the baseline results—without using our method. The comparison results as shown in Fig. 58.1. The accuracy we used in this paper is defined as

$$p_{accuracy} = 0.5 * p_{miss} + 0.5 * p_{FA}$$

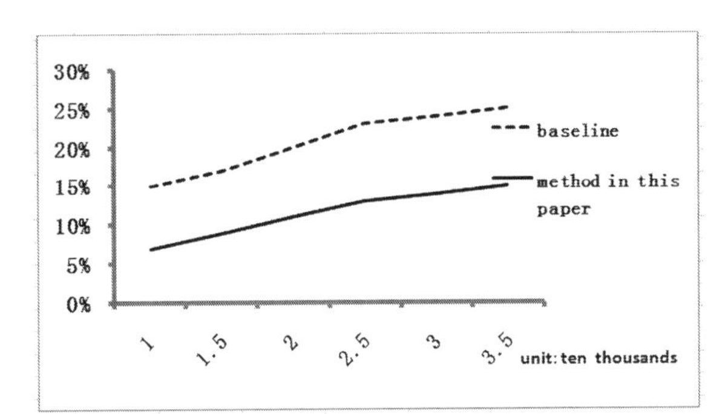

Fig. 58.1 Comparation on accuracy

As can be seen from Fig. 58.1, the method in this paper perfects better than the method without using our algorithm. The reasons are as follows, firstly, the proposed method in this paper could extract the useful keywords effectively before clustering, but the other methods cluster a huge number of words directly, which is poor efficiency. Secondly, our method could remove the excess of redundant words. Besides, the baseline method is a traditional method based on word frequency statistics, which statistics word frequency after the text was pretreated. If the word frequency is high, it is thought to be hot keywords.

The size of window influences the accuracy of topic detection largely. For example, the Fig. 58.2 shows the word frequency distribution when the size of the window is 25000. We can see from the figure, only a few words appear multiple times, many words appear only in a minority.

As can be seen from the above, there are only a few words appeared frequently, and most of the words appear only very few times. Because micro-blog is a big platform without much limitation, so it is difficult to gather the users together, unless the topic is very hot. Therefore, it is very difficult to cluster a huge number of words directly and it would be very difficult to find hot topics. In order to cluster the words easily, we first define many windows with specific size, and then filter the words using threshold T. As shown in Figs. 58.3 and 58.4, respectively shows the miss rate and false detection rate of the different size of window and the threshold T (relative to the artificial mark).

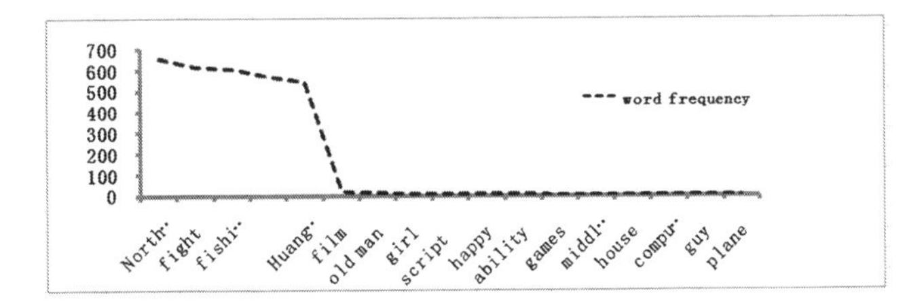

Fig. 58.2 Word frequency distribution when the size of window is 25000

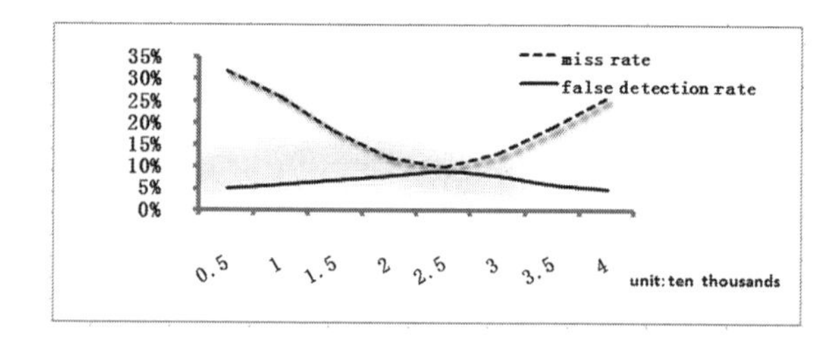

Fig. 58.3 The influence of different windows on miss rate and false detection rate

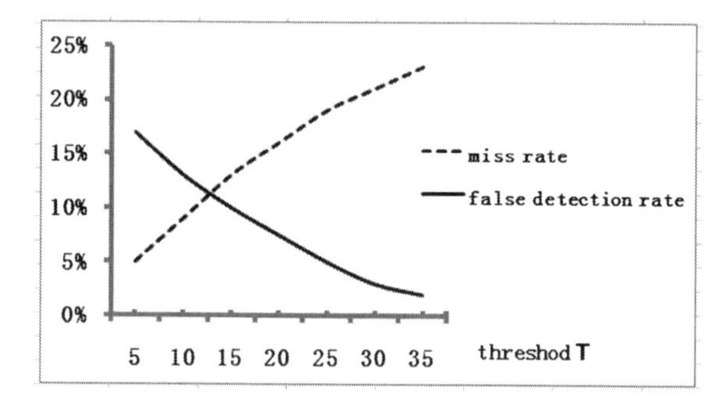

Fig. 58.4 The influence of different T on miss rate and false rate

As can be seen from the Fig. 58.3, when the size of window is small, the ratio of noise content is larger, and false detection rate is higher, the reason is that the size of window is small and most of the words spread, two related reports are more likely to be detected as two different topics mistakenly. But the topic number that would be detected is more, so the miss rate is relatively low; When the size of window is larger, most of words together within a window, so the miss rate is higher, but the false detection rate is relatively low, because the window is too wide, and most reports was contained in a window, two unrelated reports are more likely to be detected as the same topic mistakenly.

As can be seen from the Fig. 58.4, when the threshold T is set to be 5, the miss rate is the lowest, but it contains much noise. Increases as the T value, miss rate will rise, but the false detection rate reduces. Thus, the threshold T play an important role in keywords extraction. Besides, considering the growth rate of words is closely related to the growth rate of relevant users, we take a = b = 0.5.

Comprehensive above two figures, when we extract hot keywords, the size of window is set to be 25000 or so, and the threshold T is about 15.

For keywords clustering, we discussed the effect of T1 for clustering (relative to the artificial tagging). Figure 58.5 shows the miss rate and false detection rate in different values of T1.

As can be seen from the above, the best value of T1 is 0.6 or so.

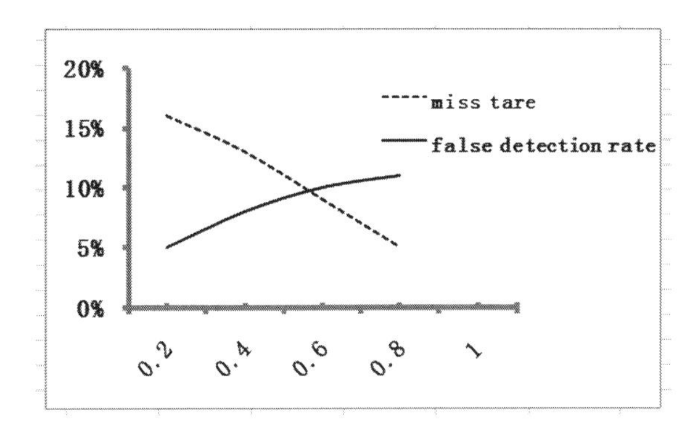

Fig. 58.5 The influence of T1 on clustering

58.6 Conclusion

In this paper, an approach based on speed growth was proposed to detect hot topics on micro-blog. First, micro-blogs are sorted in chronological order and divided into several windows; second, calculate the growth speed of each word and extract the keyword whose growth speed is larger than a certain T; lastly, cluster the keywords to get hot topics. We have done experiment on micro-blog, it proves that the approach proposed in this paper performs well. However, the miss rate and false detection rate is still much room for improvement. Therefore, we will further improve the precision of the algorithm and simplify algorithm process, make the algorithm has a better future.

Acknowledgments This research was supported by the National Natural Science Foundation of China (No. 60873247), the Natural Science Foundation of Shandong Province of China (No. ZR2009GZ007, ZR2011FM030), and National Social Science foundation of China (12BXW040).

References

1. Shi L, Zhang C, Wei L (2012) A mechanism of micro-blog users ranking introduced active index. J Chin Comput Syst 33(5):110–114
2. Zheng FR, Miao DQ, Zhang ZF, Gao C (2012) A method of topic detection on Chinese micro-blog. J Comput Sci 39(1):138–141
3. James A, Courtney W, Alvaro B (2003) Retrieval and novelty detection at the sentence level. In: SIGIR, pp 314–321
4. Yang GC (2011) Research of hot topic discovery strategy on microblogging platforms. Zhejiang University
5. Giridhar K, James A (2004) Text classification and named entities for new event detection. In: SIGIR, pp 297–304
6. Mario C, Luiqi DC, Claudio S (2010) Emerging topic detection on Twitter based on temporal and social terms evaluation. In: MDMKDD 10 proceedings of the tenth International workshop on multimedia data mining. Washington, pp 1–10

7. Swit P, Tsuyoshi M (2010) Breaking news detection and tracking in Twitter. In: Web intelligence and intelligent agent technology (WI-IAT), 2010 IEEE/WIC/ACM international conference on Toronto, ON, pp 120–123
8. Qi H, Chang K, Lim E-P (2007) Analyzing feature trajectories for event detection. In: Proceedings of the 30th annual international ACM SIGIR conference, pp 207–214
9. Nish P, Neel S (2008) Scalable and near real-time burst detection from ecommerce queries. In: Proceedings of the 14th ACM SIGKDD international conference on knowledge discovery and data mining, pp 972–980

Chapter 59
Computational Fluid Dynamics Simulation of Air Flow in the Human Symmetrical Six-Generation Bifurcation Bronchial Tree Model

Shouliang Qi, Zhenghua Li and Yong Yue

Abstract The present study aims to reveal the velocity and pressure distributions of air flow in the human symmetrical six-generation bifurcation bronchial tree model, to determine the influences of homothetic ratio, the angle of branching, and the branching plane rotation angle on the air flow. The 3D bronchial tree model is built up using SolidWorks based on optimal parameters from the references at first. And then it is transferred into ANSYS, one computational fluid dynamics software, to simulate the air flow and get the velocity and pressure distributions. Similarly, three different models are established by varying homothetic ratio, the angle of branching, and the branching plane rotation angle. Their impacts on the air flow are clarified through comparing the results. It is found the velocity and pressure distributions are symmetical genrally, but they start uneven from the fourth generation bronchus. The velocities in the inner and inferior bronchi are smaller than in the outer and superior ones. The pressure drop will decrease with the homothetic ratio, but it also increases the tree volume. The variations of the branching angle and the branching plane rotation angle will increase the pressure drop. The simulation results can reveal the air flow patterns in the models, and work as the benchmark for the future ventilation assessment of realistic human lung.

Keywords Bronchial tree · Computational fluid dynamics · Respiratory

---

S. Qi (✉) · Z. Li
Sino-Dutch Biomedical and Information Engineering School, Northeastern University, No. 3-11, Wenhua Road, Shenyang, China
e-mail: qisl@bmie.neu.edu.cn

Y. Yue
Radiology Department, Shengjing Hospital of China Medical University, No. 36, Sanhao Street, Shenyang, China

S. Li et al. (eds.), *Frontier and Future Development of Information Technology in Medicine and Education*, Lecture Notes in Electrical Engineering 269,
DOI: 10.1007/978-94-007-7618-0_59,

59.1 Introduction

Human airways are dichotomous, and consist of approximately 23 generations of branches from the trachea to the alveoli [1]. There are 2^{17} conducting bronchi or bronchioles, and each of which is followed by about 6 generations of alveolar ducts that constitute the acini for gas exchange.

Through minimizing the viscous dissipation for a finite tree volume, an ideal or optimal structure of the bronchial tree can be deduced [2]. It is an approximate fractal structure with the fractal dimension of 3. The diameter and length of the successive bronchial segments decrease gradually, and are homothetic with a size ratio. The ratio of diameter between generation *i-1* (child) and generation *i* (parent) is called h_D, and it is h_L for the length. For the optimal model, $h_D = h_L = (1/2)^{1/3} = 0.7937$ [2]. Meanwhile, the angle of branching, θ, is equal to 37.5°, and the branching plane rotation angle, β, is 90° [3].

Usually the flow in the ideal bronchial tree is assumed to be fully developed laminar flow and obey the Poiseuille law. However, the flow cannot develop fully in such a short duct, e.g., 9.45 mm for the sixth generation bronchus. Turbulence eddy and the flow disturbance caused by the bifurcations easily propagate to the bronchi [4]. The importance of study on the flow characteristics in the ideal model lies on it provides a benchmark for evaluate the ventilation efficiency of the realistic human airway. Previous studies are mainly limited to 2D dimensional or less generations (e.g. three-generation [5]) airway, and 3D multi-generation research is rarely and necessary.

In fact, the realistic human bronchial tree is far away from the optimal. h_D and h_L are about 0.85 [6, 7]. Tawhia et al. [8] also found the the branching plane rotation angle is about 79°, and the branching angle is larger for the distal bronchi. These three parameters definitely have important influences on the flow patterns and resistance. For the laminar flow, the flow resistance can be deduced theoretically. It is strongly dependent on h_D and h_L, and a 4 % reduction results in an increase of resistance by two times [2]. Bokov et al. [9] also found the resistance increases with the decrease of the h_D. But the quantitative analysis on the influence of θ and β on the flow characteristics is not found.

Computational fluid dynamic based on finite element method has been used for the flow simulation in both ideal and realistic human bronchial tree models [5, 9–11]. The feasibility and accuracy of computational fluid dynamic simulation have been proved by Rochefort et al. [11] using hyperpolarized ^{3}He magnetic resonance phase-contrast velocimetry. They found the flow distribution agreed within 3 %.

59.2 Materials and Methods

59.2.1 Geometry Model of Bronchial Tree

Human symmetrical bifurcation bronchial tree models are established by one 3D computed aided design (CAD) software, SolidWorks. The sketch is given in Fig. 59.1a. There $D_0 = 16.0$ mm, $L_0 = 30.0$ mm, the segments of 0.2 L_0 from the bifurcation interaction are used for the smoothing chamfer. In Fig. 59.2b, the 3D model is shown in the up view. Five cross section areas from CSR1 to CSR5 are marked for further analysis.

For all the four models, varying h_D, h_L, θ and β, four models can be obtained. Specific parameter values are listed in Table 59.1. The volumes of four models are 75556, 36500, 36764, and 36501 mm^3, respectively. For Model II, larger $h_D = h_L = 0.85$ increases the volume two times more than the other three models for its three-power dependence.

59.2.2 Mesh

The meshing method is set as Tetrahedrons, and the algorithm is Patch Conforming. The element size is determined to be 0.4 mm. For the inflation options, the first layer height, maximum layer and growth rate are 0.2 mm, 5 and 1.1, respectively. The mesh quality is measured by the parameters of the skewness based on the equilateral volume deviation < 0.9, the minimum of orthogonal

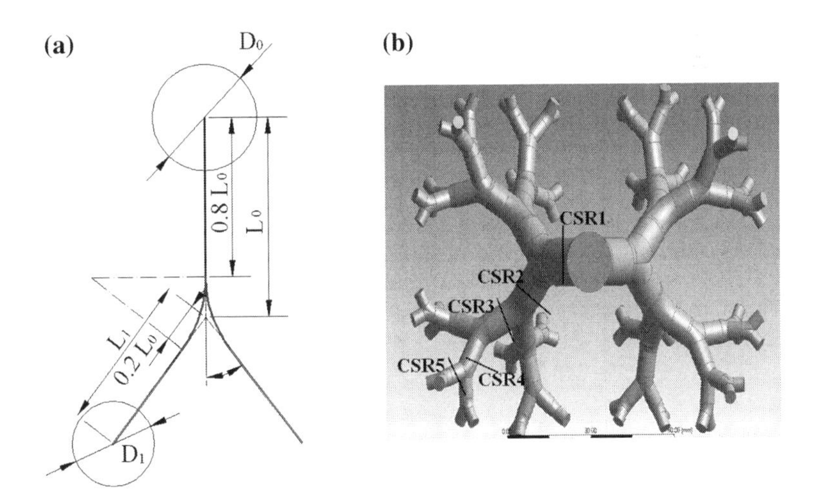

Fig. 59.1 Ideal human symmetrical bifurcation bronchial tree model: **a** sketch; **b** 3D six-generation model

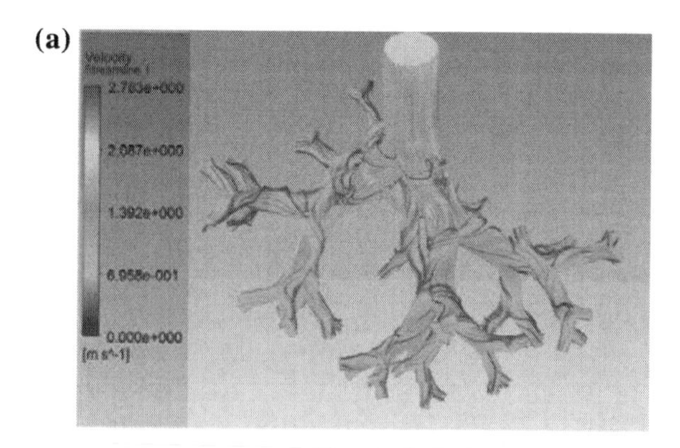

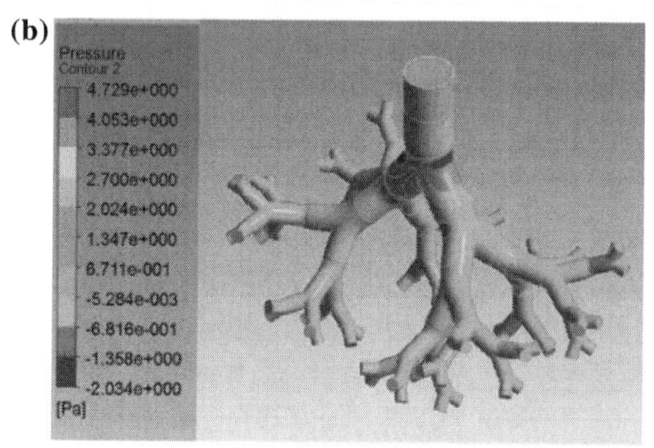

Fig. 59.2 Velocity and pressure distributions in an ideal human symmetrical bifurcation bronchial tree model (Model I): **a** velocity distribution; **b** pressure distribution

Table 59.1 Parameters for the four models

NO./Para	h_D	h_L	θ	β
Model I	0.7937	0.7937	37.5°	90°
Model II	0.85	0.85	37.5°	90°
Model III	0.7937	0.7937	40.0°	90°
Model IV	0.7937	0.7937	37.5°	79°

quality >0.1, and Wall YPlus value > 30. Finally, about 8.5×10^6 elements are obtained for Model II due to larger volume, and rough 4.2×10^6 element for the others.

59.2.3 Solution

For the CFD, the fluid was assumed incompressible (Mach number << 1), and Newtonian. The airway flow is in laminar conditions because Re was <1,000. The walls simulating branches were considered as the rigid and dry surfaces.

In present study, pressure-based (segregated) solver is used. Meanwhile, the algorithm of SIMPLE is selected to cope with the pressure–velocity coupling problem. Second-Order Upwind is applied as the interpolation scheme for the convection term. The interpolation methods for gradients of solution variables and pressure are determined using Green-Gauss Cell-Based and Standard scheme, respectively. For the boundary conditions, the velocity-inlet of 2.0 m/s and pressure-out of 1.0 atm are adopted according to methods in [5, 10].

While the scaled energy residual is $<10^{-6}$ and scaled species residual $<10^{-5}$, the convergence is considered to be reached. The mesh is refined to obtain a gird-independent solution. Present CFD is conducted by a HP 64-bit workstation with Window 7 system, Intel Xeon E5-2620 2.0 GHz processor and 32 Go RAM. 00.

59.3 Results and Discussion

59.3.1 Velocity and Pressure

Globally, the velocity and pressure distributions in an ideal human symmetrical bifurcation tree (Model I) are shown in Fig. 59.2. It can be seen that the velocity reduces gradually from the trachea to the distal bronchi. The maximum value reaches 2.79 m/s at the center of trachea. The distributions are symmetrical generally, but they start uneven from the fourth generation bronchus. The velocities in the inner and inferior bronchi are smaller than in the outer and superior ones. The streamlines show the inverse flow at the bifurcation, which mainly result from the local geometries variation and agree with the finding in [10, 12]. As shown in Fig. 59.2b, pressure is lower with the increase of the generations. But the total pressure drop only has about 7.0 pa due to optimal structure. Significant low pressure region is found especially at the first bifurcation, which means the eddy my occur.

It is noted that the maximum airway resistance exists up to fourth generation at resting conditions. In present model, there are not the upper airways features, such as glottis and larynx, which play important impact on the flow pattern in trachea. However, it is known that the flow profiles after the first bronchial bifurcation are affected moderately.

Figure 59.3 shows the details of velocity and pressure at CSR1-CSR5. It is found that the pressure and velocity patterns match well. For CSR1, one high velocity region is available, correspondingly there is a high pressure region near the wall. While the generation increases, the gradients or variations of pressure and velocity decrease. For CSR5, the highest velocity is only about 1.1 m/s.

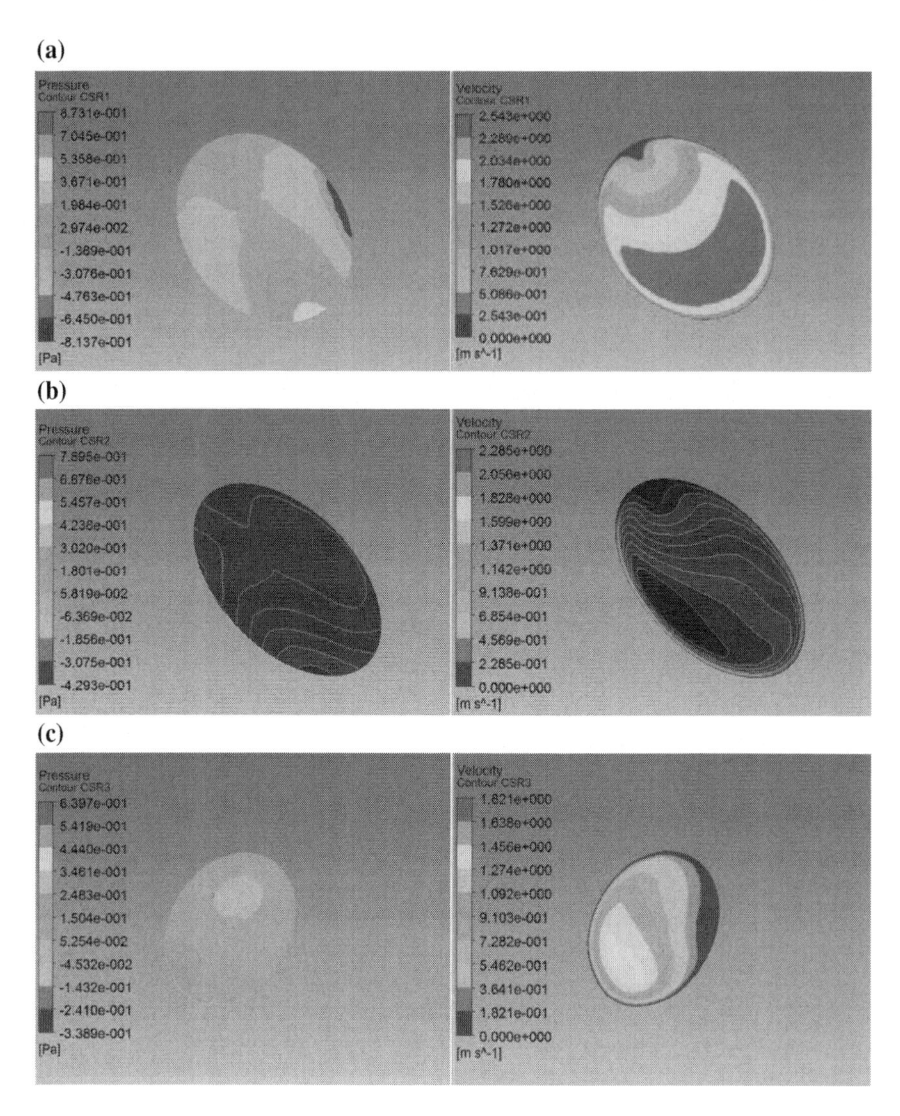

Fig. 59.3 Velocity and pressure distributions at CSR1–CSR5: **a** CSR1; **b** CSR2; **c** CSR3; **d** CSR4; **e** CSR5

59.3.2 Influence of Parameters

The influences of three parameters of h_D, θ and β are given in Fig. 59.4. It is found that with the pressure drop decreases while h_D increases, but it takes more volume. The branching angle has significant role on the flow, as shown in Fig. 59.4b. The branching plane rotation angle shows moderate impact on the flow.

(d)

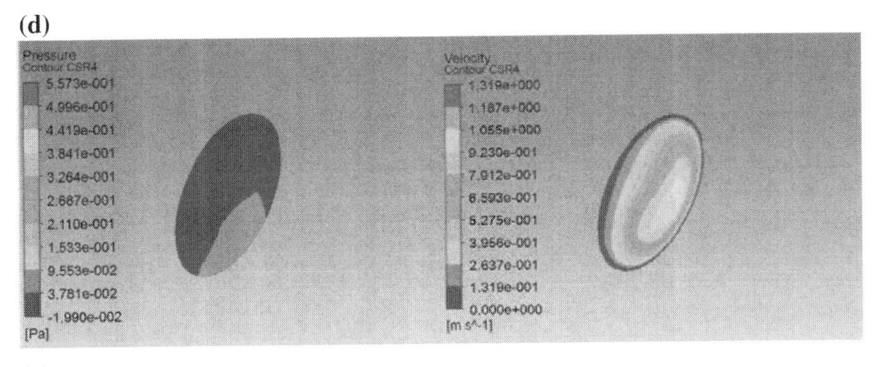

(e)

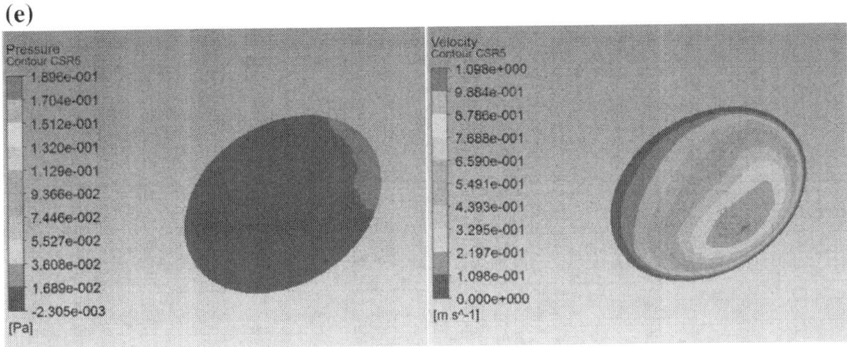

Fig. 59.3 (continued)

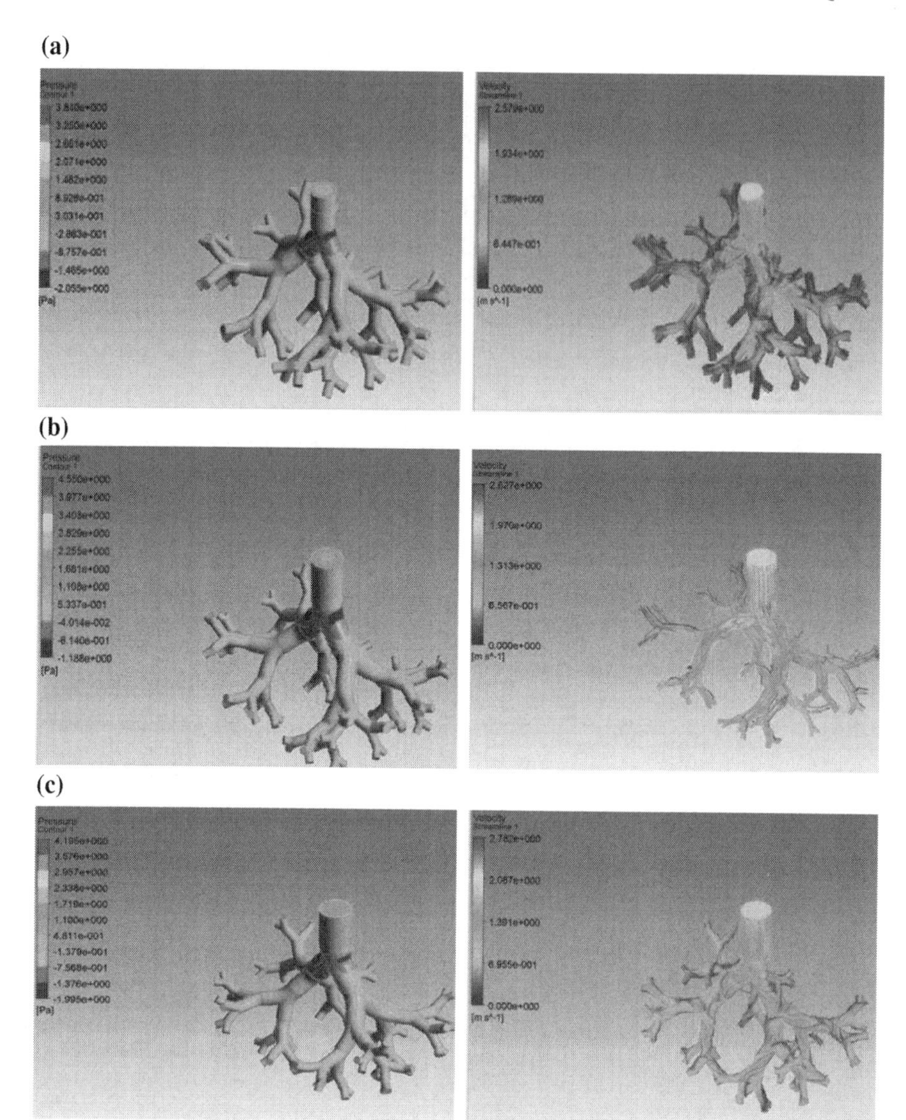

Fig. 59.4 Influence of parameters: **a** Model II with $h_D = h_L = 0.85$; **b** Model III with = 40°; **c** Model IV with = 79°

59.4 Conclusion

In present study, the computational fluid dynamics simulation has been done to reveal the air flow in the human symmetrical six-generation bifurcation bronchial tree model. The main conclusions are given as follows.

(1) The simulation results can reveal the air flow patterns in the models, and work as the benchmark for the future ventilation assessment of realistic human lung.
(2) The velocity and pressure distributions are symmetrical generally, but they start uneven from the fourth generation bronchus. The velocities in the inner and inferior bronchi are smaller than in the outer and superior ones. The pressure drop will decrease with the homothetic ratio, but it also increases the tree volume. The variations of the branching angle and the branching plane rotation angle will increase the pressure drop.

Acknowledgments This work was financially supported by the National Science Foundation Council (No. 51006021), the Fundamental Research Funds for the Central Universities (N110419001), and the Scientific Research Fund of Liaoning Provincial Education Department (L2012080).

References

1. Naidich DP, Webb WR, Harkin TJ et al (2005) Imaging of the airways: functional and radiological correlations. Lippincott Williams & Wilkins/Wolters Kluwer Health Inc., Philadelphia
2. Mauroy B, Filoche M, Weibel ER et al (2004) An optimal bronchial tree may be dangerous. Nature 427(6975):633–636
3. Horsfield K, Cumming G (1967) Angles of branching and diameters of branches in the human bronchial tree. Bull Math Biol 29(2):245–259
4. Tawhai MH, Hoffman EA, Lin CL (2009) The lung physiome: merging imaging-based measures with predictive computational models of structure and function. Wiley Interdiscip Rev Syst Biol Med 1(1):61–72
5. Liu Y, So RMC, Zhang CH (2002) Modeling the bifurcating flow in a human lung airway. J Biomech 35:465–473
6. Weibel ER (1997) In: Crystal RG, West JB, Weibel ER, Barnes PJ (eds) The lung: scientific foundations, vol. 1, 2nd edn. Lippincott-Raven, Philadelphia, pp 1061–1071
7. Montaudon M, Desbarats P, Berger P et al (2007) Assessment of bronchial wall thickness and lumen diameter in human adults using multi-detector computed tomography: comparison with theoretical models. J Anat 211(5):579–588
8. Tawhai MH, Hunter P, Tschirren J et al (2004) CT-based geometry analysis and finite element models of the human and ovine bronchial tree. J Appl Physiol 97(6):2310–2321
9. Lin CL, Tawhai MH, McLennan G et al (2007) Characteristics of the turbulent laryngeal jet and its effect on airflow in the human intra-thoracic airways. Respir Physiol Neurobiol 157(2):295–309
10. Vial L, Chet D, Fodil R et al (2005) Airflow modeling of steady inspiration in two realistic proximal airway trees reconstructed from human thoracic tomodensitometric images. Comput Methods Biomech Biomed Eng 8(4):267–277
11. Gemci T, Ponyavin V, Chen Y et al (2008) Computational model of airflow in upper 17 generations of human respiratory tract. J Biomech 41:2047–2054
12. Rochefort L, Vial LR, Fodil et al (2007) In vitro validation of computational fluid dynamic simulation in human proximal airways with hyperpolarized ^{3}He magnetic resonance phase-contrast velocimetry. J Appl Physiol 102:2012–2023
13. Bokov P, Mauro B, Revel MP et al (2010) Lumen areas and homothety factor influence airway resistance in COPD. Respir Physiol Neurobiol 173(1):1–10

Chapter 60
Discrimination of Solitary Pulmonary Nodules on CT Images Based on a Novel Automatic Weighted FCM

Zhang Xin, Jiaxing Li, Wang Bing, Ming Jun, Yang Ying and Zhang Jinxing

Abstract A novel automatic feature assessment and weighting Fuzzy C-Means (FCM) algorithm was proposed for the classification of solitary pulmonary nodules (SPN). Six pulmonary nodule features were extracted from computed tomography (CT) images, which were normalized and combined into feature sequence. The feature assessment method was used to calculate discriminative criterion of categories, where the sensitive features were selected and weighted to discriminate between benign and suspicious malignant pulmonary nodules. Forty CT slices of twenty three patients are selected to evaluate the proposed method. The experimental results show that the accuracy of discrimination is 86.3 %, the sensitiveness is 87.5 %, and the specificity is 80 %, which illustrate that the method is feasible, and have good accuracy and sensitivity.

Keywords Classification · CAD · Automatic weighted preference · FCM

60.1 Introduction

In the field of lung nodules detection, many of the developed methods propose optimal feature selection techniques before the classification stage. Hence, feature selection and classification appear as two separate stages in the CAD system.

Z. Xin (✉)
College of Electronic Information Engineering, Hebei University, Wusi East Rd.180, Baoding 071002, China
e-mail: zhangxin@hbu.edu.cn

W. Bing · M. Jun
College of Mathematics and Computer Science, Hebei University, Wusi East Rd.180, Baoding 071002, China
e-mail: wangbing@hbu.edu.cn

M. Jun
e-mail: 511099781@qq.com

S. Li et al. (eds.), *Frontier and Future Development of Information Technology in Medicine and Education*, Lecture Notes in Electrical Engineering 269,
DOI: 10.1007/978-94-007-7618-0_60,

The accurate extraction and analysis of lung nodules have been an important procedure in CAD, where specific difficulties lie in: (1) The interference of each organization's lung CT image gray value distribution is great, and the overlap of a lot of tissue or organ is serious, which resulting confusion among soft tissue, blood vessels and the nodules need to be observed; (2) The lung tumors have different shapes and complex growth environment, there is no rules at all, so the primary screen of the nodular is relatively easy, but the further screening and analysis is very difficult to achieve a higher accuracy rate. Domestic and foreign scholars have done a lot of research in this respect, proposed a number of methods, such as segmentation and template matching method based on gradient operator and shape operator, based on N-loop-filter and so on, another common method is multistage the gray-scale transformation, it can well separate the tissue like the blood vessels that connect with the tumor. The widely used methods are linear classifiers and neural network in the classification work. However, the linear classifier and neural network requires a lot of prior knowledge, and artificially set rules, which make them powerless when dealing with the new and unknown classification problem of nodules.

Cluster analysis is a summarized process, and need not determine the classification criteria before analyzing the data object, and does not consider the known class mark, which makes the cluster analysis more universal and flexible. Only extract the nodule characteristics and input cluster analysis system, the results will be obtained.

In this paper, a new combination of six features of nodules was applied, comprehensively analyzing the features' differences between the benign and suspicious malignant nodules without increasing the test dose. At the same time, a new automatically weighted FCM algorithm was applied on this complex classification problem. The experiments show that this method is clear and feasible, and have good accuracy and sensitivity.

60.2 Imaging Characteristics of Pulmonary Nodules

The base of distinction is the different characteristics between benign and suspicious malignant pulmonary nodules. There are many characteristics can be used, but it is not the more characteristics were used the better a result will be show. Now, six kinds of pulmonary nodules features are selected to test.

60.2.1 Feature Extraction

(1) The mean density, using the gray average to express in the iconography. The value of malignancy is medium and the value of the benign is medium or

higher. That is, the value of benign is larger than the suspicious malignancy, usually.

$$Ave = \frac{1}{N} \sum_{(x,y) \in R} I(x, y) \tag{60.1}$$

(2) Whether the density is uniform, using gray average variance to express in the iconography. The density of the benign tumors and inflammatory is more uniform, but suspicious malignant tumors can be empty or calcification which make the density uneven.

$$Var = \frac{1}{N} \sum_{(x,y) \in R} [I(x, y) - Ave]^2 \tag{60.2}$$

(3) Whether fat can be found In CT image, fat' CT value is in the range of [−90, −50 HU]. Usually there are no fat in suspicious malignant tumor.
(4) Compactness

$$F = \frac{4\pi.A}{P^2} \tag{60.3}$$

A is the area of nodules, and P is the perimeter. F is on behalf the similar degree between nodules and circular. When F = 1, that's to say, the nodule is a perfect circle. The rougher a boundary is, the less F value is. The smaller shape is flat, the less F value also is. And the smaller the F value is, the greater probability for suspicious malignant nodules is.

(5) Flattening: S

$$S = \frac{a}{b} \tag{60.4}$$

Draw two Perpendicular lines in a nodules, the longer length is a, and another length is b. The greater the S is, the larger the possibility of benign is.

(6) Texture feature
Shape moment descriptor: Based on that regional outline border moment can characterize the outline of the boundary P. Boundary moment m_p and boundary central moment M_p can be expressed as follows:

$$m_p = \frac{1}{N} \sum_{i=1}^{N} [z(i)]^p \tag{60.5}$$

$$M_{\mathrm{p}} = \frac{1}{N}\sum_{\mathrm{i}=1}^{N}[z(i) - m_1]^p \tag{60.6}$$

in which, z(f) is the Euclidean distance between the points on the boundary and the regional center of mass.

The regional center of mass can be calculated by:

$$\mathrm{x}_c = \frac{\sum_{x\in R_{\mathrm{x}}}\sum_{y\in R_{\mathrm{y}}} xI(x,y)}{\sum_{x\in R_{\mathrm{x}}}\sum_{y\in R_{\mathrm{y}}} I(x,y)} \qquad y_c = \frac{\sum_{x\in R_{\mathrm{x}}}\sum_{y\in R_{\mathrm{y}}} yI(x,y)}{\sum_{x\in R_{\mathrm{x}}}\sum_{y\in R_{\mathrm{y}}} I(x,y)} \tag{60.7}$$

Shape moment descriptor: △F is used to describe the roughness of the contour

$$\Delta F = F_3 - F_1 = \frac{(M_4)^{1/4}}{m_1} - \frac{(M_2)^{1/2}}{m_1} \tag{60.8}$$

60.3 Automatic Weighted FCM

FCM is a data clustering technique in which each data point belongs to a cluster to some degree that is specified by a membership grade. It achieves a classification of the collection though iterative best to the objective function, the iterative process using hill-climbing technique to find best solution. The objective function is based on the weighted measure between each date of clustering.

Each Candidate nodule has six features. The FCM clustering algorithm separates sample set into two classes using FCM theory, and find the group of each fuzzy clustering center with the objective function achieving the minimum. A Fuzzy C-division of X is a $C*N$ matrix. $U = [u_{ik}]$, where u_{ik} is the membership degrees of $\mathrm{x_k}$ to the i-class, subject to $0 < u_{ik} < 1$ and $\sum u_{ik\cdot} > 0$. FCM algorithm requires that the sum of membership degrees of every pixel to each cluster center must be 1 That's.

$$\sum_{i=1}^{c} u_{ik} = 1 \quad k = 1, 2, \ldots, n \tag{60.9}$$

The objective function of FCM,

$$J_m(_{U,V}) = \sum_{k=1}^{n}\sum_{i=1}^{c}(u_{ik})^m(d_{ik})^2 \tag{60.10}$$

where $d_{ik} = (x_k\text{-}v_i)^2$ represents the standard Euclidean v_i distance; v_i is the clustering center of the i-division; m∈[1, +∞) is the weighted index, which is used to control fuzzy degree of cluster results. In order to get the minimum value of $J_m(u,v)$, let:

$$\frac{\partial J_m(u,v)}{\partial u_{ik}} = 0 \tag{60.11}$$

$$\frac{\partial J_m(u,v)}{\partial v_i} = 0 \tag{60.12}$$

Following equation can be deduced from (60.9) and (60.10).

$$u_{ik} = \frac{1}{\sum_{j=1}^{c} \left(\frac{d_{ik}}{d_{jk}}\right)^{\frac{2}{m-1}}} \tag{60.13}$$

$$v_i = \frac{\sum_{k=1}^{n} (u_{ik})^m x_k}{\sum_{k=1} (u_{ik})^m} \tag{60.14}$$

FCM clustering algorithm is iterative process. Firstly, initialize the membership matrix U, and use (60.13, 60.14) to calculate the cluster centers; then calculate the objective function is less than a determined threshold value or the relative change to the objective function value is less than a certain threshold value, the algorithm stops; otherwise, calculate the new matrix U on the basis of (60.10) to continue.

FCM classification implicitly assumed uniform contribution for each parameter, and every parameter is equal. But, in fact, each feature is inequitable when judging nodule properties. In this paper, we take a quick feature weighting algorithm for classification. This article take the following steps: Step 1 determines the number of classification in 2. Step 2 normalizes all the characteristics. Step 3 FCM clustering and getting clustering results and two groups of clustering centers:

M (m_1, m_2, m_3, m_4, m_5, ...) N (n_1, n_2, n_3, n_4, n_5, ...).

This paper only select six characteristics, so, We take M (m_1, m_2, m_3, m_4, m_5, m_6) N (n_1, n_2, n_3, n_4, n_5, n_6). A new vector is given: $T(t_1, t_2, t_3, t_4, t_5, t_6)$, $t_1 = |m_1 - n_1|$, $t_2 = |m_2 - n_2|$...$T(t_1, t_2, t_3, t_4, t_5, t_6)$ is on behalf of the average distance apart between the two groups after the normalization of characteristics. The larger the distance is, the larger of the difference of the characteristics between the two groups is. If t_i is too small, the features' difference between the two groups is not obvious.

This article use $I(i_1, i_2, i_3, i_4, i_5, i_6)$ as weight vector.

$$I(i_1, i_2, i_3, i_4, i_5, i_6) = T(t_1, t_2, t_3, t_4, t_5, t_6) + K(1, 1, 1, 1, 1, 1) \tag{60.15}$$

All the raw data were normalized, again, and then, multiplied by this matrix and $I(i_1, i_2, i_3, i_4, i_5, i_6)$, a new matrix can be get. We use this new matrix to carry out FCM again.

60.4 Experiment

This article used all lung images made publicly available by the Lung Image Database Consortium (LIDC), the biggest publicly available collection of annotated CT. The diagnosis of benign and malignancy by artificial is finished by three radiologists. Nodules with diameters $\leq$ 5 mm, the possibility of malignancy $\leq$ 1 %; nodules with 5 $\leq$ diameters $\leq$ 10 mm, the possibility is between 6 and 28 %. Nodules with diameters $\geq$ 20 mm, the possibility are between 64 and 82 %. When nodules' diameters are too small, early diagnosis is difficult. However, when diameters are too big, there is meaningless to diagnose. So, we

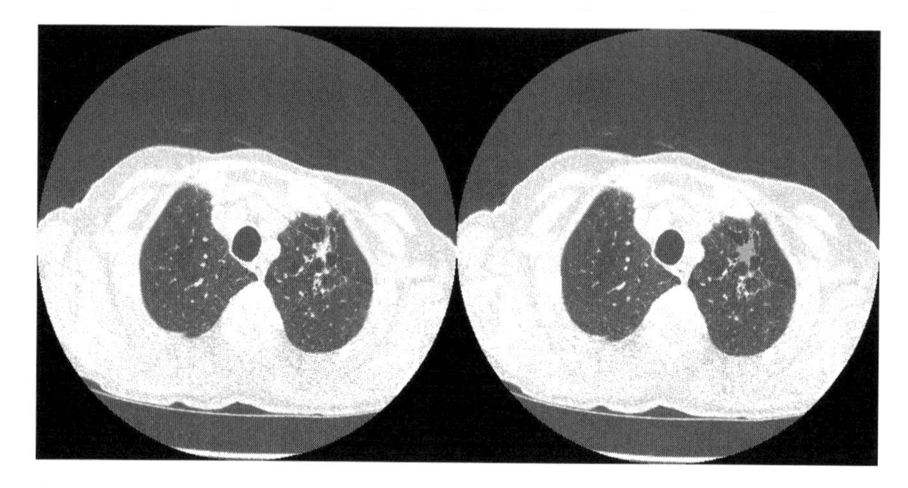

Fig. 60.1 CT image with suspicious malignant nodule and mark this nodule

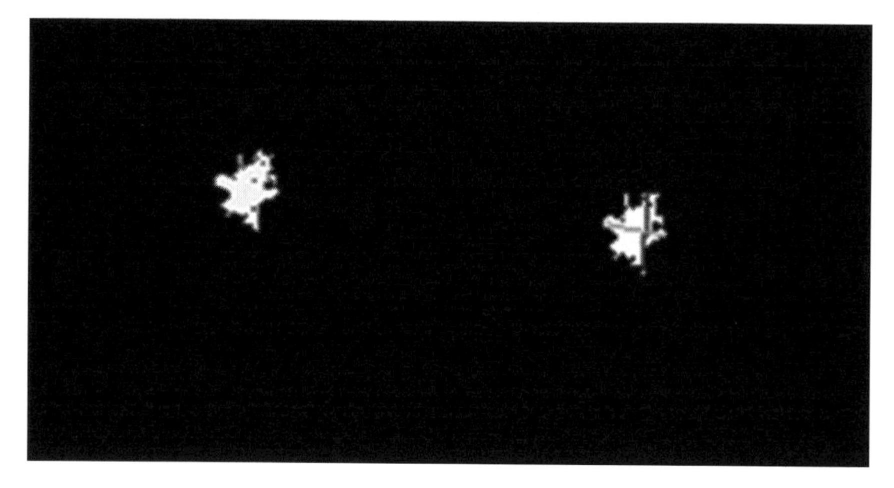

Fig. 60.2 Extract the suspicious malignant nodule and draw two perpendicular lines

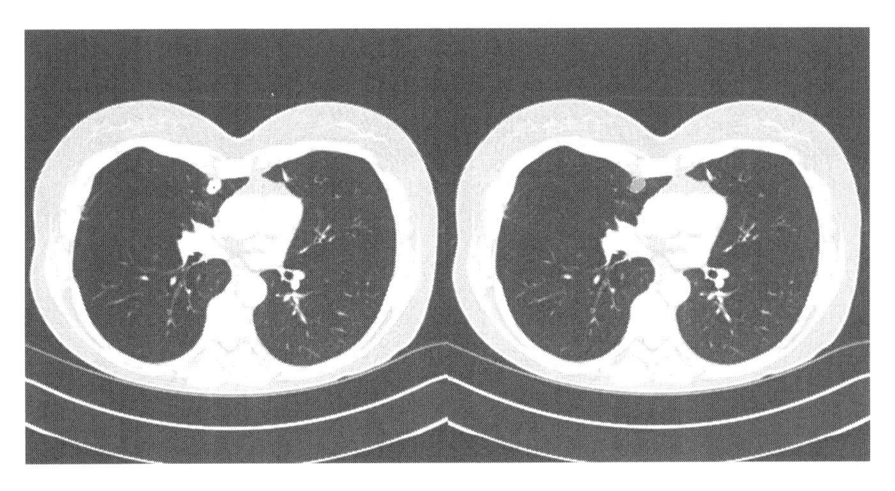

Fig. 60.3 CT image with benign nodule and mark this nodule

choose 44 isolated nodules with diameters between 4 and 20 mm, which is form 23 patients' 40 CT slices. There are 23 suspicious Malignant Solitary Pulmonary Nodules, and 21 benign nodules.

There is an example: There are two pulmonary nodules were extracted, and their characteristic values were calculated (Figs. 60.1, 60.2, 60.3, 60.4).

Now we get the characteristics values of two nodules:

These examples showed that not every nodule comply with the above characteristics. So we can summarize this problem as an uncertain and part of the characteristics of implicit classification. The solution is using FCM clustering in this article.

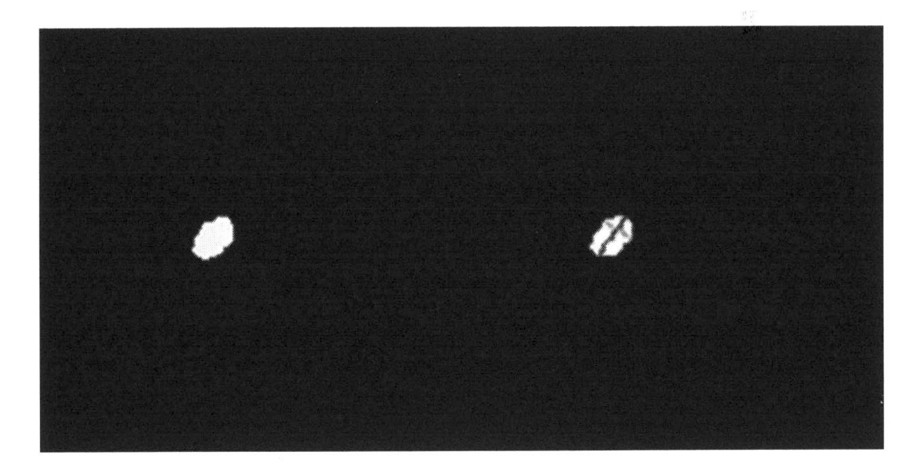

Fig. 60.4 Extract the benign nodule and draw two perpendicular lines

Table 60.1 This table is a comparison of the two nodules' different parameters

Parameters	Ave	Var	Fat	F	S	$\triangle$F
The first	210.1729	897.7018	0	0.1960	1.4975	23.3764
The second	208.1089	981.3146	1	0.9529	1.4733	16.7929

Table 60.2 This table is the result of the two algorithms

Result	Suspicious malignancy	Same as doctor' judge	Benign	Same as doctor' judge
Common FCM	27	20	17	13
Automatic weighted preference FCM	24	21	20	17

Table 60.3 This table is a comparison of the two algorithms' different performances

Performance comparison	Accuracy (%)	Sensitiveness (%)	Specificity (%)
Common FCM	75	83.3	61.9
Automatic weighted preference FCM	86.3	87.5	80

On the condition that doctor's judgment is right. That's to say, doctors: accuracy: 100 % sensitiveness: 100 % specificity: 100 %. After Experimental Verification: we can get the result and performances of two algorithms (Tables 60.1, 60.2, 60.3).

60.5 Conclusions

This paper presented a new automatic weighted preference FCM, various performances has been improved significantly. With a combination of six parameters, this experiment shows a good effect. Due to weighting parameters can be automatically obtained, this algorithm can adapt to parameter changes. So, it not only can be used in the classification of pulmonary nodules, but also can be used in all experiments of Classification about C-means and FCM clustering. This algorithm can play a supplementary role for the doctor. If a better normalization method can be found, which allow various parameters more evenly distributed between 0 and 1, this algorithm will achieve a new breakthrough.

Acknowledgments This research work is partially supported by the Hebei province science and technology pillar program (12275528D), the Chinese NSFC research fund (61190120, 61190124 and 61271318), the Hebei University BM Research fund (BM201110) and Technological Innovation of Undergraduate research fund (201210075008).

References

1. Retal B (2007) Distributed medical images analysis on a GRID infrastructure. Future Gener Comput Syst 23:475–484
2. Brem R, Baum J, Lechner M et al (2003) Improvement in sensitivity of screening mammography with computer-aided detection: a multi institutional trial. Am Roentgen Ray Soc 181:687–693
3. Das M et al (2006) Small pulmonary nodules: effect of two computer-aided detection systems on radiologist performance. Radiology 241:564–571
4. Doi K (2007) Computer-aided diagnosis in medical imaging: historical review, current status and future potential. Comput Med Imag Graph 31(4–5):198–211
5. Fukunaga K (1990) Introduction to statistical pattern recognition. Academic Press, New York
6. Kitasaka T, Mori K, Hasegawa J, Toriwaki J (2000) Lung area extraction from 3-D chest X-Ray CT images using the shape model generated by variable bezil surface. IEICE Trans Inf Syst J 83-D-2(1):165–174
7. Li Q, Li F, Doi K (2005) Computerized nodule detection in thin-slice CT using selective enhancement filter and automated rule-based classifier. In: Proceedings of SPIE, San Diego, 104–112
8. Dehmeshki J, Ye X, Lin X, Valdivieso M, Amin H (2007) Automated detection of lung nodules in CT images using shape-based genetic algorithm. Comput Med Imag Graph 31:408–417
9. Schmitt H, Grass M, Rasche V, Schramm O, Haehnel S, Sartor K (2002) An X-ray-based method for t he determination of t he contrast a gent propagation in 3-D vessel structures. IEEE Trans Med-Imag 21(3):251–262
10. Sluimer I, Schilham A, Prokop M et al (2006) Computer analysis of computed tomography scans of the lung: a survey. IEEE Trans Med Imag 25(4):385–405
11. Teverovskiy L, Carmichael O, Aizenstein H et al. (2006) Feature-based cs. intensity-based brain image registration: voxel level and structure level performance evaluation. Carnegie Me lion University, CMU-ML-06–118
12. Zheng B, Leader J, McMurray J et al (2007) Automated detection and quantitative assessment of pulmonary airways depicted on CT images. Med Phys 34(7):2844–2852

Chapter 61
Investigation of Demands on On-Campus Health Information Education Services

Zhao-feng Li, Xuan Li, Xi-peng Han, Xing Tu, Tong Li and Wen-bin Fu

Abstract Objective: To promote the provision of on-campus health information education services to college students by conducting a survey exploring the attitudes and perceptions of college students toward on-campus health information education services. Methods: The questionnaire was completed by 523 college students through internet, email and face-to-face interview. Results: 34.4 % of survey participants used internet as a major tool to seek health information and 83.7 % reported it helpful. Only 5.9 % reported getting health information service (HIS) from on-campus student health centers and only 11.1 % were satisfied. Conclusions: The on-campus HIS is lagging behind current attitudes and demands

Z. Li
Second School of Clinic Medicine, Guangzhou University of Chinese Medicine, No. 12, Jichang Road, Guangzhou 510405, China
e-mail: qdlzfcmd@126.com

X. Li
Department of Economic Management, Hai Du College of Qingdao Agricultural University, Yantai 265200, China
e-mail: qdxxwn@126.com

X. Han
School of Journalism and Communication, Xiamen University, Xiamen 361005, China
e-mail: hanxp@stu.xmu.edu.cn

X. Tu
First School of Clinic Medicine, Guangzhou University of Chinese Medicine, Guangzhou 510405, China
e-mail: 125001066@qq.com

T. Li
Department of Education, Shandong Normal University, Jinan 250014, China
e-mail: st07litong@126.com

W. Fu (✉)
Department of Acupuncture and Moxibustion, Guangdong Provincial Hospital of Traditional Chinese Medicine, Guangzhou 510120, China
e-mail: fuwenbin@139.com

S. Li et al. (eds.), *Frontier and Future Development of Information Technology in Medicine and Education*, Lecture Notes in Electrical Engineering 269,
DOI: 10.1007/978-94-007-7618-0_61,

of university students. Although many students can get HIS from internet, their knowledge about health information is still limited. Since most of the students are not satisfied with the on-campus HIS, providing effective and confidential on-campus HIS to college students by on-campus student health is necessary.

Keywords On-campus health information service · Internet · Survey

61.1 Introduction

The Internet has become a popular source of health information [1]. However, the information is lacking oversight and regulation due to its free and open information source structure; the traditional on-campus student health centers are still playing an important role in HIS and education.

Young adults, especially college students aged 18–28, usually experience optimal levels of health, typically perceive themselves to be insusceptible to infirmity and also suffer from academic stress that they tend to neglect health information education service themselves. And many health researchers are also relatively tended to neglect the demands of these students [2]. However, there are also many students who are not only concerned with their health, but feel vulnerable/susceptible concerning certain aspects of their health and in need of intervention [3]. So, some researchers have suggested that the health of university and college students is an "important and neglected public health problem" [2].

The on-campus student health center can serve as a critical setting for health services for these young adults. For example, the university, as a defined community, can conduce community health promotion polices and educational programs. Surveys in the United States reported that students received health information on specific topics from their colleges or universities [4, 5]. However, to some degree, on-campus HIS is lack and the resources are not available to college students. The goal of this survey is to provide guidance for on-campus student health centers and educators who are interested in promoting both their offline and online HIS.

61.2 Method

61.2.1 College Sample

We used an anonymous survey completed by a sample of college students from 2 universities from January to March 2013 to collect data. The questionnaire was administered as either an anonymous paper survey during face-to-face interview or online. Students participated in the study after they read an informed-consent letter.

61.2.2 Measures

The survey consisted of 12 demographic, attitudinal and behavioural items. For demographic information, respondents provided details on their genders, ages, academic background (medical background or non-medical background) and years of college (undergraduate students or graduate students).

We assessed the students' general health condition: "Are you physically and mentally healthy?" and then we asked which aspect of HIS they mainly concerned with.

We assessed the students' channel of access to health information and their attitude toward using internet for health information from responses to 2 questions. Respondents were asked, "How do you get health information?" The response options were *from parents and friends, from medical professionals (doctors, nurses and so on), from internet and from traditional media (magazines, newspapers, television, broadcasting and so on)*. We then asked "Do you think internet is helpful in getting health information?" The response options were *helpful, not helpful at all and I never tried to use network technology to get health information*.

The questionnaire asked respondents about their knowledge about on-campus health center: "Is there any on-campus health center on your campus?" Those who responded yes were to another question: "Have you ever got health information from on-campus health center?" and "How do you communicate with medical professionals about the health information that interests you?" The response options were *face-to-face visits, electronic communication (email) and never visit*.

To assess the students' attitudes about on-campus health centers in providing HIS, respondents were asked about their concerns with health education activities organized by school, about whether they read health information posters, pamphlets provided by the school health education centers and about whether they visit websites of the school health centers to get health information. The response options were *always, never, my school health center does not provide this service and no care*.

And at last, we asked if the students were satisfied with the HIS provided by on-campus health centers.

61.2.3 Data Analysis

We recorded all data into Epidata 3.0 and then imported the data into SPSS 16.0 for analysis. We calculated descriptive statistics for (1) demographics, (2) general self-rating health condition, (3) HIS concerned aspect, (4) access to HIS, (5) internet use in seeking health information and (6) satisfaction with on-campus HIS. We used Chi square test to assess differences by gender, year in college and academic background. Describe quantitative data to mean $\pm$ standard deviation (M $\pm$ SD). The alpha level of significance for all tests was 0.05.

61.3 Results

The 523 college students completed the survey were predominately 20-year-old, non-medical and undergraduate (Table 61.1). More than half (51.2 %) of the students reported both physically and mentally healthy. 41.1 % of students reported themselves slight mentally unhealthy, however, only 24.3 % mainly concerned with mental HIS. Two thirds (61.4 %) concerned with infectious diseases HIS. None respondent concerned with HIV/AIDS information and only about 10 % concerned with reproductive health information. (Table 61.2, Fig. 61.1) More than one third (34.4 %) got health information by internet and one third (33.5 %) got it from medical professionals. Male and graduate students preferred internet and medical professionals than female and undergraduate students. (Table 61.2, Fig. 61.2) 83.7 % ($n = 438$) considered internet helpful in seeking health information. Among them, more male, undergraduate students considered internet helpful in seeking health information (Table 61.2, Fig. 61.3). 98.3 % ($n = 514$) of the students knew on-campus health centers existed, while only 5.9 % ($n = 31$) got HIS from the centers. Half of the students communicated with medical professionals in face-to-face visits. Only 11.9 % students prefer to use electronic communication (email) in communication with medical professionals. (Table 61.3, Fig. 61.4) Nearly half of the students (48.4 %) did not concern with health education activities organized by school. More students read pamphlets (61 %) than posters (43 %) provided by on-campus health centers. (Table 61.4, Fig. 61.5) 22.9 % students visited websites of on-campus health centers to seek health information and 23.3 % complained none access to the websites. We examined college students' attitude about on-campus HIS. Only 11.1 % ($n = 58$) were satisfied, while 32.9 % ($n = 172$) were not and 35 % ($n = 183$) complained the poor access to it. More male, medical, graduate students unsatisfied than female, non-medical, undergraduate students. (Table 61.4, Fig. 61.6)

There were significant differences considering the gender difference. More female students reported healthy or only slight mentally unhealthy (Pearson Chi Square = 42.192, $P = 0.000$) and concerned with on-campus HIS (Pearson Chi Square = 29.589, $P = 0.000$). 44.5 % and 44.2 % ($n = 118$ and 117) of male students preferred to seek health information from medical professionals and through internet, while 43 % ($n = 111$) of female students preferred traditional media (Pearson Chi Square = 0.011, $P = 0.000$). All male students considered internet helpful while 20.9 % female students ($n = 54$) considered internet not helpful (Pearson Chi Square = 86.977, $P = 0.000$). More female students never communicated with medical professionals (Pearson Chi Square = 28.837, $P = 0.000$) and not visited website of on-campus health centers (Pearson Chi Square = 74.017, P = 0.000). More female did not read posters (Pearson Chi Square = 70.496, $P = 0.000$) but read pamphlets (Pearson Chi Square = 87.145, $P = 0.000$). More male students ($n = 116$, 43.8 %) were not satisfied with on-campus HIS than female ($n = 110$, 21 %), Pearson Chi Square = 47.4249, $P = 0.000$.

Table 61.1 Demographic characteristics of students (N = 523)

	n	%	M	SD
Age(y)			21.93	2.76
18	34	6.5		
20	229	43.8		
21	61	11.7		
22	27	5.2		
23	12	2.3		
24	17	3.3		
25	28	5.4		
26	84	16.1		
27	31	5.9		
Gender				
Male	265	50.7		
Female	258	49.3		
Academic background				
Medical	258	49.3		
Non-medical	265	50.7		
Year in college				
Undergraduate	370	70.7		
Graduate	153	29.3		

Table 61.2 Attitude about health information and internet in seeking health information of students (N = 523)

	n	%
Self-relating health condition		
Both physically and mentally healthy	268	51.2
Physically healthy but slight mentally unhealthy	215	41.1
Physically healthy but severe mentally unhealthy	33	6.3
Physically unhealthy but mentally healthy	7	1.3
Main concern aspect of health information		
Infectious diseases information (flu and etc.)	321	61.4
Mental health information	127	24.3
Reproductive health information	47	9
No care	28	5.4
Main source of health information		
Social channels (parents, friends, etc.)	27	5.2
Medical professionals (doctors, nurses, etc.)	175	33.5
Internet	180	34.4
Traditional media (newspapers, magazines, TV, radio, etc.)	141	27
Use of internet in seeking health information		
Helpful	438	83.7
Not helpful	54	10.3
Never use internet	31	5.9

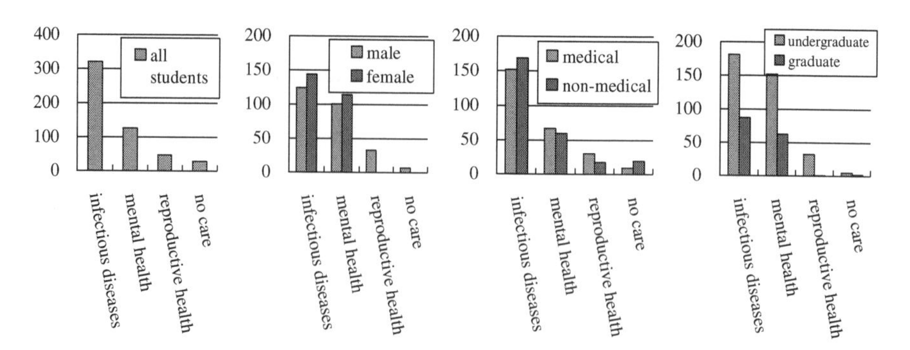

Fig. 61.1 Main concern aspect of HIS of all students, different genders, different academic backgrounds and different years in college

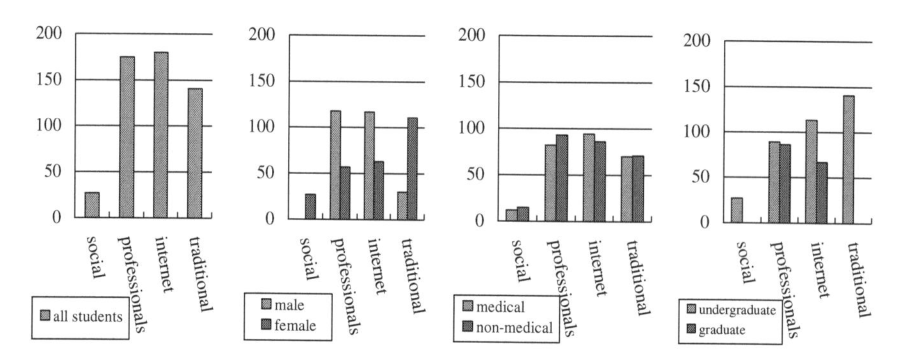

Fig. 61.2 Main source of health information of all students, different genders, different academic backgrounds and different years in college

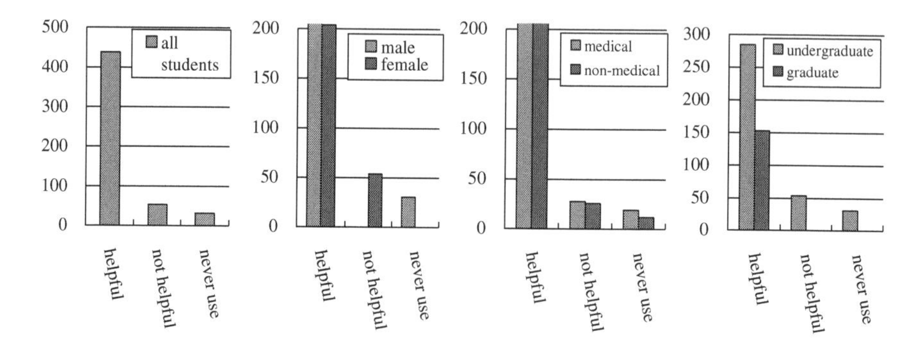

Fig. 61.3 Use of internet in seeking health information of all students, different genders, different academic backgrounds and different years in college

Table 61.3 Knowledge about on-campus health center of students (N = 523)

	n	%
Existence of on-campus health center		
Yes	514	98.3
No	0	0
Not know	9	1.7
Get HIS from on-campus health center		
Yes	31	5.9
No	281	53.7
Service not provide	60	11.5
No care	151	28.9
Communication with medical professionals		
Face-to-face visits	291	55.6
Electronic communication (email)	62	11.9
Never visit	170	32.5

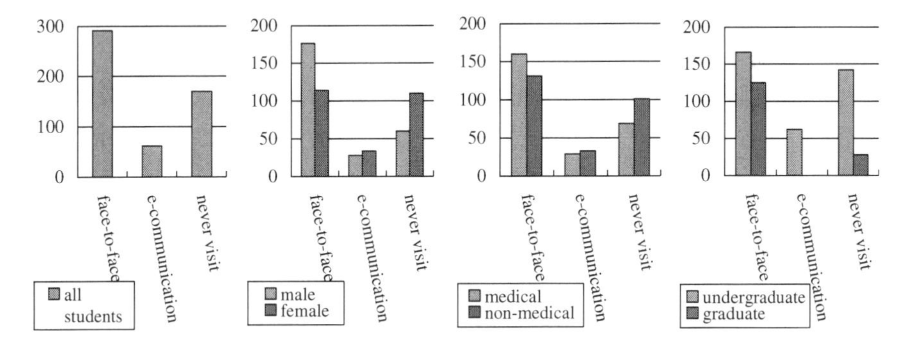

Fig. 61.4 Communication with medical professionals of all students, different genders, different academic backgrounds and different years in college

Table 61.4 Attitudes about On-campus HIS of students (N = 523)

	Yes		No		Service not provided		No care	
	N	%	n	%	n	%	n	%
Health education activities participation	86	16.4	253	48.4	64	12.2	120	22.9
Posters reading	180	34.4	225	43	59	11.3	59	11.3
Pamphlets reading	319	61	31	5.9	145	27.7	28	5.4
Centers' websites visit	120	22.9	198	37.9	122	23.3	83	15.9
Satisfaction about services	58	11.1	172	32.9	183	35	110	21

Considering the academic background differences, there was no difference in self-rating general health condition (Pearson Chi Square = 0.864, $P = 0.834$), main source of health information (Pearson Chi Square = 1.294, $P = 0.731$) and the use of internet in seeking health information (Pearson Chi Square = 2.146,

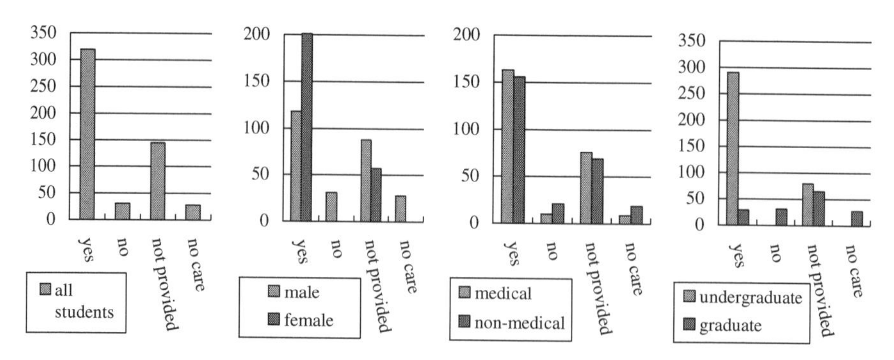

Fig. 61.5 Reading of pamphlets of all students, different genders, different academic backgrounds and different years in college

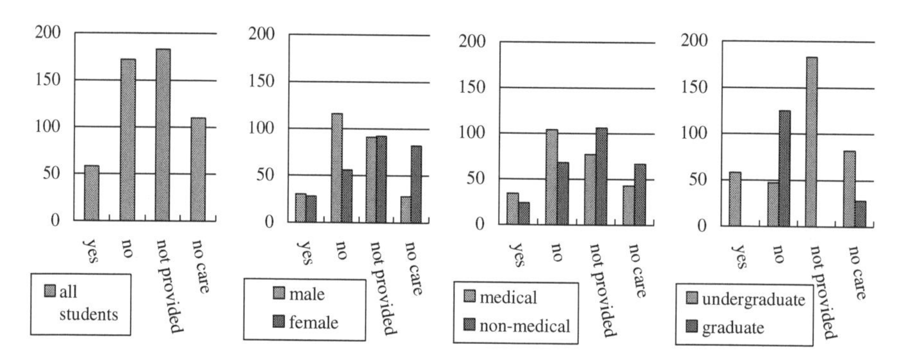

Fig. 61.6 Satisfaction about HIS of all students, different genders, different academic backgrounds and different years in college

$P = 0.342$). But, non-medical students tended to less communicate with medical professionals (Pearson Chi Square = 9.080, $P = 0.011$), less participate in health education activities (Pearson Chi Square = 58.421, $P = 0.000$), less read health information posters (Pearson Chi Square = 21.557, $P = 0.000$) and less care about on-campus HIS (Pearson Chi Square = 19.001, $P = 0.000$).

More undergraduate students ($n = 32$, 8.6 %) reported severe mentally unhealthy than graduate students ($n = 1$, 0.7 %), Pearson Chi Square = 12.3000, $P = 0.006$. All graduate students sought health information either from medical professionals ($n = 86$, 56.2 %) or through internet ($n = 67$, 43.8 %), while 45.4 % undergraduate students got information from parents, friends or traditional media (Pearson Chi Square = 0.011, $P = 0.000$). All graduate students recommended internet helpful, while 14.6 % ($n = 54$) undergraduate students recommended it useless (Pearson Chi Square = 41.970, $P = 0.000$). More undergraduate students not read posters (Pearson Chi Square = 15.062, $P = 0.002$), but preferred to read pamphlets (Pearson Chi Square = 0.022, $P = 0.000$) and to visit websites of on-campus health centers (Pearson Chi Square = 0.016, $P = 0.000$).

61.4 Discussion

Nearly one third of the students were not satisfied with the on-campus HIS, which suggests that on-campus health center should provide health information more diversified and flexible according to students' gender, academic backgrounds and ages.

No matter of their age, gender, or academic background, students preferred to read health information pamphlets than posters. This suggests it is better to provide health information by printing pamphlets.

More than one third of the students did not visit websites of on-campus health centers and there were also complain about poor access to the websites. More male students sought information by internet than female, graduate students. This is different from the previous research in the US [6–8]. It is interesting that though non-medical students considered internet more helpful in seeking health information, but more medical students use internet as their main source of health information than non-medical students. These finding suggest that we need to provide students of different academic backgrounds with more suitable health information on websites of on-campus health centers.

Students seldom got HIS from on-campus health center though nearly all of them knew it existed. Electronic communication (email) has become popular and available for decades, but students still preferred face-to-face visits to use it. Electronic communication is not as popular as we thought in communication with medical professionals. These findings may suggest that on-campus health centers should provide more flexible HIS to students who tend to be shy or unwilling to visit a medical professional.

More students reported mentally unhealthy than concerned with mental HIS. Most students mainly concerned with infectious diseases. Although former survey showed students' attitudes towards sexual matters are liberal [9], concerning with HIV/AIDS and reproductive health information are not enough. This may due to our survey time when flu is most common and wild spread or Chinese students may still be too shy to talk about their mental suffers or sexual matters in public. The students' knowledge about reproductive health and HIV/AIDS is still limited. Providing effective and confidential reproductive health services to young students is necessary, as well as infectious diseases and psychiatric disorders.

Our results suggest the great potential for using the pamphlets and internet for health education on campus. Specially, our findings suggest the following recommendations for college and university health centers: (1) incorporate more powerful and effective web-based education and programs into university student health, (2) train and encourage health staff and students to search internet and communicate through electronic communication for health information, (3) Augment effective and confidential HIS for common college health issues through pamphlets and internet.

This study also has some limitations. The study population was a convenience sample of students. The findings may not be generalizable to other college students. The number of college students whose main concern aspect of health services and their attitude of internet in seeking health information may be an overestimation because a percentage of the study sample used the internet and email to complete the survey. The rates of such internet use and recommendation of on-campus health services may not be directly comparable to those found in other studies because other researchers may have different questions about students' satisfaction about on-campus HIS and about internet or electronic communication used in seeking health information.

Future study should build on these findings to explore additional factors related to satisfaction about on-campus HIS among college students. In-depth research might be useful in exploring the barriers to health information students seek, the search strategies they use, their credibility of health information and the factors that make websites of on-campus health centers accessible and credible for students.

61.5 Authors' Contribution

Wen-bin Fu and Zhao-feng Li contributed to the conception and design of the study. Xing Tu and Tong Li contributed to the design of the survey questionnaire. Xuan Li, Zhao-feng Li and Xi-peng Han contributed to the study and data collection. Zhao-feng Li wrote the manuscript. All authors read and approved the final manuscript.

Conflicting Interests
The author(s) declared no potential conflicts of interests.

References

1. Vord de Vord R (2010) Dissertation abstracts international section a. Hum Soc Sci 70(11-A):4106
2. Stewart-Brown S, Evans J, Petersen S et al (2000) The health of students in institutes of higher education: an important and neglected public health problem? J Public Health Med 22:492–499
3. Boehm S et al (1993) College students' perception of vulnerability/susceptibility and desire for health information. Patient Educ Counsell 21:77–87
4. Fox KR, Harris J (2003) Promoting physical activity through schools. In: McKenna J, Riddoch C (eds) Perspectives on health and exercise. Basingstoke, Palgrave-Macmillan, pp 181–202
5. Brener ND, Gowda VR (2001) US college students' reports of receiving health information on college campuses. J Am Coll Health 49:223–228
6. Escoffery C, Miner KR, Adame DD et al (2005) Internet use for health information among college students. J Am Coll Health 53:183–189
7. Fox S, Raine L (2000) The online health care revolution: how the web helps americans take better care of themselves. Pew Charitable Trust, Washington
8. Houston TK, Allison JJ (2002) Users of Internet health information: differences by health status. J Med Internet Res 4(20):e7

9. Chen Bin Lu, YongNing Wang HongXiang et al (2008) Sexual and reproductive health service needs of university/college students: updates from a survey in Shanghai. China Asian J Androl 10(4):607–615

Chapter 62
Suicidality in Medication-Native Patients with Single-Episode Depression: MRSI of Deep White Matter in Frontal Lobe and Parietal Lobe

Xizhen Wang, Hongwei Sun, Shuai Wang, Guohua Xie, Shanshan Gao, Xihe Sun, Yanyu Wang and Nengzhi Jiang

Abstract The objective of this study was to investigate the changes of NAA, Cho, Cr and the metabolism ratios of deep white matter of frontal lobe and parietal lobe of those who had suicidality in medication-native with single-episode depression. Eighteen healthy control subjects (10 males and 8 females) and eighteen patients with suicidal depression were recruited from the local area. Conventional MRI and 3D-PRESS MRSI was performed in all subjects. All patients were in a depressive state on the day of MR examination with a HAM-D total score higher than 18. NAA/Cr and Cho/Cr ratios on both sides of the striatum were calculated automatically. Relative concentrations of N-acetylaspartate (NAA), choline (Cho) and creatine (Cr) were estimated from their peak area. The regions of interest (ROI) calculated in each subject included right frontal lobe, left frontal lobe, right parietal lobe and left parietal lobe. The MRSI features of depression and healthy volunteers were high and steep peak of NAA, relatively low peak of Cho and Cr. According to the peaks of NAA, Cho and Cr, no obvious differences were found in the images. The differences between depression group and control group in relative concentrations of NAA, Cho and Cr were not significant ($P > 0.05$). The same situations were found in the analyzing of NAA/Cho and NAA/Cr ratio. In frontal and partial white matter, there were no significant hemispheric differences in metabolite concentrations and ratios. The result in our study hindered that the metabolisms changes in early stage was not obvious in MRSI. The changes of metabolisms will be potential to evaluate of suicidal depression.

X. Wang · S. Gao · X. Sun
Medical Imaging Center of the Affiliated Hospital, Weifang Medical University, Weifang, China

H. Sun (✉) · Y. Wang · N. Jiang
Department of psychological, Weifang Medical University, Weifang, Shandong Province, China
e-mail: sunhw@wfmc.edu.cn

S. Wang · G. Xie
Department of Radiology, The People's Hospital of Liaocheng, Liaocheng, China

S. Li et al. (eds.), *Frontier and Future Development of Information Technology in Medicine and Education*, Lecture Notes in Electrical Engineering 269,
DOI: 10.1007/978-94-007-7618-0_62,

Keywords Magnetic resonance imaging · Magnetic resonance spectroscopy · Suicidality · Depression · Deep white matter

62.1 Introduction

Depression was common and disabling psychiatric illnesses which affect individuals worldwide and cause significant negative impact on public health. 10–30 % of patients with depression coupled with functional impairment, poor quality of life, suicide ideation and attempts, self-injurious behavior, and a high relapse rate. Treatment failures are common with existing therapies, adding urgency to the need for better understanding of the biology of mood disorders. The interaction of genetic susceptibility and environmental factors were considered to play a key role in the development of depression. However, Intervention treatment at early stage of major depression is important to improve the quality of life of patients with the disorder. Although the phenomenon of mental diseases was studied for several centuries ago, the precise mechanisms associated the development of depression remain unclear. In routine clinical practice, CT and routine MRI have been used to exclude structural diseased in the brain. Proton magnetic resonance spectroscopy (1H-MRS) is a non-invasive neuroimaging technique that allows in vivo quantification of metabolites, including glutamate-related ones.

1H-MRS provides metabolic assay of neuronal cells, cell energetics, density, membrane turnover, gliosis, and glycolysis through their respective surrogate markers, N-acetylaspartate, creatine, choline, myo-inositol, and lactate levels. Myo-Inositol/creatine and choline/creatine ratios were significantly higher in the frontal white matter in the major depression group than in the comparison group. Lower the level of N-acetylaspartate/creatine was observed in the deep white matte in the late-onset group compared with those in the early-onset group. With the age of onset as the covariate, the patients with moderate deep white matter lesions had more pronounced cognitive impairment and clinician-rated depressive symptoms than those with none and/or mild lesions. These results suggested that 1H-MRSI was a useful indicator of neuronal/axonal loss in the white matter of the frontal lobes which precedes cognitive impairment. As we all known, Suicidal depression was the reflection of reaction of biological chemicals in the brain. The underlying detailed knowledge of fundamental biology has not been clarified. Due to the difficulties in recruiting of subjects in medication-native patients with single-episode depression, most studies about MRS and depression focused on the patients in later stages. The purpose of this study was to investigate MRSI features of deep white matter in frontal lobe and parietal lobe of those suicidality medication-native patients with single-episode depression. In this way, the results of MRSI may bring more information in the mechanism of suicidal depression.

62.2 Methods

62.2.1 Subjects

The study was approved by the local research ethics committee, and written informed consents were obtained from all participants. Eighteen healthy control subjects (10 males and 8 females) were recruited from the local area with average age of 26.2 years (from 21 years old to 35 years). Healthy control subjects belonged to control group. All the subjects in this study were assessed with the Structured Clinical Interview for DSM-IV, Non-patient Edition. Exclusion criteria for healthy subjects were a history or present diagnosis of any DSM-IV axis I diagnosis, any neurological illness, history of head trauma with loss of consciousness, and a history of psychiatric disorders or suicide among first-degree relatives.

Eighteen patients (10 males and 8 females) with depressive disorder were of Han Chinese ethnicity and recruited from the Department of Psychiatry at the Liaocheng Peopole's Hospital (Shandong, China). The average of patients was 33.6 years (from 23 years old to 45 years). All patients were medication-native and suicidal tendency. They were assessed by an experienced psychiatrist and met the diagnostic criteria for major depressive disorder as determined using DSM-IV. The criteria of suicidal tendency were: (1) no history or any behavior of suicide attempt; (2) have the idea of hurting themselves repeatedly to commit suicide or want to die. Severity of depression was quantified using the 17-item Hamilton Depression Rating Scale (HAM-D). All patients were in a depressive state on the day of MR examination with a HAM-D total score higher than 18. All the patients belonged to depression group.

62.2.2 MRI Protocols

All MRI examinations were performed with a 3.0-T system (Achieva X-series 3.0T, Philips, Holland). An eight-channel birdcage head coil was used for excitation and signal reception. All subjects were imaged in supine head first position. Axial images were oriented to be perpendicular to the long axis of head, which was guided by the sagittal images. The MR imaging protocol consisted of the conventional MRI sequences to exclude the structural diseases of brain: The parameters of T2WI-FLAIR were: Repetition Time = 7000 ms, Echo Time = 120 ms, Flip Angle = 90°, matrix = 228 × 224, field of view = 23 cm × 23 cm, Thickness/gap = 6.0 mm/1.0 mm and nex = 2. The parameter of FSE-T1WI was: Repetition Time = 250 ms, Echo Time = 2 ms, Flip Angle = 90°, matrix = 228 × 224, field of view = 23 cm × 23 cm, Thickness/gap = 5.0 mm/1.0 mm and nex = 2. The data of MRSI was acquired with 3D-PRESS sequence and the parameters were listed as followed: Repetition Time = 1000 ms, Echo Time = 144 ms, size of voxel = 10 mm × 10 mm × 10 mm, Thickness = 10 mm, bandwidth = 140 MHz and nex = 6. The acquisition time of 3D-PRESS was 10 min and 44 s.

62.2.3 MRS Post-Processing

The MRS data were processed using in-house software. The water suppressed time domain data were analyzed between 1.0 and 4.35 ppm. Residual water was removed from the free induction decays in the time domain. Spectra were automatically corrected for frequency and zero-order phase shifts in reference to the N-acetylaspartate peak in each voxel. After phase correction and baseline adjustment on the spectrum, NAA/Cr and Cho/Cr ratios on both sides of the striatum were calculated automatically. Relative concentrations of N-acetylaspartate (NAA), choline (CHo) and creatine (Cr) were estimated from their peak area. The regions of interest (ROI) calculated in each subject included right frontal lobe, left frontal lobe, right parietal lobe and left parietal lobe.

62.2.4 Statistical Analysis

All the statistical analyses were performed using SPSS ver. 11.5 (SPSS Inc., Chicago, IL). The relative concentrations of NAA, Cho, Cr, NAA/Cr and Cho/Cr ratios of two groups were analyzed using an independent-sample t test. The relative concentrations of NAA, Cho, Cr, NAA/Cr and Cho/Cr ratios of right frontal lobe, left frontal lobe, right parietal lobe and left parietal lobe were compared using a paired t-test. A P value of less than 0.05 was considered to indicate a statistically significant difference.

62.3 Results

All the subjects were examined successfully by MRI. No structural diseases were found in these subjects. The MRSI features of depression and healthy volunteers were high and steep peak of NAA, relatively low peak of Cho and Cr. According to the peaks of NAA, Cho and Cr, no obvious differences were found in the images (Figs. 62.1, 62.2, 62.3.). The differences between depression group and control group in relative concentrations of NAA, Cho and Cr were not significant ($P > 0.05$). The same situations were found in the analyzing of NAA/Cho and NAA/Cr ratio. However, there was a trend that the means of NAA, Cho and NAA/Cho and NAA/Cr ratio of depression group were higher than those of control group. In frontal and partial white matter, there were no significant hemispheric differences in metabolite concentrations and ratios (Figs. 62.4, 62.5, 62.6, 62.7; Tables 62.1, 62.2).

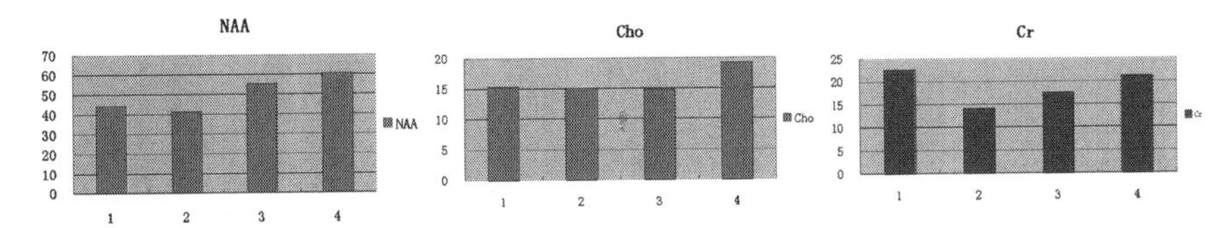

Fig. 62.1 The inner group's comparison of NAA, Cho and Cr of deep white matter in frontal and parietal lobe. *1* left frontal lobe; *2* left parietal lobe; *3* right frontal lobe; *4* right parietal lobe

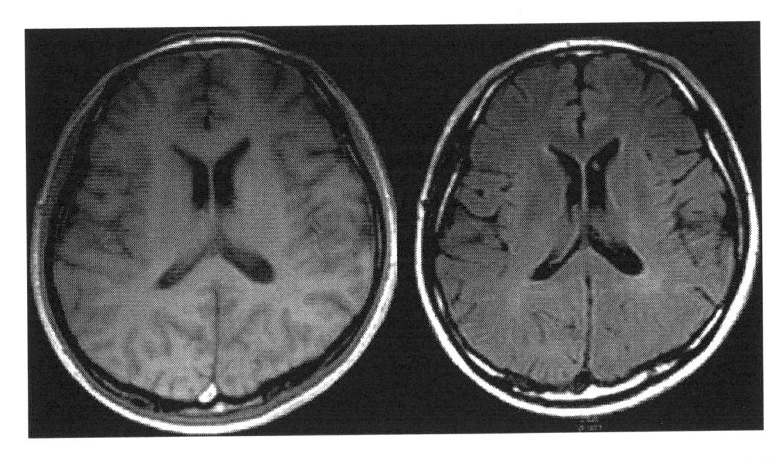

Fig. 62.2 T1WI and T2WI-FLAIR image of normal healthy subject shows no structural diseases were observed

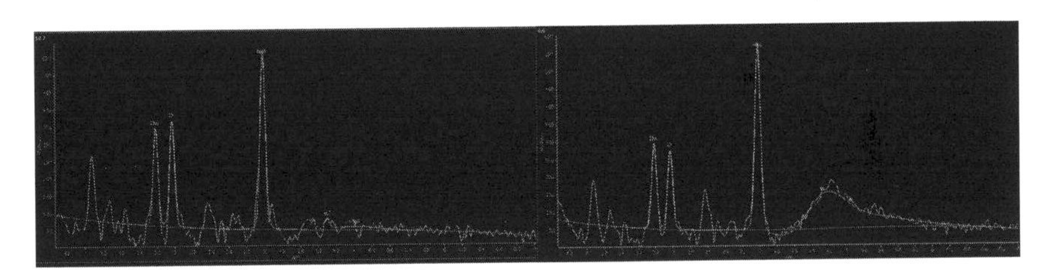

Fig. 62.3 MRSI of deep white matter in right and left frontal lobe of normal healthy subject show no difference between left and right parietal lobe

62.4 Discussion

Proton magnetic resonance spectroscopy (1H-MRS) in vivo is a noninvasive technique which can provide in vivo assessment of tissue composition and metabolic processes. With the development of MR technologies, such as water suppression, signal localization sequences and automatic data acquisition and processing, the 1H-MRS of the brain became more reliable than ever before.

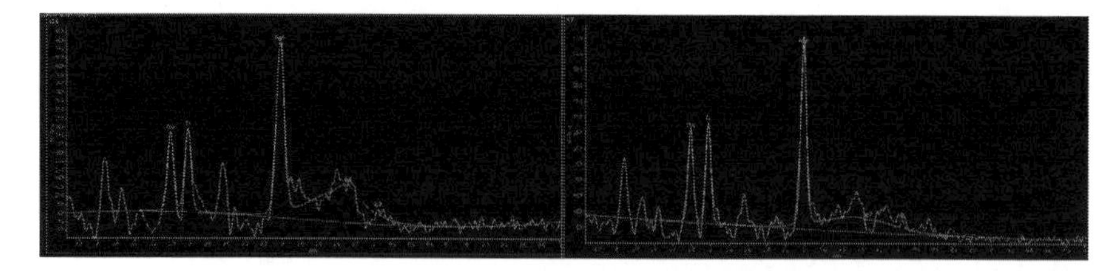

Fig. 62.4 MRSI of deep white matter in right and left frontal lobe shows no difference between left and right parietal lobe. All the MRS pictures showed steep and high peak of NAA and relatively low peak of Cho and Cr

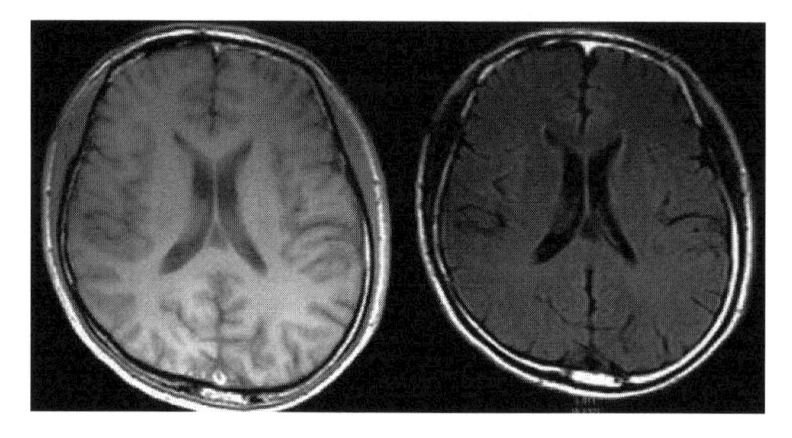

Fig. 62.5 T1WI and T2WI-FLAIR image of subject with suicidal depression. No structural diseases were observed

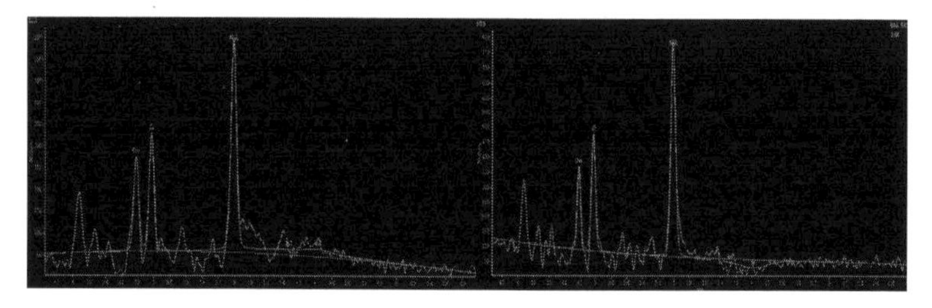

Fig. 62.6 MRSI of deep white matter in right and left frontal lobe of suicidal depression show no difference between left and right parietal lobe

Nowadays, MRSI had been considered as a routine modality in the diagnosis and differential diagnosis of diseases in brain, breast, prostate and skeletal system. It's easy to perform a MRSI n a routine clinical examination as a single session with MR imaging. Biochemical information about local cellular metabolism may provide an important clue to the patho-physiologic status in depression in the spectra,

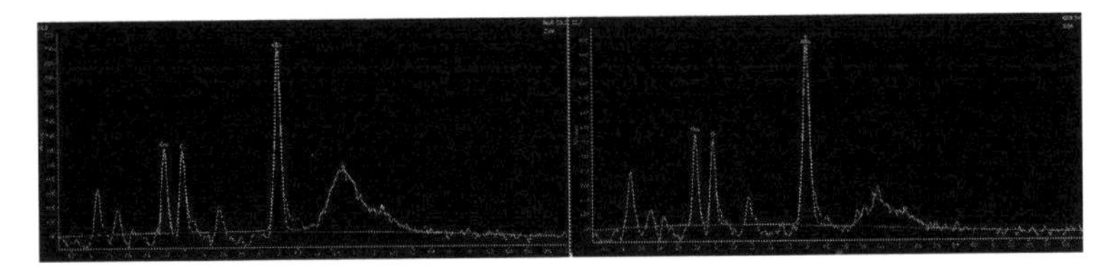

Fig. 62.7 MRSI of deep white matter in right and left frontal lobe of suicidal depression shows no difference between left and right parietal lobe. All the MRS pictures showed steep and high peak of NAA and relatively low peak of Cho and Cr. All the MRS pictures showed steep and high peak of NAA and relatively low peak of Cho and Cr

because the spectra are determined by metabolite ratios of the neurochemicals detected.

N-acetylaspartate is the second most abundant amino acid derivative in the mammalian brain. It is almost exclusive to neurons and their processes and is therefore regarded as a surrogate marker for their viability. Our hypothesis that N-acetylaspartate levels would be decreased in patients with suicidal depression was not supported by our data. Choline was an essential component of membrane lipids, phosphatidylcholine, and sphingomyelin. The 1H-MRS choline peak comprises mostly the quaternary N-methyl groups of glycerophosphocholine breakdown products (cytosolic compounds) and phosphocholine, the membrane precursors of phosphatidylcholine. Elevated Cho was attributed to abnormal cell membrane metabolism, myelin breakdown, or changes in glia density. Major depression has been found elevated Cho which reflected accelerated cell membrane turnover. In our study, the peak of Cho in suicidal depression did not decreased as most articles reported. The concentration of NAA, Cho and Cr did not change obviously in this study, which could be explained in two points: the subjects in our study were in the early stage of depression. (1)The process of demyelination or abnormal cell membrane metabolism was not serious enough to be detected in MRSI; (2) A trend was found that the levels of Cho were a little higher than those of control groups. In this way, a bigger sample of depression was necessary to retrieve the error.

Cr peak is a composite of overlapping creatine and phosphocreatine resonance. It represented the high-energy phosphate reserves in the cytosol of neurons and glia. Due to qualification of Cr was not an easy job, most studies of depression used ratios to creatine rather than concentrations of creatine. In this study, the relative concentration of creatine and ratios to creatine were used. Similarly, we did not find an elevation in creatine levels. While the trend of elevation of Cr in the deep white matter in the striatum as a whole, our high spatial resolution enabled us to detect a focal elevation was consistent with one prior study. The changes of creatine suggested that there were limitations of using creatine as inner reference for metabolite ratio. In the suicidal depression group, NAA, Cho and Cr of right parietal lobe were higher than those of other ROIs. Although no statistical

Table 62.1 Comparison of NAA, Cho and Cr between healthy control group and depression group

	NAA				Cho				Cr			
	LF	RF	LP	RP	LF	RF	LP	RP	LF	RF	LP	RP
HC	44.65±10.55	42.99 ± 12.83	56.71 ± 15.63	61.96 ± 16.37	14.80 ± 5.44	14.78 ± 2.57	16.24 ± 4.49	18.15 ± 3.76	14.58 ± 5.41	13.57 ± 4.71	18.34 ± 5.31	18.14 ± 4.92
DS	44.52 ± 8.62	41.56 ± 12.77	55.52 ± 6.64	60.64 ± 11.41	15.30 ± 3.53	15.11 ± 4.99	14.84 ± 2.08	19.23 ± 4.47	22.68 ± 25.75	14.27 ± 7.12	17.62 ± 4.88	21.18 ± 6.66
P	0.97	0.80	0.83	0.84	0.81	0.85	0.40	0.56	0.32	0.79	0.75	0.25

LF = left frontal lobe; RF = right frontal lobe; LP = left parietal lobe; RP = right parietal lobe

Table 62.2 Comparison of ratios between healthy control group and depression group

	NAA/CHo				NAA/Cr			
	LF	RF	LP	RP	LF	RF	LP	RP
HC	3.24 ± 0.67	3.34 ± 0.88	3.19 ± 0.71	3.53 ± 0.76	1.07 ± 0.45	1.17 ± 0.33	0.90 ± 0.21	1.05 ± 0.30
DS	3.03 ± 1.19	6.09 ± 9.44	3.37 ± 0.99	3.05 ± 0.95	1.03 ± 0.42	3.95 ± 8.87	0.91 ± 0.30	0.97 ± 0.31
p	0.65	0.41	0.66	0.24	0.84	0.37	0.98	0.58

LF = left frontal lobe; RF = right frontal lobe; LP = left parietal lobe; RP = right parietal lobe significance was found in these data, the result hindered that MRSI may reflect the metabolisms changes in early stage.

3.0T MR used in this study could guarantee the signal-to-noise ratio of MRSI. The main limitation of our study was the small sample of subjects with suicidal depression. Because that the subjects with suicidal depression was in single episode of suicidality and just a subgroups of depression. It's impossible to get large size of sample, except corporation with other institutions. However, the results of our study didn't provide ideal data to assess the mechanism of suicidal results. Some meaningful changes of metabolisms were observed in this study. Future studies should use larger cohorts. More ROIs in the brain should be included using 3D-MRSI.

Acknowledgments This study was supported by a grant from Shandong Province Science and Technology Development Plan (2010GSF10226) and Program of Committee of the Youth and Middle-aged Scientific Research Foundation of Shan Dong Province (BS2012YY038).

References

1. Caetano SC, Fonseca M, Olvera RL et al (2005) Proton spectroscopy study of the left dorsolateral prefrontal cortex in pediatric depressed patients. Neurosci Lett 384:321–326
2. Danielsen EA, Ross B (1999) Magnetic resonance spectroscopy diagnosis of neurological diseases. Marcel Dekker, New York
3. Ethofer T, Mader I, Seeger U et al (2003) Comparison of longitudinal metabolite relaxation times in different regions of the human brain at 1.5 and 3 Tesla. Magn Reson Med 50:1296–1301
4. Fekadu A, Wooderson SC, Markopoulo K et al (2009) What happens to patients with treatment-resistant depression? A systematic review of medium to long term outcome studies. J Affect Disord 116:4–11
5. First MB, Gibbon M, Spitzer RL (1997) Structured Clinical Interview for DSM-IV Axis I Disorders–Clinical Version (SCID–CV). American Psychiatric Publishing, Washington
6. Goelman G, Liu S, Hess D et al (2006) Optimizing the efficiency of high-field multivoxel spectroscopic imaging by multiplexing in space and time. Magn Reson Med 56:34–40
7. Hamilton M (1967) Development of a rating scale for primary depressive illness. Br J Soc Clin Psychol 6:278–296
8. Kumar A, Thomas A, Lavretsky H et al (2002) Frontal white matter biochemical abnormalities in late-life major depression detected with proton magnetic resonance spectroscopy. Am J Psychiatry 159:630–636
9. Kupfer DJ, Frank E, Phillips ML (2012) Major depressive disorder: new clinical, neurobiological, and treatment perspectives. Lancet 379:1045–1055
10. Lacerda AL, Nicoletti MA, Brambilla P et al (2003) Anatomical MRI study of basal ganglia in major depressive disorder. Psychiatry Res 124:129–140
11. Li BS, Wang H, Gonen O (2003) Metabolite ratios to assumed stable creatine level may confound the quantification of proton brain MR spectroscopy. Magn Reson Imaging 21:923–928
12. Loffelholz K, Klein J, Koppen A (1993) Choline, a precursor of acetylcholine and phospholipids in the brain. Prog Brain Res 98:197–200
13. Mirza Y, O'Neill J, Smith EA et al (2006) Increased medial thalamic creatine-phosphocreatine found by proton magnetic resonance spectroscopy in children with obses-

sive-compulsive disorder versus major depression and healthy controls. J Child Neurol 21:106–111
14. Murata T, Kimura H, Omori M et al (2001) MRI white matter hyper-intensities, (1)H-MR spectroscopy and cognitive function in geriatric depression: a comparison of early- and late-onset cases. Int J Geriatr Psychiatry 16:1129–1135
15. Sheehan DV, Lecrubier Y, Sheehan KH et al (1998) The Mini-International Neuropsychiatric Interview (MINI): the development and validation of a structured diagnostic psychiatric interview for DSM-IV and ICD-10. J Clin Psychiatry 59:22–33, quiz 34–57
16. Uranova NA, Vostrikov VM, Orlovskaya DD, Rachmanova VI (2004) Oligodendroglial density in the prefrontal cortex in schizophrenia and mood disorders: a study from the Stanley Neuropathology Consortium. Schizophr Res 67:269–275
17. Vythilingam M, Charles HC, Tupler LA et al (2003) Focal and lateralized subcortical abnormalities in unipolar major depressive disorder: an automated multivoxel proton magnetic resonance spectroscopy study. Biol Psychiatry 54:744–750
18. Wong ML, Licinio J (2001) Research and treatment approaches to depression. Nat Rev Neurosci 2:343–351

Chapter 63
Relating Research on ADC Value and Serum GGT, TBil of Lesions in Neonatal Hypoxic Ischemic Encephalopathy

Yue Guan, Anhui Yan, Yanming Ge, Yanqi Xu, Xihe Sun and Peng Dong

Abstract *Objective* Combined with neonatal hypoxic-ischemic encephalopathy (HIE) lesions' images in DWI, the ADC value, serum GGT, and the TBil content to provide the basis for the early diagnosis and treatment of HIE. *Materials and Methods* To detect serum GGT and TBil of 27 cases of HIE patients who were born in 24–48 h and adept MRI examination in one week, and measure the ADC value of the lesion. 30 healthy newborns were chosen randomly as control group. *Result* (1) Lesions' ADC value in neonatal HIE patients was significantly lower than that in normal neonatal ($P < 0.05$). There are no difference between mild and moderate HIE patient's ADC value ($P > 0.05$). ADC value of the severe lesions was lower than that in mild and moderate patients ($P < 0.05$). (2) Serum GGT values of severe HIE patients were higher than those of mild and moderate patients. NSE of moderate HIE patients was higher than that of mild patients ($P < 0.05$). Serum TBil of severe HIE were lower than that of mild and moderate patients ($P < 0.05$). Serum TBil of moderate HIE were lower than that of mild patients ($P < 0.05$). (3) the severe HIE patients' DWI images with high signal lesions were more than in mild and moderate patients, moderate HIE patients' DWI images with high signal lesions were more than mild patients ($P < 0.05$). *Conclusion* we can combine HIE patients' DWI images, lesion's ADC values and serum GGT, TBil level to use for early diagnosis of neonatal hypoxic-ischemic encephalopathy.

Keywords Hypoxic-ischemic encephalopathy · Valley GGT · Bilirubin · ADC value

Y. Guan · A. Yan · Y. Ge · Y. Xu · X. Sun · P. Dong (✉)
Medical Imaging Center of the Affiliated Hospital, Weifang Medical University, Weifang, Shandong Province, China
e-mail: dongpeng01502@yahoo.com.cn

S. Li et al. (eds.), *Frontier and Future Development of Information Technology in Medicine and Education*, Lecture Notes in Electrical Engineering 269,
DOI: 10.1007/978-94-007-7618-0_63,

63.1 Introduction

Neonatal hypoxic-ischemic encephalopathy (hypoxic ischemic encephalopathy, HIE) is due to a neonatal brain injury disease, it is due to neonatal asphyxia, resulting in brain blood supply and energy metabolism. The clinical diagnosis is based on history, biochemical markers and imaging examination. Valley of acyl transfer peptide enzymes and total bilirubin were common indicators of reflecting liver function, serum glutamic acid transfer peptide enzymes and total bilirubin levels were associated with HIE severity of the disease [1]. DWI is important magnetic resonance technology to study brain diseases. The performance of DWI about HIE were rare in Literature, no clinical research about HIE of serum GGT, TBi1 levels's and DWI performance of brain. In this study, we explore this issue.

63.2 Materials and Methods

63.2.1 The Clinical Data

We chose 27 cases of HIE patients in our hospital from June 2011 to June 2012 as the study group, including 14 male and 13 female. They were full-term infants with abnormal born history. Then we chose 30 normal full-term newborns with no abnormal obstetric history, as control group randomly, including 18 males and 12 females (Figs 63.1, 63.2, 63.3).

63.2.2 Methods

Using 1.5 T MRI instrument (Netherlands Philips Achieva Nova Dual 1.5T superconducting gradient MRI system), we examined 27 cases HIE patients' serum GGT and TBil 24–48 h after borning and knowledging MRI examination in a week, the patient supine, using a head coil signal acquisition. The main scanning parameters: a cross-sectional routine examination (1) T1WI: TR/TE = 406/15 ms, thickness 5.0 mm interval 1 mm FOV 230 cm; matrix 256 × 512, NSA = 2; (2) T2WI: TR/TE = 4600/110 ms, thickness 5.0 mm, interval 1 mm, FOV 230 cm matrix of 256 × 512, NSA = 2; (3) DWI: TR/TE = 3500/61 ms thickness 5 mm interval 1 mm FOV 230 cm, b = 0, 800 mm^2/s, matrix 256 × 160, NSA = 2. Outlining the area of being interested, measuring ADC values of the lesions, taking three regions from each lesion of being interested, measuring ADC value, we got average value at last. At the same time we counted the number of lesions with high signal which was corresponding to DWI images.

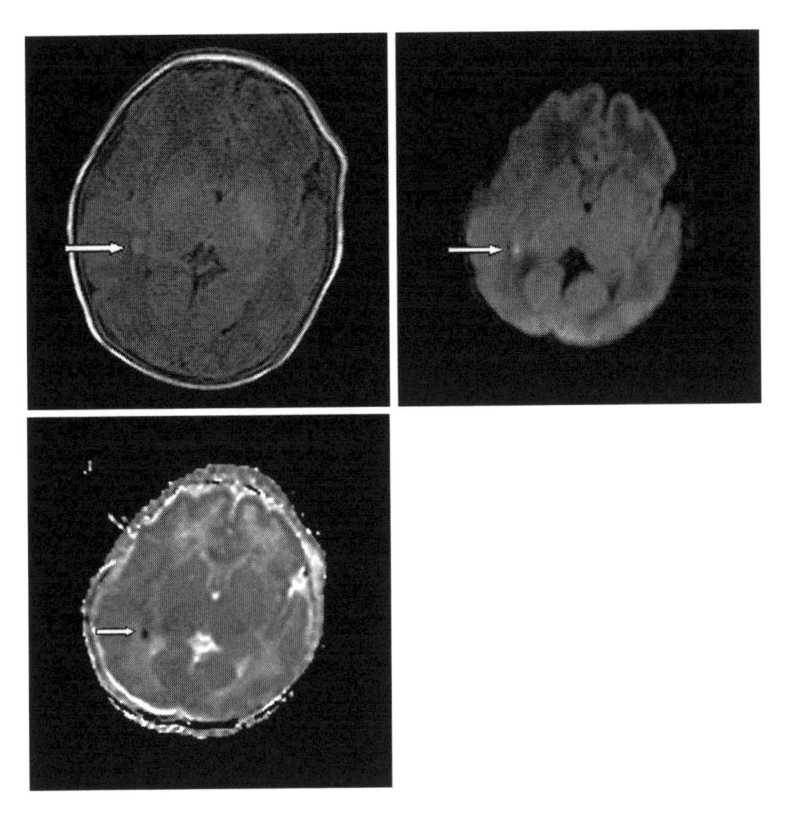

Fig. 63.1 Figures of the patients with mild HIE. Short T1 signal was seed on skin medullary junction of right temporal lobe (*white arrow shows*), high signal on DWI and signal is reduced on ADC chart

63.2.2.1 GGT, TBil Value Determination: Statistical Methods

Data were expressed as mean ± standard deviation (x (_) ± s). Use two-sample t' test and rank sum test which was compared between any two samples, q test. Using SPSS16.0 software packages to analysis statistic, $P < 0.05$ was considered statistically significant.

63.3 Results

MRI: MRI findings about HIE was divided into three degrees referring to the literature [2, 3]: (1) mild: dotting and lining high signal were showed in cortical and subcortica on T1WI, accompanied or not accompanied subarachnoid hemorrhage that under the curtain or upper the curtain. (2) Moderate: besides mild performance, we can find symmetry punctate high signal in bilateral frontal white

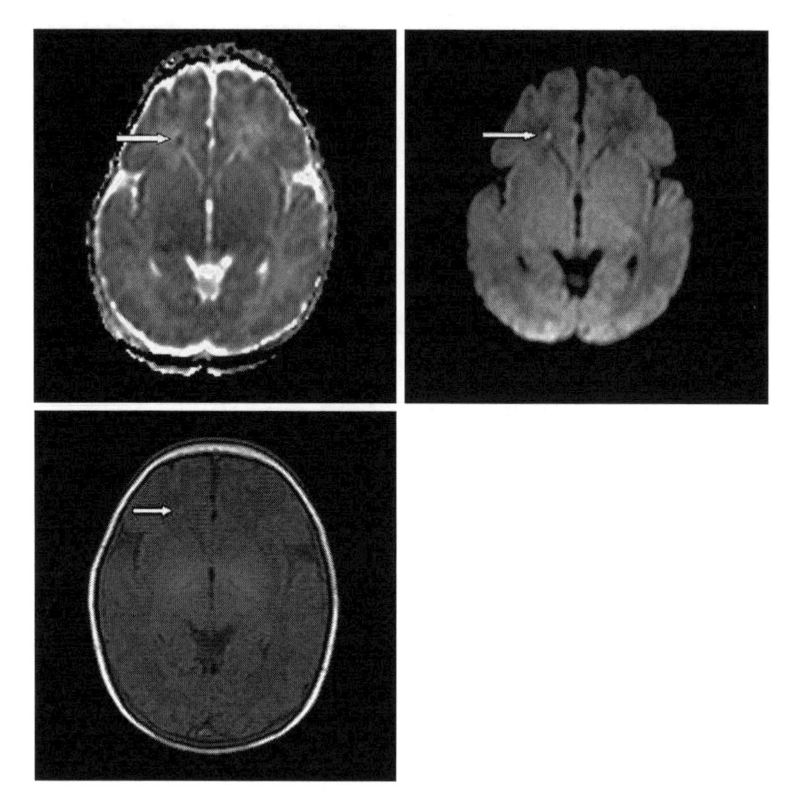

Fig. 63.2 Figure of the patients with moderate HIE. Short T1 signal was seed on the right frontal lobe (*white arrow shows*), high signal was showed on DWI, the signal is reduced on ADC chart

matter and (or) banded high signal distributed along the lateral ventricle wall, and may have limitations cerebral edema. (3) Severe: besides moderate performance, high signal can be find in basal ganglia, thalamus area and accompanied with relatively low signal in PLIC and subcortical cystic necrosis. This group of patients, 10 cases was mild, 9 patients were moderate, 8 cases were severe.

ADC value between HIE lesions with normal neonatal brain tissue. According to Table 63.1, ADC values in HIE lesion was less than ADC values in normal brain tissue by t' test ($P < 0.05$). ADC value for HIE patients staying in different degree: ADC value in the HIE patients who were mild and moderate was no significant difference. ADC value in mild HIE was greater than that in moderate HIE. And ADC value in moderate HIE was greater than that in severe HIE by Rank Sum test (Table 63.2).

Serum GGT value were for HIE patients staying in different degree: Serum GGT value in the HIE patients who were mild were less than moderate HIE, serum GGT value in mild HIE was less than that in severe HIE, serum GGT value in moderate HIE was less than that in severe HIE by Q test (Table 63.3). TBil values for HIE patients staying in different degree: TBil values in the HIE patients who

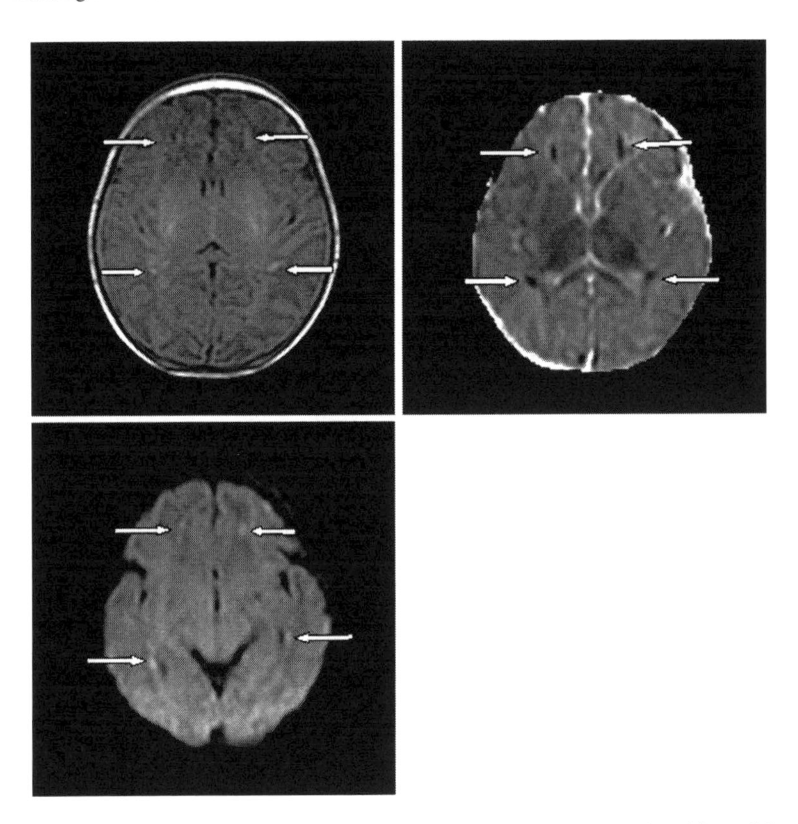

Fig. 63.3 Figure of the patients with severe HIE. Short T1 signal was seed on bilateral frontal, two lateral posterior horn (*white arrow shows*) around, high signal was showed on DWI, the signal is reduced on ADC chart

Table 63.1 ADC value were compared between HIE lesions with normal neonatal brain tissue

Group	Number	Mean ADC value(10–3 mm^2/s)
HIE patients	27	0.9698 ± 0.3363
Normal newborn	30	1.8179 ± 0.0985

According to t′test, $t' = 12.6255$, $t'(0.05) = 2.0548$, $P < 0.05$

Table 63.2 ADC value were compared for HIE patients staying in different degree

Severity	Number	Mean ADC value(10–3 mm^2/s)
Mild	10	1.2702 ± 0.2358
Moderate	9	0.9770 ± 0.1846
Severe	8	0.5863 ± 0.1119

According to Rank Sum test, $p > 0.05$ (mild and moderate), $p < 0.05$ (mild and severe), $p < 0.05$ (moderate and severe)

Table 63.3 Serum GGT value were compared for HIE patients staying in different degree

Severity	Number	Mean GGT value(nmol/L)
Mild	10	75.3100 ± 25.0877
Moderate	9	139.7222 ± 22.5234
Severe	8	313.6125 ± 124.4829

According to Q test, $p < 0.05$(mild and moderate), $p < 0.05$(mild and severe), $p < 0.05$ (moderate and severe)

Table 63.4 TBil values were compared for HIE patients staying in different degree

Severity	Number	Mean TBil value(nmol/L)
Mild	10	289.5400 ± 61.5890
Moderate	9	117.5778 ± 33.0398
Severe	8	55.0000 ± 21.2659

According to Q test, $p < 0.05$ (mild and moderate), $p < 0.05$ (mild and severe), $p < 0.05$ (moderate and severe)

Table 63.5 High signal lesions' number were compared on DWI images

Severity	Number	Mean lesions' number of high signal on DWI images
Mild	10	0.60000 ± 0.5164
Moderate	9	3.8889 ± 1.2693
Severe	8	14.8750 ± 4.0861

According to Q test, $p < 0.05$ (mild and moderate), $p < 0.05$ (mild and severe), $p < 0.05$ (moderate and severe)

were mild were greater than moderate HIE. TBil values in mild HIE was greater than that in severe HIE. TBil values in moderate HIE was greater than that in severe HIE by Q test (Table 63.4).

High signal lesions' number on DWI images: High signal lesions' number on DWI images in mild HIE were less than that in moderate HIE. High signal lesions' number on DWI images in mild HIE were less than that in severe HIE. High signal lesions' number on DWI images in moderate HIE were less than that in severe HIE (Table 63.5).

63.4 Discussion

63.4.1 Neonatal Hypoxic-Ischemic Encephalopathy

HIE is due to neonatal asphyxia, resulting in the decrease in cerebral blood flow that caused brain parenchymal damage. It is one of the main reasons for neonatal death or chronic neurological sequelae and is particularly important to the early diagnosis and treatment of HIE so far. The routine with sequence judging the cerebral infarction had difficulties, because neonatal brain development is not mature yet and it contents more water. Magnetic resonance diffusion weighted imaging (diffusion weighted imaging, DWI) have a considerable advantage in the diagnosis of early brain changes.

63.4.2 Pathophysiology of Neonatal Ischemic and Hypoxic Encephalopathy

When brain tissue was hypoxia, there was a series of harmful reaction: cell membrane ion pump dysfunction resulting in cytotoxic and cerebral edema; calcium channel to open abnormal, permeability of cell membranes increased, causing irreversible cell damage; Cerebral blood reperfusion and brain tissue re-oxygen. This process produced large amounts of oxygen radicals causing cell damage; inadequate energy supply, cell edema, apoptosis and necrosis [4].

63.4.3 Magnetic Resonance Imaging with Diffusion Weighted in HIE

DWI imaging techniques reflect the irregular movement of the water molecules in the organization and the parameters of describing the degree of diffusion was called the apparent diffusion coefficient (apparent diffusion coefficients for most sub ADC), which reflects the degree of the limited diffusion of water molecules within the organization. It was low signal on the ADC images in diffusing hypokinetic area. The experiments show that the ADC values between the mild HIE patients and moderate was no significant difference, the ADC values of mild and moderate HIE patients were significantly greater than that in severe HIE patients. ADC values of mild and moderate patients had no differences maybe relating to DWI examination time.

Some researches show HIE had cytotoxic edema in early time. With high signal on DWI, lower ADC values can be showed within hours of the injury. The minimum value performed within hours after injury 1–2 day, then gradually increased. False normal value shown on the eighth days and high-value on the tenth days [5]. Therefore, DWI detection is sensitive to early lesions of HIE. In addition, DWI has a high negative predictive value for excluding the after-effects judgment of early HIE [6, 7]. This study found that high signal lesions' number on DWI images in mild HIE were less than that in moderate and severe HIE, high signal lesions' number on DWI images in moderate HIE were less than that in severe HIE. This study shows that the DWI image as well as lesions ADC value can be used for the diagnosis and judging severe HIE.

In addition, foreign scholars said DWI sensitivity in the detection of neonatal HIE was affected by ischemia model. Compared with isolated cortical injury, deep gray matter damage was less sensitive. The study compared DWI signal intensity and ADC value of cortical injury and deep gray matter damage, found 100 % of cortical lesions DWI signal increased mildly and ADC values decrease. But only within 14 % of the deep gray matter injury, DWI signal increased mildly and ADC values decreased [8]. Research in this area was due to the limitation of the number of cases and remained to be in-depth.

63.4.4 The Significance of Serum GGT, TBil in the Diagnosis of HIE and the Relativity with ADC Value of Lesions

HIE besides cause varying degrees of brain damage and often involved multiple systems, causing multiple organ damage and accompanied by liver damage. Intracellular enzyme release increased resulted in its activity increased after liver cell damage. The study found that, serum GGT content increase with the aggravation of disease. Patients with severe HIE GGT content were higher than the mild and moderate, the moderate HIE GGT content higher than mild.

Bilirubin has a role in scavenging oxygen free radicals directly, and its mechanism of action is that when the cell membrane's fatty acids are changed into fatty acid radical formation in the role of oxygen free radicals, bilirubin would react with the later to form non-radical products and prevent unsaturated the fatty acid radicals further to form peroxidation lipid. Because HIE occurs to produce large amounts of oxygen free radicals, bilirubin are consumed as an antioxidant or oxygen free radical scavengers at the same time. The more severe the HIE were, the more oxygen free radicals produced, as well as bilirubin. This study confirms that the severe HIE patients' TBil value were less than the mild and moderate, moderate HIE patients' TBil value were less than mild.

The study found that we can initially determine the extent of brain damage by measuring the ADC values of the lesions, but not completely meet with clinical symptoms. The HIE serum GGT was Significantly elevated within 24 h after birth, while TBil was Significantly reduced, but cannot diagnose intracranial hemorrhage. Combining with them, comprehensive analysis can be helpful for diagnosis. The smaller ADC value, the higher serum GGT value, the smaller TBil value, the more severe brain damage.

In summary, the ADC values of the lesions and the number of high signal found on DWI images, combining GGT and TBil value can be used as objective indicators for HIE early diagnosis. It can further guide clinical treatment to reduce the mortality and disability rate of HIE patients.

Acknowledgments This study was supported by Research Weifang science and technology project (20111142,201104091); Shandong provincial natural science foundation of china (ZR2010HM078).

References

1. Barkovich AJ, Westmark K, Partidge C et al (1995) Perinatal asphyxia: MR findings in the first 10 days. AJNR 16:427–438
2. Dag Y, Firat AK, Karakas HM et al (2006) Clinical outcomes of neonatal hypoxic ischemic encephalopathy evaluated with diffusion-weighted magnetic resonance imaging. Diagn Interv Radiol 12:109–114
3. Forbes KP, Pipe JG, Bird R et al (2000) Neonatal hypoxic-ischemic encephalopathy: detection with diffusion-weighted MR imaging. AJNR 21:1490–1496
4. Hu L, Lin Z, Lin N et al (2005) Clinical analysis of neonatal hypoxic-ischemic encephalopathy with multiple organ damage. J Clin Res 22:26–29
5. Mao J (2003) Serum bilirubin changes and significance of neonatal hypoxic-ischemic encephalopathy. Mod Tradit Chin Med 12:362–363
6. McKinstry RC, Miller JH, Snyder AZ et al (2002) A prospective, longitudinal diffusion tensor imaging study of brain injury in newborns. Neurology 59:824–833
7. Takeda K, Nomura Y, Sakuma H et al (1997) MR assessment of normal brain development in neonates and infants: comparative study of T1 and diffusion-weighted images. J Comput Assist Tomogr 21:1–7
8. Trange EL, Saeed N, Cowan FM et al (2004) MR imaging quantification of cerebellar growth following hypoxicischemic injury to the neonatal brain. AJNR 25:463–468
9. Wang H et al (2008) HIE patients' mechanism of brain edema and its correlation between DWI, DTI characteristics and AQP-4. Chin Med Imaging Technol 24:622–625

Chapter 64
Design and Implementation of the Regional Health Information Collaborative Platform

Kong Hua-Ming, Qin Yao, Peng-Fei Li and Jing-Song Li

Abstract With the development of medical health, regional health information sharing has become the inevitable trend of the development of medical information. However, due to the regional medical information construction, it hinders the exchange and sharing of clinical data for some disadvantages like low-level degree of system integration, low real-time of information exchange, poor reliability, etc. According to the existing problems of the regional health, this paper constructs a regional health information collaborative platform, utilizes information integration to form patient as core of clinical data, uses clinical document architecture (CDA) as data exchange standard, and implements the data exchange and sharing between medical institutions and the regional medical center.

Keywords Clinical data exchange · Information integration · CDA · HL7 · Regional health

64.1 Introduction

With the social development and the implementation of the policies of the national healthcare reform, the model of hospital management which is independent cannot meet the demand at this stage, information sharing is an important way to maximize the value of information, and the regional health information sharing is the inevitable trend of the development of information technology. Regional health's goal is to make comprehensive use of the computer, communication and network technology, established in an area within the administrative department of health

---

K. Hua-Ming · Q. Yao · P.-F. Li · J.-S. Li (✉)
Healthcare Informatics Engineering Research Center, Key Laboratory for Biomedical Engineering of Ministry of Education, Zhejiang University, No 38 Zheda Road, Hangzhou 310027, China
e-mail: ljs@zju.edu.cn

S. Li et al. (eds.), *Frontier and Future Development of Information Technology in Medicine and Education*, Lecture Notes in Electrical Engineering 269,
DOI: 10.1007/978-94-007-7618-0_64,

coverage throughout the region at all levels of medical health administration and medical service institutions, to form an integrated, safe and efficient regional medical service platform, with the support of the platform, form a modern medical services and a new supervision model, and the platform full supports to the regional medical service and management decision-making, improves the level of healthcare and the performance of public health service [1]. Although the construction of regional health information has made certain achievements by present, still it still faces some problems as the absence of mechanisms, management thinking lag; careful coordination difficult; weak foundation, uneven development; lack of standards, difficult integration; high investment, multi-channel financing difficult, etc. [2].

Regional health information collaborative platform is the core content of the regional health [3], the collaborative platform in this paper can achieve the interconnection, share exchanging between heterogeneous systems, implement to save and handle the patient-centered medical procedure information, and regional information integration platform as the core, can realize the centralized management of clinical data and information sharing, ultimately improve the quality and efficiency of healthcare services.

64.2 Design of the Platform

The regional health information collaborative platform mainly includes three parts: edge gateway, access gateway and integrated regional information platform (Fig. 64.1).

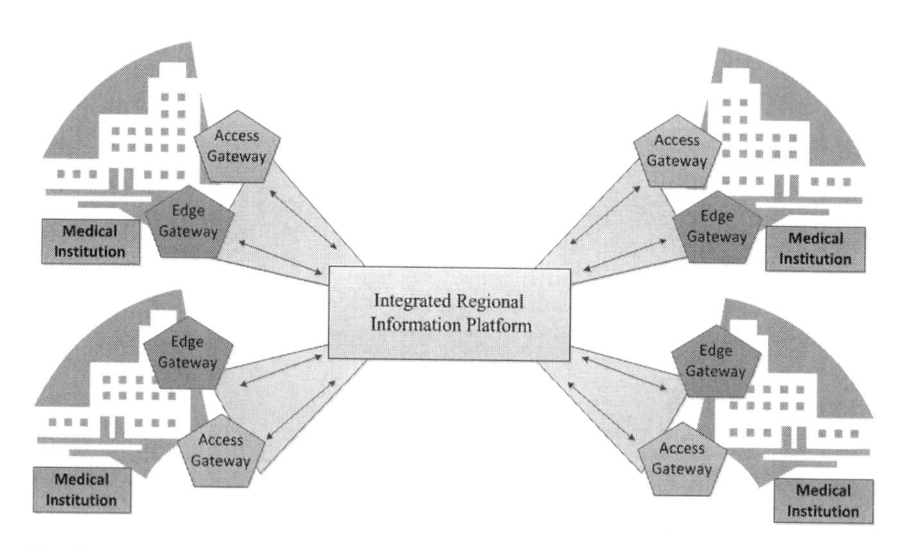

Fig. 64.1 Framework of the regional health information collaborative platform

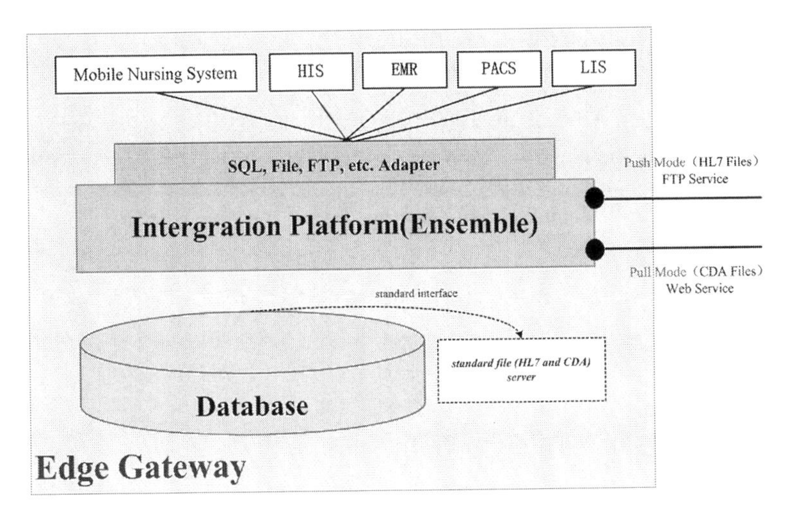

Fig. 64.2 Framework of the edge gateway

64.2.1 Edge Gateway

The function of the edge gateway is integrating the information and standardizing data, the framework as Fig. 64.2. It can realize to acquire, organize and encapsulate the data which from electronic medical record (EMR), hospital information system (HIS), picture archiving and communication system (PACS), laboratory information system (LIS), pharmacy management system and mobile-nursing system, etc. through the integration platform (Ensemble), and form the clinical metadata which is patient-centered and can meet the clinical data exchanging in the regional health. At the same time, through the data standardized interface in the integration platform, use health level 7 (HL7) and (CDA) 2.0 to do the standardized processing of medical information metadata, and exchange data between edge gateway and regional integrated information platform by both push and pull mode.

The push mode is to achieve the data exchange of patient, document and order information when some medical institution generates new registered patients or documents information. Then the adapter of integration platform is triggered, grabs the necessary medical information, standardizes the data by using messages (2.4: ADT_A01 and 2.4: MDM_T02) in HL7, and saves the main index information of patient, document and order to data repository in regional health information collaborative platform. The pull mode is to realize the standardized clinical data, when some services in the integrated regional information platform need to visit the data in some medical institutions (such as all the documents, orders of the patient within a certain period), the integrated platform uses some adapters such as SQL adapter to grab the clinical data and saves in a clinical document using CDA standard.

64.2.2 Access Gateway

Access gateway is a file server where the files (such as images, videos, reports, etc.) generated by medical information systems stored by a certain rule, it can open the appropriate access rights by configuring the FTP. When some services in integrated regional information platform need to access these parts of the data, it can provide data support.

64.2.3 Integrated Regional Information Platform

The integrated regional information platform includes clinical data standard parser interface, clinical data repository, some services, etc. The structure is shown in Fig. 64.3. In this figure, the interface realizes to get the standard files (HL7 and CDA) from various medical institutions, parses the information and saves the data in a clinical data repository. The clinical data repository mainly stores master index of patients (including basic patient information, clinical types of information, etc. in each medical institution), index information of orders and documents, the index of institution and the configuration of informed consent management, also includes the storage and management of personal health records (PHR). The system application services is made up of registration, routing and querying, which

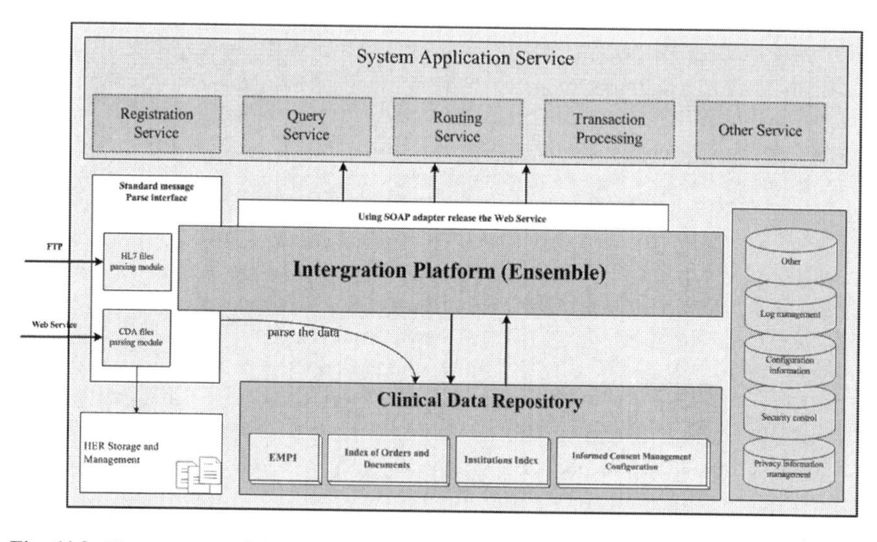

Fig. 64.3 The structure of the integrated regional information platform

is published by Simple Object Access Protocol (SOAP) adapter in Ensemble and orients to the application client. Besides, it also includes privacy information and log management, security control, configuration information, etc.

64.3 Implementation of the Platform

Regional health's main objective is to achieve sharing-and-exchanging, interconnection between different information systems, and regional medical collaboration platform is to complete the integration of heterogeneous systems, then achieves to share information by using data standards [4]. Ensemble gathers data server, integration server, application server and portal development software in one, can achieve the coordination of heterogeneous data and business process reengineering, quickly build new business solutions, reduce the complexity of integrating, complex the application integration [5]. HL7 standard as an important criterion of the application and implementation of medical information system, can achieve the standards of the data transmission by using message, standardize business processes, restrain the medical practices, ensure the quality of medical care, make the authenticity and validity of information [6]. And CDA provides the transmission and exchange of patient medical records for documents exchange.

64.3.1 Information Integration

Before exchanging data between medical institutions and regional medical center, we must need to collect data that can ensure the integrity of the data, and record the critical information throughout the patient's total medical process. The

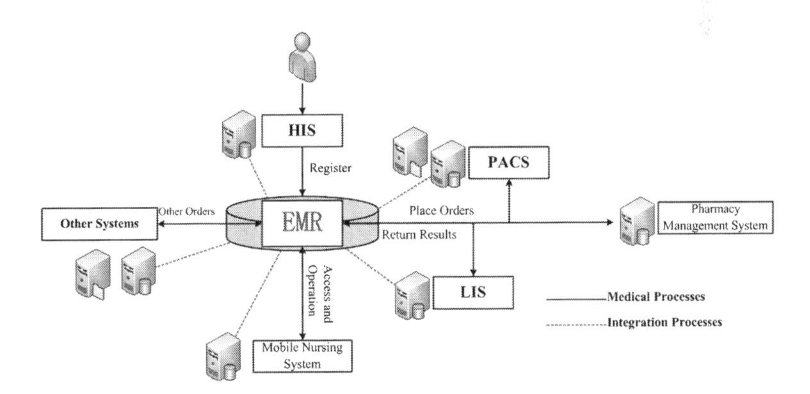

Fig. 64.4 Framework of the information integration

information integration achieves to acquire, organize and package the patients, orders, documents and other information which generated by the heterogeneous information systems through the integration platform, and gather the discrete data (such as the data from HIS, EMR, PACS, LIS, Mobile Nursing, etc. heterogeneous information systems), store in the EMR database and provide data support for data exchange. The Framework of the Information Integration is shown in Fig. 64.4.

64.3.2 Data Exchange

We adopt the CDA standard as data exchange's main carrier, because CDA is a document markup standard which base on the exchange of clinical documentation for the purpose, describes the structure and semantics of clinical documents. It is a part of the HL7 standard set which follows the XML standard and HL7 reference information model (RIM) [7, 8]. CDA document contains a header and a body, the Fig. 64.5 is a structural diagram and schema of the CDA.

The header lies between the <ClinicalDocument> and <structuredBody> elements, identifies and classifies the document and provides information on authentication, the encounter, the patient, and the involved providers. The body is wrapped by the <structedBody> , and contains some clinical reports information like insurance, diagnosis, medications, lab results, etc. [9, 10].

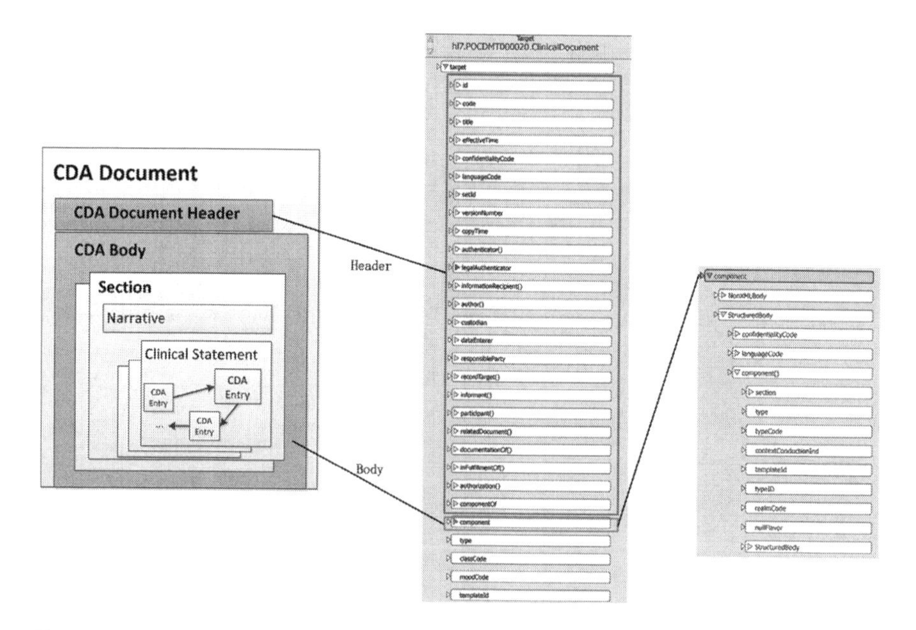

Fig. 64.5 Structure and schema of the CDA

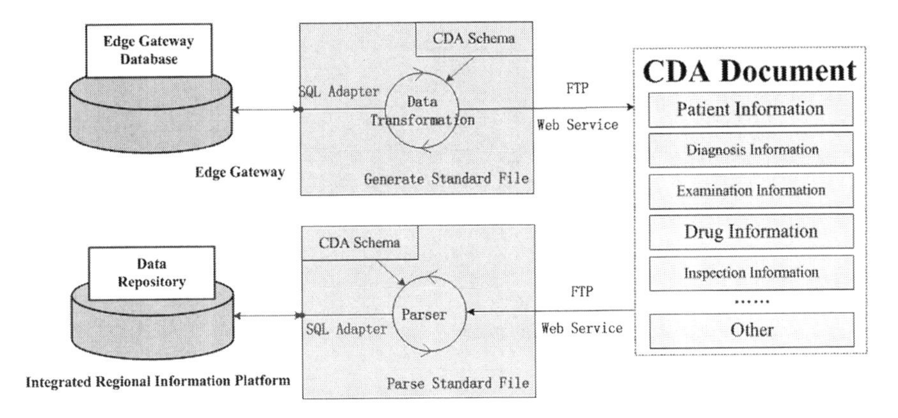

Fig. 64.6 The mechanism of data exchange

The realization process of the entire data exchange includes generating the standard file and parsing the standard file, the realization mechanism is shown in Fig. 64.6.

When a service in regional integrated information platform needs to query a patient's clinical information in a period, it can call the service interface in web service deployed on the edge gateway. This interface uses the SQL adapter to obtain the patient and clinical information from the database formed by the information integration, does the data conversion according to the CDA schema and saves this information in the standard CDA document. When the document is sent to the regional information integration platform through the network, the information can be resolved from the CDA document by using the schema mapping mechanism, stored in a clinical data repository, and ultimately shown the data through the client application.

64.3.3 Result of the Implementation

The regional health information collaborative platform is implemented through edge gateway, access gateway and integrated regional information platform, it integrates the data from heterogeneous medical information that can be the base for clinical data exchange, then uses the CDA standard to standardized the patient, diagnostic, inspection, testing and drug information, finally achieves data standardization sharing between medical institutions and regional medical center. When patient's medical information is generated after a series of diagnosis and examination, the edge gateway integrates the medical information generated by the various medical practices in the EMR's database and standardizes the data. Then through the network, the platform synchronizes the medical information to the Regional Medical Center, achieves to save the patient's registration and clinical

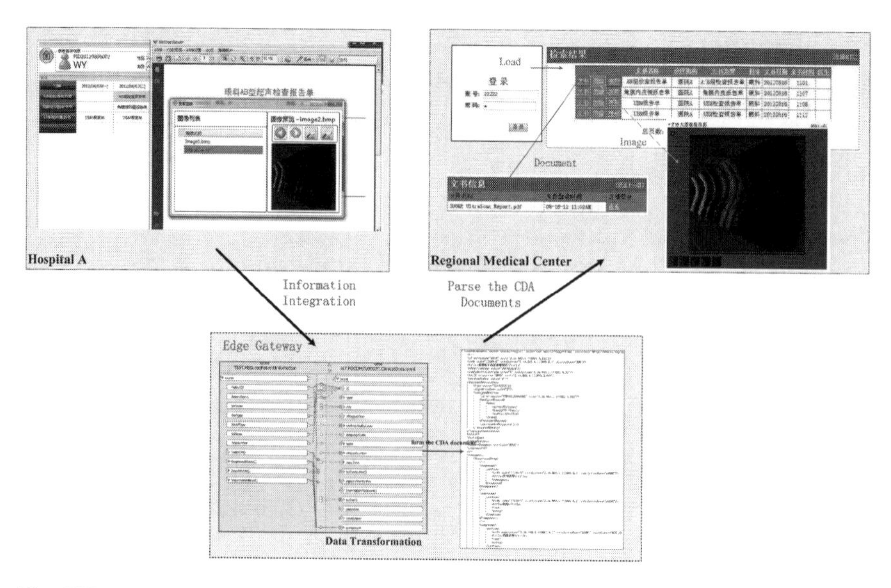

Fig. 64.7 The client interface implementation of regional health information collaborative platform

information. At last, doctors and patients can review the reports (such as documents, images, video, etc.) created during a certain period of time from the regional medical website, as shown in Fig. 64.7.

64.4 Conclusion and Discussion

The main objective of regional health is to achieve interconnection and shared between different information systems. The platform in this paper includes edge gateway, access gateway and integrated regional information platform, it uses the edge gateway to achieve information integration of heterogeneous systems (data acquisition, organization and packaging), form the regional medical metadata which is patient-centered, has highly integrated features and meets the needs of the medical information. Based on the medical information metadata, the edge gateway uses the CDA standard to standardize it, and realizes the data exchanging of patients, diagnostic, inspection, testing, drug, etc. Ultimately achieves data sharing in medical institutions and regional medical center.

Although there are various of regional medical solutions, most of the systems are not patient-centered medical and low data integration, and also lack of a certain standard. This paper presents the design and implementation of regional health information collaborative platform, which eliminates information silos between different information systems through information integration, completes the interconnection between heterogeneous systems by using CDA, solves the current regional medical problem and achieves data exchange and sharing for regional health.

Acknowledgment This work was supported by the National Natural Science Foundation (Grant No. 61173127) and Zhejiang University Top Disciplinary Partnership Program (Grant No. 188170*193251101).

References

1. Chen YM (2010) The exploration and study of constructing regional medical information plaform. Med Inf 23(3):25–26
2. Wang S, Su W (2010) The current situation and existing problems for the Chinese regional medical informatics and its corresponding strategies. Mod Prev Med 37(22):4241–4243
3. Tang K, Guan SJ, Huang Z, Li JS (2010) Medical data exchange platform in regional health care information technology. Chinese Med Equip J 31(5):35–37
4. Fontaine P, Zink T, Boyle RG, Kralewski J (2010) Health information exchange: participation by Minnesota primary care practices. Arch Intern Med 170(7):622
5. Wang Y, Zhou TS, Kong HM, Zhao JP, Li JS (2012) Clinical data exchange based on ensemble integration platform. Chin Digital Med 7(1):71–75
6. HL7. HL7 Reference Information Model[EB/OL]. http://www.hl7.org/
7. Hurrell MJ, Monk TG, Nicol A, Norton AN, Reich DL, Walsh JL (2012) Implementation of a standards-based anaesthesia record compliant with the health level 7 (HL7) clinical document architecture (CDA). J Clin Monit Comput 26(4):295–304
8. Dolin RH, Alschuler L, Boyer S, Beebe C, Behlen FM, Biron PV, Shvo AS (2006) HL7 clinical document architecture, release 2. J Am Med Inform Assoc 13(1):30–39
9. Muller M, Frankewitsch T, Ganslandt T, Bürkle T, Prokosch HU (2004) The Clinical Document Architecture (CDA) enables electronic medical records to wireless mobile computing. Medinfo 11:1448–1452
10. Müller ML, Ückert F, Bürkle T, Prokosch HU (2005) Cross-institutional data exchange using the clinical document architecture (CDA). Int J Med Informatics 74(2–4):245–256

Chapter 65
A Multi-objective Biogeography-Based Optimization with Mean Value Migration Operator

Xiang-wei Zheng, Kai-ge Gao, Xiao-guang Wang and Chi-zhu Ma

Abstract: Considering its successful application in solving discrete single objective problems, biogeography-based optimization (BBO) is considered as a new promising intelligent algorithm. Therefore, many studies are conducted to apply it to solve multi-objective optimization problems (MOPs). However, these improved BBOs are not always effective because of the complexity of MOPs. A multi-objective biogeography-based algorithm with mean value migration operator named MVBBO is proposed in this paper. In MVBBO, mean value theory and new boundary constraint rule are adopted to extend the range of feasible domain. Meanwhile, mutation operator and ε-dominance-based archive strategy are employed to achieve better convergence and diversity. Simulation on benchmark functions shows that the proposed MVBBO's final Pareto solution set is better than NSGA-II and other improved multi-objective BBOs in convergence and distribution of Pareto solutions.

Keywords: BBO · Mean value theory · ε-dominance relation · Archive strategy

X. Zheng · K. Gao · X. Wang
School of Information Science and Engineering, Shandong Normal University, Jinan, China

K. Gao (✉)
Shandong Provincial Key Laboratory for Distributed Computer Software Novel Technology, Jinan, China
e-mail: kaige_high@163.com.cn

C. Ma
School of Communication, Shandong Normal University, Jinan, China

S. Li et al. (eds.), *Frontier and Future Development of Information Technology in Medicine and Education*, Lecture Notes in Electrical Engineering 269,
DOI: 10.1007/978-94-007-7618-0_65,

65.1 Introduction

Many optimization problems in engineering applications are multi-objective optimization problems (MOPs) which have more than one conflict objective. In solving MOPs, it is likely to lead to performance decline of the others when to improve an objective. The basic and traditional method to solve MOPs is to transform multiple objectives into single objective by assigning each objective a predefined weight and then all objectives are summed up. The disadvantages of the traditional methods are that the multi-objective nature will be omitted and each cycle only achieves an "optimal" solution. Generally speaking, it is difficult to achieve the best result for all objectives of MOPs at the same time, so there is a demand for new methods of solving MOPs. Evolutionary algorithms (EAs) demonstrate their advantages to solve MOPs since 1990. EAs are inspired by nature and evolution and they are a class of random search techniques and simulation of biological evolution processes. They simulate the population's collective learning process, where individuals learn information from their neighbors. To efficiently solve MOPs, researchers have proposed many evolutionary mechanisms and strategies and developed many multi-objective EAs called MOEAs based on GA, DE and so on, and they can achieve more than one solution in a generation in solving MOPs [1].

In 2008, Dan Simon proposed a new evolutionary algorithm called biogeography-based optimization (BBO) and published in IEEE Transactions on Evolutionary Computation [2]. BBO is based on biological population and its evolution process simulates biological population's dynamic changes, including distribution, migration, mutation, reproduction and extinction process. Compared with other EAs, BBO has its unique mechanism. It uses a coding way and migration operator (migration operator is based on an immigration rate) to realize information sharing between individuals. Meanwhile, its mutation operator realizes the mutation of some worst individuals where each individual has its mutation rate. Researches show that although original BBO has simple structure, many improved BBOs have good performance in solving single objective problems. Therefore, it's possible to apply BBO to solve MOPs.

In this paper, a multi-objective biogeography-based optimizer named MVBBO is proposed to solve MOPs, which is constructed with mean value theory, new boundary constraint rule and ε-dominance-based archive strategy. Section. 65.2 reviews the basis and related work of BBO. Section. 65.3 details MVBBO's several elements and its formal description. Section. 65.4 demonstrates and discusses some simulation results by comparing MOBBO with classic NSGA-II on four test functions. Section. 65.5 presents the concluding remarks of the paper and future work.

65.2 Related Work

Since BBO's appearance in 2008, BBO has been further studied from many aspects. There are several studies on single objective optimization and their applications. Ma [3] explored the behavior of six different migration models in BBO and investigated the performance through benchmark functions with a wide range of dimensions and diverse complexities. The study showed that each model's performance is different from others and sinusoidal migration curves provide the best performance among the six models. Dawei et al. [4] applied features from evolutionary strategy (ES) to BBO modification, and a new immigration refusal approach was added to BBO. *T* test results on the modified BBO showed that features from ES has a big effect on BBO, but the effect of using immigration refusal is not that large. GONG et al. [5] proposed a hybrid DE with BBO (DE/BBO) for the global numerical optimization problem, which combined the exploration of DE with the exploitation of BBO effectively and a new hybrid migration operator was proposed. It demonstrated that DE/BBO has a good trade-off between the exploration and the exploitation.

Recently, some studies on multi-objective optimization based on BBO are conducted. Bhattacharya and Chattopadhyay [6] proposed a methodology based on BBO, which takes care of economic dispatch problems involving constraints such as transmission losses, ramp rate limits, valve point loading, multi-fuel options and prohibited operating zones. Zhidan and Hongwei [7] proposed a biogeography-based multi-objective evolutionary algorithm called BBMOEA. The migration operator of original BBO is developed and perturbation factor is introduced to increase the diversity of population. Costa et al. [8] proposed a multi-objective BBO with adopting a predator–prey approach named PPBBO and it was validated in the constrained design of a brushless dc wheel motor. Jamuna and Swarup [9] proposed a multi-objective biogeography based optimization (MO-BBO) algorithm. In MO-BBO, the Pareto optimal solution is obtained using the non-dominated sorting and crowding distance. The compromised solution is chosen using a fuzzy based mechanism from the Pareto optimal solution.

Although there are some developments of BBO, most of these studies only do better in solving single objective optimal problems, and their effectiveness is not good enough in solving MOPs. In this paper, a new algorithm called MVBBO is proposed and it is efficient to solve MOPs.

65.3 Mvbbo

Compared with the original BBO, MVBBO is improved in the following aspects, including adopting real-coding way, mean value migration operator and ε-dominance-based archive strategy.

65.3.1 Migration Operator

In MVBBO, the replacement way of selected variable is different from original BBO. In the following description, x refers to each solution vector in X (X is n-dimension space) and x_i is the i-th variable of x. As is shown in Figs. 65.1, 65.2 and 65.3, where axis $\boldsymbol{x}$ shows variable's range, we take solution vectors a and b for example, assume that a_i is selected to be updated with b_i's guidance ($a_i > 0$, $b_i > 0$ and $a_i < b_i$). (Attention: Here is b_i's guidance, not only is b_i, and we use x_i to represent the possible number.)

(1) Original BBO's migration operatorIn original BBO's migration operator, a_i will be replaced only by b_i with a_i's fixed immigration rate (λi) of this generation, as is shown in Fig. 65.1.
(2) MVBBO's new migration operatorIn MVBBO's new migration operator, x_i's search range is ideally extended, and a_i can be replaced with the random real number in search range. According to the relation of x_i's ideal search range (a_i, $2b_i - a_i$) and x_i's real limits range (the range is (L_i, U_i)), there are two circumstances: Normal and Special.

Normally as shown in Fig. 65.2, x_i's ideal search range (a_i, $2b_i - a_i$) is completely contained by x_i's real limits (L_i, U_i). Therefore, x_i can be any real number in (a_i, $2b_i - a_i$), and each has equal probability to be selected to replace a_i.

Specially as shown in Fig. 65.3, x_i's ideal search range (a_i, $2b_i - a_i$) is not completely contained by x_i's real limits (L_i, U_i). That's saying, there is a subset of (a_i, $2b_i - a_i$) which is out of (L_i, U_i). So the newly generated variable x_i have the possibility to be beyond x_i's real limits (L_i, U_i). The special x_i can described as a set X_o shown as (65.1).

$$X_0 = \{xi | xi \in (ai, 2bi - ai) \cap xi \notin (Li, Ui)\} \tag{65.1}$$

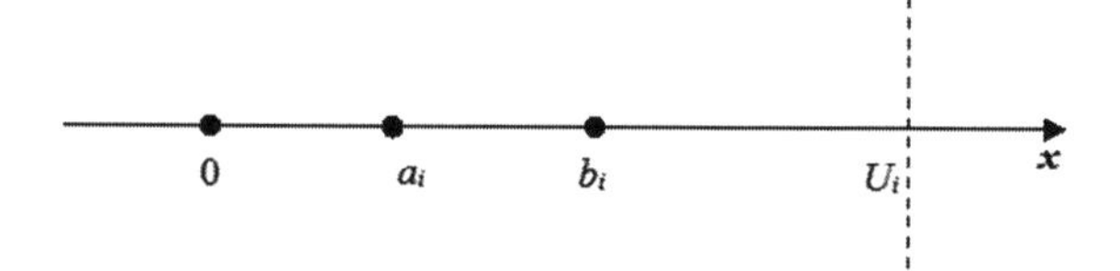

Fig. 65.1 Original migration operator

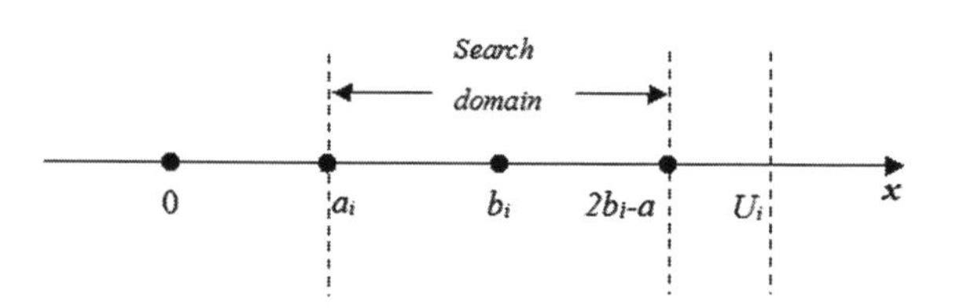

Fig. 65.2 New migration operator (Normal, $2b_i - a_i \leq U_i$)

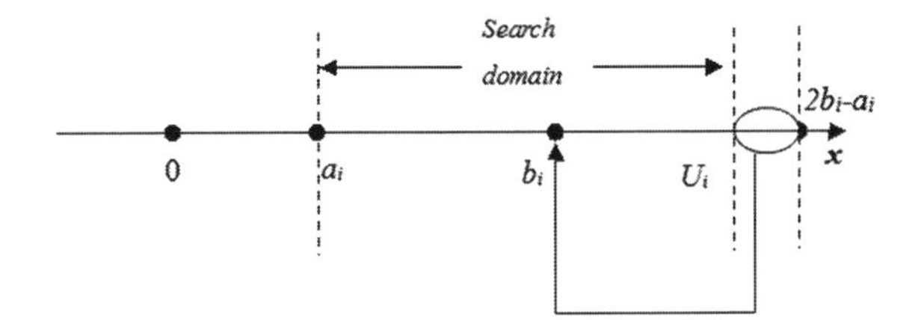

Fig. 65.3 New migration operator (Special, $2b_i - a_i > U_i$)

To guarantee x_i's feasibility, when x_i is not belongs to (L_i, U_i). the following boundary constraint rule defined in (65.2) is employed to replace x_i with x^*.

$$x^* = bi \tag{65.2}$$

Where U_i is the upper bound and L_i is the lower bound. When x_i is out of the range, $x^* = b_i$ is used to replace x_i, where b_i is the variable which is selected to guiding a_i's update. The rule ensures that each variable in vector is feasible and the selected guiding variable b_i will be selected with higher probability.

In conclusion, the new migration operator can extend search range, and the selected shared variable will be introduced to immigration variable with a relative higher probability than original migration operator and this improves the diversity of population.

65.3.2 Mutation Operator

Mutation refers to biological survival environments change sharply because of natural disaster or other uncontrollable conditions' occurrence. In BBO, mutation operator can enhance the diversity of population, and non-excellent individuals will have possibility to be better. Here a new mutation operator combining with Cauchy distribution is proposed, which means that the random number obtained in mutation process obeys Cauchy distribution.

Cauchy distribution's feature can be described as follows: closer to horizontal axis, change less, and the whole distribution is unlimited. The possibility of Cauchy distribution to generate a random number away from origin is higher than Normal distribution. Therefore, mutation operator with Cauchy distribution in mutation operator can extend random number's distribution and enhance the algorithm's ability to escape from local optimal. Take solution vector x for example, if x is selected to be mutated, the mutation operator is defined in (3.3).

$$x^* = x + x_* Cauchy(0, 1) \tag{65.3}$$

Where *Cauchy (0,1)* is the standard Cauchy distribution.

65.3.3 Description of MVBBO

MVBBO can be simply described as follows.

(1) Define parameters. Internal population Np, external archive Ne, solution dimension d, max immigration rate I, max emigration rate E, max mutation rate M, max generation times G.
(2) Initialize population. Set generation timer $t = 0$ and external archive $Ne_0 = \Phi$, initialize internal population Np_0.
(3) Evaluate solutions. Calculate each solution's fitness(HSI) in Np_t and Ne_t.
(4) Select non-dominated solutions. Sort solutions according to their HSI, achieve new external archive Ne_{t+1}. Ne_{t+1} includes all non-dominated solutions in the previous generation.
(5) Calculate λ, μ, p and HSI of each solution in Ne_{t+1}.
(6) Immigration process. Immigrate variable to selected solution with the new migration operator. Achieve new Ne_{t+1}.
(7) Mutation process. Mutate solution with mutation operator and employ boundary constraint rule to achieve new Ne_{t+1}. Merge Ne_{t+1} to Np_{t+1} with ε-dominance archive strategy. Set $t = t+1$.
(8) If $t <= G$, go to step (3), else output final Ne and exit.

65.4 Simulation and Discussion

In this paper, the selected benchmark functions are ZDT1, ZDT2, ZDT4 and ZDT6, which were designed by Deb et al. To evaluate MVBBO's performance quantitatively, two metrics for MOPs, Generational Distance (GD) and Spacing(SP) are employed [10].

In our study, MVBBO's parameters are setted as follows: initial population size $N_p = 100$, external archive size $N_e = 100$, solution dimension $d = 10$, max generations $G = 200$, max immigration rate $I = 1$, max emigration rate $E = 1$, max mutation rate $M = 0.1$. According to Deb et al. [11], NSGA-II's parameters are setted as follows: population size $N_p' = 100$, solution dimension $d' = 10$, max generations $G' = 200$, crossover rate $P_c = 1$, mutation rate $P_m = 0.1$, distribution index for crossover operator $\eta c = 20$, distribution index for mutation operator $\eta m = 20$. MVBBO and NSGA-II are both programmed and implemented in Matlab 7.0. For each benchmark function, algorithms are repeatedly run 20 times.

Table 65.1 shows MVBBO and NSGA-II's average performance on ZDT1, ZDT2, ZDT4 and ZDT6 respectively [12, 13].

The optimal Pareto fronts and true Pareto fronts of the ZDT4 and the ZDT6 achieved by MVBBO and NSGA-II, are shown in Figs. 65.4 and 65.5.

As can be seen from Table 65.1, Figs. 65.4 and 65.4. On GD, from the data in Table 65.1, the GD of MVBBO on all test functions are smaller than NSGA-II,

Table 65.1 MVBBO and NSGA-II's performance

Metrics	Algorithm	ZDT1	ZDT2	ZDT4	ZDT6
GD	MVBBO	0.0024	0.0014	0.0020	0.0008
	NSGA-II	0.0023	0.0015	0.0737	0.0167
SP	MVBBO	0.0020	0.0011	0.0029	0.0012
	NSGA-II	0.0028	0.0039	0.9005	0.0250

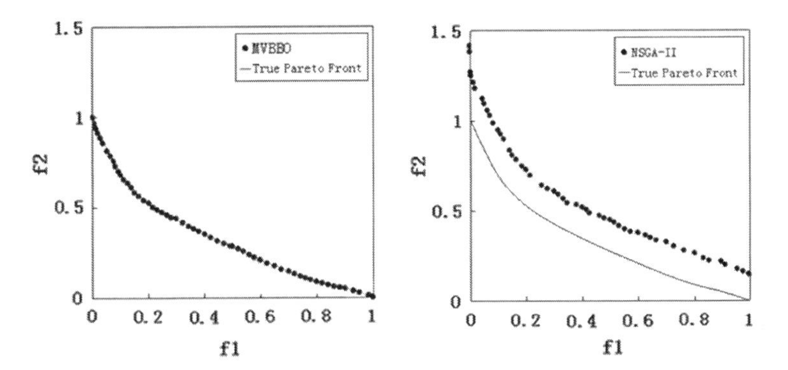

Fig. 65.4 Pareto-front of ZDT4

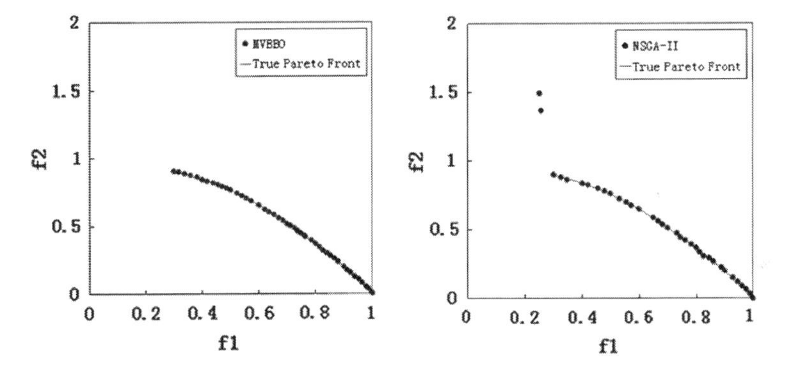

Fig. 65.5 Pareto-front of ZDT6

that means final solutions of MVBBO are more closer to the true Pareto optimal front which also can be seen from Figs. 65.4 and 65.5. On *SP*, from the data in Table 65.1, it's obviously that MVBBO's *SPs* are smaller or similar to NSGA-II. Meanwhile, final solutions of MVBBO are more uniformly distributed than NSGA-II as shown in Figs. 65.4 and 65.5.

All in all, on most test functions, the Pareto optimal set achieved by MVBBO is better than NSGA-II.

65.5 Conclusions

In this paper, a multi-objective biogeography-based algorithm with mean value migration operator is proposed. In MVBBO, mean value theory and new boundary constraint rule are adopted to extend the range of feasible domain and ε-dominance-based archive strategy is employed to achieve better convergence and diversity. The simulation results on benchmark functions show that most metrics on MVBBO are better than NSGA-II. Generally speaking, MVBBO is effective and efficient in solving MOPs. However, our study is primary and more work will be conducted in the future. On the one hand, the migration operators of MVBBO should be elaborated and tested to improve its performance. On the other hand, MVBBO will be applied in practical applications to further test its performance.

Acknowledgments We are grateful for the support of the Promotive Research Fund for Excellent Young and Middle-aged Scientists of Shandong Province (BS2010DX033) and a Project of Shandong Province Higher Educational Science and Technology Program (J10LG08).

References

1. Zheng X, Liu H (2010) A scalable coevolutionary multi-objective particle swarm optimizer. Int J Comput Intell Syst 3(5):590–600
2. Simon D (2008) Biogeography-based optimization. IEEE Trans Evol Comput 12(6):702–713
3. Haiping MA (2010) An analysis of the equilibrium of migration models for biogeography-based optimization. Inf Sci 180(18):3444–3464
4. Dawei Du, Simon D, Ergezer M (2009) Biogeography-based optimization combined with evolutionary strategy and immigration refusal systems. In: IEEE International Conference on Man and Cybernetics, pp 997–1002
5. Gong W, Cai Z, Ling CX (2010) DE/BBO: a hybrid differential evolution with biogeography-based optimization for global numerical optimization. Soft Comput 15(4):645–665
6. Bhattacharya A, Chattopadhyay PK (2010) Biogeography-based optimization for different economic load dispatch problems. IEEE Trans Power Syst 25(2):1064–1077
7. Zhidan XU, Hongwei MO (2012) Improvement for migration operator in biogeography-based optimization algorithm. Pattern Recognit Artif Intell 25(3):544–549 (In Chinese with English Abstract)
8. Costa E, Silva MA, Coelho LS, Lebensztajn L (2012) Multiobjective biogeography-based optimization based on predator-prey approach. IEEE Trans Magn 48(2):951–954
9. Jamuna K, Swarup KS (2012) Multi-objective biogeography based optimization for optimal PMU placement. Appl Soft Comput 12(5):1503–1510
10. Zheng X, Liu H (2009) A hybrid vertical mutation and self-adaptation based MOPSO. Comput Math Appl 57(11):2030–2038
11. Deb K, Pratap A, Agarwal S et al (2002) A fast and elitist multiobjective genetic algorithm: NSGA-II. IEEE Trans Evol Comput 6(2):182–197
12. Zhang M, Luo W, Wang X (2009) A normal distribution crossover for ε-MOEA. J Software 20(2):305–314. (In Chinese with English Abstract)
13. Chen M, Zhang C, Luo C (2009) Adaptive evolutionary particle swarm algorithm for multi-objective optimization. J Syst Simul 21(22):7061–7065 (In Chinese with English Abstract)

Chapter 66
Observation of Curative Effect on 200 Cases of Myasthenia Gravis Treated with Traditional Chinese Medicine

Wang Di and Wang Zhenqiu

Abstract Aim: To observe the curative effect of applying a patented traditional Chinese medicine, namely "a traditional Chinese medicine for treating myasthenia gravis" (assigned Chinese Patent of Invention in 2007), to myasthenia gravis. Methods: 200 cases of myasthenia gravis were collected during 1988–2010. One single course of treatment takes 3 months when using the above-mentioned patented medicine. Such changes of clinical symptoms are noticed before and after treatment: eyelid ptosis, diplopia, weakness, dysarthria, dysphagia, choke cough. We compile scorings according to the quantitative myasthenia gravis (QMG) score system of Myasthenia Gravis Foundation of America. Curative effect: (1) Short-term: the shortest treatment course of this group of cases was 1 month and the longest was 30 months with an normal distribution of 7.21 ± 6.23 months. Among the 200 cases, 104 cases were fully recovered (52 %), 58 cases had obvious effect (29 %), 31 cases (15.5 %) were effective and 7 cases were ineffective (3.5 %), hence the total effective rate was 96.5 % (Table 66.1 in the text). There is a huge difference ($P < 0.001$, Table 66.2 in the text) between QMG scores of various symptoms before and after treatment (paired-t test). (2) Long-term curative effect: through following up part of the recovered patients (24 cases) for at least half a year and at most 19 years with an average period of 5.72 years, the patients can still participate in normal work or housework without recurrence. Conclusion: The curative effect of 200 cases of myasthenia gravis treated by this patent traditional Chinese medicine was satisfied during 1988–2010.

Keywords Myasthenia gravis · Chinese medicine

W. Di (✉)
Traditional Chinese Medicine, China Changchun University, Changchun 130117, China
e-mail: wangdi0606@yahoo.com.cn

W. Zhenqiu
Shenyang Research Institute of Traditional Chinese Medicine, Shenyang 110005, China

S. Li et al. (eds.), *Frontier and Future Development of Information Technology in Medicine and Education*, Lecture Notes in Electrical Engineering 269,
DOI: 10.1007/978-94-007-7618-0_66,

Table 66.1 Curative effect of all classes (case, %)

Classification	*N*	Cured	Markedly effective	Effective	Ineffective
Class I	78(39)	47(23.5)	17(8.5)	12(6)	2(1)
ClassII					
ClassIIa	19(9.5)	10(5)	7(3.5)	2(1)	0(0)
ClassIIb	23(11.5)	11(5.5)	9(4.5)	3(1.5)	0(0)
ClassIII					
ClassIIIa	14(7)	6(3)	6(3)	2(1)	0(0)
ClassIIIb	48(24)	26(13)	14(7)	6(3)	2(1)
ClassIV					
ClassIVa	5(2.5)	1(0.5)	1(0.5)	3(1.5)	0(0)
ClassIVb	13(6.5)	3(1.5)	4(2)	3(1.5)	3(1.5)
Total	200(100)	104(52)	58(29)	31(15.5)	7(3.5)

Table 66.2 Comparison of scores of all symptoms before and after treatment (Paired t-test)

Symptom		Case	Average	Standard deviation	*t* value	*P* value
Left ptosis	Before therapy	174	2.94	0.33	41.37	<0.001
	After therapy	174	0.42	0.75		
Right ptosis	Before therapy	165	2.95	0.29	40.55	<0.001
	After therapy	165	0.42	0.77		
Diplopia	Before therapy	90	1.00	0.00	43.74	<0.001
	After therapy	90	0.04	0.21		
Dysarthria	Before therapy	66	1.00	0.00	20.29	<0.001
	After therapy	66	0.14	0.35		
Dysmasesis	Before therapy	70	1.00	0.00	39.26	<0.001
	After therapy	70	0.04	0.20		
Dysphagia	Before therapy	63	1.00	0.00	24.27	<0.001
	After therapy	63	0.10	0.30		
Suffocated by water	Before therapy	47	1.00	0.00	46.00	<0.001
	After therapy	47	0.02	0.15		
Difficulty in raising one's head	Before therapy	19	1.00	0.00	18.00	<0.001
	After therapy	19	0.05	0.23		
Dyspnea	Before therapy	16	1.00	0.00	15.00	<0.001
	After therapy	16	0.06	0.25		
Lassitude	Before therapy	69	1.00	0.00	47.73	<0.001
	After therapy	69	0.03	0.17		

Myasthenia gravis (MG for short) is a chronic disease of neurotransmitters transmission dysfunction at neuromuscular junctions caused by autoimmunity [1]. Epidemiological survey indicates that the annual incidence rate of MG is 7.4/100, 000 [2]. Although the incidence rate is not high, but MG is difficult to treat and the duration is much longer. Its treatment has always been a major problem in the medical area. Clinical manifestations of MG is that part or the whole body shows skeletal muscle pathological fatigue. If the throat and respiratory muscles have been involved, the patient is prone to difficulty in breathing which is the leading cause of death of the patient. It shows that until 1995, the mortality of MG can be as high as 80 % [3], cited by the World Health Organization (WHO) as a refractory disease. For the treatment of MG, the common treatment including the removal of the thymus, cholinesterase inhibitors, immunosuppressive agents, plasmapheresis, immunoglobulin's, hematopoietic stem cell transplantation. But there are many side effects, high dependence and high recurrence rate with the methods mentioned above [4]. From years of clinical observation, Chinese medicine treatment of MG has the advantage of fewer side effects and low recurrence rate. The satisfactory curative effect has been achieved through applying this 2007-issued patent traditional Chinese medicine—"a traditional Chinese medicine for treating myasthenia gravis" to clinical treatment for many years. This article only summarizes the 200 cases of this disease, which are treated by this medicine during 1988–2010, as follows.

66.1 Clinical Data

These 200 cases are all confirmed case of MG prior to this treatment, among which 170 cases were confirmed by hospitals above provincial and municipal level, which occupy 85 % of total cases. The remaining 15 % were positive during neostigmine test or electromyogram changes consistent with MG. And in the meantime, features of these 15 % all consistent with the characteristics of MG, such as alleviation in the morning and aggravation in the afternoon, alleviation after rest, aggravation after activity and the symptoms are temporarily alleviated after taking Pyridostigmine Bromide tablets out. Prior to this treatment among the patients, the shortest duration of MG was 1 month and longest was 20 years and the average was 36.35 months; 92 (46 %) patients were male and 108 patients were female (54 %); the youngest patient was only 1.5 years old and the eldest was 85 years old and the average age was 36.49 years old. There are 78 cases of Class I, 42 cases of Class II (including 19 cases of Class Ilia, 23 cases of Class Ibis), 62 cases of Class III (including 14 cases of Class Ilia, 48 cases of Class Iamb), 18 cases of Class IV (including 5 cases of Class Ivan, 13 cases of Class Ivy) and no case of Class V.

66.2 Methods of Treatment and Observation

The MG was treated by this patent medicine. Composition of prescription: Codonopsis, Poria, Atractylodes, yams, arrowroot, Rehmannia, Eucommia, velvet, medlar, Cyperus rotundus, astragalus, dogwood, Bupleurum, Angelica, Loranthaceae, Cimicifuga, Achyranthes, fleece-flower root, Dendrobium. Take one dose a day after boiling the medicine with water. One course of treatment takes 3 months. Outcome measures and methods of statistics: Outcome measures: The clinical symptoms before and after treatment (including eyelid ptosis, diplopia, limb weakness, dysarthria, dysphagia, cough etc.) were observed. The statistical scorings were compiled according to the quantitative myasthenia gravis (QMG) score system of Myasthenia Gravis Foundation of America. The curative effect is judged according to Curative effect standard; Method of statistics: all data were shown in the form of mean ± standard deviation ($\bar{X} \pm S$); all scores before and after treatment should receive paired-*t*-test by SAS6.12.

66.3 Observation of Curative Effect

66.3.1 Classification Criteria

Classification is according to the classification system raised in 2000 by Myasthenia Gravis Foundation of America (MGFA) [5]:

(1) Class I: Any eye muscle weakness, possible ptosis, no other evidence of muscle weakness elsewhere
(2) Class II: Eye muscle weakness of any severity, mild weakness of other muscles

Class IIa: Predominantly limb or axial muscles
Class IIb: Predominantly bulbar and/or respiratory muscles

(3) Class III: Eye muscle weakness of any severity, moderate weakness of other muscles

Class IIIa: Predominantly limb or axial muscles
Class IIIb: Predominantly bulbar and/or respiratory muscles

(4) Class IV: Eye muscle weakness of any severity, severe weakness of other muscles

Class IVa: Predominantly limb or axial muscles
Class IVb: Predominantly bulbar and/or respiratory muscles (Can also include feeding tube without intubation)

(5) Class V: Intubation needed to maintain airway

66.3.2 Curative Effect Criteria

It was established in accordance with the Directional principle for clinical research of new Chinese medicine of MG, which was enacted by Ministry of Health of the People's Republic of China in 1995 [6].

(1) Cured: clinical symptom and physical symptom completely disappeared; return to normal life without recurrence in 3 months.
(2) Markedly effective: most of clinical symptom and physical symptom disappeared; restoring part of the work or light work.
(3) Effective: clinical symptom and physical symptom are improved; to be able to manage their own daily life but unable to work again.
(4) Ineffective: No improvement of clinical symptom and physical symptom or death.

66.3.3 Therapeutic Outcomes

66.4 Discussion

66.4.1 Analysis of Curative Effect

(1) Short-term curative effect: the shortest treatment course of this group of patients was 1 month and the longest was 30 months with an average curative month of 7.21 months. Among the 200 cases, 104 cases were fully cured (52 %), 58 cases had obvious effect (29 %), 31 cases (15.5 %) were effective and 7 cases were ineffective (3.5 %), hence the total effective rate was 96.5 % (Table 66.1). The difference between QMG scores of various symptoms before and after treatment (paired-t-test) was rather statistically obvious ($P < 0.001$, Table 66.2).
(2) Long-term curative effect: Some partial cured patents in this group (24 cases) were followed up for at least half a year and at most 19 years with an average period of 5.72 years. These follow-up patients can still participate in normal work or do housework without recurrence. For example: in Wuhan, two cured patients who were respectively 7 years old and 3 years old when they were attacked by this disease have been enrolled in university now.
(3) Analysis of curative effect of 50 cases associated with thymic diseases: In this group of cases, there were 10 patients associated with thymus hyperplasia in which 2 patients had taken surgery; the other 40 patients had thymoma, in which 27 patients had taken surgery. Both have different degrees of recurrence after surgery and even severe respiratory muscle involvement. Among 8

patients of thymus hyperplasia without surgery, 6 patients were fully cured and 2 patients had obvious effect after taking this patent traditional Chinese medicine; and among 13 patients of thymoma without surgery, 9 patients were fully cured and 4 patients had obvious effect. It shows that it is also effective to only take this traditional Chinese medicine for those associated with thymic diseases.

66.4.2 Discussion of Relevant Problems

(1) Principal drug with large dose and special purpose treatment: this disease is neurotransmitters transmission impediment at neuromuscular junction. Chinese medicine holds the view that "spleen governs the flesh or muscles" and "kidney determines the conditions of the bone and marrow", therefore "kidney" has certain relation with nerve of encephala and spinal cord. Traditional Chinese doctors treat hemiplegia with traditional Chinese medicine Bu-Yang-Huan-Wu-Tang and use milk veteh to treat deficiency of vital energy. And being fatigued without strength of myasthenia gravis also belongs to deficiency of vital energy, thus take large doses (120 g) of milk veteh and spleen-strengthening and kidney-invigorating drugs as the principal drug to cure this disease completely.
(2) Sticking out relatively long treatment course: according to therapeutic features of this disease, this patent traditional Chinese medicine can only be effective after taking it for a long time with a total course of treatment covering 1 year preferred. After recovery, it is also necessary to continue to take it for a period of time alternately, namely, taking for 1 week and then stop taking for 1 week to consolidate curative effects. Take care to be calm and avoid being overtired, especially, preventing cold to avoid recurrence.
(3) Avoiding recurrence: during treatment, few patients' symptoms deteriorate repeatedly but they can be fully recovered at last if continuing to take medicine. The reasons for recurrence include: (a) interruptions in treatment: since the best course of treatment is about 1 year, if the treatment time is relatively short and drug is discontinued immediately after symptoms have disappeared, it is easy to have a relapse, for example, there are two cases with recurrence rate as high as four times; (b) mood fluctuations and anger: one case relapsed because of spiritual attack due to failure of promotion due to his disease; (c) tiredness: one case has a relapse because of working in the field; (d) catching cold or upper respiratory tract infection: this is the most common cause for which there are three patients died of severe respiratory muscle involvement caused by cold. Therefore, it is essential to prevent and cure cold during treatment.
(4) Attaching importance to ocular muscle involvement: in this group of cases, type I patients occupy 39 %, but occurrence rate of ptosis of upper eyelid reaches up to 97.5 %. We found that the time when ptosis of upper eyelid

appears after getting up in the morning is gradually extended with favorable turn of treatment from initial several minutes to half an hour, one hour, all morning, all the afternoon to evening at last or even to disappearance of this symptom. If patients' conditions are with frequent fluctuations, the time when ptosis of upper eyelid appears will be advanced again. In a word, ocular muscle involvement plays an importance role in diagnosis and curative effect observation of this disease.

This paper is only preliminary brief summary for clinical treatment of this disease. Since this patent traditional Chinese medicine is still a compound prescription, it requires discarding the dross and selecting the essential and finding out real effective treatment constituents. And causes of this disease and mechanism of treatment are required to be determined, therefore, this paper is made with a hope that people in medicine circle can make further research and exploration on this basis.

Acknowledgments This work was supported by Jilin province science and technology development plan No.20080718.

References

1. Skeie GO, Aarli JA (2003) Muscle autoantibodies in subgroups of myasthenia gravis pstients. J Neurol 247: 369–375
2. Thanvi BR, Lo (2004) TCN.Update on myasthenia gravis. Fellowship Postgrad Med 80(950):690–700
3. Juel VC (2004) Myasthenia gravis: managementof myasthenic crisis and perioperative care. Semin Neurol 24:7581
4. Li L, Zhang L (2008) Diagnosis and treatment of myasthenia gravis. Chin Arch Tradit Chin Med 26:2375–2377
5. Jaretzki A, Barohn RJ, Ernstoff RM et al (2000) Myasthenia gravis: recommendations for clinical research standards. Task force of the medical scientific advisory board of the myasthenia gravis foundation of america. Neurology 55(1):16–23
6. Ministry of Health of the People's Republic of China, Guiding principles for clinical study of new Chinese medicines, Ministry of Health of the People's Republic of China, Beijing, China 1995:213–216

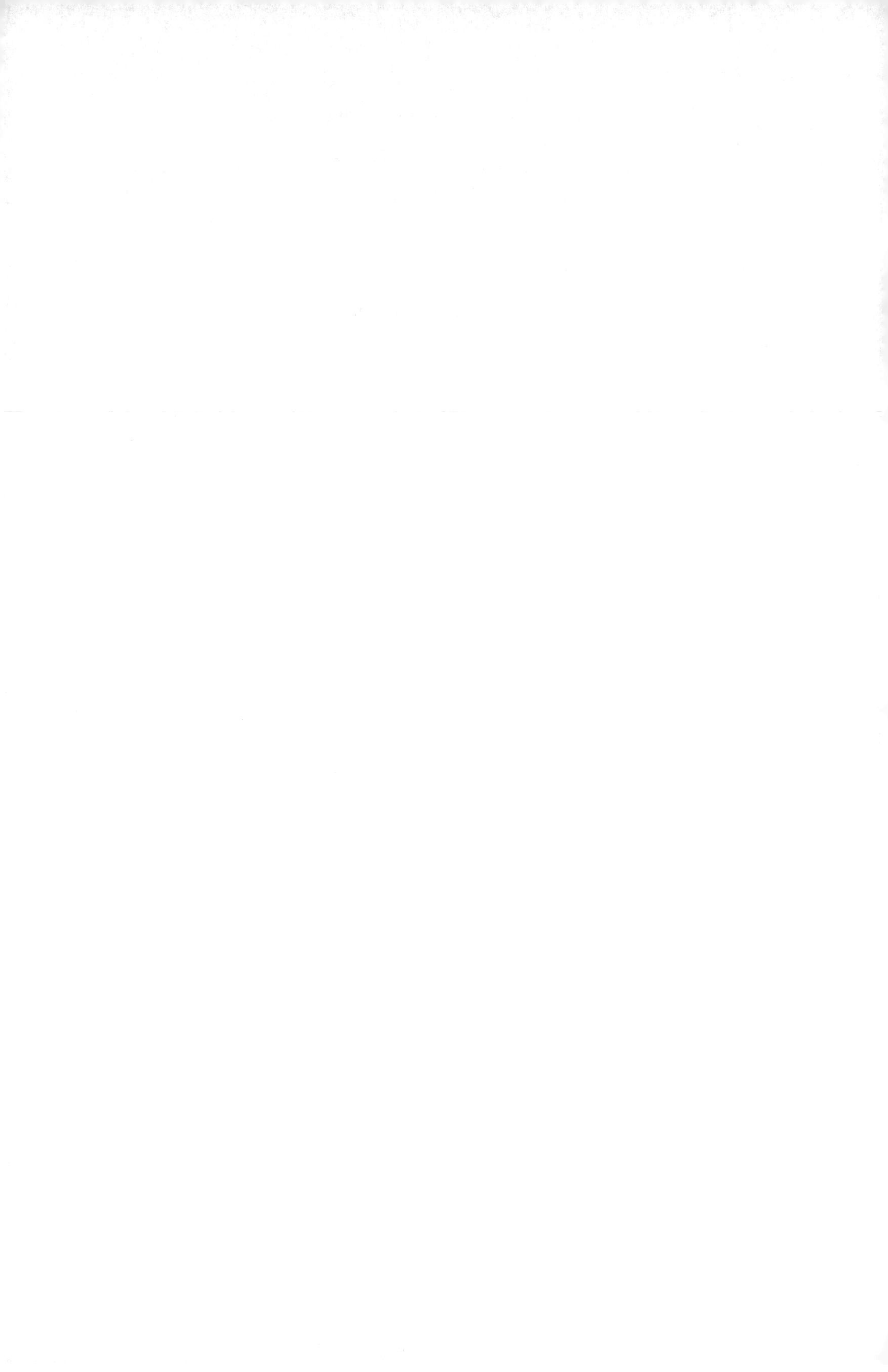

Chapter 67
Integrating Social Question–Answer Sites in Learning Management System

Yongqi Liu, Zhao Du, Lantao Hu and Qiuli Tong

Abstract Learning Management System (LMS) has been widely used for delivering course materials or training to learners in most educational institutions. To provide collaborative learning activities, LMSs, such as Moodle and Claroline, provide students discussion forums. With discussion forums, students participate in discussions as if they were in real classrooms. However, traditional discussion forums have two main drawbacks: knowledge cannot be accumulated and students have no social contacts. As a result, students cannot review the topics in forums after the end of a semester. What's more, students interact only with classmates in a course, which is bad for knowledge sharing. In this paper, we integrate social social Question and Answer sites (Q&A sites) in LMS to achieve better interaction and collaboration. Unlike traditional forum or BBS, a Q&A forum is a social network. Users in a Q&A sites achieve knowledge by following other users, following experts, following topics. They post questions, give answers and vote for or against answers. Users can also participate in discussion after they graduate from school. With these benefits, social Q&A site is meaningful for knowledge sharing and accumulation.

Keywords Social Question–Answer sites · Social network · Learning management system · Knowledge sharing · Knowledge accumulation

Y. Liu (✉) · L. Hu
Department of Computer Science and Technology, Tsinghua University,
Beijing 100084, China
e-mail: lyq@cic.tsinghua.edu.cn

Z. Du · Q. Tong
Information Technology Center, Tsinghua University, Beijing 100084, China

S. Li et al. (eds.), *Frontier and Future Development of Information Technology in Medicine and Education*, Lecture Notes in Electrical Engineering 269,
DOI: 10.1007/978-94-007-7618-0_67,

67.1 Introduction

Learning Management System (LMS) is a software application based on the state-of-the-art Internet and WWW technologies [1]. It is used by colleges, universities and corporate training departments for the purpose of enhancing and supporting teaching and learning processes. Studies show that, in America more than 90 % colleges and universities are using LMSs [2], while the ratio is 95 % in UK [3]. LMS has been an essential object these days.

Knowledge accumulation and sharing are of great importance in LMS. With the aim of improving the cooperation between students or between students and teachers, LMS typically integrates some tools to promote social software inside their platforms, such as discussion forums, blogs, wikis, email, chat, etc. [4] With these tools, students can make discussions on topics and share knowledge or materials; teachers can interact with students and check students' learning status and realize what students need.

Online learning forums are set up for students to communicate and collaborate more easily and efficiently. Nowadays, LMSs such as Moodle and Claroline provide students online learning forums for presenting content and receiving feedback from their peers and faculty. In forums, students can ask questions and participate in discussions on various topics, as if they were in real classrooms.

Although online learning forums bring social features in LMSs, there are some drawbacks:

- Students' access to forum normally ends when the course ends. Since a forum is closed at the end of a semester, knowledge and experiences in the forum are cleared, which is bad for knowledge accumulation and reuse.
- Only participants in a course can join the discussion forum. So students who are interest in the domain but not members of the course have no access to participate in discussion, which is bad for knowledge sharing.
- It is difficult for users to find people with similar interests. Since traditional forums are question-centered, not user-centered, students meet with each other only when they are focusing on the same question. There is a lack of communication and interaction between students.

Several research efforts have been made for changing traditional forums in LMS. Li et al. [5] explore the role of Social Networking Sites (SNS) in e-learning by investigating the attitudes, behaviors, knowledge and views of computing students towards the use of SNS in e-learning. Nygard et al. [6] evaluate the potential benefits of a social networking tool for collaboration within teams while carrying out a major course project. Na et al. [7] identify limitations of current Q&A board system and propose a new Q&A board which is based on WIKI concept, to improve the limitations.

Our work is focused on integrating social Question–Answer site in LMS. Social Q&A site is a place for users to ask and answer questions. "Q&A" should not be confused with Question Answering, a research area in natural language processing.

Social Q&A sites often provides users personalized homepage of everything they want to know about by following topics, questions, people and boards. It is convenient for users to manage knowledge and share knowledge with friends. With social Q&A site, LMS can present a solution to:

- Enhance lifelong interaction and collaboration between students
- Promote knowledge sharing
- Accumulate knowledge of a certain course so that new students can inherit experience of graduate students
- Manage knowledge for individuals.

This paper is structured as follows: Sect. 67.2 explains the concept of social Q&A site and the difference between the traditional discussion forum and social Q&A site; Sect. 67.3 provides details of our proposal and describes how Q&A site works in LMS; Sect. 67.4 analyses the privacy and authority which is of great importance in work related to social networks; Sect. 67.5 shows the integration of Q&A sites in LMS and gives the system architecture; Sect. 67.6 presents some concluding remarks.

67.2 Social Q&A Sites Versus Discussion Forums

In this section, we will show what social Q&A site is like. Then we will talk about the difference between traditional discussion forums used in LMS nowadays and social Q&A sites.

67.2.1 Social Q&A Sites

Social Q&A sites combine traditional Q&A sites (like BBS, discussion forum in LMS, etc.) and social networks (like Face book, twitter, etc.). On one hand, Users ask and answer questions on a broad range of topics. They not only seek information, but also gather opinions, seek advice, share experiences and satisfy one's curiosity about various things [8]. On the other hand, the social element is what makes it different from other discussion forums. Social Q&A site focuses on leveraging social connections to get questions answered [9].

Social Q&A sites have turned out to be very popular these years. One of them is Quora (http://www.quora.com/). It is co-founded by two former Face book employees in June 2009 [10] and achieves lots of users till now. Users can ask any question; get real answers from people with firsthand experience and blog about what they know. What's more, users can follow certain topics and person that interest them. If someone follow posts a question, answers a question or votes an answer up or down, this activity appears on his Quora homepage, which can be viewed by friends. It is simple for users to share questions in their social networks.

As a social network site, users voluntarily ask and answer questions from fellow users. All users in the site have equal status and there are no authorities. Although there are experts in some domain, their opinions have no priority. All users can vote "best answers", so that the answers agreed by most users will be selected as the best answer. This can ensure the correctness of answers.

67.2.2 Social Q&A Sites Versus Discussion Forums

Traditional forum is question-centered. The most common pattern is that one person post a question and others give their answers. Most LMSs offer discussion forums. However, the discussion forums are separated by courses. Students who have ten courses may have ten different discussion forums. This is inconvenient for knowledge management since the information is fragment. Another question is that students can only communicate with classmates in a course but cannot get advice from other students and teachers outside the course.

The main difference between social Q&A sites and traditional forums is that social Q&A sites are user-centered web service. Every user has personal homepage, recording his history of questions and answers. So knowledge accumulates automatically. Users follow friends with same interests. They can also follow experts in certain domain to know their opinions and get advice directly from experts.

Based on above, we focus on integrating social Q&A sites in LMS. The social Q&A sites may have following functions:

- Allowing users to publish questions and give answers
- Allowing users to ask question to a certain user
- Allowing users to follow topics, friends or experts
- Providing "best answer" by means of students' voting for or against answers
- Providing personal homepage to manage knowledge
- Allowing users to check friends' homepage

67.3 Social Q&A Site in LMS: In Detail

Unlike common Q&A sites such as Yahoo Answers, social Q&A site used for assisting education must consider the particularity of education. In this section, we introduce social Q&A sites in education and show details about questions, personal homepage and user relationship, which are three main elements of social Q&A sites.

67.3.1 Questions

In LMSs, questions can be divided into two groups, teaching affairs and specialized knowledge. Teaching affairs are notice or announce from teachers, such as "When should students hand in homework?" or "How many students are there in the course?" Specialized knowledge questions are about content of courses, such as "What does NLP stands for?" or "What is the difference between C and C++ ?"

Usually, teaching affairs are effective during a course, while they are no longer meaningful after the course ends. So there is no necessity to keep teaching affairs after a semester. On the contrary, specialized knowledge is useful all the time. So it should be stored for users to review at any time. Based on above, we design the content architecture of our social Q&A site in Fig. 67.1.

Tags are used in social Q&A site to classify questions. With tags, we can class questions of different subject easily. For example, if someone posts a question "What are the advantages of using C++ over C?" and tags it with "Programming language", we can easily find that the question is about programming language. Anyone who is interest in this domain can find the question through tags and give answers. Recommendation system could be added in this system to find users' hobby and recommend questions to them by means of tags. Considering privacy, a special tag "public" or "private" is used, which we may talk about in Sect. 67.4.

Since teaching affairs are time-sensitive, we concern only about courses which a user takes during a semester. Therefore, the first level tags of teaching affairs are course names and lower level tags can be any other events such as "homework", "examination" or anything else.

Contrasts to teaching affairs, specialized knowledge is not time-sensitive. So organization of specialized knowledge is different from that of teaching affairs. Since many courses in higher education are about same topics, we use subject instead of course names. Many organizations have their discipline classification. For example, U.S. Department of Education published CIP: 2000 to provide a

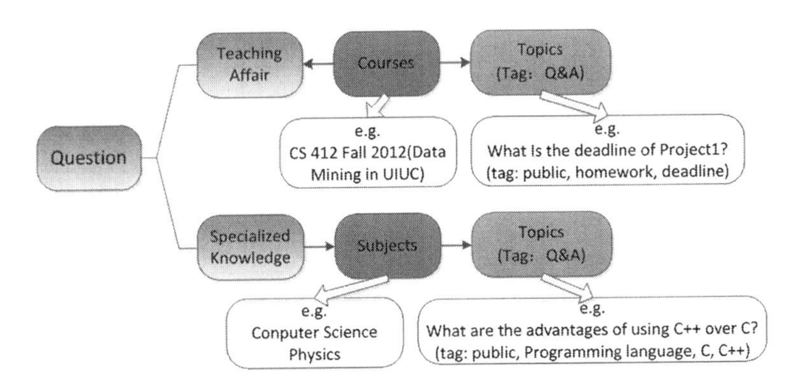

Fig. 67.1 Q&A content in LMS

taxonomic scheme that will support the accurate tracking, assessment and reporting of fields of study [11]. With this classification, tremendous course names can be categorized into little subjects. We use these subjects as the first level tag while course names as the second level tags. For instance, we use "Computer Science" as the first level tag while "Computer System", "Computer Language" and others as lower level tags.

67.3.2 Personal Homepage

A user in social Q&A site has his personal homepage. The homepage contains mainly five parts of items: collected knowledge, discussion space, history of questioning and answering, private space and friend space.

If a user sees anything of great value, he can follow it and add it to his homepage; Discussion space is used for communicating with others. Visitors to the homepage can ask questions or make comments in discussion space; any questions and answers of the user are recorded in his homepage; if a user doesn't want visitors to see any knowledge that he collected, he can put it in private place; a user can see questions and answers that his friends made recently at friend space.

Homepage is used for knowledge management. A user may have many courses during his life. If no tools to management knowledge are provided, he may forget it easily. With homepage, one can review any knowledge stored easily.

67.3.3 User Relationship

Users in social Q&A sites form a network. They ask questions, give answers, vote for or against answers and find friends in the network Fig. 67.2. shows the social relationship of a user and how a user gets knowledge from the network.

In our system, there are three roles: stranger, friend and expert. Experts can be teachers or other scientists. Their opinions may be of great value, but have no priority. Users can follow them and make discussions with them.

Green arrows in Fig. 67.2 mean that a user has some tags. Users in social Q&A site are labeled with tags. If he shows interests in a subject and follows it, the tag is added to his attribute. The tags of a user can be seen by other users. A user can find friends or experts with same interests through tags. So it is convenient for users to find friends with same interests.

Blue arrows mean asking and answering questions. If User A has any question, he can post it on the Q&A site. Anyone who sees this question can give it an answer. If User A wants to seek help from a certain person, he can visit the person's personal homepage and leave a message. Furthermore, he can discuss with that person.

Fig. 67.2 User relationship in social Q&A site

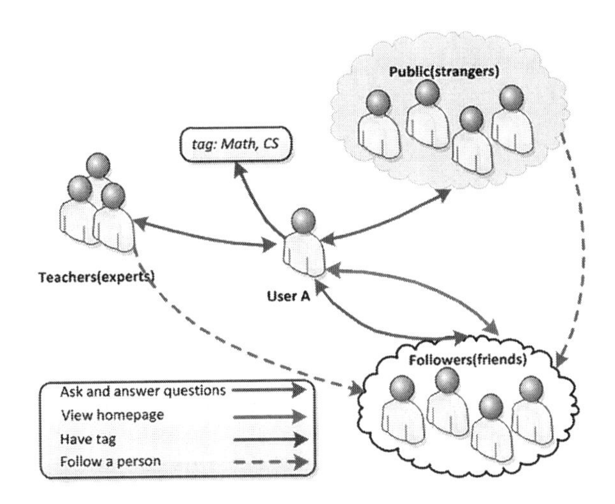

Red arrows mean the privilege to view other's personal homepage. If User A shares interests with any other user, A can follow and make friends with him. Brown arrows in Fig. 67.2 show the status changing from strangers or experts to friends. Friends can visit each other's homepage. Since they share same interests, knowledge collected by friends may inspire the each other in a sense.

67.4 Privacy and Authority

This issue of protecting privacy is of great importance in work related to social networks. When posting information to a social network, a user probably expects authorized contacts to be able to view it.

In our system, we have a two level privacy protection method. First, visitors are divided into two kinds: friends and strangers. If user A follows user B and B follows back, they become friends. If two people are not friends, they are strangers. Both friends and strangers can visit one's homepage, but their authorities are not the same. Friends can check the knowledge that the owner collected, while strangers cannot. If a stranger wants to ask someone a question, he can leave a message on one's homepage, but he cannot see more information. The second privacy protected method is that, in our system, knowledge can be tagged with "public" or "private". If a user follows many topics, but he doesn't want everyone knows what he is interested in, he can tag the knowledge with "public", the knowledge can be seen by visitors to his homepage; if some knowledge is tagged with "private", only the owner can see it.

Another problem in knowledge sharing system is copyright. For the convenience of discussion, someone (like a teacher) may post some articles with copyright on the site. He can only enable a certain group of users to achieve them. In this way, copyright is protected.

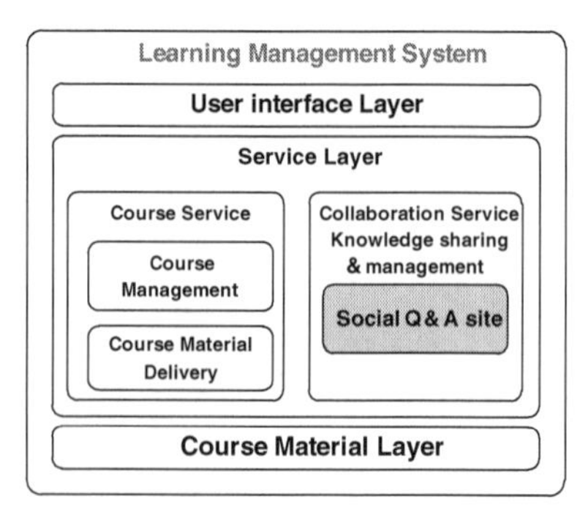

Fig. 67.3 Architecture of LMS integrated with social Q&A site

67.5 System Architecture

In this section, we integrate social Q&A site in LMS. Figure 67.3 shows the architecture of our proposal.

LMS normally contains three layers, course material layer, service layer and user interface layer. Social Q&A site is integrated in service layer to support interaction and collaboration of students. It can benefit knowledge management and knowledge sharing. It replaces the position of discussion forum, which has less social features.

67.6 Conclusion

With the development of internet, students nowadays are accustomed to communicate with others on social networks. So it is helpful to integrate some social network features in LMS. In this paper, we work on integrating social Q&A site in learning management system to replace the traditional discussion forum. With social Q&A site, users achieve knowledge by following specific questions, following individuals, or following topics and manage knowledge in personal homepage. The integration of social Q&A site in LMS makes it more convenient for students to share and manage knowledge.

Acknowledgments This work is supported by the Beijing Education and Science "Twelfth 5-Year Plan" (No. CJA12134) and the Joint Fund of Ministry of Education and China Mobile (No. MCM20121032).

References

1. Avgeriou P, Papasalouros A, Retalis S et al (2003) Towards a pattern language for learning management systems. Educ Technol Soc 6(2):11–24
2. Hawkins BL, Rudy J (2007) Educause core data service

3. Brown T, Jenkins M (2006) A longitude prospective regarding the use of VLEs by higher education institutions in the United Kingdom. Interact Learn Environ 14(2):177–192
4. Vidal JC, Lama M, Sueiro MR et al (2012) Semantic integration of social information in learning systems. 2012 IEEE 12th international conference on advanced learning technologies (ICALT), IEEE,pp 676–677
5. Li X, Ganeshan K, Xu G (2012). The role of social networking sites in E-learning. In: Frontiers in education conference (FIE) pp 1, 6, 3–6 Oct. 2012
6. Nygard KE, Bender L, Walia G et al (2011) Collaboration using social networks for team projects. The international conference on frontiers in education: computer science and computer engineering (FECS'11), pp 86–92
7. Na S-H, Choi O-H, Lim J-E, Kim C -H (2008) Investigating Q&A system requirements for effective instructor-learner interaction in e-Learning service environment. Adv Softw Eng Appl 108–110
8. Lada A, Adamic, Zhang J, Bakshy E, Ackerman MS (2008) Knowledge sharing and yahoo answers: everyone knows something. In: Proceeding of the 17th international conference on World Wide Web, pp 665–674
9. Ovadia S (2011) Quora.com: another place for users to ask questions. Behav Soc Sci Librarian 30(3):176–180
10. http://en.wikipedia.org/wiki/Quora
11. http://nces.ed.gov/pubs2002/cip200
12. Quantcast profile for Yahoo! Answers. Quantcast.com. Retrieved 1–30 Dec

Chapter 68
The Study of Dynamic Threshold Strategy Based-On Error Correction

Zhimin Yang, Jie Li, Gaofeng Han, Yue Wang and Songnan Zhao

Abstract Currently, the threshold control for the monitor and management of network equipment functionality adopts both static and dynamic threshold strategies. In traditional dynamic threshold computation methods, there is no support for error data correction and data sampling time interval is long. With these methods, the computed baseline value keeps unchanged within each sampling time interval. Hence, the calculated baseline value is not good at describing the changing trend of network equipment functionality. In other words, it has worse support to applications with real time and dynamic requirement. In this paper, a novel approach for computing dynamic threshold is proposed based on error correction. It improves the traditional dynamic threshold computation model. With the developed system for the monitor and management of network equipment functionality, we prove the feasibility of the dynamic threshold computation based on error correction. Through the experiment, we demonstrate that the dynamic threshold computation based on error correction can improve the threshold predicting accuracy with better support to real time and dynamic requirement. It has excellent performance in describing the changing trend of network equipment functionality.

Keywords Dynamic threshold · Network equipment functionality · Development trend · Error correction · Linear regression

Z. Yang (✉) · Y. Wang · S. Zhao
Department of Computer Science, Shandong University at Weihai, Weihai 264209, People's Republic of China
e-mail: yangzhimin@sdu.edu.cn

J. Li · G. Han
Department of Computer Science, Anhui Wenda Information and Technology College, Hefei 231201, People's Republic of China

S. Li et al. (eds.), *Frontier and Future Development of Information Technology in Medicine and Education*, Lecture Notes in Electrical Engineering 269,
DOI: 10.1007/978-94-007-7618-0_68,

68.1 Problem Description

At present, the monitor and management of network equipment functionality adopts static threshold strategy or dynamic threshold strategy to control the threshold value [1–13]. Both the above two strategies cannot perfectly describe the network equipment functionality and its changing trend timely and dynamically.

Dynamic threshold is determined by the computation based on baseline value [3–6]. When carrying out the monitor and management for network equipment functionality, the monitor and management system samples a set of monitoring values to calculate a value of baseline, and evaluates whether the network equipment is busy or not. Then, the baseline value is used as a threshold standard for a future period. This method for dynamic threshold computation costs longer data sampling time interval and postpones the data processing capability of network monitor and management system [7–13]. Hence, the traditional dynamic threshold method has weak performance in terms of real time processing and sampling frequency is also a factor of real time processing [11–19].

The functionality data of network equipment has the periodic characteristics. Sampling data changes with the time. Especially, error data has significant influence to the accuracy of the baseline value for the dynamic threshold. In traditional approach, there is no support for error data correction. Furthermore, the baseline value in each sampling interval is static. The baseline has no capability of prediction and real time. It can not accurately describe the changing trend of network equipment functionality.

In order to improve the capability of real time, dynamic processing and prediction, we propose a dynamic threshold computation method based on error correction to upgrade the previous dynamic threshold processing model. The new processing model aims to offer more precision in describing the changing trend of network functionality according to the periodic changing characteristics of network equipment functionality.

68.2 Improved Strategy of Threshold Control

In our improved strategy of threshold control, the data sampling frequency of network equipment functionality is increased to calculate the baseline value. It defines and updates the standard of dynamic threshold value timely to support real time applications. When a certain measurement for network equipment functionality exceeding the ranging of the threshold value, the monitor and management system sends alarming signal immediately.

The monitor equipment for data sampling calculates the baseline value according to the usage data of CPU in one day with both the traditional and the improved strategies. Through the experiment of different threshold control strategies, we can get two sets of monitoring control results. The result and comparison are shown in Fig. 68.1.

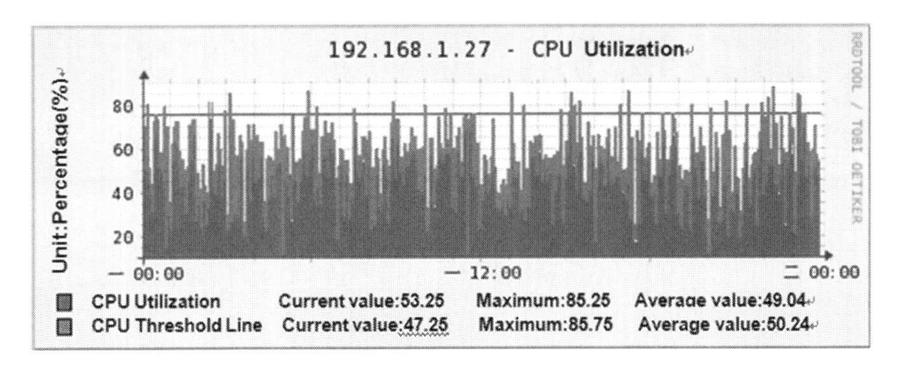

Fig. 68.1 Comparison of Two Dynamic Threshold Strategies Results

In Fig. 68.1, the flat line keeps the value around 75 % is the CPU usage percentage under the traditional strategy for calculating the baseline. Due to the low sampling frequency, the calculating period is one day. The threshold has a change in one day. So, under the theme of traditional dynamic threshold calculation for baseline, the result is a flat line without change within one day.

The curve in Fig. 68.1 stands for CPU usage percentage threshold calculated with the improved dynamic threshold computation. The adopted threshold control strategy is as follows. The sampling frequency is 5 min. From the 0 o'clock to 24 o'clock, there are $24 \times 60 \div 5 + 1 = 289$ sampling points. With these points, we can connect and draw a dynamic threshold curve for a day. Due to the improved sampling frequency within a day and the real time processing for data, the baseline appears to be a dynamic changing curve according to real time.

With the comparison between two curves of dynamic threshold, the traditional threshold strategy has its threshold unchanged with a certain period. In other words, it cannot precisely depict the real time feature of dynamic threshold. However, our proposed improved dynamic threshold strategy can better describe the value for measuring networks functionality changes.

When monitoring network equipment functionality, if a sampled functionality data exceeds the threshold line, this sampled data is abnormal data. If we don't correct the abnormal data and directly use it, the predicted value based on the threshold will introduce error and inaccuracy. So, we adopt the error correction in our improved dynamic threshold control. Further, we introduce the computation method for dynamic threshold based error correction.

In our computation method for dynamic threshold based error correction, the historical network equipment functionality data will only be used after the real time abnormal correction. The processing method is as follows. We use linear regression to set up a functionality prediction model. This model has the capability of correcting abnormal data and predicting the data trend. With that, the calculated dynamic threshold can be used as a norm for determine whether a functionality exceeds the standard limitation. Furthermore, it can be used for predicting the development trend. More sampling data is gathered for analysis, more accurate the calculated dynamic threshold is.

With the above introduction, the computation method for dynamic threshold based error correction has following features:

1. Increased sampling frequency, reduced waiting time interval, increased real time characteristic for dynamic threshold, improved real time monitoring capability for network equipment functionality.
2. Set up a prediction model with regression. Increase the real time correction and prediction capability for abnormal data. Hence, the accuracy of network equipment functionality dynamic threshold is increased. It effectively control and limit the functional trend deviation and torture.

68.3 Computing Model of Dynamic Threshold Based on Error Correction

Linear regression is as follows. When the graph with scattered points pairs appears the trend of a linear relationship, the least square is used to find the relationship between the two points. In other words, linear regression is adopted. Based on the changes of argument, the changing trend of the parameter can be predicted.

68.3.1 Setting up Computation Model of Dynamic Threshold

In the computation method for dynamic threshold based error correction, the linear regression prediction model is set up for network functionality to compute the dynamic threshold of baseline.

The regression model is as follows:

$$y_i = a + bx_i + \varepsilon_{i(i=1,2,\ldots,n)}. \tag{68.1}$$

In the above model (68.1), x is the sampling point and y is the sampled data at each sampling point. y is the function of x. a and b is the regression factors. ε is the total influence from all random factors which sometimes can be ignored. Without considering all that influence, the regression model can be set up as follows:

$$\hat{y}_i = a + bx_i. \tag{68.2}$$

The regression factor of the model can be estimated with the least square. According to the error principle of lease square decomposition, there are 2 conditions which should be satisfied. (Σ represents $\sum_{i=1}^{n}$).

$$\sum (y_i - \hat{y}_i)^2 = Minimumvalue \tag{68.3}$$

$$\sum (y_i - \hat{y}_i) = 0 \tag{68.4}$$

Denote

$$Q = \sum (y_i - \hat{y}_i)^2 = \sum (y_i - a - bx_i)^2. \tag{68.5}$$

According to the principle of limitation theory, in order to achieve the minimum value, we can calculate the partial derivative and set its result as 0. In other words:

$$\frac{\partial Q}{\partial a} = -2\sum (y_i - a - bx_i) = 0 \tag{68.6}$$

$$\frac{\partial Q}{\partial b} = -2\sum (y_i - a - bx_i)x_i = 0. \tag{68.7}$$

They can be further transformed into (68.8, 68.9):

$$na + b\sum x_i = \sum y_i \tag{68.8}$$

$$a\sum x_i + b\sum x_i^2 = \sum x_i y_i. \tag{68.9}$$

With the above (68.8, 68.9), we can calculate the estimated value for the regression factor as (68.10, 68.11):

$$\hat{b} = \frac{n\sum x_i y_i - n\sum x_i \sum y_i}{n\sum x_i^2 - (\sum x_i)^2} \tag{68.10}$$

$$\hat{a} = \frac{\sum y_i}{n} - \hat{b}\frac{\sum x_i}{n}. \tag{68.11}$$

68.4 Implementation on Abnormal Correction for Dynamic Threshold

The error checking approach for dynamic threshold is as follows. Specifically, at a time stamp, the information of a dynamic threshold can be replaced with the predicted data of the regression for the functionality data four weeks ago.

For example, if we denote the sampling four weeks ago as d_{1i}, d_{2j}, d_{3k}, d_{4l}.

When put $(1,d_{1i})$, $(2,d_{2j})$, $(3,d_{3k})$, $(4,d_{4l})$, $n = 4$ into formula (68.10, 68.11), we can calculate the regression factors of $\hat{a}$, $\hat{b}$. When input them to formula (68.2), we can get the function of linear regression:

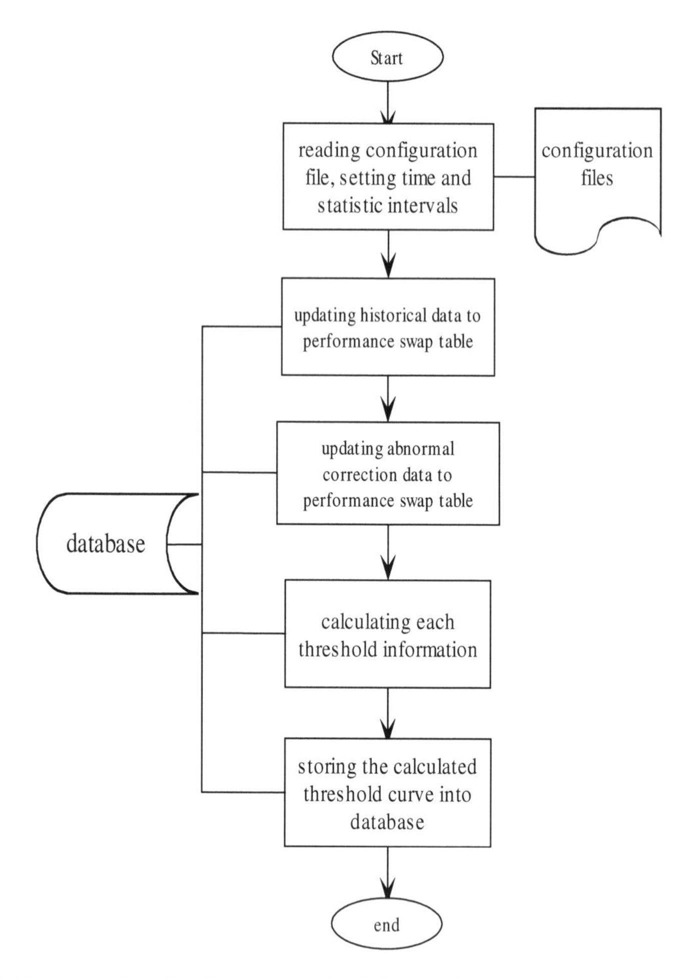

Fig. 68.2 The processing flow for dynamic threshold based error correction

$$\hat{y}_i = a + bx_i$$

If we set the x = 5, the parameter y should be multiplied with floating percentage +1 which is the dynamic threshold for the current time stamp.

The processing flow for dynamic threshold based error correction is as follows. Through the linear regression prediction model which calculates all the threshold of the sampling points, the threshold curve can be drawn based on all the points.

All the abnormal data participating the calculation will be replaced with $\widehat{y}$ for calculating threshold statistic analysis. The processing flow for dynamic threshold based error correction is demonstrated in Fig. 68.2.

The experiment of the network functionality monitoring and management system demonstrates that our dynamic threshold based error correction has both real time and dynamic features as shown in Fig. 68.3. It can reflect the

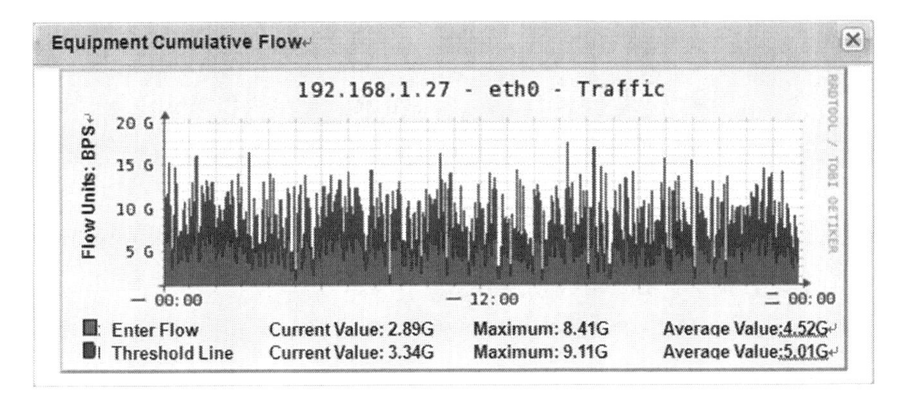

Fig. 68.3 Trend curve of dynamic threshold based error correction for network equipment functionality

functionality trend of network equipment with a more scientific and efficient manner. Hence, we can monitor the network much better.

68.5 Conclusion

This paper offers an approach for implementing dynamic threshold in network functionality management. It compares the disadvantages and advantages between the traditional static threshold method and improved dynamic threshold method. Based on that comparison, we proposed the method of dynamic threshold computing based on error correction. It improves the sampling frequency and sets up the linear regression prediction model to calculate the dynamic threshold.

In contrast to the traditional method, our proposed dynamic threshold computing based on error correction can better describe the real world situation for network running environment. It is more scientific to the threshold information and benefits the network service standard.

References

1. Wang Y, Yang Z (2012) Study and implementation of network performance management system based on the dynamic threshold. In: Master Thesis of Shandong University
2. James FK, Keith WR (2004) Computer networking a top-down approach featuring the internet, Addison-Wesley, Boston
3. Qing H (2008) Study and implementation of network performance management system based on SNMP. J Neimenggu Univ
4. Hu M (2009) Design and implementation of an adaptive SNMP System. J SE Normal Univ

5. Wang S (2008) Study of abnormal network functional data checking technique based on SNMP. Harbin Eng Univ
6. http://www.eclipse.org/birt/phoenix/intro
7. http://zh.wikipedia.org/zhcn/SNMP#SNMP.E5.9F.BA.E6.9C.AC.E5.85.83.E4.BB.B6
8. http://wenku.baidu.com/view/d853793467ec102de2bd8915.html
9. Xie X (2004) Computer networks (the 4th version)
10. Yunsheng L (1994) Real Time database systems. Comput Sci 21(3):42–46
11. Owens M (2006) The definitive guide to SQLite. Apress, New York
12. Walls C, Breidenbach R (2005) Spring in action. Dreamtech Press, New Delhi
13. Elliott J, O'Brien TM, Fowler R (2008) Harnessing hibernate. O'Reilly Media, New York
14. Holdener III AT (2008) Ajax: the definitive guide. O'Reilly Media, New York
15. Wu Y (2007) Management monitoring and malfunction prediction based on statistic analysis. J Zhongshan Univ
16. Vivek C, Bakore A, Eaves J (2004) Professional Apache Tomcat 5
17. Advanced Mathematics (2007) Department of Tongji University, 6th edn. Advanced Education Publishing House, New Delhi
18. Fredrick S, Ramsay C, Blades S (2008) Learning Ext JS. Packt Publishing Limited, Mumbai
19. Weathersby J, Bondur T, Chatalbasheva I (2011) Integrating and extending birt. Addison-Wesley Professional, Boston

Chapter 69
Identification of Evaluation Collocation Based on Maximum Entropy Model

LingYun Zhao, FangAi Liu and Zhenfang Zhu

Abstract In the process of analyzing the orientation of hotel comment, some opinion-bearing words may cause ambiguity. In this paper a method of evaluation collocation identification based on maximum entropy is proposed. This method designed a sentiment word table, mined the category of opinion-bearing words as semantic feature, combined this feature with lexical, part-of-speech, position and negative adverbs to construct a compound template, and then employed maximum entropy model to implement evaluation collocation identification. Experimental results show that the accuracy is higher when using the compound template constructed in this paper to identify evaluation collocation.

Keywords Orientation · Evaluation collocation · Maximum entropy · Sentiment word table · Semantic feature

69.1 Correlational Research

In the process of analyzing the orientation of hotel comments, some words of the comments have no orientation, and the same word has different meanings when it evaluates different objects, in other word, some opinion-bearing words may cause ambiguity. Finding out the opinion-bearing words accurately and establishing the

L. Zhao (✉)
Business School, Shandong Jianzhu University, Jinan 250101, China
e-mail: zhaoly@sdjzu.edu.cn

F. Liu
School of Information Science and Engineering, Shandong Normal University, Jinan 250014, China

Z. Zhu
School of Information Science and Electric Engineering, Shandong Jiaotong University, Jinan 250357, China

S. Li et al. (eds.), *Frontier and Future Development of Information Technology in Medicine and Education*, Lecture Notes in Electrical Engineering 269,
DOI: 10.1007/978-94-007-7618-0_69,

relationship with its evaluation objects, namely evaluation collocation, is the hot issue researched at home and abroad.

The evaluation collocation research abroad mainly based on the syntactic relationships templates, such as literature [1], it acquires evaluation collocations by using dependency syntax to extract templates, but need to build a large number of dependency syntaxes manually; literature [2] proposed that, get evaluation objects first and then find out the adjective which is nearest to the evaluation object, but it ignores opinion-bearing words like verbs and nouns.

The domestic research mainly focuses on Chinese text, Because the formats of comments are not standard in the methods of literature [3], so they get high error proportion, and finally effects recognition accuracy.

The methods researched above achieved the analysis of orientation of hotel comments in a certain extend, but they lack the analysis of semantic relationship between evaluation collations. According to this problem, this article proposed a evaluation collation recognition method based on maximum entropy model which introduced semantic features, that is, classify the evaluation words which have the same or similar meaning to a category as semantic feature, and then establish feature module of maximum entropy model from comments corpus which includes these words, this method improved the performance of evaluation collocation recognition, and it also provides a effective method to evaluate and judge the orientation of comments.

69.2 Automatic Evaluation Collocation Recognition Based on Maximum Entropy

Judging whether the evaluation objects and evaluation words in comments corpus have collocation relationship, is a binary classification problem, that is, collocated or not. In this paper, classify the evaluation collocations by maximum entropy model, and establish polarity word list to extend the maximum entropy feature module, to improve the classification accuracy.

69.2.1 Establish Sentiment Word List

In the hotel comments “clear”, “clean”, “neat” appear in different comments, but they have the close meaning, and they express the positive evaluation to the hotel. So, this article classifies evaluation words which have the same meaning to a category by < Synonyms Dictionary(extended) > , and establishes evaluation word categories(E Type). Through the manipulations such as word segmentation, speech tagging, extracting adjectives, verbs, and nouns, manual screening, semantic extension to < CILIN(extended) > and classification and so on, this

Table 69.1 Sentiment word table

EType sentiment words
C01 not bad, good, ok, beautiful
C02 clear, neat, clean
C03 comfortable, cosy
C04 sweet, temperate, warm
C05 large, roomy
C06 tiny, small
C07 cheap, moderate, profitable, economy
C08 conveniency, convenience
D01 old-fashioned, old, worn, shabby
D02 bad, not good, dark
D03 mouldy, mildew
D04 ordinary, common
D05 dirty, soiled, stain
……

article establishes evaluation word category list(below is called "sentiment word table")which is frequently used in hotel comment field. Part of the word categories are presented in Table 69.1.

In Table 69.1, E Type is listed as category code, and present with the combination of letters and numbers, C indicates that the words of this category is commendatory, D indicates derogatory sence, and differentiate them with numbers. Due to the length of the article, only list the top 13 categories which have the high representation and word frequency in hotel comments corpus.

69.2.2 Maximum Entropy Recognition

69.2.2.1 Basic Theory

The maximum entropy principle is proposed by E.T.Jaynes in 1957, Della Pietra et. applied it to natural language processing model for the first time in 1992. Its basic thought is, through the given training data, choose a proper statistical model, make it correspond with all known facts, and make no hypothesis to the unknown facts.

In the practical problems, use feature function to represent a moderate number of known constraint conditions, make the helpful information from analyzing evaluation collocations as the feature of maximum entropy model f,and use binary representation function about (w, c) to represent feature function as follow:

$$f(w,c) = \begin{cases} 1, if \quad cp(w) = ture \quad and \quad c = c' \\ 0, \qquad\qquad\qquad\qquad other \end{cases} . \tag{69.1}$$

In the above formula, c′ is whether they are collocated in training set.

Obviously, feature functions could be irrelevant, and classification problem becomes optimal solution problem which satisfy a group of constraint conditions, and that is, utilize maximum entropy frame model to get optimal probability distribution under the condition that every candidate collocation restricts the context as follow:

$$p^* = \arg\max H(p) \tag{69.2}$$

In above formula, $H(p)$ expresses the entropy of probability distribution, on the basis of maximum entropy principle, the values of $p(c|w)$ correspond with the exponent model as follow:

$$p(c|w) = \frac{1}{Z_\lambda}\exp(\sum_{i=1}^{k}\lambda_i f_i(c,w)) \tag{69.3}$$

$$Z_\lambda(x) = \sum_{c}\exp(\sum_{i=1}^{k}\lambda_i f_i(c,w)) \tag{69.4}$$

λ_i is parameters, could be regarded as the weight of feature function, and it indicates the importance of feature f_i to the model. $Z_\lambda(x)$ is normalized factor. Through training from the training set, get the known values, and then acquire probability distribution function, accomplish the establishment of maximum entropy model, and make the model from looking for probability value to parameter λ_i. The frequently used parameter estimate method includes GIS algorithm, IIS algorithm, L-BFGS algorithm and so on. Darroch and GIS (Generalized Iterative Scaling) is frequently used to calculate λ_i.

69.2.2.2 Constructing Maximum Entropy Feature Template

For the features in the hotel comments area, use the context information of evaluation objects and evaluation words, that is, part of speech feature, distance, prefix negative words, dependency structure features, combine with the Evaluation of Words Types (EType) this semantic features in Table 69.1 to determine the atom feature template of the maximum entropy, see Table 69.2. The scope of this article is recognizing evaluation collocation in a sentence, E to evaluation words, O to evaluation objects.

Atomic template 1–6 are parts of speech features, This paper introduced the atomic template11 basing on the following reasons:

According to the principle of maximum entropy, constructed the maximum entropy features model which is suitable for training sets of templates is the crux of the problem. But these fundamental characteristics such as word, parts of speech is not able to better reflect the relationships between evaluation objects and evaluation words. Therefore, through corpus analysis and data mining, took categories of evaluation words this semantic feature as semantic features of maximum entropy model.

Table 69.2 Atomic feature template

Template number	Atomic template	Template significance
1	O	Evaluation objects
2	OPos(−1)	Part of speech of the previous word of evaluation objects
3	OPos(+1)	Part of speech of the next word of evaluation objects
4	E	Evaluation words
5	EPos(−1)	Part of speech of the previous word of evaluation words
6	EPos(+1)	Part of speech of the next word of evaluation words
7	Distance	The number of words between O and E
8	N	The negative adverbs
9	ORelate	The dependence structures of evaluation objects
10	ERelate	The dependency structures of evaluation words
11	EType	The type of evaluation words
12	Y	Observed values

Atomic template 1–6 are parts of speech features, This paper introduced the atomic template11 basing on the following reasons:

According to the principle of maximum entropy, constructed the maximum entropy features model which is suitable for training sets of templates is the crux of the problem. But these fundamental characteristics such as word, parts of speech is not able to better reflect the relationships between evaluation objects and evaluation words. Therefore, through corpus analysis and data mining, took categories of evaluation words this semantic feature as semantic features of maximum entropy model.

When there is a higher frequency of some evaluation objects and evaluation words which come along at the same time, such as < room, clean and tidy > or < room, clean > , inevitably, these co-occurrence words have combination relations, so the possibility of evaluation collocation is great. However, for certain combinations of low rate, extended and classify the evaluation words can improve the frequency of such combinations occurrence. Formulas (69.1, 69.3) can be proved by the maximum entropy model that, when calculated conditional probabilities in use of the characteristic functions, which is equivalent to increasing the weight of the characteristic function, then when the entropy get the maximum, corresponding to the set of probability distributions, will be advantageous, the accuracy rate of recognition of the maximum entropy model will also improve, which established by joining features of words classification, it means that under the constraint of the join of the evaluation category of words to achieve the maximum entropy distribution, can make more rational judgement to the test evaluation collocation.

Judging from the comments itself, hotel comments corpus in a category of evaluation often contrapose a class of evaluation objects, such as "cheap, low-priced, effective, economic" usually for the price, and "clean, neat, clean" usually decorate room, evaluation categories of words not only mine the potential relationship between evaluation objects and evaluation words, but also link the evaluation words, makes relationship in the hotel comments field, provides a favorable way to analyse the orientation of comments after identify the match.

Table 69.3 Composite feature template

Composite template	Composite template
1	OPos(−1), OPos(+1), EPos(−1), EPos(+1), Y
2	OPos(−1), O, OPos(+1), EPos(−1), E, EPos(+1), N, Y
3	OPos(−1), O, OPos(+1), EPos(−1), E, EPos(+1), N, Distance, Y
4	OPos(−1), O, OPos(+1), EPos(−1), E, EPos(+1), N, Distance, ORelate, ERelate, Y
5	OPos(−1), OPos(+1), EPos(−1), EPos(+1), EType, Y
6	OPos(−1), O, OPos(+1), EPos(−1), E, EPos(+1), N, EType, Y
7	OPos(−1), O, OPos(+1), EPos(−1), E, EPos(+1), N, Distance, EType, Y
8	OPos(−1), O, OPos(+1), EPos(−1), E, EPos(+1), N, Distance, ORelate, ERelate, EType, Y

69.2.2.3 Mix Templates

Using the 12 atomic feature templates in Table 69.2, the context information cannot be covered adequately, cannot take advantage of the maximum entropy model, so according to the features of hotel comments corpus, the atom templates are combined to composite templates to represent the complex contexts, such as Table 69.3:

The composite templates 1 in Table 69.3 only think about parts of speech; composite templates 2 joined words with negative adverbs, the negative adverb is taken into account, because it can change the polarity of evaluation words; composite templates 3 considered the distance between evaluation objects and evaluation words, the closer of the two the greater likelihood of the matches; composite templates 4 using the Chinese syntax parser of Harbin Institute of Technology for parsing, the dependencies between evaluation objects and evaluation words indirectly reflected the potential modification of relationships between them, extracted the dependencies of evaluation objects and evaluation words into composite templates, added semantic information; composite templates 5–8 corresponding to composite templates 1–4, added atomic features 11 into composite templates, experimental verification of the effectiveness of the category of evaluation words.

69.3 Experiment and Result

69.3.1 Data Set

The experimental corpus was provided by the Hotel comment cropus from Tan Songbo, the pros and cons 600 articles, a total of 1200 articles, including the training expected to 900 articles, test is expected to 300 articles. From which to randomly select the containing Table 69.1 13 types of polarity words category of the sentence, in these sentences, polarity words are likely to be used with a relationship to the noun, from which to select and rate the evaluation words combination with all the nouns as a candidates match in this sentence. Evaluation of candidate match, with its context after artificial identification, mark is used with a 1 instead of 0 as an experimental standard.

69.3.2 Evaluation Index

This experiment uses a Northeastern University Dr Zhang Le implementation of C ++ ME Model and GIS Training algorithms. For the evaluation of test data and identify performance as a whole, mainly use the following evaluation:

$$recall = \frac{a}{b} \times 100\,\%,\ precision = \frac{a}{c} \times 100\,\%,\ F = \frac{2 \times rp}{r+p} \times 100\,\%.$$

$a$correctly identify the match in the test corpus; b real matches in the test corpus; c collocation of recognition matches in the test corpus.

69.3.3 Experimental Results and Analysis

Due to the experimental corpus of domain-specific, depending on the selection of composite templates, take two sets of comparison, evaluation of word categories is not included in Tables 69.4, 69.5 contained in the evaluation word category. Experimental results are as follows:

Table 69.4 Experimental data indicate that, with increasing characteristic features in the template, accuracy and F Value is also rising, evaluation of collocation recognition performance in growing. When Word, speech, distance, prefix when negative Word feature is applied to the model, accurate rates have reached 64.25 %, F values reached 63.98 %. For example "hotel is not stylish enough" by adverb of negation prefix can identify < Hotel, not style > . On the basis of these four characteristics, according to the syntactic analysis adding dependencies to a semantic feature, making composite template 4 than composite

Table 69.4 Experimental results of template 1–4(category of evaluation words not included)

Composite templates	Accurate rates (%)	Recall rates (%)	Recognition properties F(%)
1	61.12	48.38	54.01
2	63.81	63.54	59.04
3	64.25	63.72	63.98
4	67.78	65.32	66.53

Table 69.5 Experimental results of template 5–8 (category of evaluation words included)

Composite templates	Accurate rates (%)	Recall rates (%)	Recognition properties F(%)
5	61.21	48.56	54.16
6	64.37	63.89	64.13
7	65.69	64.12	64.89
8	67.86	65.91	66.87

template 3 recognition accuracy and performance respectively of about 3 percentage points. Which in "service does not like is HaoSheng group management of, comparatively poor", the polarity Word "poor" in this sentence and two a noun "service" and "group" constitute candidate evaluation pairs, composite template1, 2 and 3 are to this two group recognition for match, however in composite template 4 will be < service, poor > callout for 1, < Group, poor > callout for 0, results correct.

Table 69.5 on the basis of the Table 69.4, the categories of evaluation words added to the model, The accurate rates of composite templates 5 slightly increased than composite templates 1, but less obvious, mainly because the term itself is not added to the template, affecting the accuracy; observation of complex template 6 and composite templates 2 proved that the combination of polarity words and word category can improve recognition performance largely; composite templates 7 and composite templates 3 further illustrates the importance of the polarities word category to the accuracy and recognition. For example, "this hotel is so dark" in this sentence, composite template 3 does not have the correct recognition < Hotel, dark > this match, in fact the evaluation of test data is the collcation match, and composite template 7 gives the correct judgment. Main is because, here of "dark" has "bad, not good, disappointing" of meaning, Table 69.1 takes its for the same class, turn in recognition of process, the model using this features of polarity word category made correct of recognition; composite template 8 contains all atomic templates, eventually of accurate rate for 67.86, recognition performance reached has 66.87 %.

69.4 Summary

This paper proposed a method of evaluation collocation identification based on maximum entropy in the process of analyzing the orientation of hotel comment. By synonym classifying and extending the polarity words in corpus, category as semantic information features of evaluation, while the words itself, and context information, the distance between evaluation objects and evaluation words, dependent relationship as atomic features, be combined in a common application to maximum entropy model to obtain evaluation of collocation in comments. Automatic identification for comment text orientation of evaluation matches with analysis and opinion mining research has a point of great significance. Next, the comment text will be deeper semantic analysis of mining more effective features and comments in the text of a large number of tests in different areas, and continually enhance the general evaluation of collocation recognition performance.

References

1. Popescu AM, Etzioni O (2007) Extracting product features and opinions from reviews. In: Natural language processing and text mining, Springer, London, pp 9–28
2. Liu B et al (2005) Opinion observer: analyzing and comparing opinions on the web. In: Proceedings of the 14th international conference on World Wide Web. ACM. New York. pp 342–351
3. Zhao YY et al (2010) A survey of sentiment analysis. J Softw 21(8):1834–1848
4. FAN N et al (2010) Extraction of subjective relation in opinion sentences based on maximum entropy model. Comput Eng 36(2):4–6
5. Della Pietra S et al (1992) Adaptive language modeling using minimum discriminant estimation. In: HLT '91 proceedings of the workshop on speech and natural language. pp 103–106
6. Darroch JN, Ratcliff D (1972) Generalized iterative scaling for log-linear models. Ann Math Statist 43(5):1470–1480

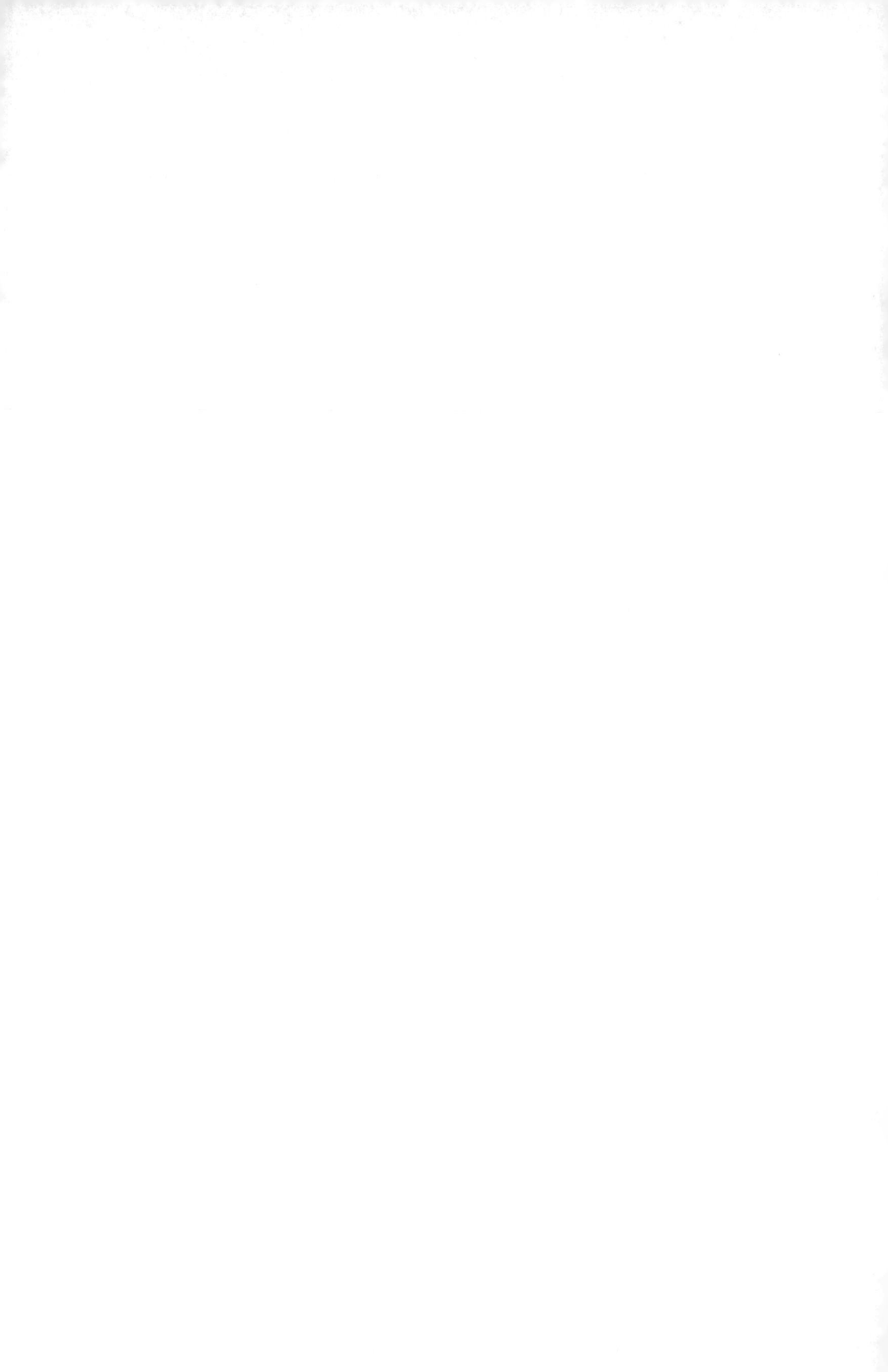

Chapter 70
Comparison of Beta Variable Gene Usage of T Cell Receptor in Peripheral Blood and Synovial Fluid of Rheumatoid Arthritis Patients

Jianwei Zhou, Cui Kong, Xiukui Wang, Zhaocai Zhang, Chengqiang Jin and Qin Song

Abstract *Objective* To compare the beta variable (Vβ) gene usage of T cell receptor (TCR) in peripheral blood (PB) and synovial fluid (SF) of the patients with rheumatoid arthritis (RA). *Methods* The total RNAs were extracted from PB and SF of 12 RA patients and reverse-transcribed and amplified by polymerase chain reaction (PCR), then the TCR Vβ gene usages were detected with real-time fluorescence quantitative PCR with DNA melting curving technique. *Results* For the four patients with acute RA, Vβ1 and Vβ13.1 were the key advantage usage genes in PB, while in SF that were Vβ10 and Vβ13.1. Except for Vβ11, there were no other genes found to be restrictively used both in PB and SF. For the eight patients with chronic RA, in PB, the main advantage usage genes were Vβ1, Vβ5.1, Vβ7 and Vβ13.1, the limited usage genes were Vβ2, Vβ11, Vβ21 and Vβ22. In SF, the predominant usage genes were Vβ1, Vβ6, Vβ7, Vβ13.1 and Vβ18, the limited usage genes were Vβ2, Vβ10, Vβ11, Vβ12, Vβ17, Vβ22, Vβ23 and Vβ24. *Conclusions* TCR Vβ gene usages in PB are similar to that in SF of RA patients, and this is probably an indication for the further studies of the pathogenesis and therapy of RA in future.

Keywords Rheumatoid arthritis · T cell receptor · Variable beta gene · Peripheral blood · Synovial fluid · Advantage usage · Limited usage

---

J. Zhou (✉) · Z. Zhang · C. Jin
Clinic Laboratory, The Affiliated Hospital of Jining Medical College, Jining 272029, China
e-mail: immunolife@126.com

C. Kong
Department of Cardiovascular Disease, The Affiliated Hospital of Jining Medical College, Jining, China

X. Wang
Department of Stomatology, The Affiliated Hospital of Jining Medical College, Jining, China

Q. Song
Department of Immune Rheumatic Disease, The Affiliated Hospital of Jining Medical College, Jining, China

S. Li et al. (eds.), *Frontier and Future Development of Information Technology in Medicine and Education*, Lecture Notes in Electrical Engineering 269,
DOI: 10.1007/978-94-007-7618-0_70,

70.1 Introduction

Rheumatoid arthritis (RA) is one of the most common chronic inflammatory diseases, characterized by chronic inflammation of synovium of the peripheral joints. To date, the complete mechanism is unclear, increasing evidence suggests that autoimmune mechanisms involving autoreactive T cells contribute to the pathogenesis of RA. [1–5] T cells recognize antigens by their T cell receptor (TCR), a process that involves molecules of the human leukocyte antigen (HLA). Mature T cells express one of two types of TCR: a heterodimer of α and β chains or γ and δ chains. By animal experiments, Corthay [6] found that $\alpha\beta$ T cells play a more important role in the occurrence of RA than that of $\gamma\delta$ T cells. In animal experiments, researchers [7, 8] found that, in collagen-induced arthritis (CIA) rats, there were TCR variable beta (Vβ) gene overexpressed, moreover, companying the development of the disease, some Vβ families turned to hold certain clone types. While in human patients with RA, T lymphocytes may undergo expansion in the synovium, several groups have studied TCR gene expression in the joints and blood of RA patients. [9, 10] If biased TCR Vβ was associated with the pathogenic T cell populations, the corresponding TCR elements could be targeted by TCR-specific immunotherapies, such as TCR peptide vaccination or T-cell vaccination. [11, 12] Unfortunately, many contradictory findings have been reported, moreover, although there are several reports relate to TCR Vβ clone in RA patients, few reports focused on the comparison of TCR Vβ gene usage of peripheral blood (PB) and synovial fluid (SF) of RA patients.

Currently, the techniques, such as Southern blot analysis, [13] staining with TCR V-gene-specific antibodies, [14] PCR-ELISA, [15] immuoscope spectratyping technique [16] and so on, were applied to detecting expansion of TCR gene. More presently, the real-time florescence quantitative polymerase chain reaction (FQ-PCR) and DNA melting curve analysis technique was successfully modified and used to detect skewness of TCR. [17, 18] In this study, we applied this technique to analyze the TCR Vβ gene usages in PB and SF of acute and chronic RA patients, to compare the clone characteristics of these two sample groups, and intend to provide information for the further studies of mechanism and therapy of RA.

70.2 Patients and Methods

70.2.1 Patients

PB and SF lymphocytes were collected from four acute RA patients and eight chronic RA patients (the detail information were listed in Table 70.1), who were determined according to the American Rheumatism Association diagnostic criteria, [19] and had not been treated with immunomodulating drugs in the previous 6 months prior to the study and were seronegative for markers of hepatitis viruses,

Table 70.1 The clinical materials of all the RA patients

Patients	Age	Sex	Diagnosis	Duration (yr)	Sample
1	39	Male	Acute RA	<1	PB, SF
2	42	Female	Acute RA	<1	PB, SF
3	51	Female	Acute RA	<1	PB, SF
4	46	Male	Acute RA	<1	PB, SF
5	48	Female	Chronic RA	5	PB, SF
6	62	Male	Chronic RA	8	PB, SF
7	67	Male	Chronic RA	11	PB, SF
8	45	Female	Chronic RA	7	PB, SF
9	55	Female	Chronic RA	9	PB, SF
10	58	Female	Chronic RA	13	PB, SF
11	47	Male	Chronic RA	6	PB, SF
12	66	Male	Chronic RA	14	PB, SF

HIV and other pathogenic infections. Excluded from the study were patients with tumors and immunological disorders. This study protocol was approved by the hospital Ethics Committee.

70.2.2 Extraction of RNAs and Synthesis of the First cDNAs

The sense primer, anti-sense primer and specific primers for 26 TCR Vβ gene families (both of Vβ5 and Vβ13 include two subfamilies: Vβ5.1 and Vβ 5.2, Vβ13.1 and Vβ13.2) were previously described [20] and synthesized by the Guang-zhou Daangene Corporation of China. A total of 5 ml of blood and 2 ml SF were taken from each of the RA patients, 5 ml of blood was taken from twelve healthy controls respectively. Lymphocytes were isolated from PB and SF by Fcoll-Hypaque density centrifugation. Using an Omega RNA extraction kit according to the manufacturer's instructions, total RNAs were extracted from PB and SF respectively, and 1 μg total RNA was reverse transcribed with 250 pm olig (dT), 200 U Moloney murine leukemia virus (M-MuLV) reverse transcriptase, and 2 μl of 10 mM dNTP mix (cDNA Synthesis Kit; MBI-Fermentas), in a total volume of 20 μl (six reactions for every sample). The cDNAs were stored at −80 °C.

70.2.3 Determination of TCR Vβ Gene Usage in SF and PB RA Patients

According to the previous study, [21] the 26 TCR Vβ gene usages were detected by real-time FQ-PCR with DNA melting curve analysis technique. The progress was showed as following: the PCR for each of 26 gene families were carried out in

40 μl mixtures that contained 2 μl sense primer and anti-sense primer, 2 μl MgCl2 (2.0 μM), 4 μl dNTP (10 mM), 5 μl 10 × buffer, 1.2 U Taq-polymerase, and 1 μl cDNA template. The experimental conditions were 94 °C for 3 min, 94 °C melting for 1 min, primer annealing at 56 °C for 1 min, and 72 °C for 1 min, 35 cycles; then extension at 72 °C for 10 min. Finally, each of 26 TCR V*β* genes usage was analyzed by the melting curve analysis technique.

70.2.4 Calculation of Usage Frequency and Coincidence Rate of TCR Vβ Genes Between PB with SF

In order to explore the relationship or difference of TCR V*β* gene usage in PB and SF of each RA patient, the usage frequency and coincidence rate for advantage genes and limited genes were calculated respectively. I. The formula for usage frequency: usage frequency (%) = A/B × 100. A represented the number of advantage (limited) genes existing in PB or SF; B represented the total number of the same genes in the same sample. II. The formula for coincidence frequency: coincidence rate (%) = 2n/N × 100. n represented the number of common advantage (limited) genes existing in PB and SF; N represented the number of the total number of advantage (limited) genes in the both samples.

70.2.5 Statistical Analysis

Chi square test was used to the comparison of coincidence rates of the TCR V*β* gene usage between in PB and SF of RA patients. The level of 0.05 was taken as the criteria for significance.

70.3 Results

70.3.1 The Overall View of TCR Vβ Gene Usages in PB and SF of all RA Patients

In all of PB samples of the twelve healthy volunteers, there were no biased TCR V*β* gene families, while in PB and SF samples of RA patients, except for V*β*5.2 and V*β*8, the skewed TCR V*β* genes, including advantage and limited usage genes, covered all other 24 TCR V*β* genes (Table 70.2). In all the advantage usage genes of PB and SF, V*β*1 and V*β*13.1 were the most predominant ones, V*β*7 and V*β*18 were next to them (Fig. 70.1); Compared with advantage V*β* genes, the number of limited usage gene families was lower, such as V*β*2, V*β*10, V*β*11, V*β*17, V*β*21,

Table 70.2 The TCR Vβ usage in PB and SF of RA patients

Patients	PB		SF	
	Advantage usage	Limited usage	Advantage usage	Limited usage
1	Vβ1, Vβ13.1	–	Vβ1, Vβ5.1, Vβ13.1	–
2	Vβ7, Vβ18	–	Vβ4, Vβ7, Vβ9,	–
3	Vβ1, Vβ16	–	Vβ1, Vβ13.1,	Vβ11
4	Vβ13.1, Vβ15, Vβ18	–	Vβ10, Vβ13.1	–
5	Vβ1, Vβ4, Vβ7, Vβ23,	Vβ2	Vβ1, Vβ4, Vβ7, Vβ13.1	Vβ2
6	Vβ5.1, Vβ6, Vβ14	Vβ22	Vβ6, Vβ15, Vβ20	Vβ10, Vβ22
7	Vβ1, Vβ2, Vβ9, Vβ12	Vβ11	Vβ1, Vβ9, Vβ18	Vβ23
8	Vβ1, Vβ10, Vβ13.1	–	Vβ1, Vβ14, Vβ13.1	Vβ12
9	Vβ5.1, Vβ6, Vβ13.1, Vβ16, Vβ13.2	Vβ11	Vβ3, Vβ5.1, Vβ6, Vβ13.2, Vβ18, Vβ20	–
10	Vβ7, Vβ13.2	–	Vβ4, Vβ7, Vβ9, Vβ13.1	Vβ22
11	Vβ1, Vβ5.1, Vβ11, Vβ22	–	Vβ1, Vβ5.1, Vβ12, β22	Vβ24
12	Vβ7, Vβ13.1, Vβ18, Vβ19	Vβ21	Vβ6, Vβ7, Vβ16, Vβ18	Vβ11, Vβ17

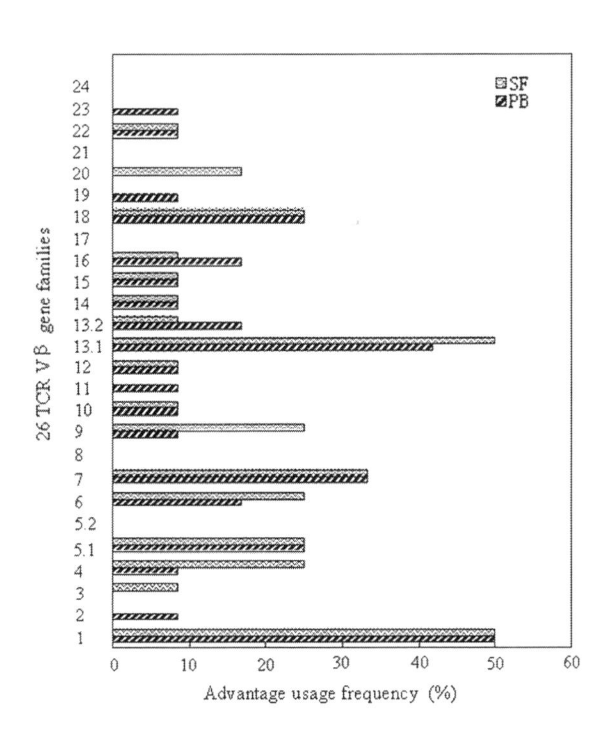

Fig. 70.1 Advantage usages of TCR Vβ in PB and SF of twelve RA patients. In PB, except for Vβ3, Vβ5.2, Vβ8, Vβ17, Vβ20, Vβ21 and Vβ24, all of the other TCR Vβ gene families were predominantly used with different levels. Vβ1 was the advantageously used genes with the highest level; Vβ13.1, Vβ7, Vβ5.1 and Vβ18 were second to it. In SF, except for Vβ2, Vβ5.2, Vβ8, Vβ11, Vβ17, Vβ19, Vβ21, Vβ23 and Vβ24, all of the other TCR Vβ genes were predominantly used with different levels. Vβ13.1 was the advantageously used genes with the highest level; Vβ4, Vβ5.1, Vβ6, Vβ18 and Vβ20 were next to it subsequently

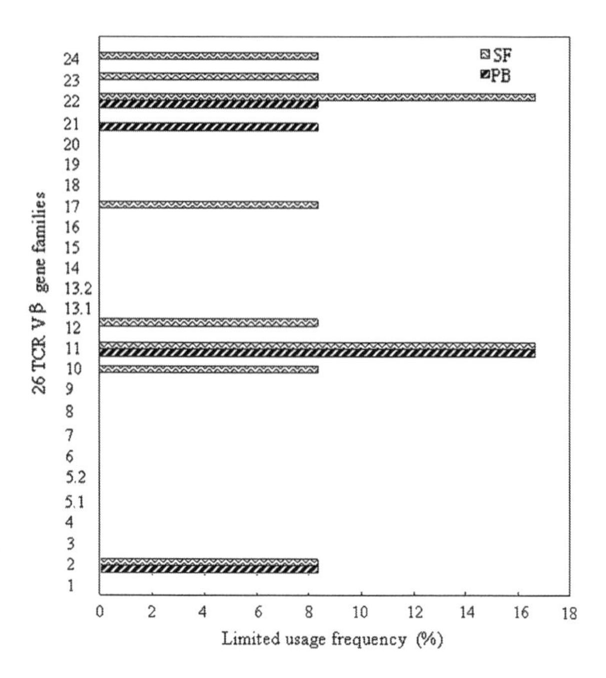

Fig. 70.2 Limited usages of the TCR Vβ in PB and SF of twelve RA patients. In PB, there were four TCR Vβ gene families exhibited limited usage: Vβ1, Vβ11, Vβ21 and Vβ22. Vβ11 was the one with the highest level, Vβ1, Vβ21 and Vβ22 were next to it. In SF, there were eight TCR Vβ gene families exhibited limited usage: Vβ2, Vβ10, Vβ11 Vβ12, Vβ17, Vβ21, Vβ22, Vβ23 and Vβ24. Vβ11 and Vβ22 were the ones with the highest level; the others were next to them

Vβ22 and Vβ23. Among them, the usage frequencies of Vβ11 and Vβ22 were relatively higher (Fig. 70.2).

70.3.2 TCR Vβ Gene Usages in PB and SF of Acute RA Patients

In PB of the four patients with acute RA, the TCR Vβ gene families which exhibited advantage usage were Vβ1, Vβ7, Vβ13.1, Vβ15, Vβ16 and Vβ18, Vβ1, Vβ13.1 and Vβ18 were the highly biased ones which usage frequencies were all 50 %; in the SF samples, that advantage usage gene were Vβ1, Vβ4, Vβ5.1, Vβ7, Vβ9, Vβ10 and Vβ13.1, Vβ1 and Vβ13.1 were also the ones with the highest usage frequencies, which were 50 and 75 % respectively (Table 70.3, Fig. 70.3). There was no restrictively used TCR Vβ gene in PB of the acute RA patients, while in the SF samples, there was only Vβ11 exhibited limited usage in patient-11 (Fig. 70.5).

70.3.3 TCR Vβ Gene Usages in PB and SF of Chronic RA Patients

In PB of the eight patients with chronic RA, except Vβ3, Vβ5.2, Vβ8, Vβ15, Vβ17, Vβ20, Vβ21 and Vβ24, the other gene families were all predominantly used

Table 70.3 TCR Vβ gene usage frequencies in PB and SF of RA patients

Vβ	Usage frequency for acute RA (%)				Usage frequency for chronic RA (%)			
	PB		SF		PB		SF	
	A	L	A	L	A	L	A	L
1	50	0	50	0	50	0	50	0
2	0	0	0	0	12.5	12.5	0	12.5
3	0	0	0	0	0	0	12.5	0
4	0	0	25	0	12.5	0	25	0
5.1	0	0	25	0	37.5	0	25	0
5.2	0	0	0	0	0	0	0	0
6	0	0	0	0	25	0	37.5	0
7	25	0	25	0	37.5	0	37.5	0
8	0	0	0	0	0	0	0	0
9	0	0	25	0	12.5	0	25	0
10	0	0	25	0	12.5	0	0	12.5
11	0	0	0	25	12.5	25	0	12.5
12	0	0	0	0	12.5	0	12.5	12.5
13.1	50	0	75	0	37.5	0	37.5	0
13.2	0	0	0	0	25	0	12.5	0
14	0	0	0	0	12.5	0	12.5	0
15	25	0	0	0	0	0	12.5	0
16	25	0	0	0	12.5	0	12.5	0
17	0	0	0	0	0	0	0	12.5
18	50	0	0	0	12.5	0	37.5	0
19	0	0	0	0	12.5	0	0	0
20	0	0	0	0	0	0	25	0
21	0	0	0	0	0	12.5	0	0
22	0	0	0	0	12.5	12.5	12.5	25
23	0	0	0	0	12.5	0	0	12.5
24	0	0	0	0	0	0	0	12.5

A represented advantage gene usage; L represented limited gene usage

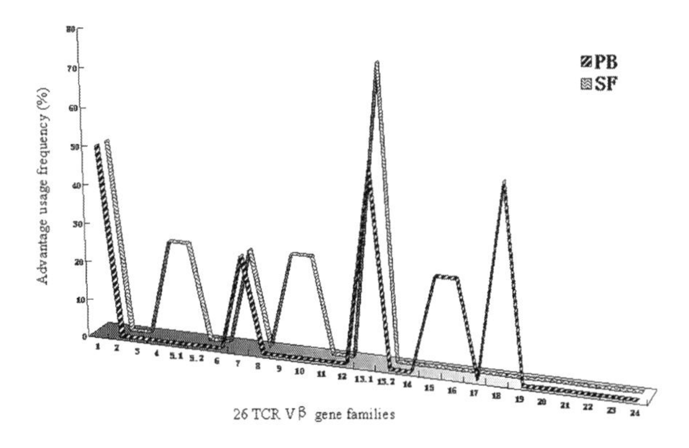

Fig. 70.3 Advantage usages of TCR Vβ genes in PB and SF of the four acute RA patients. In PB of the four patients with acute RA, the advantage usage TCR Vβ gene families were Vβ1, Vβ7, Vβ13.1, Vβ15, Vβ16, Vβ18, Vβ1, Vβ13.1 and Vβ18, all their usage frequencies were 50 %; in SF, that advantage usage gene were Vβ1, Vβ4, Vβ5.1, Vβ7, Vβ9, Vβ10 and Vβ13.1, Vβ1 and Vβ13.1 were also the ones with the highest usage frequencies, which were 50 and 75 % respectively

more or less, Vβ1 was the highest one which advantage usage frequency was 50 %, Vβ5.1, Vβ7 and Vβ13.1 were second to it, their usage frequency were all 37.5 %. In the SF samples, the advantage usage genes were Vβ1, Vβ6, Vβ7, Vβ13.1, Vβ18 and so on, the frequency of Vβ1 (50 %) was higher than that of other four gene families (37.5 %) (Table 70.3, Fig. 70.4).

Vβ2, Vβ11, Vβ21 and Vβ22 exhibited restrictedly used in the PB samples of chronic RA patients, Vβ11 was the highest one which usage frequency was 25 %; while in the SF samples, the limited usage genes were Vβ2, Vβ10, Vβ11, Vβ12, Vβ17, Vβ22, Vβ23 and Vβ24, the limited usage frequency of Vβ22 was 25 % which was higher than the other genes (Fig. 70.5).

70.3.4 The Coincidence Rate of TCR Vβ Gene Usage of PB with SF of RA Patients

As Table 70.4 showed, the lowest coincidence rate of TCR Vβ gene usage between PB and SF existed in RA patient-10, it was 16.7 %, while the highest rate was 75.0 %, which existed in RA patient −5 and −11. The average value of Vβ advantage gene families for acute and chronic RA patients were 46.8 and 53.5 % respectively, there was no significant difference between the two samples ($P > 0.05$); the average value of Vβ limited genes for acute and chronic RA patients were 0 and 16.7 %, the difference was significant ($P < 0.05$).

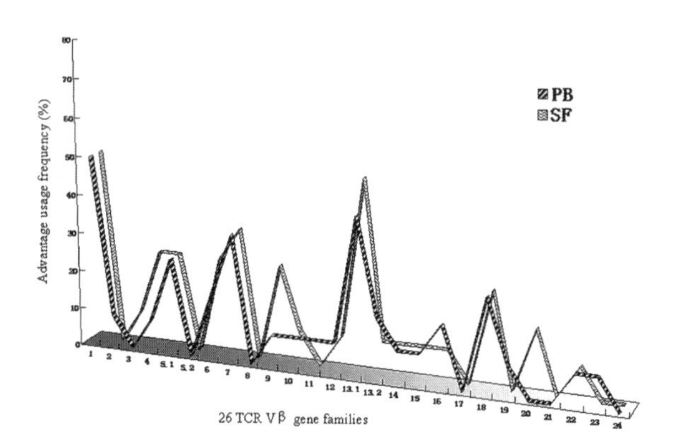

Fig. 70.4 Advantage usages of TCR Vβ genes in PB and SF of the eight chronic RA patients. In PB of the eight patients with chronic RA, except Vβ3, Vβ5.2, Vβ8, Vβ15, Vβ17, Vβ20, Vβ21 and Vβ24, the other gene families were all predominantly used more or less, Vβ1 was the highest one which advantage usage frequency was 50 %, Vβ5.1, Vβ7 and Vβ13.1 were second to it, their usage frequency were all 37.5 %. In SF, the key advantage usage genes were Vβ1, Vβ6, Vβ7, Vβ13.1 and Vβ18, the frequency of Vβ1 (50 %) was higher than that of the other four gene families (37.5 %)

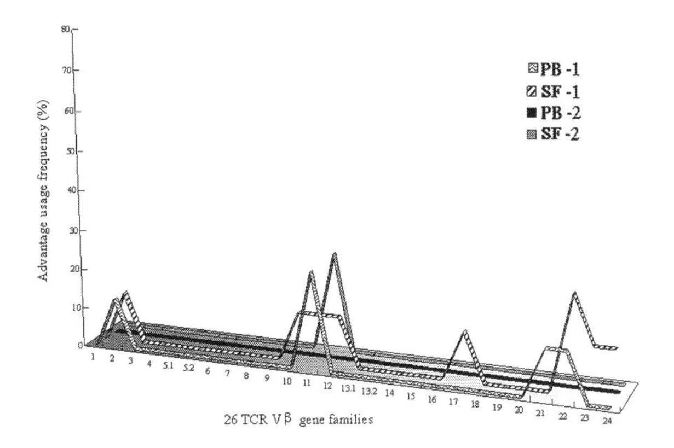

Fig. 70.5 Limited usage of TCR Vβ genes in PB and SF of the acute and chronic RA patients. There was no limited usage TCR Vβ gene in PB of the acute RA patients, while in SF, there was only Vβ11 which showed restrictedly used in patient-11. Vβ2, Vβ11, Vβ21 and Vβ22 exhibited restrictedly used in PB of chronic RA patients, Vβ11 was the highest which usage frequency was 25 %; while in SF, the limited usage genes were Vβ2, Vβ10, Vβ11, Vβ12, Vβ17, Vβ22, Vβ23 and Vβ24, the limited usage frequency of Vβ22 was 25 % which higher than other genes

Table 70.4 The coincidence rates of TCR Vβ gene usages in PB and SF of RA patients

Patients	Coincidence number/total number (advantage genes)	Coincidence rate (%)	Coincidence number/total number (limited genes)	Coincidence rate (%)
1	4/7	57.1	0/0	0
2	2/5	40.0	0/0	0
3	2/4	50.0	0/0	0
4	2/5	40.0	0/0	0
5	6/8	75.0	1/1	100
6	2/6	33.3	1/3	33.3
7	4/7	57.1	0/0	0
8	4/6	66.7	0/0	0
9	6/11	54.5	0/0	0
10	1/6	16.7	0/0	0
11	6/8	75.0	0/0	0
12	4/8	50.0	0/0	0
Mean for the acute	—	46.8	–	0
Mean for the chronic	—	53.5	–	16.7
Mean for total	—	51.3	–	11.1

70.4 Discussion

In this study, we used FQ-PCR with DNA melting curve analysis technique to detect the TCR Vβ usage in PB and SF of RA patients, and found that, not only in the acute but also thechronic RA patients, or not only in the PB but also the SF samples, Vβ5.2 and Vβ8 were not selectively used, which including predo-minant and restricted usage. This was very different from the results of animal experiments, [22, 23] which showed that TCR Vβ5.2 and TCR Vβ8.2 clonotypes predominated in the T lymphocytes infiltrating in the joints of CIArats. Further, with the constructed recombinant eukaryotic expression vectors pTARRGET-TCRVβ5.2-/Vβ8.2-HSP70, researchers [24, 25] found that the arthritic systems of CIA rats were significantly alleviated, that is, the recombinants could protect effectively for CIA rats. Controversially, Haqqi [26] found the predominant usage families were not Vβ5.2 and Vβ8.2 but Vβ3 and Vβ10 in BUB mice, and using the antibodies specific to each of genes simulta- neously, they also achieved a successful result for effectively treating CIA. These data probably indicated that, between human RA patients and other animals with RA, or between different species of animals with RA, the skewness of TCR Vβ genes are different.

No matter acute or chronic patients, there were some advantageously used Vβ genes in PB and SF, the gene families with highest frequency in PB were Vβ1 and Vβ13.1, this differed from Zhang's [27] study, which showed that Vβ17 was the gene with high level of expression. While in SF, they report that the advantage genes were Vβ12 and Vβ13.1, which were partly similar to this study (predominant usage gene were also Vβ1 and Vβ13.1). In another reports, Paliard [28] observed that the expression of Vβ14 in the peripheral blood of 6 out 9 RA patients was undectable or substantially diminished in comparison to peripheral blood of normal donors, namely, Vβ14 was a restrictive expression gene. Interestingly, in the results of this experiment, Vβ14 was no longer the limited expression gene family, it just was the overexpressed gene family in PB of patient-6 and in SF of patient-8. These conflict results probably lie in the different methods for detecting the biases of TCR Vβ genes.

As Fig. 70.3 showed, for the four patients with RA, the mainly advantage usage genes were Vβ1, Vβ13.1 and Vβ18 in PB, while in SF, except for Vβ18, the former two genes were still overexpressed. As far as the number of advantage Vβ genes was concerned, the gene number of PB (9 genes families) was little less than that of SF (12 gene families). This was similar to the study of VanderBorght, [29] he reported that the average number of overexpressed Vβ genes was higher in synovial tissue (ST) than that in PB. Besides, he found that the dominant genes in PB were Vβ3, Vβ10, Vβ10 and Vβ18, while in SF Vβ2 and Vβ4 were predominant. Coincidently, Vβ18 was the common advantage gene in his and our studies. Then, whether Vβ18 was just the TCR Vβ gene families to diagnosis or therapy target point for the acute patients with RA? This needs further deep studies to unclose. Except for the predominately expressed genes, we also found the limited genes—Vβ11 in SF of patient-4, and there was no restricted gene in other samples of the four acute RA patients. This maybe due to short-time antigen stimulation, the limited usage gene families did not formed. However, the restricted TCR Vβ gene usage in the acute RA patients has not been seen to be reported. What is the meaning of appearance of limited TCR Vβ in the pathogenesis? It dose remain unclear.

For the patients with chronic RA, we found that the PB and SF sample mainly shared the common advantage usage genes: Vβ1, Vβ7 and Vβ13.1; and the common limited usage genes: Vβ2, Vβ11, Vβ21 and Vβ22. The existence of the common biased genes indicated that there are the similar antigen peptides in PB an SF, and under the stimulation of the peptides specific to rheumatoid arthritis, T cell recognized the common antigen peptides presented by antigen presenting cells (APC), so PB and SF hold the common skewness of TCR Vβ families. The same phenomenon, which the advantage TCR Vβ gene usage in PB was similar to that in SF, also existed in the report of VanderBorght, [30] they found that Vβ2 and Vβ4 were predominantly expressed in SF samples, these expansions accounted for the vast majority of CDR3-region sequences identified among these subsets in the joints. The similar skewness also occurred in the blood, because the biased Vβ2 and Vβ4 were detected as well. Hence, the predominant genes in PB and SF all differed from that of this study. However, probably due to the different microenvironments in PB and SF, the number and type of antigens were not exactly identical in the two samples, so the TCR Vβ usages of PB were different from that of SF. In Roessner's study, [31] the frequencies of Vβ2 and Vβ6 were remarkable higher than that of other gene families in SF; Sun [32] also found the differences, and he thought this because the HLA background of Chinese RA patients differs from that of other countries. In Sun's report, [32] Vβ14 and Vβ16 were overexpressed and Vβ17 was restricted-expressed in ST, while in PB samples, there was no obviously over-/low-expressed Vβ families. Dramatically, Both Alam [33] and Zagon [34] found that Vβ17 was not the restricted but advantage usage gene in their studies respectively, this is just opposite to the former study. These conflict results probably not only caused by the HLA background, but also due to the methodological differences for detecting TCR Vβ usage.

In this study, we also calculated the coincidence rate of PB and SF in the same RA patients. As Table 70.4 showed, for advantage usage TCR Vβ genes, the average coincidence rate for acute RA patients was 46.8 %, while that for chronic RA patients was 53.5 %, there was no significant difference between the two samples ($P < 0.05$), so from this angle of view point, there are very similarity between PB and SF in the PA patients. However, for the limited usage TCR Vβ genes, the difference of coincidence rate of limited usage in PB and SF was significant ($P < 0.05$). But because the cases for acute RA patients were low, does this difference exit between the two samples in fact? It is remained to be proved by further more experiments with large number of acute RA cases.

In summary, TCR Vβ usage in PB is similar to that in SF of RA patients, however, even in the same patient, there are still difference between the two samples. Hence, in PB and SF, TCR Vβ usage not only holds the common characters, but also has the property of personalization. These results are probably helpful for the further studies of the pathogenesis and therapy of RA in future.

Acknowledgments The article is supported by the Provincial Science and Technology Development Project (Grant 2012YD18054), the Provincial Nature Science Foundation (Grant ZR2012HL29), the High School Science and Technology Plan Project (Grant J11LF18), the Population and Family Planning Commission (Grant [2011]13), and the Development Plan Project of Jining Science and Technology Bureau of Shandong Province (Grant [2011]57), the Youth Foundation of Jining Medical College (Grant [2011]).

References

1. Svelander L, Erlandsson H, Lorentzen JC, Trollmo C, Klareskog L, Bucht A (2004) Oligodeoxynucleotides containing CpG motifs can induce T cell-dependent arthritis in rats. Arthritis Rheum 50:297–304
2. Maffia P, Brewer JM, Gracie JA, Ianaro A, Leung BP, Mitchell PJ et al (2004) Inducing experimental arthritis and breaking self-tolerance to joint-specific antigens with trackable, ovalbumin-specific T cells. J Immunol 173:151–156
3. Lee DM, Weinblatt ME (2001) Rheumatoid arthritis. Lancet 358:903–911
4. Bardos T, Mikecz K, Finnegan A, Zhang J, Glant TT (2002) T and B cell recovery in arthritis adoptively transferred to SCID mice: antigen–specific activation is required for restoration of autopathogenic CD4 + Th1 cells in a syngeneic system. J Immunol 163:6013–6021
5. Singh K, Deshpande P, Pryshchep S, Colmegna I, Liarski V, Weyand CM, Goronzy JJ (2009) EPK-dependent T-cell receptor threshold calibration in rheumatoid arthritis. J Immunol 183:8258–8267
6. Corthay A, Johansson A, Vestberg M, Holmdahl R (1999) Collagen-induced arthritis development requires T cells but no T cells: studies with T cell-deficient (TCR mutant) mice. Int Immunol 11:1065–1073
7. Kobari Y, Misaki Y, Setogunbi K, Zhao W, Komagata Y, Kawahata K et al (2004) T cells accumulating in the inflamed joints of a spontaneous murine model of rheumatoid arthritis become restricted to common clonotypes during disease progression. Int Immunol 16:131–138
8. Zhao WM, Yamamoto K (2004) Analysis of the change in clonotypes of T cells accumulated in 4 feet joints of SKG mice. Xi Bao Yu Fen Zi Mian Yi Xue Za Zhi 20:70–72
9. Fox DA (1997) The role of T cells in the immunopathogenesis of rheumatoid arthritis: new perspectives. Arthritis Rheum 40:598–609
10. Kinne RW, Palombo-Kinne E, Emmrich F (1997) T cells in the pathogenesis of rheumatoid arthritis villains or accomplices? Biochim Biophys Acta 1360:109–141
11. Moreland LW, Heck LW, Koopman WJ, Saway PA, Adamson TC, Fronek Z et al (1995) Vβ 17 T-cell receptor peptide vaccine. Results of a phase I dose-finding study in patiets with rheumatoid arthritis. Ann N Y Acad Sci 756:211–214
12. Breedveld FC, Struyk L, Van Laar JM, Miltenburg AM, de Vries RR, Van den Elsen P (1995) Therapeutic regulation of T cells in rheumatoid arthritis. Immunol Rev 144:5–16
13. Howell MD, Diveley JP, Lundeen K, Esty A, Winters ST, Carlo DJ, Brostoff SW (1991) Limitied T cell receptor β chain heterogeneity among interleukin-2 receptor-positive synovial T cells suggests a role for superantigen in rheumatoid arthritis. Proc Natl Acad Sci USA 88:10921–10925
14. Bröker B, Korthäuer U, Heppt P, Weseloh G, de la Camp R, Kroczek RA et al (1993) Biased T cell receptor V gene usage in rheumatoid arthritis. Oligoclonal expansion of T cells expressing V alpha 2 genes in synovial fluid but not in peripheral blood. Arthritis Rheum 36:1234–1243
15. VanderBorght A, Van der Aa A, Geusens P, Vandevyver C, Raus J, Stinissen P (1999) Identification of overrepresented TCR genes in blood and tissue biopsies by PCR-ELISA. J Immunol Methods 223:47–56
16. Yao XS, Diao Y, Sun WB, Luo JM, Qin M, Tang XY (2007) Analysis of the CDR3 length repertoire and diversity of TCR α chain in human peripheral blood T lymphocytes. Xi Bao Yu Fen Zi Mian Yi Xue Za Zhi 4:215–220
17. Zhou JW, Ma R, Tang WT, Luo R, Yao XS (2011) Primary exploration of the third complementarity determining region spectratyping and molecular features of T cell receptor alpha chain in the peripheral blood and tissue of patients with colorectal carcinoma. ACTA Med Mediterranea 27:23–30

18. Zhou J, Kong C, Luo J, Cao J, Shi Y (2013) Comparaing TCR beta chain variable gene skewness between children with tuberculosis and BCG-vaccinated children. Arch Iranian Med 16:104–108
19. Chogle AR, Desai BH, Jhankaria GR (1996) American Rheumatism Association 1958 and 1987 revised criteria for rheumatoid arthritis–how useful to the clinician. J Assoc Phys India 44:93–97
20. Yao XS, Xiao ZJ, Li M, Sun WB, Zhang WY, Wang Q et al (2006) Analysis of the CDR3 region of alpha/beta T-cell receptors (TCRs) and TCR BD gene double-stranded recombination signal sequence breaks end in peripheral blood mononuclear cells of T-lineage acute lymphoblastic leukemia. Clin Lab Haemat 28:405–415
21. Zhou J, Ma R, Luo R, He X, Sun W, Tang W et al (2010) Primary exploration of molecular and spectratyping features of CDR3 of TCR β chain in the peripheral blood and tissue of patients with colorectal carcinoma. Cancer Epidemiol 34:733–740
22. Zhang XM, Zhao WM, Li Y, Liu ZL (2005) Analysis of TCR Vβ clonotypes of T lymphocytes infiltrating in the joints of rat with collagen-induced arthritis. Xi Bao Yu Fen Zi Mian Yi Xue Za Zhi 21:538–540
23. Honda A, Ametani A (2004) Matsumoto Ta, Lwaya A, Kano H, Hachimura S, et al. Vaccination with an immunodominant peptide of bovine type II collagen induces an anti-PCR response, and modulates the onset and severity of collagen-induced arthritis. Int Immunol 16:737–745
24. Xiao J, Li ST, Wang W, Li Y, Zhao WM (2007) Protective effects of overexpression TCR Vβ5.2–HSP70 and TCR Vβ8.2-HSP against collagen-induce arthritis in rats. Xi Bao Yu Fen Zi Mian Yi Xue Za Zhi 6:439–445
25. Ge PL, Ma LP, Wang W, Li Y, Zhao WM (2009) Inhibition of collagen-induced arthritis by DNA vaccines encoding TCR Vβ5.2 and TCR Vβ8.2. Chin Med J 122:1039–1048
26. Haqqi TM, Qu XM, Anthony D, Ma J, Sy MS (1996) Immunization with T cell receptor Vβ chain peptides deletes pathogenic cells and prevents the induction of Collagen-induced arthritis in mice. Immunoltherapy of Collagen-induced arthritis 97:2849–2858
27. Zhang ZL, Zhang GZ, Dong Y (2002) T cell receptor Vβ gene bias in rheumatoid arthritis. Chin Med J 115:856–859
28. Paliard X, West SG, Lafferty JA, Clements JR, Kappler JW, Marrack P et al (1991) Evidence for the effects of a superantigen in rheumatoid arthritis. Science 235:325–329
29. VanderBortht A, Keyser FD, Geusens P, Backer MD, Malaise M, Baeten D et al (2002) Dynamic T cell receptor clonotype changes in synovial tissue of patients with early rheumatoid arthritis: effects of treatment with cyclosporine (Neoral). J Rheumat 29:416–426
30. VanderBorght A, Geusens AP, Vandvyver C, Raus J, Stinissen P (2000) Skewed T-cell receptor variable gene usage in the synovium of early and chronic rheumatoid arthritis patients and persistence of clonally expanded T cells in a chronic patient. Rheumatology 39:1189–1201
31. Roessner K, Trived H, Gaur L, Howard D, Aversa J, Cooper SM et al (1998) Biased T-cell antigen receptor repertoire in lyme arthritis. Infect Immun 66:1092–1099
32. Sun W, Nie H, Li N, Zang YC, Zhang D, Feng G et al (2005) Skewed T-cell receptor BV14 and BV16 expression and shared CDR3 sequence and common sequence motifs in synovial T cells of rheumatoid arthritis. Genes and Immun 6:248–261
33. Zagon G, Tumang JR, Li Y, Friedman SM, Crow MK (1994) Increaseed frequency of V beta 17-positive T cells I patients with rheumatoid arthritis. Arthritis Rheum 37:1431–1440
34. Alam A, LuléJ, Coppin H, Lambert N, Maziéres B, De Préval C, Cantagrel A (1995)T-cell receptor variable region of the beta-chain gene use in peripheral blood and multiple synovial membranes during rheumatoid arthritis. Hum Immunol 42:331–339

Chapter 71
New Impossible Differential Cryptanalysis on Improved LBlock

Xuan Liu, Feng Liu and Shuai Meng

Abstract LBlock is a 64-bit lightweight block cipher which can be implemented in both hardware environments and software platforms. It was proposed by Wu Wenling and Zhang Lei at ACNS2011. We studied the security of LBlock found that the permutation layer can getting better on security in the internet of things. In order to assure it can achieve enough security, we gave an improvement on permutation layer of LBlock. By analyzing the property of the diffusion transformation, it has shown that a new kind of 11-round impossible differential was presented. To the best of our knowledge, this is the first paper that proposes this way analysis on improved LBlock.

Keywords LBlock · Impossible differential · Improved design

71.1 Introduction

Cryptographic techniques are seen as an essential method for the confidentiality, protection of the privacy and the data integrity. Recently, the research of the lightweight cryptography has been attracted much attention. Specially, A series of lightweight block ciphers have been proposed in the literature, such as PRESENT [1], HIGHT [2], mCrypton [3], DESL [4], KATAN and KTANTAN [5], CGEN [6], MIBS [7], TWIS [8] etc.

X. Liu (✉) · F. Liu · S. Meng
School of Information Science and Engineering, Shandong Normal University,
Jinan 250014, China
e-mail: liuxuan0309@126.com

X. Liu · F. Liu · S. Meng
Shandong Provincial Key Laboratory for Novel Distributed Computer Software Technology,
Jinan 250014, China

S. Li et al. (eds.), *Frontier and Future Development of Information Technology in Medicine and Education*, Lecture Notes in Electrical Engineering 269,
DOI: 10.1007/978-94-007-7618-0_71,

LBlock [9] is a 64-bit lightweight block cipher which can be implemented in both hardware environments and software platforms. It was proposed by Wu Wenling and Zhang Lei at ACNS2011. In this paper, we studied the security of LBlock found that the Permutation Layer can getting better on security in the internet of things, if the permutation layer transform word-wise to bit-wise. By analyzing the property of the diffusion transformation, it has shown that a new kind of 11-round impossible differential with 8-round impossible differential distinguisher was presented.

This paper is organized as follows. In Sect. 71.2, the detailed description and some properties of LBlock are presented. Then, the proposed improved LBlock is introduced in Sect. 71.2.3, and Sect. 71.3 shows result on impossible differential cryptanalysis of reduced-round improved LBlock. The concluding remarks is drawn in the last section.

71.2 Prelimimaries

We first introduce some notations used throughout this paper and then give a simple description of the LBlock.

71.2.1 Notations

The following notations are used throughout this paper.

M	64 bits plaintext
C	64 bits ciphertext
K	80 bits master key
K_r	32 bits round subkey
F	Round function
s	4×4 S-box
S	Substitution layer consists of eight 4×4 S-box in parallel
P	Permutation
$\oplus$	Bit-wise XOR
$\lll 7$	7 bits cyclic left shift
$\|\|$	Two binary strings concatenation
$[i]_2$	Binary form of an round counter i

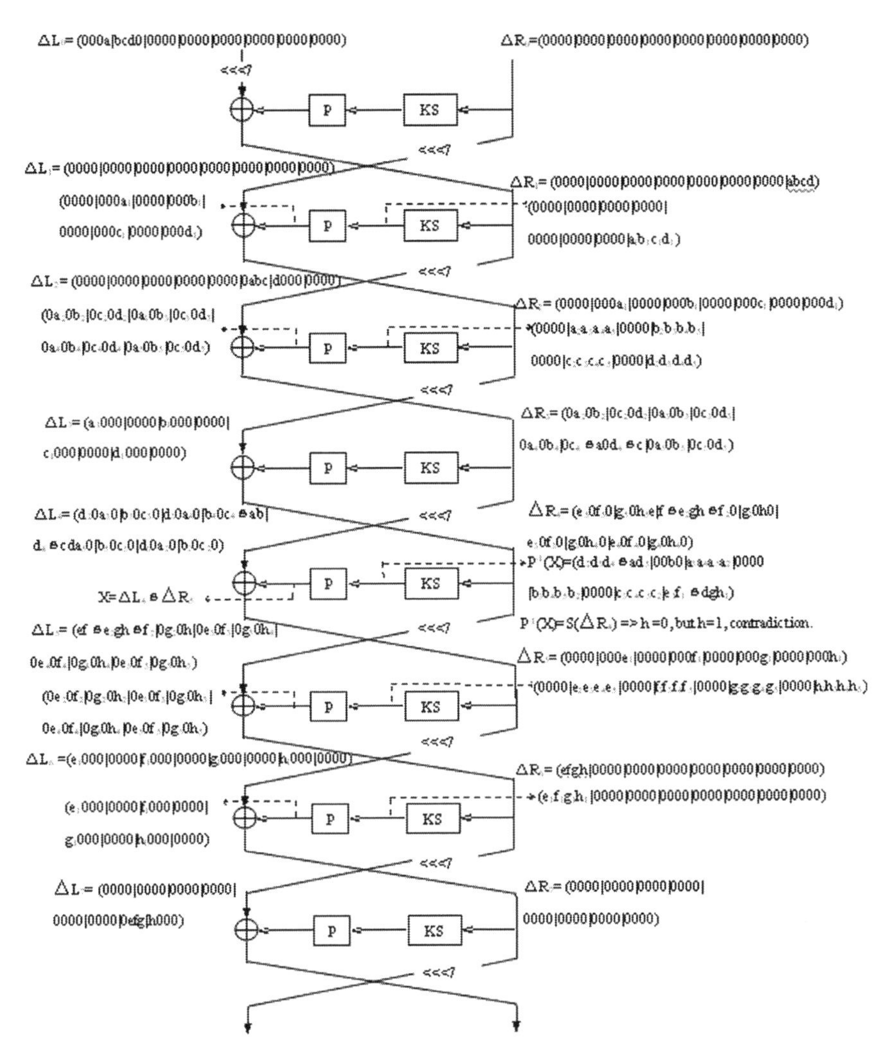

Fig. 71.1 8-round impossible differential of improved LBlock

71.2.2 Description of LBlock

Encryption Algorithm. The general structure of LBlock is a variant of Feistel network and consists of a 32-round iterative structure. Let $M = X_1 \| X_0$ denote a 64-bit plaintext, and then the data processing procedure can be expressed as follows.

1. For $i = 2, 3, \ldots, 33$, do $Xi = F(Xi-1, Ki-1) \oplus (Xi-2 \lll 8)$
2. Output $C = X32 \| X33$ as the 64-bit ciphertext.

Table 71.1 Permutation bit-wise mapping

i	0	1	2	3	4	5	6	7
P[i]	0	8	16	24	1	9	17	25
i	8	9	10	11	12	13	14	15
P[i]	2	10	18	26	3	11	19	27
i	16	17	18	19	20	21	22	23
P[i]	4	12	20	28	5	13	21	29
i	24	25	26	27	28	29	30	31
P[i]	6	14	22	30	7	15	23	31

Key Schedule. To reduce the cost of hardware and to decrease key set-up time, the key schedule of LBlock is rather simple. The 80-bit master key K is stored in a key register and denoted as $K = k_{79}\, k_{78}\, k_{77} \cdots k_1\, k_0$. Output the leftmost 32 bits of current content of register K as round subkey K_1, and then operate as follows:

For i = 1, 2, ..., 31, update the key register K as follows:

1. $K \lll 29$.
2. $[k_{79}\, k_{78}\, k_{77}\, k_{76}] = S_9[k_{79}\, k_{78}\, k_{77}\, k_{76}]$; $[k_{75}\, k_{74} k_{73}\, k_{72}] = S_8[k_{75}\, k_{74}\, k_{73}\, k_{72}]$.
3. $[k_{50}\, k_{49}\, k_{48}\, k_{47}\, k_{46}] \oplus [i]_2$.
4. Output the leftmost 32 bits of current content of register K as round subkey K_{i+1}.

71.2.3 Improvement on LBlock

We employ on bit-wise permutation layer. The inputs and outputs are 32 bits, respectively. We denote input one bit as i, each bit moved to the bit P[i] new position as output by permutation layer, which is given by Table 71.1 in detail.

Since bit-wise permutation provides fast diffusion without hardware implementation cost and enhances security against impossible differential, saturation, meet-in-the-middle etc. Especially, we focus on hardware efficiency and achieve simplicity demands a linear layer that can be implemented with a minimum number of processing elements. Therefore, we have chosen a bit-wise permutation instead of word-wise.

71.3 Result on Impossible Differential Cryptanalysis of Reduced-Round Improved LBlock

71.3.1 8-Round Impossible Differential Distinguisher

We search for the impossible differential characteristic of improved LBlock using the impossible differential cryptanalysis, and present an impossible differential cryptanalysis on 11-round improved LBlock, which is based on the following 8-round impossible differential.

(000a|bcd0|0000|0000|0000|0000|0000|0000|0000|0000|0000|0000|0000|0000|0000|0000)

$\nrightarrow$(0000|0000|0000|0000|0000|0000|0000|0000|0000|0000|0000|0000|0000|0000-|0efg|h000), where a, b, c, d, e, f, g are not all zero and h is 1, and we indicate one impossible differential of 8-round improved LBlock as shown in Fig. 71.1.

The second 3-round differential ends with difference $(\triangle L_8, \triangle R_8) =$ (0000|0000|0000|0000|0000|0000|0000|0000|0000|0000|0000|0000|0000|0000|0efg|h000), when rolling back this difference through 2-round transformation, we get the difference $(\triangle L_6, \triangle R_6) = (e_1000|0000|f_1000|0000|g_1000|0000|h_1000|0000|efgh$ $|0000|0000|0000|0000|0000|0000|0000)$, where e, f, g, e_1, f_1, g_1 and h_1 are not all zero, and h is 1. After the subkey addition and S layer, $\triangle R_5 = \triangle L_6 \ggg 7$ becomes $(0000|000e_1|0000|000f_1|0000|000g_1|0000|000h_1)$. Where e_1, f_1, g_1 and h_1 are not all zero. Further, after the linear transformation P this difference evolves to $(0e_20f_2|0g_20h_2|0e_30f_3|0g_30h_3|0e_40f_4|0g_40h_4|0e_50f_5|0g_50h_5)$. Thus we get $(\triangle L_5, \triangle R_5) = (ef \oplus e_2gh \oplus f_2|0g_20\ h|0e_30f_3|0g_30h_4|0e_40f_4|0g_40h_4|0e_50f_5|0g_50h_5|0000|$ $000e_1|0000|000f_1|0000|000g_1|0000|000h_1)$. Where e_i, f_i, g_i and h_i $(2 \le i \le 5)$ denote not all zero, and h is 1. If the first 3-round differential and second 3-round differential can built up the 8-round differential, then L_4, L_5 and R_5 must satisfy the following: $R_4 = L_5 \ggg 7$, $P(S(K(R_4))) = L_4 \oplus R_5$.

Hence, we have $S(R_4)=S(K(R_4))=P^{-1}(R_3 \oplus R_5)$. Because P^{-1} is a linear transformation, we have $P^{-1}(\triangle L_4 \oplus \triangle R_5) = P^{-1}(\triangle L_4) \oplus P^{-1}(\triangle R_5)=P^{-1}$ $(d_20a_30|b_30c_30|d_30a_40|b_40c_4 \oplus ab|d_4 \oplus cda_50|b_50c_50|d_50a_20|b_20c_20) \oplus P^{-1}$ $(0000|000e_1|0000|000f_1|0000|000g_1|0000|000h_1)=P^{-1}(d_20a_30|b_30c_30|d_30a_40|b_40c_40|$ $d_40a_50|b_50c_50|d_50a_20|b_20c_20) \oplus P^{-1}(0000|0000|0000|000ab|cd00|0000|0000|0000)$ $\oplus$ $P^{-1}(0000|000\ {}_1|0000|000f_1|0000|000g_1|0000|000h_1)=(d_2d_3d_4d_5|0000|a_3a_4a_5a_2|$ $0000|b_3b_4b_5b_2|0000|c_3c_4c_5c_2|0000|) \oplus (00a0|00b0|0000|0000|0000|0000|0c00|0d00)$ $\oplus$ $(0000|0000|0000|0000|0000|0000|0000|\ e_1f_1g_1h_1)=(d_2d_3d_4 \oplus ad_5|00b0|a_3a_4a_5a_2|$ $0000|b_3b_4b_5b_2|0000|c_3c_4c_5c_2|e_1f_1 \oplus dgh_1)$.

Since, $S(\triangle R_4) = S(e_50f_50|g_50h_5e|f \oplus e_2gh \oplus f_20|g_20h0|e_30f_30|g_30h_40|$ $e_40f_40|g_40h_40) \Rightarrow h_4 = 0$, this is h = 1 contradiction. The S-boxes of improved LBlock are permutation, so we can get the fourth and sixth words difference in $\triangle R_4$ equal zero, h = 0, This contradicts with h = 1.

71.3.2 Impossible Differential Cryptanalysis of 11-Round Improved LBlock

Based on above 8-round impossible differential with additional three rounds at the beginning and one round at the end as in Fig. 71.2, we can mount a key recovery

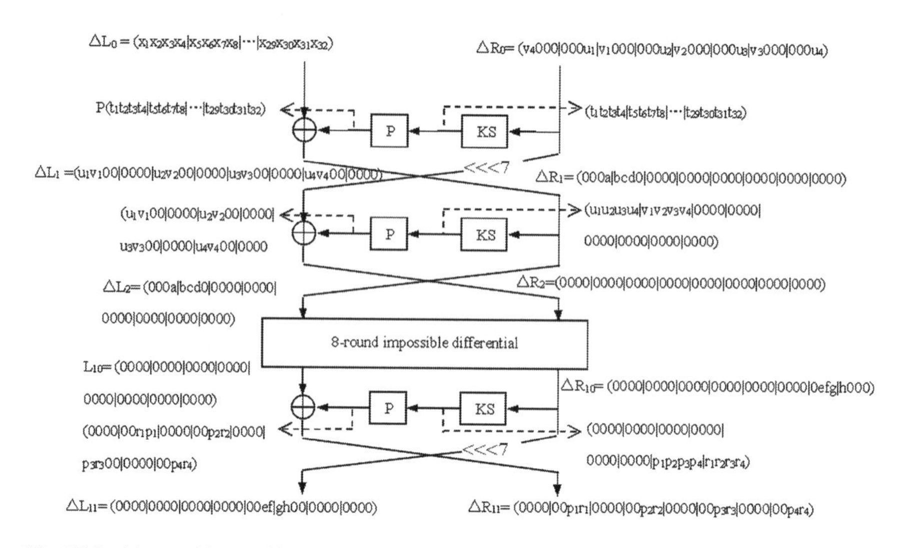

Fig. 71.2 11-round impossible differential attack to improved LBlock

attack on 11-round improved LBlock. The attack procedure can be described as follows.

Step 1 Choose structure of plaintexts as follows.

$L_0 = (x_1x_2x_3x_4|x_5x_6x_7x_8|\ldots|x_{29}x_{30}x_{31}x_{32})$,
$R_0 = (y_1\alpha_2\alpha_3\alpha_4|\alpha_5\alpha_6\alpha_7y_8|y_9\alpha_{10}\alpha_{11}\alpha_{12}|\alpha_{13}\alpha_{14}\alpha_{15}y_{16}|y_{17}\alpha_{18}\alpha_{19}\alpha_{20}|\alpha_{21}\alpha_{22}\alpha_{23}y_{24}|y_{25}\alpha_{26}\alpha_{27}\alpha_{28}|\alpha_{29}\alpha_{30}\alpha_{31}y_{32})$.

where x_i $(1 \le i \le 32)$ and y_i (i = 1, 8, 9, 16, 17, 24, 25, 32) take all possible values in F, α_i is constants in F. For each possible value of x_i $(1 \le i \le 32)$ and y_i (i = 1, 8, 9, 16, 17, 24, 25, 32), we can get a unique 64–bit string $((x_1x_2x_3x_4|x_5x_6x_7x_8|\ldots|x_{29}x_{30}x_{31}x_{32})$ $(y_1\alpha_2\alpha_3\alpha_4|\alpha_5\alpha_6\alpha_7y_8|y_9\alpha_{10}\alpha_{11}\alpha_{12}|\alpha_{13}\alpha_{14}\alpha_{15}y_{16}|y_{17}\alpha_{18}\alpha_{19}\alpha_{20}|\alpha_{21}\alpha_{22}\alpha_{23}y_{24}|y_{25}\alpha_{26}\alpha_{27}\alpha_{28}|\alpha_{29}\alpha_{30}\alpha_{31}y_{32}))$ Also, for different value of x_i $(1 \le i \le 32)$ and y_i (i = 1, 8, 9, 16, 17, 24, 25, 32), the corresponding 64-bit string is also different. Hence, a structure includes 2^{40} plaintexts, one structure proposes $2^{40} \times 2^{40} \times 2^{-1} = 2^{79}$ pairs of plaintexts.

Step 2 Take 2^N structures (2^{N+79} pairs of plaintexts). Choose pairs whose ciphertext difference $(\triangle L_{11}, \triangle R_{11})$ satisfy the following:

$\triangle L_{11} = (0000|0000|0000|0000|00ef|gh00|0000|0000)$,

$\triangle R_{11} = (0000|00p_1r_1|0000|00p_2r_2|0000|00p_3r_3|0000|00p_4r_4)$ where e, f, g and p_i, r_i $(1 \le i \le 4)$ are not all zero, and h is 1, there are 2^{12} $(\triangle L_{12}, \triangle R_{12})$, so the probability is about $2^{12} \times 2^{-64} = 2^{-52}$. Hence, the expected number of such pairs is $2^{N+79} \times 2^{-52} = 2^{N+27}$.

Step 3 Guess the 4-bit value at the $k_{11,26}$, $k_{11,27}$, $k_{11,28}$, $k_{11,29}$ of subkey k_{11}, for every remaining pair, calculate $s_7(L_{11,26} \oplus k_{11,26}) \oplus s_7(L^*_{11,26} \oplus k_{11,26})$, $s_7(L_{11,27} \oplus k_{11,27}) \oplus s_7(L^*_{11,27} \oplus k_{11,27})$, $s_7(L_{11,28} \oplus k_{11,28}) \oplus s_7(L^*_{11,28} \oplus k_{11,28})$, $s_8(L_{11,29} \oplus$

$k_{11,29}) \oplus s_8(L^*_{11,29} \oplus k_{11,29})$ and choose pairs which satisfy $s_7(L_{11,26} \oplus k_{11,26}) \oplus s_7(L^*_{11,26} \oplus k_{11,26}) = R_{11,26} \oplus R^*_{11,26}$, $s_7(L_{11,27} \oplus k_{11,27}) \oplus s_7(L^*_{11,27} \oplus k_{11,27}) = R_{11,27} \oplus R^*_{11,27}$, $s_7(L_{11,28} \oplus k_{11,28}) \oplus s_7(L^*_{11,28} \oplus k_{11,28}) = R_{11,28} \oplus R^*_{11,28}$, $s_8(L_{11,29} \oplus k_{11,29}) \oplus s_8(L^*_{11,29} \oplus k_{11,29}) = R_{11,29} \oplus R^*_{11,29}$. Since the probability is about 2^{-4}, the expected number of the remaining pairs is $2^{N+27} \times 2^{-4} = 2^{N+23}$.

Step 4 Guess the 32-bit value of the first round key k_1, for every remaining plaintext pair (L_0, R_0) and (L^*_0, R^*_0).

$L_0 = (x_1x_2x_3x_4|x_5x_6x_7x_8|\ldots|x_{29}x_{30}x_{31}x_{32})$,

$R_0 = (y_1\alpha_2\alpha_3\alpha_4|\alpha_5\alpha_6\alpha_7y_8|y_9\alpha_{10}\alpha_{11}\alpha_{12}|\alpha_{13}\alpha_{14}\alpha_{15}y_{16}|y_{17}\alpha_{18}\alpha_{19}\alpha_{20}|\alpha_{21}\alpha_{22}\alpha_{23}y_{24}|y_{25}\alpha_{26}\alpha_{27}\alpha_{28}|\alpha_{29}\alpha_{30}\alpha_{31}y_{32})$.

$L^*_0 = (x^*_1x^*_2x^*_3x^*_4|x^*_5x^*_6x^*_7x^*_8|\ldots|x^*_{29}x^*_{30}x^*_{31}x^*_{32})$,

$R^*_0 = (y^*_1\alpha_2\alpha_3\alpha_4|\alpha_5\alpha_6\alpha_7y^*_8|y^*_9\alpha_{10}\alpha_{11}\alpha_{12}|\alpha_{13}\alpha_{14}\alpha_{15}y^*_{16}|y^*_{17}\alpha_{18}\alpha_{19}\alpha_{20}|\alpha_{21}\alpha_{22}\alpha_{23}y^*_{24}|y^*_{25}\alpha_{26}\alpha_{27}\alpha_{28}|\alpha_{29}\alpha_{30}\alpha_{31}y^*_{32})$.

Compute (L_1, R_1) and (L^*_1, R^*_1), and choose pairs whose difference satisfy $R_1 \oplus R^*_1 = (000a|bcd0|0000|0000|0000|0000|0000|0000)$ where a, b, c and d are not all zero. Since the probability is about $(2^4-1) \times 2^{-32} = 2^{-28}$, the expected number of the remaining pairs is $2^{N+23} \times 2^{-28} = 2^{N-5}$.

Step 5 Guess the 4-bit value of the second round key k_2 at the four bits (4, 5, 6, 7), perform the following:

Step 5.1 For every remaining pair (L_0, R_0) and (L^*_0, R^*_0), and the corresponding output of the first round (L_1, R_1) and (L^*_1, R^*_1).

$L_1 = (y_1y_2\alpha_3\alpha_4|\alpha_5\alpha_6\alpha_7\alpha_8|y_9y_{10}\alpha_{11}\alpha_{12}|\alpha_{13}\alpha_{14}\alpha_{15}\alpha_{16}|y_{17}y_{18}\alpha_{19}\alpha_{20}|\alpha_{21}\alpha_{22}\alpha_{23}\alpha_{24}|y_{25}y_{26}\alpha_{27}\alpha_{28}|\alpha_{29}\alpha_{30}\alpha_{31}\alpha_{32})$,

$R_1 = (\gamma_1\gamma_2\gamma_3z_4|z_5z_6z_7\gamma_8|\gamma_9\gamma_{10}\gamma_{11}\gamma_{12}|\gamma_{13}\gamma_{14}\gamma_{15}\gamma_{16}|\gamma_{17}\gamma_{18}\gamma_{19}\gamma_{20}|\gamma_{21}\gamma_{21}\gamma_{23}\gamma_{24}|\gamma_{25}\gamma_{26}\gamma_{27}\gamma_{28}|\gamma_{29}\gamma_{30}\gamma_{31}\gamma_{32})$.

$L^*_1 = (y^*_1y^*_2\alpha_3\alpha_4|\alpha_5\alpha_6\alpha_7\alpha_8|y^*_9y^*_{10}\alpha_{11}\alpha_{12}|\alpha_{13}\alpha_{14}\alpha_{15}\alpha_{16}|y^*_{17}y^*_{18}\alpha_{19}\alpha_{20}|\alpha_{21}\alpha_{22}\alpha_{23}\alpha_{24}|y^*_{25}y^*_{26}\alpha_{27}\alpha_{28}|\alpha_{29}\alpha_{30}\alpha_{31}\alpha_{32})$,

$R^*_1 = (\gamma^*_1\gamma^*_2\gamma^*_3z^*_4|z^*_5z^*_6z^*_7\gamma^*_8|\gamma^*_9\gamma^*_{10}\gamma^*_{11}\gamma^*_{12}|\gamma^*_{13}\gamma^*_{14}\gamma^*_{15}\gamma^*_{16}|\gamma^*_{17}\gamma^*_{18}\gamma^*_{19}\gamma^*_{20}|\gamma^*_{21}\gamma^*_{21}\gamma^*_{23}\gamma^*_{24}|\gamma^*_{25}\gamma^*_{26}\gamma^*_{27}\gamma^*_{28}|\gamma^*_{29}\gamma^*_{30}\gamma^*_{31}\gamma^*_{32})$.

Compute $s_1(z_4 \oplus k_{2,4}) \oplus s_1(z^*_4 \oplus k_{2,4}) = v_4$, $s_2(z_5 \oplus k_{2,5}) \oplus s_2(z^*_5 \oplus k_{2,5}) = v_5$, $s_2(z_6 \oplus k_{2,5}) \oplus s_2(z^*_6 \oplus k_{2,6}) = v_6$, $s_2(z_7 \oplus k_{2,7}) \oplus s_2(z^*_7 \oplus k_{2,7}) = v_7$. Choose pairs whose difference and check whether its can satisfy above these conditions. Since the probability is about $(2^{-1})^4 \times (2^4-1)/2^4 = 2^{-4}$, the expected number of the remaining pairs is $2^{N-5} \times 2^{-4} = 2^{N-9}$.

Step 5.2 Further guess the 28-bit value of the second round key k_2 at the remaining 28 bits, for every remaining plaintext pair, calculate R_2 and R^*_2.

Step 6 For every remaining pair through compute and check whether $\triangle R_2 = (0000|0000|0000|0000|0000|0000|0000|0000)$. If yes, discard the candidate value of $(k_{11,26}, k_{11,27}, k_{11,28}, k_{11,29}, k_1, k_2)$. According to the key schedule of improved LBlock, we can get $k_1 = k_{79}k_{78\ldots}k_{48}$ and $k_2 = k_{47}k_{46\ldots}k_{16}$. Actually, we guess 64 bits key in total.

Since such a difference is impossible, every key that proposes such a difference is a wrong key. After analyzing ciphertext pairs, there remain only about $2^{64} \times (1-2^{-4})^{2N-9}$ wrong candidate value of $(k_{11,26}, k_{11,27}, k_{11,28}, k_{11,29}, k_1, k_2)$.

If we discard all wrong key, thus $2^{64} \times (1-2^{-4})^{2N-9} < 1$, $N \approx 19$, and only the correct subkey will be output.

The data and time complexities of above attack can be estimated as follows. First of all, we choose 2^{19} structures and the data complexity is $2^{19} \times 2^{40} = 2^{59}$ chosen plaintexts. The time complexity of Steps 3–6 for recovering 68 bits of key is as follows:

Step 3: $2 \times 2^4 \times 2^{2N+27} \times 4/8 = 2^{50}$
Step 4: $2 \times 2^4 \times 2^{32} \times 2 \times^{N+23} = 2^{79}$
Step 5.1: $2 \times 2^4 \times 2^{32} \times 2^4 \times 2^{2N-5} \times 4/8 = 2^{54}$
Step 5.2: $2 \times 2^4 \times 2^{32} \times 2^4 \times 2^{28} \times 2^{N-9} = 2^{60}$
Step 6: $2 \times 2^{64} \times \left\{1 + (1-2^{-4}) + (1-2^{-4})^2 + \cdots + (1-2^{-4})^{2^{N-1}-1}\right\} \times \frac{1}{8} \approx 2^{66}$

Therefore, the time complexity of the attack is about $(2^{50} + 2^{79} + 2^{54} + 2^{60} + 2^{66}) \times 1/11 \approx 2^{75.5}$ 11-round encryptions. According to the complexities of impossible differential attack on 11-round improved LBlock, we expect that the full 32-round improved LBlock has enough security margins against this attack.

71.4 Conclusion

In this paper, we gave an improvement on LBlock employed on bit-wise permutation layer by analyzing the structure of encryption. Since bit-wise permutation provides fast diffusion without hardware implementation cost and enhances security against impossible differential, saturation, meet-in-the-middle etc. Therefore, we have chosen a bit-wise permutation instead of word-wise. By analyzing the property of the diffusion transformation, it has shown that a new kind of 11-round impossible differential was presented. Our proposed attack requires approximately 2^{59} chosen plaintexts, $2^{75.5}$ 11-round encryptions. To the best of our knowledge, this is the first paper that proposes impossible differential analysis on improved LBlock.

References

1. Bogdanov A, Knudsen LR, Leander G, Paar C, Poschmann A, Robshaw M, Seurin Y, Vikkelsoe C (2007) PRESENT: an ultra-lightweight block cipher. In: Paillier P, Verbauwhede I (eds) Cryptographic hardware and embedded systems—CHES 2007, LNCS, vol 4727. Springer, Heidelberg, pp 450–466
2. Hong D, Sung J, Hong S, Lim J, Lee S, Koo B, Lee C, Chang D, Lee J, Jeong K, Kim H, Kim J, Chee S (2006) HIGHT: a new block cipher suitable for low-resource device. In: Goubin L, Matsui M (eds) CHES 2006, LNCS, vol 4249. Springer, Heidelberg, pp 46–59

3. Lim C, Korkishko T (2006) mCrypton–a lightweight block cipher for security of low-cost RFID tags and sensors. In: Song J, Kwon T, Yung M (eds) WISA 2005, LNCS, vol 3786. Springer, Heidelberg, pp 243–258
4. Leander G, Paar C, Poschmann A (2007) New lightweight DES variants. In: Biryukov A (ed) FSE 2007, LNCS, vol 4593. Springer, Heidelberg, pp 196–210
5. De Canniere C, Dunkelman O, Knezevic M (2009) KATAN and KTANTAN—a family of small and efficient hardware-oriented block ciphers. In: Clavier C, Gaj K (eds) CHES 2009, LNCS, vol 5747. Springer, Heidelberg, pp 272–288
6. Robshaw MJB (2006) Searching for compact algorithms: CGEN. In: Nguyen PQ (ed) VIETCRYPT 2006, LNCS, vol 4341. Springer, Heidelberg, pp 37–49
7. Izadi M, Sadeghiyan B, Sadeghian S, Khanooki H (2009) MIBS: A new lightweight block cipher. In: Garay JA, Miyaji A, Otsuka A (eds) CANS 2009, LNCS, vol 5888. Springer, Heidelberg, pp 334–348
8. Ojha S, Kumar N, Jain K, Sangeeta (2009) TWIS—A lightweight block cipher. In: Prakash A, Gupta I (eds) ICISS 2009, LNCS, vol 5905. Springer, Heidelberg, pp 280–291
9. Wenling W, Lei Z (2011) Applied cryptography and network security–ACNS 2011, LBlock: a lightweight block cipher. Lecture notes in computer science, vol 6715. Springer, Heidelberg, pp 327–344
10. Wu W, Zhang W, Feng D (2007) Impossible differential cryptanalysis of reduced-round ARIA and Camellia. J Comput Sci Technol 22(3):449–456
11. Chen J, Jia K, Yu H, Wang X (2011) New impossible differential attack of reduced-round camellia-192 and camellia-256. In: Parampalli U, Hawkes P (eds) ACISP 2011, LNCS, vol 6812. Springer, Heidelberg, pp 16–33

Chapter 72
Speckle Noise Reduction in Breast Ultrasound Images for Segmentation of Region Of Interest (ROI) Using Discrete Wavelets

S. Amutha, D. R. Ramesh Babu, R. Mamatha, S. Vidhya Suman and M. Ravi Shankar

Abstract Ultrasound imaging is a widely used diagnostic technique for the early detection of breast diseases. However, the usefulness of ultrasound imaging is degraded by the multiplicative speckle noise. This reduces the efficiency of diagnosis by radiologists. In order to improve the efficiency of diagnosis, we propose an algorithm for speckle denoising and edge enhancement for the segmentation of ROI. The algorithm is performed in three steps. In the first step, speckle denoising is achieved through shrinkage based on local variance matrix. The second step enhances the edges based on formation of homogenous blocks. The third steps segments the object boundaries based on K-means clustering algorithm. The results of the proposed method have been compared with the well known filters. The experimental results show that the proposed algorithm has considerably improved the image quality without providing any noticeable artifact.

Keywords Breast ultrasound · Speckle noise · Edge enhancement · Segmentation of ROI · Wavelets

72.1 Introduction

Breast cancer is the second leading cause of death among women according to cancer facts and figures 2012 [1]. Although Mammography is the primary method for breast cancer detection, it has some disadvantages. It is not accurate in detecting breast cancer [2]. As a result, approximately 65 % of cases referred to surgical biopsy are actually benign lesions [3, 4] which is stressful for patients. Ultrasound imaging is a safe noninvasive diagnostic technique [5]. It provides excellent contrast resolution, especially in differentiating the normal and malignant cells. However,

S. Amutha (✉) · D. R. Ramesh Babu · R. Mamatha · S. Vidhya Suman · M. Ravi Shankar
Department of Computer Science, Dayananda Sagar College of Engineering,
Bangalore, India
e-mail: amuthanaddhu@gmail.com

S. Li et al. (eds.), *Frontier and Future Development of Information Technology in Medicine and Education*, Lecture Notes in Electrical Engineering 269,
DOI: 10.1007/978-94-007-7618-0_72,

the main drawback of medical ultrasound image is the poor quality of images due to the speckles present in it [6]. Speckle in ultrasound B-scans is a granular structure which is caused by constructive and destructive coherent interferences of back scattered echoes [17]. To improve the human interpretation and for the image processing tasks like segmentation and registration [7], speckle denoising is very essential. To reduce speckle noise, many techniques like Kuan filter [8], Frost filter [9], Speckle Reduction Anisotropic Diffusion (srad) [10], and Wavelet thresholding [11] have been used. Temporal averaging technique increases the signal-to-noise ratio (SNR) by averaging multiple uncorrelated images that are obtained by the transducer shift. This method is good at reducing speckle noise but causes the loss of small details because of blurring [12]. Nonlinear coherent diffusion (NCD) model is effective for finding edge pixel and its orientation. But this method is difficult to find various sized edges because of the single-scale approach.

Multi-scale approach based on wavelet transform is chosen for filtering various sized edges by using both spatial and frequency information [13]. The method based on wavelet transform has three steps: First, the original image is decomposed by wavelet transform. Then, wavelet coefficients are modified. Finally, the refined image is reconstructed from the modified wavelet coefficients through the inverse wavelet transform.

72.2 Speckle Denoising and Edge Enhancement for Segmentation of ROI

The algorithm is performed in three steps sequentially. In the first step the speckle denoising is carried out using wavelet shrinkage. In the second step formation of homogenous blocks are adopted for edge enhancement. In the third step K-means clustering is used for segmenting the region of interest. Figure 72.1 shows the block diagram of the proposed algorithm.

72.2.1 Speckle Denoising

The drawback of the medical ultrasound image is its noisy nature. This is due to the multiplicative noise called speckles formed during the acquisition of the image. This degrades the visual evaluation. Daubechies wavelet is chosen for denoising due to the advantage of better representation of image semantics. First the image is decomposed into four subbands LL, LH, HL, HH where LL is low frequency subband and LH, HL, HH are the high frequency subbands. Total variation (TV) method based on Rudin-Osher-Fatemi (ROF) in Eq. (72.1) is used for denoising the LL co-efficients.

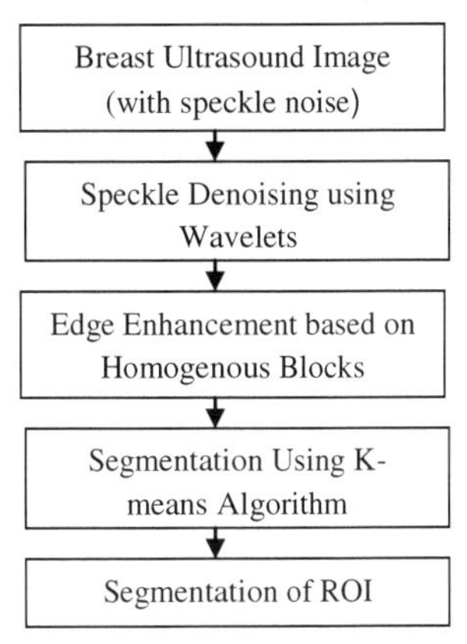

Fig. 72.1 Block diagram for the proposed methodology

$$\inf_{u}\left\{J(u)+(2\lambda)^{-1}\| f-u \|_{L^2}^{2}\right\} \tag{72.1}$$

where f is the noise image, u is the image that need to be restored from f, λ is a constant greater than zero and is a turning parameter. $J(u) = \int|\nabla_u|$ is often referred to as total variation(TV). For the higher frequency subbands, threshold is calculated using local variance using Eq. (72.2). The flowchart for speckle denoising is shown in Fig. 72.2.

$$V(i,j)=\frac{1}{L^2}\sum_{(p,q)\in Z_{ij}} C_{LH}^2(p,q)-\frac{1}{L^4}\left(\sum_{(p,q)\in Z_{ij}} C_{LH}(p,q)\right)^2 \tag{72.2}$$

where

$$Z_{ij}=\left[i-\frac{L-1}{2},i+\frac{L-1}{2}\right]\times\left[j-\frac{L-1}{2},j+\frac{L-1}{2}\right]$$

V(i, j) is the local variance applied on C_{LH} on a small window centered on (i, j), where i, j are positive integers and L is odd size of the small window. Then soft thresholding is applied to suppress the noise using equation (72.3)

$$f(x)=sign(x)(|x|-T) if |x|-T \; if \; |x|>T \; else \; 0 \tag{72.3}$$

Soft thresholding eliminates the discontinuity that is inherent in hard thresholding. In soft thresholding coefficients below a threshold 'T' are attributed to noise and are set to zero. Coefficients above the threshold 'T' are modified by subtracting the threshold from the coefficients.

72.2.2 Edge Enhancement

The denoised image from the previous stage is subjected to edge enhancement. We propose the edge enhancement based on grouping of homogeneous blocks. The image

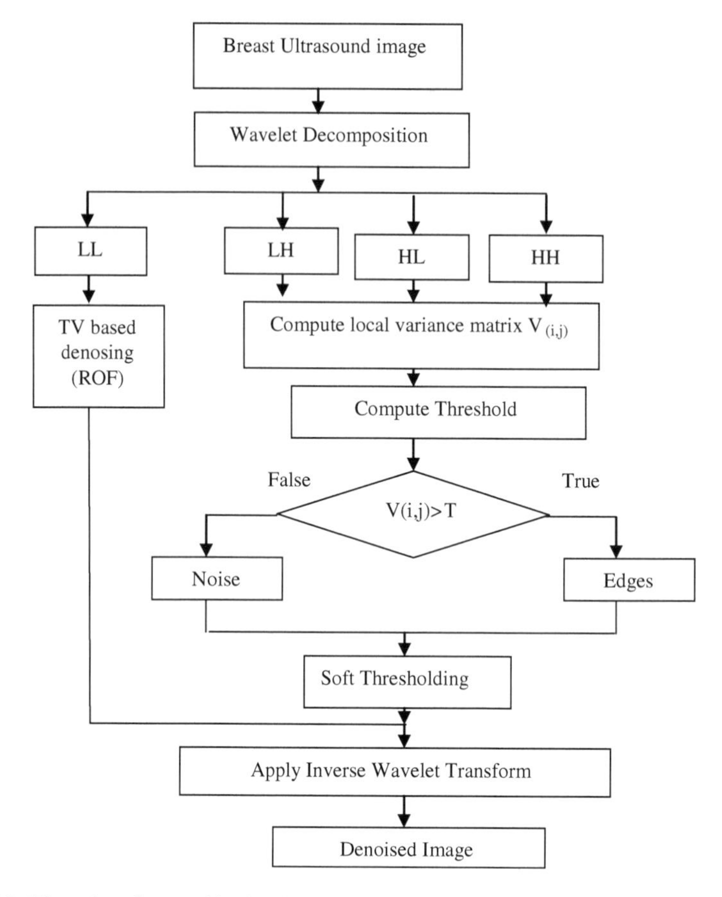

Fig. 72.2 Flow chart for speckle denoising

is divided into 2 × 2 homogenous blocks. The maximum valued pixel is selected from each block and the other pixels in the block are replaced with the maximum valued pixel. This procedure is iterated for the remaining blocks in the image.

72.2.3 Segmentation of ROI

K-means clustering [18] is used for segmenting the objects based on image features. The image features are classified based on their inherent distance from each other and the centroid. The pixels are clustered around centroids $\mu_i \forall_i = 1 \ldots\ldots\ldots k$ which are obtained by minimizing the objects using Eq. (72.4), from image S_i.

$$V = \sum_{i=1}^{k} \sum_{x_i \in s_i} \left(x_j - \mu_i\right)^2 \tag{72.4}$$

$i = 1,2 \ldots\ldots\ldots\ldots$ k and μ_i is the centroid or mean point of all the points $x_j \in s_i$.

72.3 Experimental Results and Discussions

In order to measure the performance of the proposed algorithm,breast ultrasound images are taken from the database "The Digital Database for Breast Ultrasound Image" [16]. Speckle noise with variance $\sigma_n = 0.5$ is added using the MATLAB command.The quantitative performance measures such as MSE, PSNR and Q are calculated.The subjective analysis is given in terms of visual quality of the images. The Mean square error (MSE) measures the quality change between the original and the processed image based on the Eq. (72.5).

$$MSE = \frac{1}{mn}\sum_{i=0}^{m-1}\sum_{j=0}^{n-1}[(i,j) - K(i,j)]^2 \tag{72.5}$$

The peak signal to noise ratio (PSNR) measures the image fidelity and calculated using the Eq. (72.6), The mathematically defined universal quality index Q models any distortion as a combination of three different factors: loss of correlation, luminance distortion, and contrast distortion.

$$PSNR = 20.\log_{10}(MAX_1) - 10.\log_{10}(MSE) \tag{72.6}$$

The results are compared with existing filters, Speckle reducing anisotropic diffusion filtering (srad), Wavelet shrinkage filter, Total variation filter. Table 72.1 shows the quantitative performance analysis of the proposed method, compared

Table 72.1 Image quality evaluation: MSE: mean square error, PSNR: peak signal to noise ratio, Q: universal quality ratio

Filter type	MSE	PSNR	Q
Srad	29.4551	31.6840	0.7249
Wavelet	94.5670	31.3837	0.7590
Total variation	124.2650	27.6355	0.7021
Proposed	24.1256	38.4571	0.9142

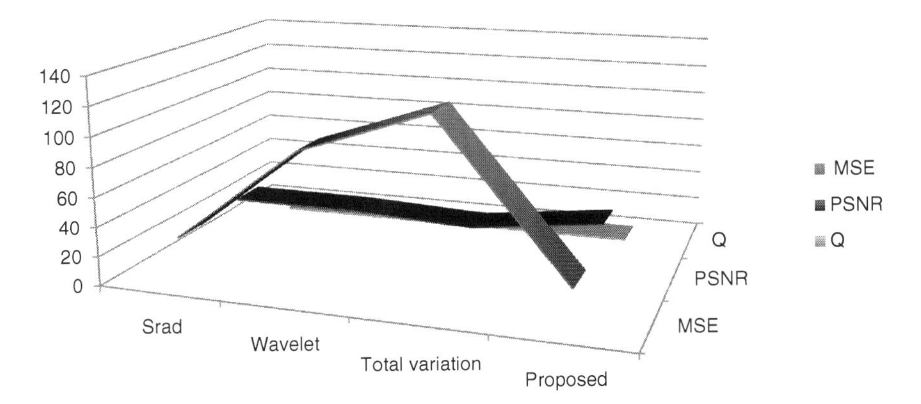

Fig. 72.3 3-D view of image quality evaluation

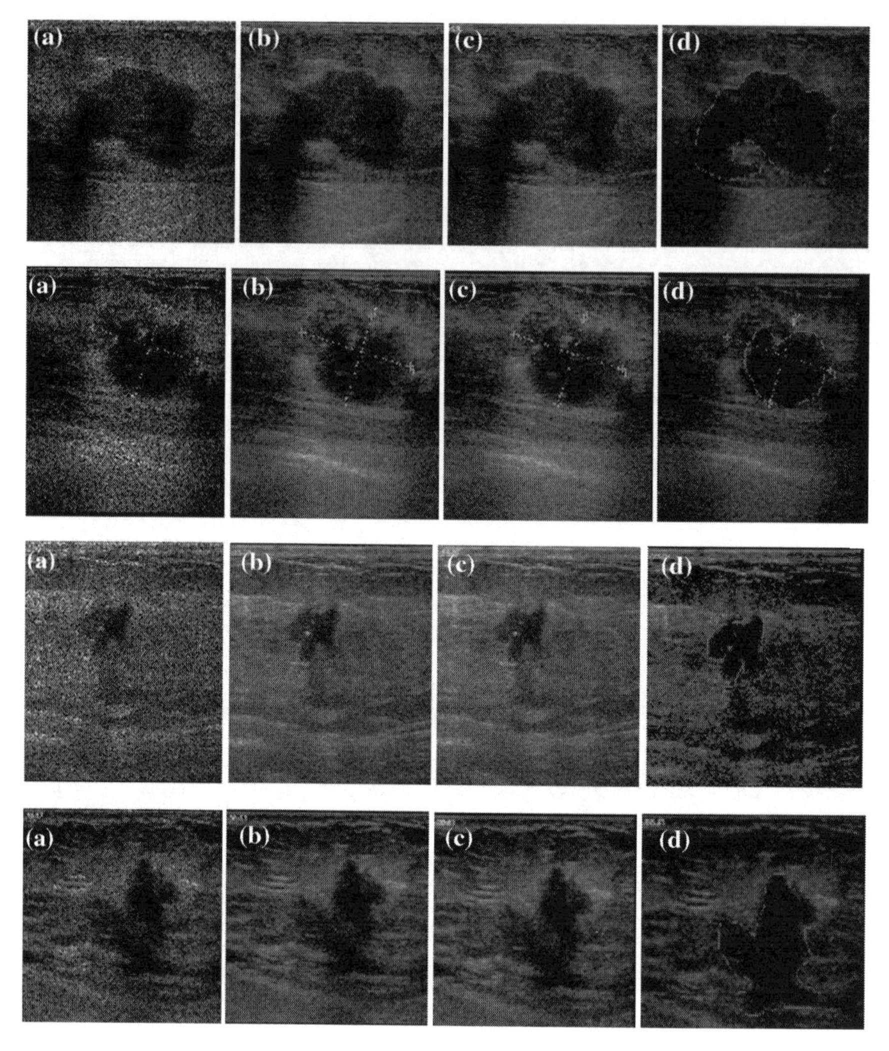

Fig. 72.4 **a** Image with speckles **b** speckle denoised **c** edge enhanced **d** segmented region

with the existing methods. The proposed method has considerably improved the image quality.

The comparative analysis of the image quality is given in Fig. 72.3. The subjective analysis is Fig. 72.4 shows the segmentation results.

72.4 Conclusions

In this study, we presented an effective algorithm which significantly reduced the speckles while preserving the resolution and the structure of the original ultrasound images. This helped in the accurate extraction of the region of interest. The algorithm was applied to the images from the database "The Digital Database for Breast Ultrasound Image". The algorithm consists of three stages which includes reduction of speckles with edge preservation, enhancement of the edges and segmentation of the ROI. The Daubechies wavelet was used for speckle denoising, grouping of homogenous pixels resulted in the edge enhancement. The proposed algorithm is more tolerant to noise than the existing ones. The experimental results shows that the proposed algorithm has considerably improved the image quality without generating any noticeable artifacts.

Acknowledgments The authors would like to thank Dr. Sairam Geethanath, HOD, Department of Medical Electronics, Dayanand Sagar College of Engineering, India for his support for the development of this work.

References

1. American Cancer Society Breast Cancer Facts and Figures (2012). Atlanta, US
2. Joseph YL, Carey EF (1999) Application of artificial neural networks for diagnosis of breast cancer. In: Proceedings of the congress of evolutionary computation, Washington, USA, 1755–1759
3. Kopans DB (1992) The positive predictive value of mammography. Am J Roentgenol 158(3):521–526
4. Knutzen AM, Gisvold JJ (1993) Likelihood of malignant disease for various categories of mammographically detected, nonpalpable breast lesions. Mayo Clinic Proc 68(5):454–460
5. Hoboken A (2003) Webb introduction to biomedical imaging. Wiley, New York, USA
6. Jain AK (1989) Fundamental of digital image processing. Prentice-Hall, NJ
7. Narayanan SK, Wahidabanu RSD (2009) A view on despeckling in ultrasound imaging. Int J Signal Process Image Process Pattern Recogn 2(3):85–98
8. Kaun DT, Sawchuk TC, Chavel SP (1987) Adoptive restoration of images with speckle. IEEE Trans Acoust Speech Signal Process. vol. ASSP-35
9. Frost VS, Stiles JA, Shanmugan KS, Hltzman JC (1982) A model for radar images and its application to adoptive digital filtering for multiplicative noise. IEEE Trans Pattern Anal Mach Intell. vol. PAMI-4
10. Yu Y, Acton ST (2002) Speckle reducing anisotropic diffijsion. IEEE Trans Image Process, 11(11) Nov 2002
11. Gupta N, Swamy MNS, Plotkin E (2005) Despeckling ofi medical ultrasoundi mages using data and rate adoptive lossy compression. IEEE Trans Med Imag 24(6) Jun 2005
12. Kim YS, Ra JB (2005) Improvement of ultrasound image based on wavelet transform: speckle reduction and edge enhancement. In: Proceedings of the SPIE Vol. 5747 (SPIE, Bellingham, WA)
13. Zhou Q, Liu L, Zhang D, Bian Z (2002) Denoise and contrast enhancement of ultrasound speckle image based on wavelet. In: Proceedings of the ICSP p 1500–1503

14. Xu Y, Nishimura T (2009) Segmentation of breast lesions in ultrasound images using spatial fuzzy clustering and structure Tensors. World Academy of Science, Engineering and Technology 53, Kitakyushu-shi, Japan
15. Wang Y-J, Lu S-X (2009) Breast ultrasound images enh ancement using fuzzy logic. doi 10.1109/DBTA.2009.90. Washington, USA
16. Tiana J-W, Wang Y, Huang J-H, Ning C-P, Wang.H-M, Liu Y, Tang X-L (2008) The digital database for breast ultrasound image. In: Proceedings of the 11th joint conference on information sciences, Harbin, China
17. Banazier AA, Kadah Y (2011) Speckle noise reduction method combining total variation and wavelet shrinkage for clinical ultrasound imaging. 978-1-4244-7000-6/11 © 2011 IEEE. Biomedical engineering department Cairo University Cairo, Egypt
18. Xinwu LI (2008) A volume segmentation algorithm for medical image based on K-means clustering. Int Conf Intell Inf Hiding Multimedia Sig Proc. 978-0-7695-3278-3/08 © 2008 IEEE doi 10.1109/IIH- MSP.2008.161

Chapter 73
Sonic Hedgehog Signaling Molecules Expression in TGF-β1-Induced Chondrogenic Differentiation of Rat Mesenchymal Stem Cells In Vitro

Yingchao Shi, Ying Jia, Shanshan Zu, Yanfei Jia, Xueping Zhang, Haiji Sun and Xiaoli Ma

Abstract Sonic Hedgehog (SHH) is involved in the induction of early artilaginous differentiation of mesenchymal cells in the limb and in the spine. Transforming growth factor beta 1 (TGF-β1) promotes chondrogenic differentiation of bone marrow mesenchymal stem cells (MSCs), while the signaling pathway by which TGF-β1 affects chondrogenic differentiation remains obscure. This study aimed to investigate expression of SHH- signaling molecules SHH and GLI1 during TGF-β1-induced chondrogenic differentiation of rat MSCs in vitro. TGF-β1 promoted chondrogenic differentiation of MSCs at 10 ng/ml from 7 to 21 days, demonstrated by enhancing cartilage markers collagen type II expression during chondrogenic differentiation. Expressions of Shh and Gli1, were tested by RT-PCR and western blot analysis during chondrogenic differentiation. Expressions of Shh and Gli1 were decreased compared to the control on both mRNA and protein level during TGF-β1-induced chondrogenic differentiation of MSCs from 7 to 21 days. Altogether, these data demonstrate that inactivation of SHH-GLI1 pathway during TGF-β1-induced chondrogenic differentiation of MSCs in vitro. These findings provide new data for the mechanistic link between TGF-β1-induced chondrogenic differentiation and Hedgehog signaling pathway.

Keywords Sonic hedgehog (SHH) · GLI1 · Chondrogenic differentiation · TGF-β1 · Mesenchymal stem cells Introduction

Y. Shi · X. Zhang · H. Sun (✉)
College of Life Science, Shandong Normal University, Jinan 250014, China
e-mail: sunhj5018@126.com

Y. Jia · S. Zu · Y. Jia · X. Ma (✉)
Medical Research and Laboratory Diagnostic Center, Jinan Central Hospital Affiliated to Shandong University, Jinan 250013, China
e-mail: mxl7125@126.com

S. Li et al. (eds.), *Frontier and Future Development of Information Technology in Medicine and Education*, Lecture Notes in Electrical Engineering 269,
DOI: 10.1007/978-94-007-7618-0_73,

73.1 Introduction

Articular cartilage (AC) is an avascular tissue composed of chondrocytes, responsible for abundant matrix synthesis and maintenance [8]. When damaged due to traumatic or pathological conditions, AC does not heal spontaneously under physiological circumstances, which results in Osteoarthritis (OA). Current treatment strategies are restricted to short-term symptomatic relief by pharmaceutical interventions and surgical procedures [10]. Therefore, treatment of cartilaginous damage poses a significant clinical challenge. Tissue engineering—based constructs to enhance OA-cartilage repair by mobilising chondrogenic cells is a promising approach for restoration of AC structure and function [1, 5].

Mesenchymal stem cells (MSCs) constitute a population of pluripotent cells within the bone marrow, which are capable of differentiating into a number of cell lineages including adipocytes, chondrocytes, myocytes and osteoblasts [3]. MSCs are considered as a promising candidate cell source for bone tissue engineering and regeneration. At present, two effective methods are used to induce the differentiation of stem cells into chondrocytes: the application of growth factors and co-culture. Recently, MSCs cultured in medium with transforming growth factor beta 1 (TGF-β1) produced a cartilage-specific matrix and showed evidence of chondrogenic potential [4, 12]. All these findings indicate that TGF-β1 has a significant effect on the chondrogenic differentiation of MSCs. However, the signaling pathway by which TGF-β1 affects chondrogenic differentiation of MSCs hasn't yet to be elucidated.

Sonic hedgehog (SHH) protein is known to be an important signaling protein in early embryonic development. Also, SHH is involved in the induction of early cartilaginous differentiation of mesenchymal cells in the limb and in the spine [6]. However, the role of SHH-GLI1 pathway in chondrogenic differentiation of MSCs induced by TGF-β1 is unclear. In this study, we study the expressions of SHH and GLI1 during chondrogenic differentiation of MSCs induced by TGF-β1 which provides the new data for engineering true hyaline cartilage in vitro.

73.2 Materials and Methods

73.2.1 Experimental Animals and Rat MSCs Isolation

All experiment animals were approved by the Local Ethics Committee for Animal Care and Use of Shandong University in China. Twenty 4-week-old Wistar male rats weighing approximately 90 $\sim$ 100 g were purchased from Shandong University Animal Center (Jinan, China). Rats were killed by cervical dislocation method. The bilateral femora and tibias were dissected under aseptic conditions. The bone marrow cells were flushed out of the femora and tibias with Dulbecco's modified Eagle's medium–low glucose (DMEM–LG, Gibco, NY, USA) by a 5-ml syringe. The marrow cells were seeded at a concentration of 5 × 10^5/cm^2 in 30 ml plastic flasks (Corning, USA) containing DMEM–LG supplemented with 10 % fetal calf serum (Gibco, Milan, Italy), 1 % glutamine (Sigma, St. Louis, MO), and 1 % penicillin–streptomycin (Sigma). The cells were then incubated in 5 % CO_2 at 37 °C, and the medium was changed every 3 days. When the cells reached 80 ~ 90 % confluency in the flasks, cells were trypsinized (0.25 % trypsin, Gibco) and expanded into plates as passage.

73.2.2 Induction of Chondrogenic Differentiation in Rat MSCs

Rat MSCs from passage 3 were seeded in 6-well plates at the concentration of 1 × 10^5/cm^2. After pre-cultured for 24 h, the MSCs were allowed to culture in chondrogenic differentiation medium (including 10 ng/ml TGF-β1, 10 mmol/L β-glycerophosphate, 50 μg/ml Vitamin C) according to the experimental requirements for 7, 14 and up to 21 days. All MSCs were incubated in 5 % CO2 at 37 °C, and the medium was replaced every 3 days before harvest [15] according to the experimental requirements for up to 21 days. All MSCs were incubated in 5 % CO_2 at 37 °C, and the medium was replaced every 3 days before harvest.

73.2.3 Immunocytochemistry

MSCs were fixed with 4 % paraformaldehyde in PBS (pH 7.4), permeabilized with 0.5 % Triton X-100 in PBS, and washed with PBS at room temperature. After blocking with 5 % non-fat dry milk in PBS, cells were incubated with the goat anti-collagen type II antibody, one of cartilage markers, (1:100, Santa Cruz Biotechnology, CA, USA) at 4 °C for 12 h. Cells were proceeded to incubate with rat anti-goat IgG HRP (1:500, Santa Cruz Biotechnology, CA, USA) at 37 °C for 1 h. Washed with PBS for three times. Then, the staining was developed with a DAB staining kit according to the manufacturer's protocol (Zhongshan Golden Bridge, Beijing, China) and visualized by using a converted microscope.

73.2.4 RT-PCR Analysis

Total RNA was isolated by using Trizol reagent (Invitrogen, CA, USA) according to the manufacturer's protocol. RT-PCR was performed by M-MLV Reverse Transcriptase (Invitrogen, CA, USA) according to the manufacturer's specifications. Briefly, first strand cDNAs were synthesized at 37 °C for 1 h in 20 μl reaction mixture using 2 μg isolated mRNA. The serially diluted first-strand cDNA samples were used as templates. β-actin was a normalization control for RT-PCR synthesis of cDNAs. The primer sequences were listed as follows: Shh: 5′-CAATTACAACCCCGACATCA-3′ (forward) and 5′-AGTCACTCGAA GCTTCACTCC-3′ (reverse); Gli1: 5′-TTCAACTCGATGACCCCACC-3′ (forward) and 5′-GGCACTAGAGTTGAGGAATT-3′ (reverse). PCR amplification was performed for 30 cycles, and the cycling conditions were as follows: 94 °C for 30 s, 59 °C (β-actin) or 53 °C (Shh and Gli1) for 40 s, 72 °C for 45 s, with a final extension at 72 °C for 10 min. PCR products were assayed by 1 % agarose gel electrophoresis and analyzed under UVI gel-image analysis system (UVI, UK). Relative density of objective mRNA was indicated by the ratio of $OD_{objective}$ to $OD_{\beta\text{-actin}}$.

73.2.5 Western Blot Analysis

Cells were suspended in standard sodium dodecyl sulfate (SDS) sample buffer. Protein concentrations were determined with a Bio-Rad protein assay kit, using bovine serum albumin (BSA) as reference. Proteins (50 ng) were separated on SDS–polyacrylamide gels electrophoresis (10 % acrylamide), transferred to nitrocellulose membranes, and then probed with goat anti-SHH (1:500, Abcam, USA), rabbit anti-GLI1(1:500, Abcam, USA) and rabbit anti-GAPDH (1:2000, Sigma, USA), followed by incubation with horseradish peroxidase-conjugated secondary antibodies (ICN, USA). Proteins were visualized with a SuperSignal West Pico chemiluminescence kit (Pierce, USA).

73.2.6 Statistical Analysis

Data were expressed as mean ± SEM. Statistical significance was assessed at $P < 0.05$. Experiments were independently triplicated and results were qualitatively identical.

73.3 Results

73.3.1 Expression of Collagen Type II in MSCs during Chondrogenic Differentiation Induced by TGF-β1

Cells in the mesenchymal condensation differentiate into chondrogenic lineage based on simultaneous expression patterns for known cartilage markers aggrecan, Sox9, CEP-68, and collagen type II and X [14]. Here, collagen type II expression

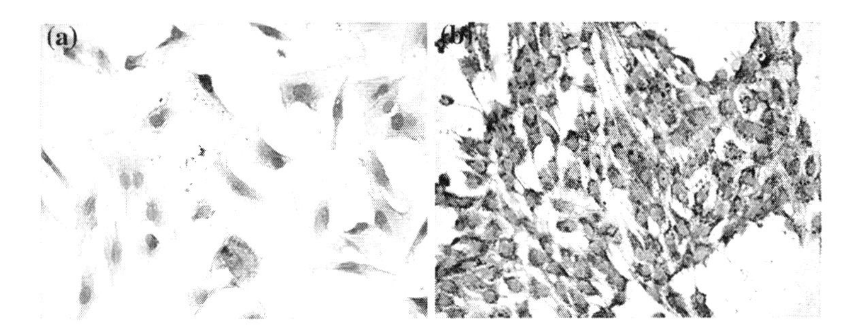

Fig. 73.1 Positive expression of type II collagen during chondrogenic differentiation in different periods ($\times$ 40). *A* MSCs;*B* induction 24d

was tested to determine chondrogenic differentiation in rat MSCs treated with 10 ng/ml TGF-β1, 10 mmol/L β-glycerophosphate, 50 μg/ml Vitamin C for 0, 7, 14 and 21 days. Treatment with TGF-β1 chondrogenic differentiation medium for 7, 14, and 21 days significantly enhanced the number of collagen type II positive cells ($P < 0.01$) (Fig. 73.1).

73.3.2 Shh and Gli1 mRNA Expression During TGF-β1-Induced Chondrogenic Differentiation in MSCs

Hedgehog signaling pathway (Hh) has been associated with the proliferation of MSCs, and played a major role in the induction of chondrogenic differentiations. However, there are little available data about the role of Hedgehog signaling molecules in chondrogenic differentiation of bone marrow mesenchymal stem cells induced by TGF-β1. In the nucleus, signaling of hedgehog is mediated by transcription factors of the Gli family, Gli1, Gli2, and Gli3. Gli transcription factors activate or repress downstream targets that mediate Hedgehog signaling. Gli3 has been shown to mainly act as a repressor of Ihh target genes in chondrocytes, but the role of other Gli isoforms is less clear [7]. Our results indicated that after 10 ng/ml TGF-β1 treatment, mRNA expression of Shh was down-regulated and expression of Gli1 was also down-regulated, as compared with that of control cells (Fig. 73.2).

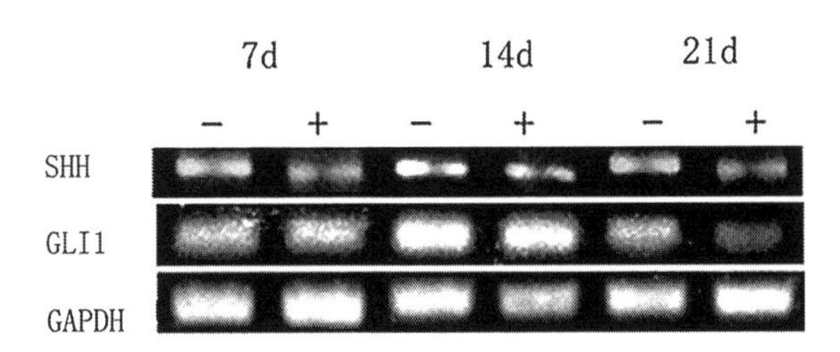

Fig. 73.2 Shh and Gli1 mRNA expression during chondrogenic differentiation of MSCs. 7d, 14d, 21d mean the time of TGF-β1 treatment

73.3.3 SHH and GLI1 Expression During TGF-β1-Induced Chondrogenic Differentiation in MSCs

To confirm that TGF-β1 changed expression of genes in the Hedgehog signaling pathway, western blot experiments were carried out on SHH and GLI1 protein expression. We analyzed SHH and GLI1 expression in rat MSCs treated with 10 ng/ml TGF-β1 for 0, 7, 14 and 21 days. This concentration of TGF-β1 significantly increased expression of collagen type II. The expression level of SHH decreased in TGF-β1 induction group compared with non-induction group (Fig. 73.3) ($P < 0.01$). Meanwhile expressions of GLI1 decreased in the induction group compared with non-induction group (Fig. 73.4) ($P < 0.01$). The expression of the hedgehog target molecule GLI1 obviously decreased after 21d TGF-β1 induction ($P < 0.01$).

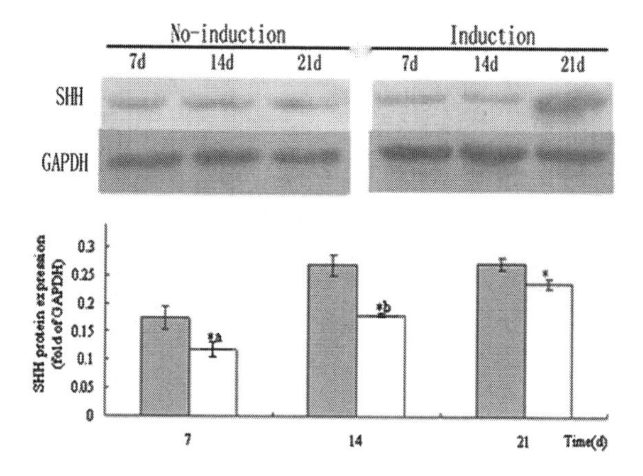

Fig. 73.3 Expression of SHH during chondrogenic differentiation in MSCs. *$P < 0.05$, induction groups versus non-induction groups. $^{a}P < 0.05$, 7d versus 14d in induction groups

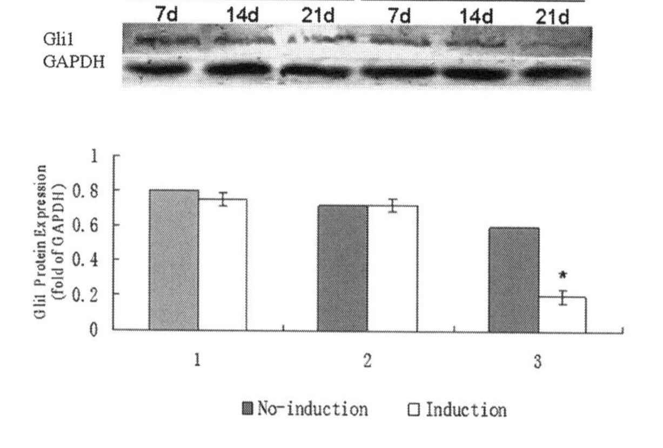

Fig. 73.4 Expression of GLI1 during chondrogenic differentiation in MSCs. *$P < 0.05$, induction groups versus non-induction groups

73.4 Discussion

TGF-β1 and TGF-β3 belong to the TGF-β super family of signaling molecules. The chondrogenic properties of TGF-β3 on MSCs in vitro are well known [2]. TGF-β1 and TGF-β3 share similar effects on mammalian cells and differ mainly in their potency. Yet the signaling pathway by which TGF-β1 affects chondrogenic differentiation remains obscure. The objectives of this study were to show the correlation between TGF-β1 induced chondrocyte differentiation and SHH-GLI1 pathway.

Sonic hedgehog (Shh) protein is known to be an important signaling protein in early embryonic development. In addition, Shh is involved in the induction of early cartilaginous differentiation of mesenchymal cells in the limb and in the spine [13, 16]. Transcription factors of the Gli family, Gli1, Gli2, and Gli3 activate or repress downstream targets that mediate Hedgehog signaling. Gli3 has been shown to mainly act as a repressor of Ihh target genes in chondrocytes, while the role of Gli1 is less clear in chondrogenic differentiation.

Present study confirmed that TGF-β1 promoted chondrogenic differentiation in rat mesenchymal stem cells at the concentration of 10 ng/ml from 7 to 21 days, demonstrated by up-regulation expression of collagen type II, one of cartilage markers. Here, we investigated the expressions of SHH and GLI1 during chondrocyte differentiation induced by TGF-β1 in MSCs. The present study showed that TGF-β1decreased Shh expression and Gli1 expression on both RNA level and protein level during chondrocyte differentiation in MSCs. The expression level of Gli1 was significantly down-regulated after 21d, suggesting that TGF-β1 decreased SHH expression via a GLI1-dependent mechanism during chondrogenic differentiation of MSCs. Our results suggested inactivation of Sonic Hedgehog-GLI1 Pathway in TGF-β1-induced chondrogenic differentiation of rat mesenchymal stem cells in vitro.

In summary, these results demonstrate that TGF-β1 can affect SHH and GLI1 expression during chondrogenic differentiation of MSCs, confirming and extending the findings of Hedgehog signaling pathway involving in chondrogenic differentiation [9, 11]. These findings provide insights into the mechanistic link between Hedgehog signaling pathway and TGF-β1-induced chondrogenic differentiation of MSCs. Since the mechanism of hedgehog signaling pathway involving in TGF-β1-induced chondrogenic differentiation of MSCs is not fully known yet, further studies will need to identify additional details about this association.

Acknowledgments This work was supported by the National Nature Science Foundation of China (No. 81272588) and the Shandong High School Science & Technology Fund Planning Project (J11LC14).

References

1. Ahmed TA, Giulivi A, Griffith M, Hincke M (2011) Fibrin glues in combination with mesenchymal stem cells to develop a tissue-engineered cartilage substitute. Tissue Eng Part A 17:323–335
2. Arévalo-Silva CA, Cao Y, Weng Y, Vacanti M, Rodriguez A, Vacanti CA et al (2001) The effect of fibroblast growth factor and transforming growth factor-β on porcine chondrocytes and tissue-engineered autologous elastic cartilage. Tissue Eng 7:81–88
3. Beyer Nardi N, da Silva Meirelles L (2006) Mesenchymal stem cells: isolation, in vitro expansion and characterization. Handb Exp Pharmacol 174:249–282
4. Gong G, Ferrari D, Dealy CN, Kosher RA (2010) Direct and progressive differentiation of human embryonic stem cells into the chondrogenic lineage. J Cell Physiol 224:664–671
5. Hattori K, Ohgushi H (2009) Progress of research in osteoarthritis. Tissue engineering therapy for osteoarthritis. Clin Calcium 19:1621–1628
6. Hong D, Chen HX, Ge RS, Li JC (2008) The biological roles of extracellular and intracytoplasmic glucocorticoids in skeletal cells. J Steroid Biochem Mol Biol 111:164–170
7. Kesper DA, Didt-Koziel L, Vortkamp A (2010) Gli2 activator function in preosteoblasts is sufficient to mediate Ihh-dependent osteoblast differentiation, whereas the repressor function of Gli2 is dispensable for endochondral ossification. Dev Dyn 239:1818–1826
8. Koelling S, Kruegel J, Irmer M, Path JR, Sadowski B, Miro X, Miosge N (2009) Migratory chondrogenic progenitor cells from repair tissue during the later stages of human osteoarthritis. Cell Stem Cell 4:324–335
9. Lin AC, Seeto BL, Bartoszko JM, Khoury MA, Whetstone H, Ho L et al (2009) Modulating hedgehog signaling can attenuate the severity of osteoarthritis. Nat Med 15:1421–1425
10. Lohmander LS, Roos EM (2007) Clinical update: treating osteoarthritis. Lancet 370:2082–2084
11. Mak KK, Kronenberg HM, Chuang P-T, Mackem S, Yang Y (2008) Indian hedgehog signals independently of PTHrP to promote chondrocyte hypertrophy. Development 135:1947–1956
12. Nakagawa T, Lee SY, Reddi AH (2009) Induction of chondrogenesis from human embryonic stem cells without embryoid body formation by bone morphogenetic protein 7 and transforming growth factor beta1. Arthritis Rheum 60:3686–3692
13. Sterling JA, Oyajobi BO, Grubbs B, Padalecki SS, Munoz SA, Story B et al (2006) The hedgehog signaling molecule Gli2 induces parathyroid hormone-related peptide expression and osteolysis in metastatic human breast cancer cells. Cancer Res 66:7548–7753
14. Vinatier C, Bouffi C, Merceron C, Gordeladze J, Brondello JM, Jorgensen C et al (2009) Cartilage tissue engineering: towards a biomaterial-assisted mesenchymal stem cell therapy. Current Stem Cell Res Ther 4:318–329
15. Zhao L, Hantash BM (2011) TGF-β1 regulates differentiation of bone marrow mesenchymal stem cells. Vitam Horm 87:127–141
16. Zunich SM, Douglas T, Valdovinos M, Chang T, Bushman W, Walterhouse D et al (2009) Paracrine sonic hedgehog signalling by prostate cancer cells induces osteoblast differentiation. Mol Cancer 8:12

Chapter 74
A FCA-Based Approach to Data Integration in the University Information System

Yong Liu and Xueqing Li

Abstract The relational database is the most widely used data access and organization model in the current system of university education information. It has positive significance for promoting the process of data integration, to be found from the database the corresponding ontology, to build a data model. In this paper, based on the theory of formal concept analysis (FCA) discovers the ontology from a relational database, and tries to establish the data integration model in domain-specific, in order to discover the concept of hierarchical relationships of the data and semantic information more objectively. This method maintains not only the original data semantic relationships of relational database tables, but also the use of the theory of FCA to automatically extract the characteristics of semantic information to improve the quality and reliability of the final data model. Combined with common MIS in the university, the paper uses the proposed method, tries to demonstrate the process of building a title appraisal system data model from relational database query result set (section), and verifies the effectiveness of the method discussed.

Keywords Formal concept analysis · Concept lattice · Data integration · Hasse diagram

74.1 Introduction

With the accelerating process of university informatization, the information systems which are using for teaching, scientific research and management are increasingly rich in universities. However, due to the university information

Y. Liu (✉)
School of Computer Science and Technology, Shandong University, Jinan 250101, China
e-mail: liuyong@sdu.edu.cn

X. Li
Department of Computer Engineering, Changji University, Changji 831100, China
e-mail: xqli@sdu.edu.cn

S. Li et al. (eds.), *Frontier and Future Development of Information Technology in Medicine and Education*, Lecture Notes in Electrical Engineering 269,
DOI: 10.1007/978-94-007-7618-0_74,

system construction with long time, the lack of unified planning and other reasons. It's led to the emergence of the so-called *islands of information* between the various systems, so that departments cannot be shared with the educational foundation information. To solve this problem, this paper presents the integrated part of the MIS system in university for accessing to data consistency and validity.

Domain-specific data model building process is actually from the existent various semantic data model which are extracted and automatic process of organization, and generate ontology. Ontology learning objects has dictionary, knowledge base, text, relational Schema, and semi-structured data (XML Schema) [5, 6]. In the current education informatization system, the relational data model is the main access and data organization model. From the database, most of concept extraction methods are to obtain a relational database schema information by reading the data dictionary. And then according to the corresponding relationship between entities to define a set of mapping rules, so as to realize the building of domain-specific data model [3]. There are also some domestic scholars dedicated to mapping from relational database to ontology research. These methods are research ontology concept extraction. Most of these methods is to study the extraction and representation of the ontology concepts and their hierarchical relationships. Relying on manual, however, from the data table or E-R model for the concept of hierarchy is too flat. Between the concepts of semantic information cannot be fully embody, in order to get more objective the concept of hierarchical and semantic information.

This paper presents a method to build domain-specific data model from a relational database based on the theory of FCA, and the paper will be in the University Information System Integration application examples to illustrate it. The focus on the ontology found in the University several independent information systems, and learns to build an integrated data model.

74.2 Formal Context and Formal Concept Analysis Theory

FCA (Formal Concept Analysis) is a mathematical tool which was first used by the German scholar Rudolf Wille. For data analysis and rule extraction from the formal context, concept lattice. It has been widely studied and applied to machine learning, software engineering, and access to information and other fields. The detail description about FCA and concept lattice can be found in references [7].

FCA is not realistic modeling, and concept lattice is given data on the basis of domain knowledge to analyze and structured. FCA is always dependent on a given formal concept, however, ontology can be established without given data. FCA in the concept of extension and intension is also primarily two aspects of ontology, however, ontology is more focus on the concept intension part. FCA and ontology have their own characteristics. They can complement each other in the following two aspects. On the one hand, FCA as a technique for ontology engineering, the concept lattice is used to extract the given data conceptual level, and as the basis of ontology applications, for manual or semi-automatic to generate ontology, and the ontology visualization and analysis tasks. On the other hand, the ontology can improve the application of the FCA. FCA attributes without any structure. If the properties of the FCA is as ontology concept, you can build the relationships and interdependencies between attributes to improve the quality of the application of the FCA.

Philipp in the literature [2] pointed out that there was a two-way interactive relationship between FCA and Ontology. FCA is a technology of the ontology theory works, by the concept lattice to aid access to structured data, or you can extract useful conceptual level from a known object data set as a basis for building ontology. Combined with FCA and ontology theory can help the domain knowledge ontology modeling in the following two aspects improved. On the one hand, FCA introduced ontology building process can improve concepts found and organizations affected by the subjective impact of development. On the other hand, Concept lattice representing the concept from the given data can help developers find all possible abstract concepts and relationships.

74.3 Based on FCA Theory to Build Domain-specific Data Model

Contrast relational model, ontology is able to express complex semantic data model. Happel and Seedorf [4] tried to work out a method to build knowledge ontology, but as he pointed out in the article, they are not to be given a set of normative guidelines. However, this method can play role in their research environment. This paper presents the main task of ontology learning based on relational database what is the use of FCA to analyze the implication of the semantic information in the relational model, and mapped into the ontology concepts and properties. This study and application background are shown in Fig. 74.1.

Title Appraisal System construction depends on the three applications of the *External data sources*, *Personnel Management MIS*, *Scientific Research MIS* and *Undergraduate Teaching MIS*. In the process of Fig. 74.1, the data integration process is divided into three stage: the relational tables pretreatment, construct formal context, through the concept lattice to ontology model mapping to establish data model.

74.3.1 The Original Data Table Pretreatment

Assume R expressed a two-dimensional relational tables. Query result set from an external data source (relational database), two situations may arise. First case, all database table is R^* after pretreatment, can pose a direct the formal concept C of

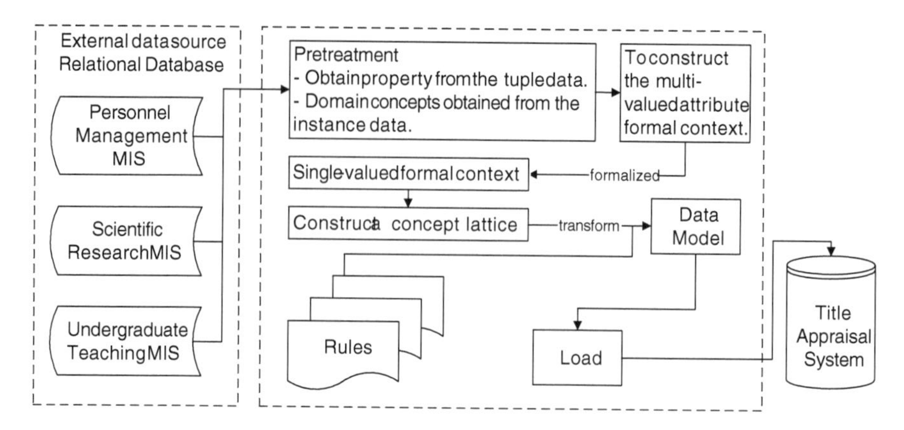

Fig. 74.1 Data integration process

the object-relational database. The second case, a number of non-defined relationship R is obtained. Finally, depending on the application purpose, by hand on R^* table merge operations to form the original formal concept C. Most of the data in the data table is multi-valued, C is also a multi-value of the object database formal concept.

We get three groups teacher information on the query result set from the three relational database in Fig. 74.1. Multi-valued formal context shown in Tables 74.1, 74.2, 74.3. Having regard to the article the reasons for the limited space and personal privacy. We select only the part of the data in the result set is used to illustrate the problem.

74.3.2 Single-Valued Formal Concept Generation Method

For multi-valued formal concept defined as follows.

Definition 1 A multi-value formal concept can be expressed using the four-tuple (O, A, W, R), it is a collection of objects O, and multi-valued attribute set A, and the attribute value range W, and several sets between a ternary relation $R(R \in$

Table 74.1 Teachers' basic information query result set (section)

Object	Degree	Professional title	Major
1	Ph. D.	Associate Professor	Applied chemistry
2	Ph. D.	Lecturer	Physical geography
3	Ph. D.	Associate Professor	Physical geography
4	M.E.	Lecturer	Inorganic chemistry
5	M.E.	Assistant	Inorganic chemistry

The data in this table from *Personnel Management MIS* as shown in Fig. 74.1

Table 74.2 Teachers' workload query result set (section)

Object	Teaching types	Semester	Definition	Teaching objects	Course hours
1	Class teaching	2010.9–2011.1	Physical geography	Bachelor,42	68
1	Class teaching	2010.9–2011.1	Environmental chemistry	Bachelor,42	68
2	Class teaching	2011.9–2012.1	Physical geography	Bachelor,45	68
2	Thesis guidance	2011.9–2012.6	Null	Bachelor,5	75
3	Thesis guidance	2011.9–2012.6	Null	Bachelor,5	60

The data in this Table *Undergraduate Teaching MIS* as shown in Fig. 74.1

Table 74.3 Teachers' scientific research query result set (section)

Object	Category	Time	Definition	Journals	Project sources
1	Published	2012.3	Effect of montmorillonite on arsenic accumulation…	African Journal of Biotechnology	Null
1	Published	2012.6	Heavy metal induced ecophysiological function …	African Journal of Biotechnology	Null
2	Project	2012.5–2013.5	South Xinjiang bilingual teachers Tepei …	Null	Xinjiang, university research projects
3	Published	2011.9	The road dust PGEs time change characteristics	Environmental Science	Null
3	Project	2012.1–2014.12	Cumulative process in arid areas … (41101497)	Null	National natural science foundation

The data in this table from *Scientific Research MIS* as shown in Fig. 74.1

$O \times A \times W)$ is constituted. When the conditions $(o, a, w) \in R$ and $(o, a, v) \in R$ is satisfied, $w = v$ was established.

If conditions comply with the set of $G(G \subseteq A)$, then all elements g in G are corresponding with w_g. Which $w_g = (w|wRg, g \in G \wedge w \in W)$ I expressed that the collection of a binary relation between A collection W. Afterwards, in order to better discover the information implicit in the formal concept. According to the vacancy situation of the property value. Attribute reduction of single-valued formal concept C^* is executed. Leaving only be able to fully determine the minimum set of attributes of the concept and the formal concept hierarchy.

In accordance with the above-described method, through each of the scanning multi-value formal concept attribute column in Tables 74.1, 74.2, 74.3, split the

Table 74.4 Single-value formal concept of teachers' basic information

Object	Professional title			Degree		Major		
	AP	LT	AT	D1	D2	M1	M2	M3
1	X			X		X		
2		X		X			X	
3	X			X			X	
4		X			X			X
5			X		X			X

AP Associate Professor, *LT* Lecturer, *AT* Assistant, *D1* Ph. D., *D2* M.E., *M1* Applied Chemistry, *M2* Physical geography, *M3* Inorganic Chemistry

text attribute columns, clustering a numeric attribute columns, filter out date types, and big data objects (binary). Finally, obtain a corresponding single value formal concept shown in Tables 74.4, 74.5, 74.6.

In the process of conversion from the formal context of the multi-valued to single-valued formal context, in order to get a clearer picture on the part of a significant single-valued attribute. Taking into account the complexity of the subsequent Hasse diagram. We streamline manual part of the concept of multi-valued attributes. For example, in Table 74.3, *Time* and *definition.*

Table 74.5 Single-value formal concept of teachers' workload

Object	Types		Semester			Teaching objects		
	CT	TG	S1	S2	S3	O1	O2	O3
1	X		X			X		
1	X		X			X		
2	X			X			X	
3		X			X			X
3		X			X			X

CT Class Teaching, *TG* Thesis Guidance, *S1* 2010.9-2011.1, *S2* 2011.9–2012.1, *S3* 2011.9–2012.6, *O1* Bachelor,42, *O2* Bachelor,45, *O3* Bachelor,5

Table 74.6 Single-value formal concept of teachers' scientific research

Object	Category		Journals			Project sources		
	C1	C2	J1	J2	J3	P1	P2	P3
1	X		X					X
1	X		X					X
2		X			X	X		
3	X			X				X
3		X			X		X	

C1 Published, *C2* Project, *J1* African Journal of Biotechnology (SCI), *J2* Environmental Science, *J3* Null, *P1* Xinjiang, university research projects, *P2* National Natural Science Foundation, *P3* Null

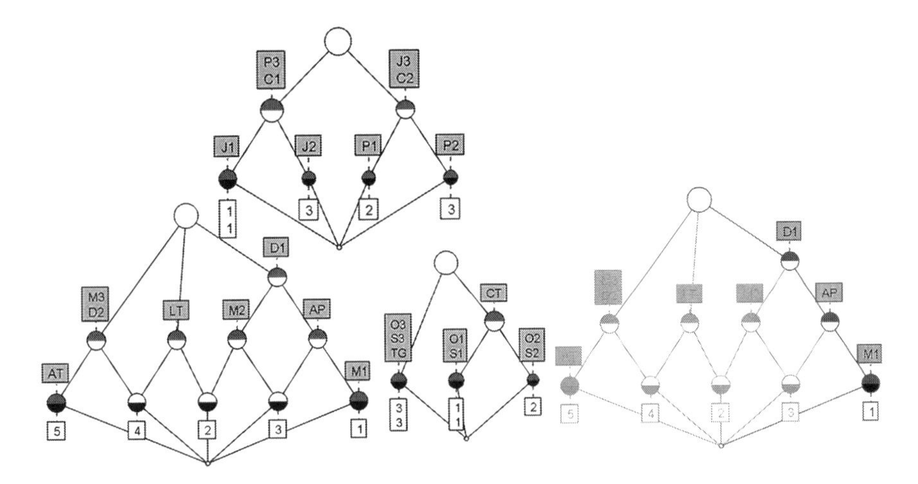

Fig. 74.2 Simplified symbols' Hasse diagram of the formal context

74.3.3 The Original Data Table Pretreatment

Generated concept lattice algorithm from the formal concept can be roughly divided into two categories. They are Batch construction algorithm and incremental construction algorithm [1]. In this paper, it is adopted a breadth first search (BFS) and bottom-up batch algorithm to construct concept lattice. The details of the algorithm, please read the literature [8]. Based on the generated concept lattice to give its corresponding Hasse diagram, as shown in Fig. 74.2. Then the Hasse diagram is re-circulating trimmed to remove the concept of unreasonable.

The Hasse diagram Fig. 74.2 is a simplified of the concept lattice numeral view. In fact, each node contains a collection of objects and a set of attributes. In this simplified Hasse diagram, all child nodes of this node object reference numeral constitute a collection of objects for each node, and all parent nodes of node attributes reference numeral constitute a collection of properties for each node. For example, the label 1 in Fig. 74.2, i.e. which means that the corresponding concept ({1}, {M1, AP, D1}).

In Hasse diagram, the hierarchical relationship between the concept lattice nodes corresponding to the relationship between the parent and child classes in the ontology, a node can be defined as a class in the ontology. Contained an object concept lattice nodes is equivalent to an instance of the class in the ontology. The concept lattice node object attribute is equivalent to the class attributes of ontology. Therefore, a concept lattice of generated by formal concept can be seen as the prototype of an ontology, yet still based on domain knowledge for further expansion. Specific conversion steps are as follows.

Step 1. First remove the Hasse diagram in concept node under the element.

Step 2. Removal under the elements of the concept for each node to add sub-concept nodes.

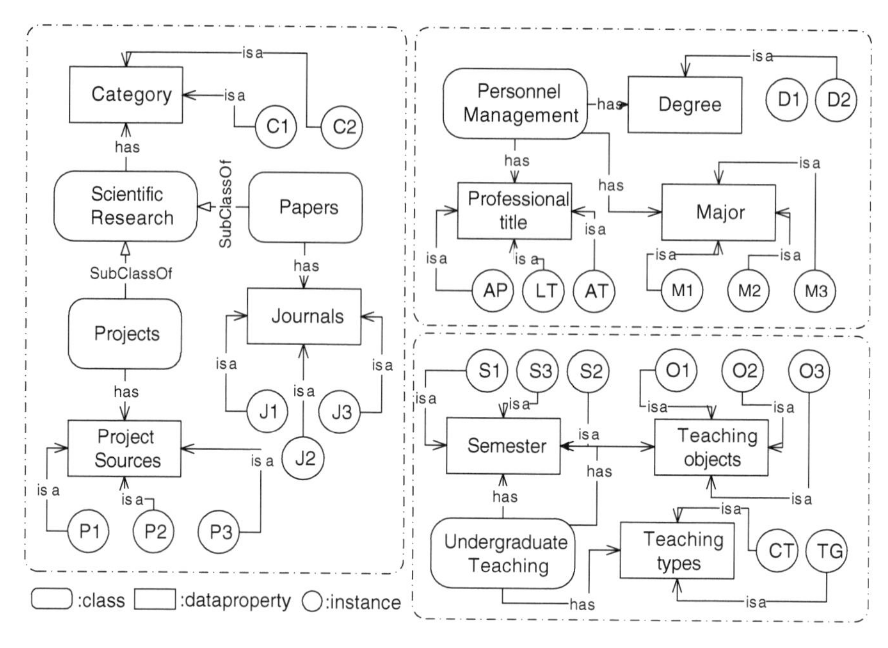

Fig. 74.3 Title appraisal system of university data model (section)

Step 3. The conceptual level model directly maps into a hierarchical model of the ontology, each concept node is mapped into a class the level relational mapping into sub class relations, the concept node properties are mapped to dataproperty.

Step 4. Each table in the collection of data pre-processing stage are mapped into an ontology class.

Step 5. The definition of the predicate and rules add a non-hierarchical relationship between the concepts. This step can be repeated by domain experts to assist, until satisfaction.

In compliance Hasse diagram towards the ontology conversion rules, and then do some appropriate combined with modifications depending on the circumstances, as shown in Fig. 74.3 is constructed of a data model on the university's Title Appraisal System. This model is independent ontology description language which is the modeling of the concepts and relationships. Of course, the ultimate use of tools or programming language to implement this data model will be also repeatedly corrected in order to achieve the real purpose of the application.

74.4 Conclusion

Data integration process, to build ontology data from a relational database model is too dependent on the subjective judgment of the rule-makers, making the resulting data model cannot be used in specific applications. In view of this problem, this paper presents the ontology learning methods based on FCA oriented relational database. After the relational data table pretreatment, and multi-value formal concept conversion to a single value formal concept, and Hasse diagram visual display of formal concept and to generate ontology model, three major steps. This paper relies on FCA method automatically learning from the relational database semantic information to guide the ontology established. This method is not only the use of automatic objective of the FCA to extract semantic features, but also increasing the semantic learning between the data and data, while maintaining the original relational database tables and table semantics, so that the eventual establishment of ontology richer semantic information. By describing a relational database for the field of education information (section) to construct an instance of the data model, the paper illustrates the feasibility of this method. This paper proposed method to build ontology or data model in other fields based on FCA provides guidance method. But in the process of dealing with multi-valued formal concept, the time complexity and space complexity will grow exponentially. Therefore, looking for a more optimized algorithms will be further research objectives.

References

1. Baixeries J, Szathmary L, Valtchev P, Godin R (2009) Yet a faster algorithm for building the Hasse diagram of a concept lattice. In: Formal concept analysis. Springer, Heidelberg, pp 162–177
2. Cimiano P, Hotho A, Stumme G, Tane J (2004) Conceptual knowledge processing with formal concept analysis and ontologies. In: Concept lattices. Springer, Berlin, pp 189–207
3. Ganter B, Wille R, Franzke C (1997) Formal concept analysis: mathematical foundations. Springer, New York
4. Happel HJ, Seedorf S (2006) Applications of ontologies in software engineering. In: Proceedings of workshop on sematic web enabled software engineering (SWESE) on the ISWC, pp 5–9
5. Hu C, Ouyang C, Wu J, Zhang X, Zhao C (2009) NON-structured materials science data sharing based on semantic annotation. Data Sci J 8:52–61
6. Liu Y, Liu S, Li P (2013) Tourism domain ontology construction method based on fuzzy formal concept analysis
7. Louie B, Mork P, Martin-Sanchez F, Halevy A, Tarczy-Hornoch P (2007) Data integration and genomic medicine. J Biomed Inform 40(1):5–16
8. Ouyang CP, Hu CJ, Li Y, Liu ZY (2011) Approach of ontology learning from relational database based on FCA. Comput Sci 38(12):167

Chapter 75
Research and Design on Agent-Based Collaborative Learning Model for Sports Students

Zhaoxia Lu, Lei Zhang and Dongming Liu

Abstract Collaborative learning is a new breakthrough to traditional education pattern. Current research results show both the intelligence and reactivity are limited in existing collaborating learning systems, hence the distributed teaching activity for students majored sports, who are more initiative, interactive, practical but poor of self-control and focus, can not be provided effectively. Aiming at problems in current learning systems, we refer to the idea of multi-agent, do research on multi-agent collaborative learning model and algorithm for sports students, and improve the adaptive capacity, decision-making capacity and response capacity. The primary experiment results showed that the multi-agent based intelligent collaborative learning system can accommodate the characteristic of sports students, realize intelligent, collaborative and individual learning.

Keywords Distributing · Collaborative learning · Multi-agent

75.1 Introduction

With rapid development of computer technology and Internet, the research and teaching in sports fields, including athletic training, game management and physical education, have been experiencing enormous changes. The most instant and prolonged influence for sports colleges is the innovation of education idea and mode. The traditional teaching pattern of theory courses become more and more

Z. Lu (✉) · L. Zhang
Computer Division, Basic Theory Department, Shandong Sport University, 250102 Jinan, China
e-mail: luzxia@sdu.edu.cn

D. Liu
Department of Materials Science and Engineering, Shandong University, 250061 Jinan, China

S. Li et al. (eds.), *Frontier and Future Development of Information Technology in Medicine and Education*, Lecture Notes in Electrical Engineering 269,
DOI: 10.1007/978-94-007-7618-0_75,

unsuited for students majoring on sports, who are more initiative, interactive, practical and fond of team work than students majoring in science and arts. The cramming education method can not create good results, but kill the learning enthusiasm and produce weariness. Hence probing for novel teaching pattern model for sports students learning theory courses became a significant research topic. Related researches [1–3] show that collaborative learning by aid of abundant virtual resources and instantly accessing information is particularly suitable for the sports students who are often good teamwork players. Nevertheless, current collaborative learning systems mostly are as supplementary tools or part of traditional teaching process. They provided simple and restricted tools for instructors and learners to organize learning, and need passive participation rather than active participation. Those systems can not develop the superiority of collaborative learning based on network for sports students who are poor of self-control and focus, debase the learning results due to lack of restrict and resource isotropy rather.

Due to the deficiency of existing systems on intelligence, individuality and instantaneity, we take advantage of the multi-agent technology in AI to build a model of distributed collaborative learning for sports students studying theory courses. The agents in the model can take effect on the implementation of supervision, teaching analysis, information filtering, collaborative learning, intelligent reasoning. The model could define the individuality of learner, customize learning rules.

75.2 Research Background and Basis

75.2.1 Multi-Agent Technology

The research on Agent belongs to artificial intelligence domain [4]. Agent [5] refers to a segment of program which possesses the ability to simulate human behavior and relations, have certain intelligence, operate autonomously under appropriate conditions provide the corresponding service. Because of the complexity of problems solving, a single Agent is difficult to independently complete a given task, so it is necessary to establish the appropriate architecture to a number of organized Agent, jointly undertaking a common task, in order to improve the ability to solve problems [6].

Application of Agent to the collaborative learning model [7] can implement information collection, organization, and filtering, collection of learning situation of learners, dynamical adjust of the content and learning strategy, perception and reaction of environment, social communication through the interaction among learners, and finally realize the intelligent and individualized collaborative learning environment.

75.2.2 Deficiency of Current Network-Based Learning Systems

Traditional distributed learning system generally possesses the following functions: implementing automatic learning through system provided tools; when coming across difficulties, learner will ask the teacher questions during learning; submitting assignment by FTP or email; interacting with other learners and instructor through instant messaging tools or through the non real-time discussion as BBS. The teacher can accomplish teaching tasks online, renew the content of courses, answer questions from learners, provide supplementary information according to the situation of learners, and correct homework. But the traditional distributed learning system exists the following shortcomings:

1. The learning method is single and content is not well targeted.
2. Tutoring is restricted to the local knowledge and online status.
3. Lack of learning intelligence, can not teach students in accordance with their aptitude.
4. Lack of effective knowledge management strategy [8].

75.3 Multi-Agent Based Collaborative Learning System

75.3.1 The Collaborative Learning Model

Multi-agent collaboration refers to the cooperation of multiple Agents in order to achieve a common goal together. Each Agent, affected by the cooperation, constantly adjusts its own state (such as knowledge, belief, intention, etc.) according to the information received.

The following presents a collaborative learning model based on multi-agent. Agent will be divided into four types according to the participating roles: student Agent, teacher Agent, collaboration group Agent, cooperative control Agent. Personalized teaching and learning can be realized through interaction and collaboration between Agents, in addition, real-time dynamic feedback, online thematic discussions, and the summary and incentive evaluation of study effect are also achieved.

Definition 1 Multi-agent Collaborative Learning Model is a quadruple: ***MCLM = {CLid,G,R,S}***,

CLid is the identification of collaborative learning activity;

G = {Ag1,Ag2,...,Agn} is a finite set of N participating Agents in the collaborative learning activities. Collaborative Agents are divided into four types:

student Agent (StuAgent), teacher Agent (TeaAgent), collaboration group Agent (CgrpAgent), cooperative control Agent (CctlAgent);

R represents collaborative learning rules and strategies, including division of team, division of collaboration task, the learning effect evaluation strategy, cooperation performance evaluation strategy;

S indicates the collaborative learning state, describing the task execution of collaborative learning group.

Definition 2 Student Agent is defined as a six tuple: ***StuAgent = {SAid, BasicInfo, Level, Knowledge, ThinkingStyle, Progress}***,

Said is the unique identification of learner;

BasicInfo is the basic information definition of the learner;

Level is the evaluation of original learning level of the learner;

Thinking Style is the learner's thinking mode;

Progress is a learning schedule description.

75.3.2 Collaborative Learning System

The intelligent learning process based on MCLM is divided into: learner registration/login, group division, task allocation, cooperative learning implementation, summary results, evaluation of learning and so on. The corresponding system architecture is showed as Fig. 75.1, which described Agents, the collaborative learning area and a set of databases including Student Model Database(SMD), Teaching Strategy Database(TSD), Teaching Resource Database(TRD), and other resource database.

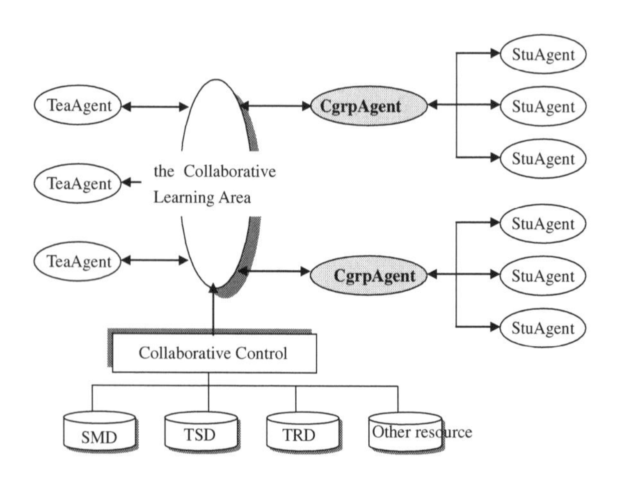

Fig. 75.1 The architecture of intelligent collaborative learning system

75.3.2.1 Intelligent Collaborative Learning Agent

There are four types of Agent that participating in the collaborating learning activities (as shown in Fig. 75.2): student Agent (StuAgent), teacher Agent (TeaAgent), collaboration group Agent (CgrpAgent), cooperative control Agent (CctlAgent). Each type of agent have their own problem solving ability according to their functions. Different types of Agent can interact according to relevant rules, in order to reach the ultimate goals. Each Agent should have had the characteristic of reactive, proactive and interactivity. Reaction is that Agent can adjust its behavior according to the dynamic environment or other Agent's behavior. Proactive is that Agent can produce the motivation and behavior of next action according to their goals. Interaction is that Agent can coordinate and cooperate with other Agent. Different types of Agent are described as follows:

- TeaAgent
  TeaAgent implements the teacher model in collaborative learning system. It is commissioned to complete the teaching activities, including intelligent decomposition of teaching task, correcting homework, selection of teaching content and teaching strategies according to the individual student model, guidance and answering, combined with the overall knowledge structure model stored in the system database and individual knowledge structure model of the StuAgent.

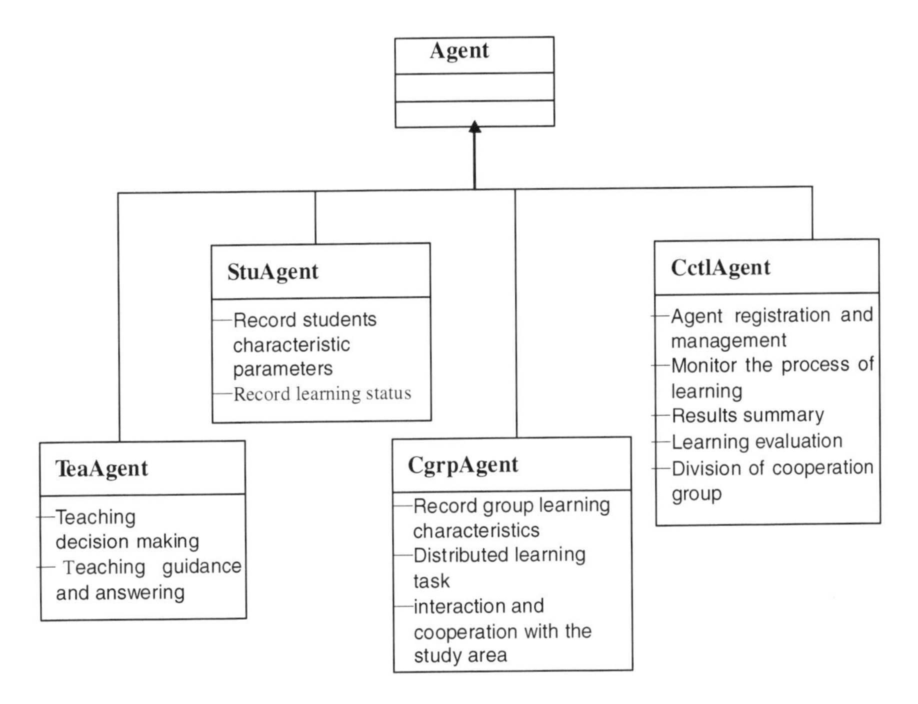

Fig. 75.2 Class diagram of intelligent agents

- StuAgent
  StuAgent implements the student model in collaborative learning system. When a learner login in, a StuAgent will be created on behalf of him. StuAgent records the personal characteristics and learning parameters of the corresponding student, such as the level of knowledge learning, ability to accept, thinking mode, cognitive style, and stores these information into the corresponding student model base. Students will be classified according to the corresponding parameters. The individual student model will be constructed, as the reference of team division, learning content selection and learning process control. With the deepening of study, various measures of learners are to be changed, StuAgent will track the learning process dynamically, and make the corresponding revision. In addition, StuAgent is also responsible for handling learners' request, submitting homework or searching the corresponding resources from the system and network.
- CgrpAgent
  The control group is partitioned based on personal characteristics and certain principles, such as the learning achievement, learning ability, learning level, thinking tendency etc. CgrpAgent is responsible for the group management, recording group learning state, task partitioning, learning results recycling, group learning result evaluation etc.
- CctlAgent
  When task was submitted to the Collaborative Learning Area, CctlAgent first analyzed the submitted task, determined the coefficient of difficulty and workload, then allocated task to a collaborative learning group according to the personality characteristic parameters. The group assigned the task further according to the characteristics of task and personality of learners. Only the task assignment meet the personality characteristics and the cognitive ability of students, can the learners complete the task with high quality.

75.3.2.2 Collaborative Learning Area

Collaborative learning area is a virtual space for learners sharing. Online learners can watch PPT, video and other learning materials in their computers or participate in the discussion, communication. Collaborative learning is divided into online and offline. When online learning, CctlAgent records presentations and discussions of all online members, analyzes the results, and stores the results information to StuAgent and TeaAgent, in order to give guidance for learners' decision-making. When asynchronous learning, CctlAgent will record the content that has been discussed and questions that has not been discussed, and offer to the member not online, to help the learners to understand the learning progress conveniently and quickly.

75.4 Experimental Results and Analysis

75.4.1 Experiment Design and Process

The survey data gathered from the 2009 sports majored undergraduates of Shandong Sport University by random cluster sampling, with 46 students in experimental group and 48 students in control group. Experiment time was from October to December in 2009.

The operation level of computer basis on the sample was evaluated before the experiment. The results showed no significant difference between the experimental group and the control group ($p > 0.05$) (see Table 75.1), which means two groups of subjects are at the same level in ability of computer operation before the experiment, and the sample is meaningful.

The experimental group was applied the distributed collaborative learning model. Students were partitioned into 6 collaborative learning groups based on their learning habits and characteristics. Each group includes 6–8 students, in which one as the group leader and others as members of the group. The control group was applied traditional teaching methods, in which teacher instructed theoretical knowledge to students and students did exercises and homework. Except the learning mode, the experimental group and the control group are the same in other conditions (teachers, teaching content, work content, test content, learning time).

Learning content: learning basic computer operation knowledge; learning editing and formatting of documents using Word; learning making, editing, data statistics, and automatic calculation of sports spreadsheet using Excel; learning to make and edit sports courseware using Powerpoint.

Test and evaluation: learning effect was tested after the experiment. Test contents include basic skills and comprehensively practical cases (see Table 75.2).

Table 75.1 Computer test results of the level of basic operation of the experimental group and the control group before the experiment

Rank	n	Computer basic operation
Experimental group	46	36.44 ± 7.33
Control group	48	36.18 ± 7.18
t		0.166
p		0.868

Table 75.2 Test content

	Test contents
Test 1	To format a dissertation by Word
Test 2	Establish a questionnaire with function of statistics and automatic calculation
Test 3	Create and edit football teaching courseware with Powerpoint

75.4.2 Experimental Results and Analysis

1. Learning Interest, Attitude, Self-confidence of Students
   94 questionnaires had been distributed, in which all have been retrieved, and 92 were effective. Survey results show that: the double samples nonparametric rank sum test, $p = 0.030$ ($p < 0.05$), which indicated that the experimental group and the control group were significantly different in learning interest, attitude and self-confidence. Students in the experimental group employed group learning and collaborative learning, which focused task-driven and team-worked pattern. Knowledge learning was looked as overcoming difficulties, and group members were cooperated to strive to achieve the target. In this way, learning enthusiasm and creativity of students were greatly stimulated, problem-solving ability was exercised and promoted, learning interest and confidence was enhanced.
2. Learning Effects of Students
   Test scores of the experimental group and the control group are shown in Table 75.3. The results showed that there existed no significant difference ($p > 0.05$) on comprehensive knowledge test, but there was a significant difference ($p < 0.05$) in the test 1 and test 2, extremely significant difference in test 3 ($p < 0.01$).

Cause analysis: (1) The comprehensive knowledge test scores of the experimental group have no outstanding performance, or even slightly lower than that of the control group, indicating that collaborative learning platform need to be strengthened on mobilizing and promoting students' learning autonomy; (2) Three test results of the experimental group are obviously better than that of the control group, indicating that the ability of problem analysis and problem solving was promoted through cooperative case study and task-driven mode, students' understanding and usability of knowledge was boosted by mutual discussion and work together, the knowledge expansion ability was also improved; (3) The experimental group students were especially outstanding in test 3, may be because the test 3 cases were comprehensive and of design, and have greater creative space, especially suitable for the teamwork model.

Table 75.3 Average test scores of the experimental group and the control group

Test content	Experimental group	Control group	t	*P*
Comprehensive knowledge	49.77 ± 4.82	50.67 ± 3.55	−1.03	0.306
Test 1	26.52 ± 1.92	25.44 ± 2.25	2.51	0.014*
Test 2	25.91 ± 2.01	24.69 ± 2.62	2.10	0.038*
Test 3	27.03 ± 1.84	25.87 ± 2.27	3.05	0.003**

?:*p < 0.05;**p < 0.01

75.5 Summary and Future Work

Traditional teaching pattern of theory courses is not suitable for students majoring on sports, who are initiative, interactive, practical and fond of team work, but poor of self-control and focus. Application of distributed collaborative learning mode is an effective solution. In this paper, a multi-agent collaborative learning model was presented and corresponding platform was built. The model was designed to solve the deficiency of existing products on intelligence, individuation and reactivity. Learning through collaboration between the Agents can adapt to the changing situation, find the optimal strategy quickly, hence intelligence, accuracy and fast response are satisfied.

Preliminary experiments have shown that, the intelligent multi-agent collaborative learning platform can well adapt to the characteristics of sports students, improve the ability to analyze and solve problems, realize intelligent personalized learning, and achieved a better learning effect. Even so, also found in the experiment, the desired objectives in mobilizing the enthusiasm and interest of students through collaborative learning platform were not achieved. Next step of the work will further expand the teaching resources, improve and perfect the collaborative learning platform.

References

1. Huang R (2001) Web-based cooperative learning system model. China Distance Educ 5:42–47
2. Yang Y, Fu Y, Liu Y (2007) Individualized distance education system based on multi-agent. Comput Sci 34(9):290–292
3. Qi C-X, Qi Z-F, Sang J-Y, Sun Y-J (2010) Web-based collaborative learning system. In: 2nd international conference on networking and digital society (ICNDS), pp 557–560
4. Lange DB, Oshima M (1999) Serven good reasons for mobile agents. Commun ACM 42(3):88–89
5. Shi Z (2002) Intelligent agent and application. Science Press, Beijing
6. Yu L, Peng D (2008) Research on an intelligent learning platform based on agent. Comput Appl Softw 25(2):99–102
7. Kumar R, Rosé CP (2011) Architecture for building conversational agents that support collaborative learning. IEEE Trans Learn Technol 4(1):21–34
8. Zhao R, Zhang C (2009) A Framework for collaborative learning system based on knowledge management. In: 2009 first international workshop on education technology and computer science, pp 733–736

Chapter 76
Toxicology Evaluation and Properties of a New Biodegradable Computer Made Medical Biomaterial

Jinshu Ma, Chao Zhang, Jingying Sai, Guangyu Xu, Xiaotian Zhang, Chao Feng, Fan Li and Fang Wang

Abstract *Background* Poly (propylene carbonate) (PPC) synthesized from carbon dioxide and propylene oxide has attracted considerable research attention recently. To explore the potential application of these new polymers for bone repair, it is necessary to use other biodegradable polymers to enhance the properties of PPC. Poly (3-hydroxybutyrate) was used in this study to modify the mechanical properties and biocompatibility of PPC. *Methods* Poly (propylene carbonate) (PPC) was melt-mixed with 30 % poly (3-hydroxybutyrate) to enhance its physical properties, while maintaining the inherently high structural integrity and ductility. The mechanical strength, porosity, morphologies and biocompatibility of porous modified-PPC (PM-PPC) were fully investigated using tensile tester, hammering method, scanning electron microscopy, cytotoxicity test for its biocompatibility. *Results* The PM-PPC was measured by mechanical tests for its compressive strength, elongation module and tensile strength, with the results being 43, 725 and 32 Mpa respectively. The data showed that the mechanical properties of PM-PPC were significantly improved compared with PPC. The mean porosity of PM-PPC was 15 %, as determined by hammering method. The biocompatibility test of PM-PPC showed that it has excellent potential for use as a biomedical material. *Conclusions* In conclusion, the PM-PPC showed improved mechanical properties, and an acceptable biocompatibility supporting its potential for use in patients. Thus, PM-PPC is a promising candidate for use as a novel medical material.

Keywords Porous modified-PPC · Composites · Mechanical properties

Abbreviation List

PPC	Poly (propylene carbonate)
M-PPC	Modified-poly (propylene carbonate)

J. Ma · C. Zhang · J. Sai · G. Xu · X. Zhang · C. Feng · F. Li · F. Wang (✉)
Department of Pathogenobiology, Norman Bethune College of Medicine, Jilin University, 126 Xinmin Street, Changchun 130021, People's Republic of China
e-mail: majs10@mails.jlu.edu.cnwf@jlu.edu.cn

S. Li et al. (eds.), *Frontier and Future Development of Information Technology in Medicine and Education*, Lecture Notes in Electrical Engineering 269,
DOI: 10.1007/978-94-007-7618-0_76,

PM-PPC	Porous modified-poly (propylene carbonate)
GTR	Guided tissue regeneration
P (3HB)	Poly (3-hydroxybutyrate)
PHB	Poly (3-hydroxybutyrate)
PCL	Poly (3-caprolactone)
PLA	Poly (lactic acid)
PHBV	Polyhydroxybutyrate Valerate
NMR	Nuclear magnetic resonance
PO	Propylene Oxide
GPC	Gel permeation chromatography
SEM	Scanning electron micrograph
OD	Optical density

76.1 Background

Porous polymer/ceramic composites have shown extraordinary promise as guided tissue regeneration (GTR) membranes and bone tissue scaffolds [1, 2]. The better osteoconductivity of the porous composites has suggested they may be an ideal clinical matrix for bone cell growth and differentiation [3, 4]. As a biodegradable polymer with ester bonds on its CO_2 backbone, Poly (propylene carbonate) (PPC) was first synthesized by copolymerization of CO_2 and PO [5]. The polycarbonate of PPC can be readily dissociated into H_2O and CO_2 [6–8]. Currently, scholars are endeavoring to improve the thermal stability, viscosity and biodegradability of PPC [9–11].

Poly (3-hydroxybutyrate) [P (3HB) or PHB] has mechanical properties similar to polypropylene [12], and it is acknowledged to be a thermoplastic polyester with good biocompatibility properties [13, 14]. However, its brittleness, high price, and poor thermal stability have hindered its commercial application.

Many methods have been developed for improving the properties of biodegradable polymers. Random and block copolymerization has succeeded in improving their biodegradation rate as well as their mechanical properties. Physical blending is another simple but effective way to prepare biodegradable composites displaying different physical characteristics.

Although, Poly (3-caprolactone) (PCL), poly (lactic acid) (PLA) and PHBV have been reported as PPC blended materials [9, 11, 15], few studies have been done on the preparation or properties of porous modified-PPC (PM-PPC). We have now developed a novel, completely biodegradable and applicable PM-PPC with new computer method, and evaluated by nuclear magnetic resonance spectroscopy (NMR), gel permeation chromatography (GPC) and tensile testing, its molecular structure and properties compared to PPC.

Currently, little is known about the biocompatibility of PM-PPC. Therefore, we have investigated the possible cytotoxicity testing of PM-PPC in vitro for its biocompatibility.

76.2 Methods

76.2.1 Preparation of PM-PPC

CO_2 (99.8 % purity) and propylene oxide (PO) (99.5 % purity) was provided by the Changchun Institute of Applied Chemistry (China). P (3HB) was purchased from the Beijing Biological Institute (China). Other chemicals used in the study were purchased from the Beijing Chemical Works (China). Toluene, benzene, 1, 4-dioxane, tetrahydrofuran, and glutaric anhydride were purified as previously described [16]. PPC was synthesized by a ternary rare-earth-metal catalyst system [17] and the chemical reaction of PO and CO_2 (Fig. 76.1) was performed as described by Li et al. [18]. The synthesized PPC were squeezed into 2 mm slices by hydrodynamic pressure, for mechanical property testing. Then we use the new computer method to design and synthesize the two materials before to make porous M-PPC. The resulting porous blends (PM-PPC) were then cut into 2 mm sheets or 1 mm cylinders at 140 °C and used in tensile and dynamic mechanical analysis [19].

76.2.2 Determination of PPC Chemical Constitution

The chemical constitution of PPC was determined by Bruker AV400 Nuclear magnetic resonance (NMR). Proton (1H) nuclear magnetic resonance spectra (1H NMR) were recorded on a Varian UNITY-plus Spectrometer at 400 MHz. 1H NMR peak areas were determined by spectrometric integration and reported as relative intensities by a given number of hydrogens [20].

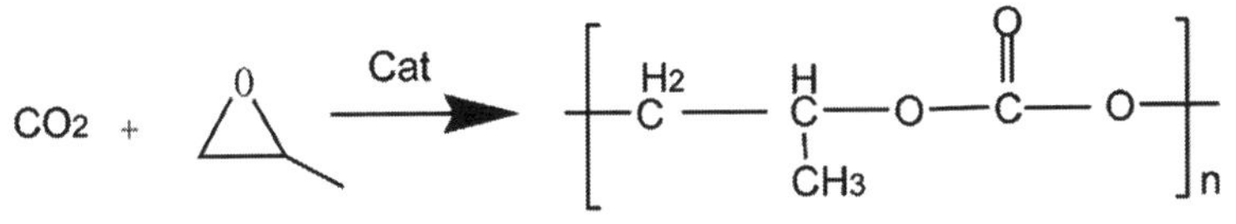

$$CO_2 + \text{PO} \xrightarrow{\text{Cat}} \left[-\overset{H_2}{C} - \underset{CH_3}{\overset{H}{C}} - O - \overset{O}{\overset{\|}{C}} - O - \right]_n$$

Fig. 76.1 Synthesis of PPC from CO_2 and PO

76.2.3 Determination of Molecular Weight of PPC

The molecular weights and polydispersities of PPC were determined using gel permeation chromatography (GPC) with a Waters Model 515 pump and a Waters Model 410 refractive index detector, with chloroform and tetrahydrofuran used as the solvent and the mobile phase respectively. Calibration was performed with 1,000–3,000,000 g/mol polystyrene standards. Number-average molecular weight (M_n) and Weight-average molecular weight (M_w) were calculated using the Waters empower software [21].

76.2.4 Detection of Mechanical Properties

PPC and PM-PPC mechanical tests were conducted according to ASTM D638 specifications [22]. The tensile properties of the samples were determined with a universal test machine (UTM, Instron 5565, Instron) at a cross-head speed of 10 mm/min at 25 °C. The mean value from at least five specimens of each sample was collected.

76.2.5 Detection of Porosity

Scanning electron micrograph (SEM) analysis was performed with a Hitachi S-450 SEM. M-PPC and PM-PPC specimens were submerged into liquid nitrogen, fractured, and then sputter-coated with a thin layer of gold before SEM observations. The distribution of PM-PPC pore sizes were analyzed by mercury intrusion porosimetry (Pascal 140-240/440, Porotec, Hofheim, Germany) [23].

76.2.6 Preparation of Leaching Liquor

PPC and PM-PPC were sterilized at 137.3 kPa, 121 °C for 30 min by steam. They were then incubated in 0.9 % physiological saline at a ratio of 6 cm^2 surface area/ml for 48 h, at 37 °C [24].

76.2.7 Cytotoxicity Test

1×10^5 mouse fibroblast L929 cells/mL (purchased from Institute of Virology Academia Sinica, Beijing, China) were seeded in 96-well plates, with DMEM containing 10 % fetal bovine serum at 37 °C with 5 % CO_2 [25]. Cells of experimental groups were treated with PPC and PM-PPC leaching liquor. Cells of the negative and positive control group were treated with DMEM medium or 0.7 % acrylamide solute respectively. The L929 fibroblast cells were treated for 24, 48 and 72 h and then added 20 μl of MTT solution (5 mg/mL in PBS) respectively. After incubation at 37 °C for 4 h, the medium was removed from the well and 150 μl of DMSO was added to dissolve any insoluble formazan crystals. The absorbance was measured at 570 nm using an ELISA analyzer (Spectra MAX 250, Molecular Devices, Sunnyvale, USA). Five cytotoxicity tests were conducted per sample.

76.2.8 Statistical Analysis

All data were collected in triplicate and expressed as means ± standard deviations. The data were analyzed using statistical analysis software SPSS 12.0. The data were compared using t-test and differences were considered significant when $p < 0.05$.

76.3 Results

76.3.1 Molecular Constitution of PPC

The 1H NMR spectra of PPC determined by Bruker AV400 NMR is illustrated in Fig. 76.2. For PPC, the peaks at 1.25–1.4 ($-CH_3$), 4.1–4.3 ($-CH_2$) and 4.95–5.05 (–CH) were attributed to methyl, methylene and methine protons. The purity quotient of PPC confirmed it was suitable for use in this study.

76.3.2 Molecular Weight of PPC

The molecular weight and polydispersity of PPC were determined using gel permeation chromatography (GPC). The M_n and M_w of PPC synthesized in the present study were 1,00,000 and 1,82,000 respectively, the polydispersity was 1.82.

76.3.3 Mechanical Properties

As shown in Fig. 76.3, the tensile strength and elongation module of PM-PPC were significant decreased compared to PPC ($p < 0.05$), conversely, the compressive strength was increased.

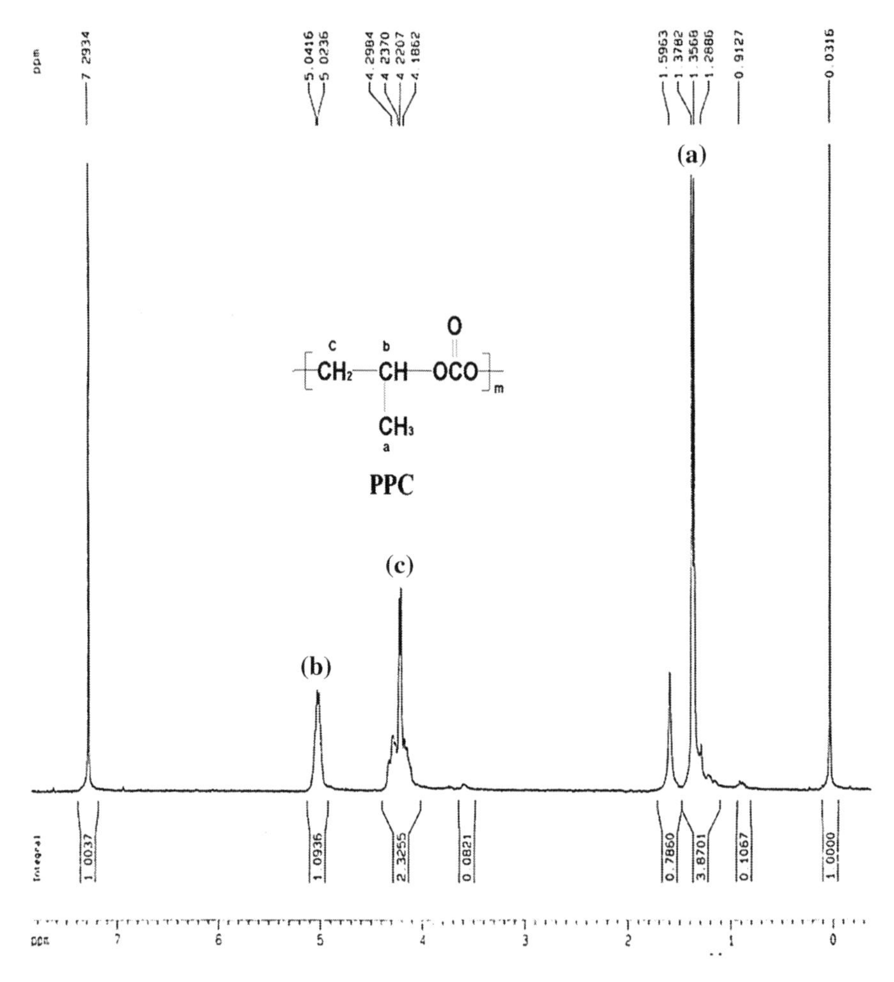

Fig. 76.2 1H NMR spectra of pure PPC. **a** stands for $–CH_3$, **b** stands for –CH, **c** stands for $–CH_2$

76.3.4 Porosity

The morphology of the M-PPC was observed by SEM as shown in Fig. 76.4a and no porous structure can be observed in M-PPC. However, the porosity of PM-PPC was observed, and is shown at different magnifications in Fig. 76.4b, c and d. The pore diameter of PM-PPC varied from 50 to 200 µm. Mean porosity of PM-PPC was 15 %, as determined by hammering method.

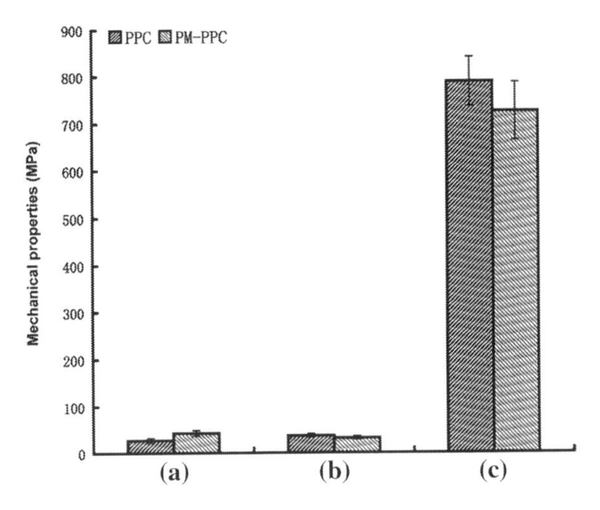

Fig. 76.3 Mechanical properties of PPC and PM-PPC. **a** compressive strength, **b** elongation module, **c** tensile strength

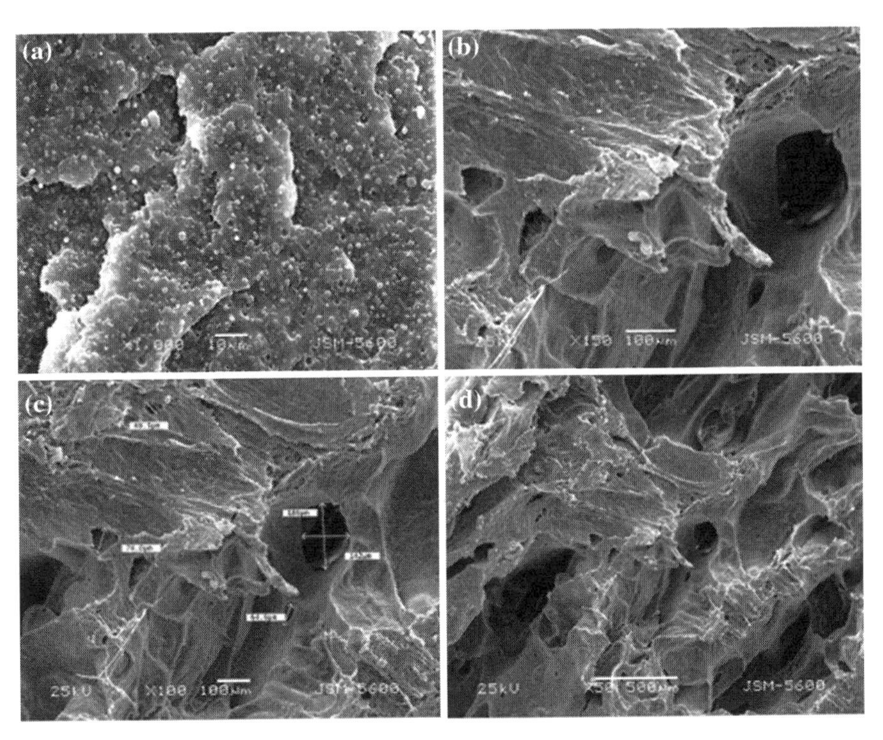

Fig. 76.4 SEM photographs of M-PPC and PM-PPC. **a** The SEM photograph of M-PPC, ×1,000, **b** pore of PM-PPC (SEM), ×150, **c** pore of PM-PPC (SEM), ×100, **d** pore of PM-PPC (SEM), ×50

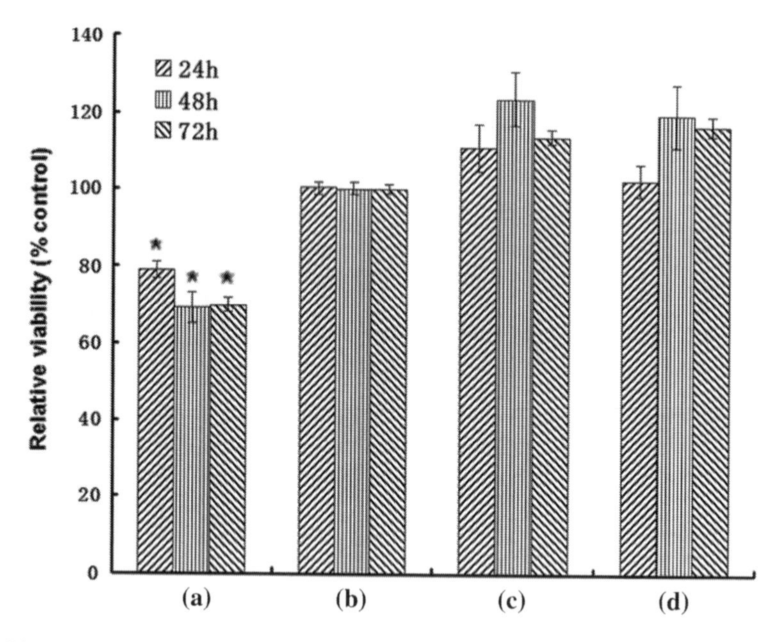

Fig. 76.5 MTT cytotoxicity of PPC and PM-PPC. Cytotoxicity effect of PPC and PM-PPC on the mouse fibroblast L929 cells were detected by MTT assay on 24, 48 and 72 h. **a** Positive control group, **b** negative control group, **c** PM-PPC group **d** PPC group. The results are presented as the mean ± standard error of the mean. * represents $p < 0.05$ compared to the negative control

76.3.5 Cytotoxicity Test

After culturing for 72 h, the relative viability of cells from the positive control group was significantly lower than from the PM-PPC treatment group ($p < 0.05$), as shown in Fig. 76.5, and there was no significant difference between the negative control and PM-PPC treatment group ($p > 0.05$), which suggests that PM-PPC is not cytotoxic.

76.4 Discussion

PPC was first synthesized from CO2 and PO with ZnEt2/H2O as catalyst [5]. However, this method had disadvantages including a low efficiency catalyst, and poor mechanical strength. Outstanding rates of CO2 and PO copolymerization have recently been achieved by adding quaternary ammonium salt as co-catalyst [26]. The PPC produced by the copolymerization of CO2 and PO exhibited excellent biodegradability, as confirmed both by soil burial and buffer-solution immersion tests [27]. Although PPC produced had good biocompatibility and biodegradability, its poor thermal and mechanical performance, and the low catalytic efficiency and long polymerization time of the method has limited its usefulness.

The mechanical properties of PM-PPC and PPC presented in Fig. 76.3 show that the ternary rare-earth-metal catalyst system used in the study has overcome these disadvantages in PPC synthesis. Our ternary rare-earth-metal catalyst system has made the combining process less costly, improving its commercial prospects for medical use. The PPC acted as a continuous phase while P (3HB) functioned as a rigid reinforcement, thereby leading to a decrease in the hardness of PM-PPC. The strong molecular interaction between PPC and P (3HB) accounted for the formation of the miscible blends. Our morphological observations have indicated that the PM-PPC shows amazing comprehensive properties.

High molecular weight PPC has become an economically viable biodegradable plastic with tens of thousands of tons produced per year, providing a new solution to overcome the problem of high costs in biodegradable plastics production [28]. The blending of different polymers is a simple and economical method to enhance the properties of a polymer matrix [29], and the mechanical properties of the polymers are strongly dependent on their composition [30]. The properties of polymeric blends are also greatly dependent on the morphology, miscibility, and possible interactions between the polymer components. Blends of PPC with poly (3-hydroxybutyrate-co-3-hydroxyvalerate) and short hildegardia populifolia fiber have been reported [31, 32]. However, the properties of those blends were only enhanced to a very limited extent [33]. In this study we have prepared PPC with a high tensile strength of 37 MPa and an elongation modulus of 788 Mpa, as well as PM-PPC with a tensile strength of 32 MPa and an elongation modulus of 725 Mpa. As a result of blending with P (3HB) the elongation module and tensile strength of PM-PPC has clearly decreased.

As a bone repair material, biodegradable polymers are now attracting considerable research attention and, as an aliphatic polycarbonate, PPC is both a non-toxic and a biodegradable material. An ideal material for bone repair should have both good strength and good conductivity, but unfortunately on its own PPC has low hardness (strength) and poor bone conductivity, limiting its usefulness in bone repair [7, 9]. Our study shows that as the P (3HB) content of the blends increases, the breaking strength of the resulting blends also increases [34]. Thus, the accession of PPC could significantly reduce the brittleness and improve the elongation capabilities of the blends. At the same time, PPC could inhibit the crystallization process of P (3HB) and reduce the melting point of P (3HB). For these reasons, we selected the P (3HB)/PPC 30/70 wt % as the optimal blend ratio, and our results prove that the PM-PPC prepared shows the appropriate physical properties.

Pore size and porosity are the main evaluators of bone repair materials. Large pores in materials will provide enough space for growth of new bone, while small pores could significantly enhance the flow and diffusion of liquids, which would be conducive to improving the microenvironment and enhancing cell metabolism [35]. The diameter of osteoblasts is about 20 μm and, therefore, it is generally accepted that material with a pore diameter less than 100 μm is not suitable for the growth of bone cells [36]. Classical methods for the preparation of porous materials include phase separation, solution casting-wash-out particle, fiber bonding, gas foaming, etc. [37]. Phase separation and solution casting-wash-out particle methodologies requires large amounts of organic solvents, and the gas foaming method might lead to a closed pore material, which would negatively affect nutrient transport and cell growth. Therefore, we prepared a PM-PPC that is more comparable to human bone compression and strength. The three-dimensional porous structure of our PM-PPC indicates that it could simulate the structure of cancellous bone, be conducive to the growth of bone cells and accelerate the processes of bone renewal.

The cytotoxicity test indicates that PM-PPC should be considered a promising candidate for use as a novel bone repair material. Any substance proposed for use in parenteral formulations must be tested for potential incompatibility with fibroblast cells in vitro cytotoxicity test. The results of this cytotoxicity test show that PM-PPC did not induce any cytotoxic response in fibroblast cells. Therefore, the biocompatibility of PM-PPC can be judged as excellent.

76.5 Conclusions

In this study we have demonstrated that it is possible to combine two materials, P (3HB) and PPC, into optimized multifunctional composites that enhance both mechanical properties and porosity. PPC is the dominant component, with the incorporation of 30 % P (3HB), and the melt blending and salting out techniques enhanced the tensile strength, ductility and compressive strength of PM-PPC. The conversion to PM-PPC not only improved the mechanical properties of PPC but also increased its porosity, which should favor bone regeneration. Thus, PM-PPC is a composite with good porosity, enhanced mechanical properties and biocompatibility, which can be regarded as a suitable candidate for use as bone repair biomaterial.

Acknowledgments This work was supported by the China National Science and Technology Support Program (grant number 2007BAE42B06). We thank Professor Rick C Nicholson at Mothers and Babies Research Center, Hunter Medical Research Institute, John Hunter Hospital, Newcastle, Australia for his language assistance and structure design in this paper.

Competing interests The authors declare that they have no competing interests.

References

1. Causa F, Netti PA, Ambrosio L (2007) A multi-functional scaffold for tissue regeneration: the need to engineer a tissue analogue. Biomaterials 28(34):5093–5099
2. Tan X, Li M, Cai P, Luo L, Zou X (2005) An amperometric cholesterol biosensor based on multiwalled carbon nanotubes and organically modified sol-gel/chitosan hybrid composite film. Anal Biochem 337(1):111–120

3. Harrison BS, Atala A (2007) Carbon nanotube applications for tissue engineering. Biomaterials 28(2):344–353
4. Valappil SP, Misra SK, Boccaccini AR, Keshavarz T, Bucke C, Roy I (2007) Large-scale production and efficient recovery of PHB with desirable material properties, from the newly characterised *Bacillus cereus* SPV. J Biotechnol 132(3):251–258
5. Inoue S, Koinuma H, Tsuruta T (1969) Copolymerization of carbon dioxide and epoxide. J Polym Sci B 7(4):287–292
6. Ge XC, Xu Y, Meng YZ, Li RKY (2005) Thermal and mechanical properties of biodegradable composites of poly(propylene carbonate) and starch-poly(methyl acrylate) graft copolymer. Compos Sci Technol 65(14):2219–2225
7. Du LC, Meng YZ, Wang SJ, Tjong SC (2004) Synthesis and degradation behavior of poly (propylene carbonate) derived from carbon dioxide and propylene oxide. J Appl Polym Sci 92(3):1840–1846
8. Guo CH, Wu HS, Zhang XM, Song JY, Zhang X (2009) A comprehensive theoretical study on the coupling reaction mechanism of propylene oxide with carbon dioxide catalyzed by copper (I) cyanomethyl. J Phys Chem A 113(24):6710–6723
9. Lu XL, Du FG, Ge XC, Xiao M, Meng YZ (2006) Biodegradability and thermal stability of poly (propylene carbonate)/starch composites. J Biomed Mater Res A 77A(4):653–658
10. Ge XC, Zhu Q, Meng YZ (2006) Fabrication and characterization of biodegradable poly (propylene carbonate)/wood flour composites. J Appl Polym Sci 99(3):782–787
11. Ma XF, Yu JG, Wang N (2006) Compatibility characterization of poly (lactic acid)/poly (propylene carbonate) blends. J Polym Sci B 44(1):94–101
12. Wang XY, Peng SW, Dong LS (2005) Effect of poly (vinyl acetate) (PVAc) on thermal behavior and mechanical properties of poly (3-hydroxybutyrate)/poly (propylene carbonate) (PHB/PPC) blends. Colloid Polym Sci 284(2):167–174
13. Valappil SP, Misra SK, Boccaccini AR, Roy I (2006) Biomedical applications of polyhydroxyalkanoates, an overview of animal testing and in vivo responses. Expert Rev Med Devic 3(6):853–868
14. Wu Q, Wang Y, Chen GQ (2009) Medical application of microbial biopolyesters polyhydroxyalkanoates. Artif Cell Blood Sub 37(1):1–12
15. Hirotsu T, Ketelaars AAJ, Nakayama K (2000) Biodegradation of poly (epsilon-caprolactone)-polycarbonate blend sheets. Polym Degrad Stabil 68(3):311–316
16. Ree M, Bae JY, Jung JH, Shin TJ (1999) A new copolymerization process leading to poly (propylene carbonate) with a highly enhanced yield from carbon dioxide and propylene oxide. J Polym Sci A 37(12):1863–1876
17. Zhang ZH, Mo ZS, Zhang HF, Zhang Y, Na TH, An YX, Wang XH, Zhao XJ (2002) Miscibility and hydrogen-bonding interactions in blends of carbon dioxide/epoxy propane copolymer with poly (p-vinylphenol). J Polym Sci B 40(17):1957–1964
18. Li XH, Meng YZ, Chen GQ, Li RKY (2004) Thermal properties and rheological behavior of biodegradable aliphatic polycarbonate derived from carbon dioxide and propylene oxide. J Appl Polym Sci 94(2):711–716
19. Ishaug-Riley SL, Crane-Kruger GM, Yaszemski MJ, Mikos AG (1998) Three-dimensional culture of rat calvarial osteoblasts in porous biodegradable polymers. Biomaterials 19(15):1405–1412
20. Li Y, Shimizu H (2009) Compatibilization by homopolymer: significant improvements in the modulus and tensile strength of PPC/PMMA blends by the addition of a small amount of PVAc. ACS Appl Mater Interfaces 1(8):1650–1655
21. Cho SW, Park HJ, Ryu JH, Kim SH, Kim YH, Choi CY, Lee MJ, Kim JS, Jang IS, Kim DI, Kim BS (2005) Vascular patches tissue-engineered with autologous bone marrow-derived cells and decellularized tissue matrices. Biomaterials 26(14):1915–1924
22. Zhang K, Wang YB, Hillmyer MA, Francis LF (2004) Processing and properties of porous poly (L-lactide)/bioactive glass composites. Biomaterials 25(13):2489–2500
23. Kasten P, Beyen I, Niemeyer P, Luginbuehl R, Bohner M, Richter W (2008) Porosity and pore size of beta-tricalcium phosphate scaffold can influence protein production and

osteogenic differentiation of human mesenchymal stem cells: an in vitro and in vivo study. Acta Biomater 4(6):1904–1915
24. Huang S, Zhou K, Huang B, Li Z, Zhu S, Wang G (2008) Preparation of an electrodeposited hydroxyapatite coating on titanium substrate suitable for in vivo applications. J Mater Sci Mater Med 19(1):437–442
25. Sun H, Qu Z, Guo Y, Zang G, Yang B (2007) In vitro and in vivo effects of rat kidney vascular endothelial cells on osteogenesis of rat bone marrow mesenchymal stem cells growing on polylactide-glycoli acid (PLGA) scaffolds. Biomed Eng Online 6:41
26. Lu XB, Wang Y (2004) Highly active, binary catalyst systems for the alternating copolymerization of CO2 and epoxides under mild conditions. Angew Chem Int Ed Engl 43(27):3574–3577
27. Meng YZ, Du LC, Tiong SC, Zhu Q, Hay AS (2002) Effects of the structure and morphology of zinc glutarate on the fixation of carbon dioxide into polymer. J Polym Sci A 40(21):3579–3591
28. Qin Y, Wang X (2010) Carbon dioxide-based copolymers: environmental benefits of PPC, an industrially viable catalyst. Biotechnol J 5(11):1164–1180
29. Chen SM, Tan L, Qiu FR, Jiang XL, Wang M, Zhang HD (2004) The study of poly (styrene-co-p-(hexafluoro-2-hydroxylisopropyl)-alpha-methyl-styrene)/poly (propylene carbonate) blends by ESR spin probe and Raman. Polymer 45(9):3045–3053
30. Pego AP, Poot AA, Grijpma DW, Feijen J (2003) Physical properties of high molecular weight 1,3-trimethylene carbonate and D, L-lactide copolymers. J Mater Sci Mater Med 14(9):767–773
31. Peng SW, An YX, Chen C, Fei B, Zhuang YG, Dong LS (2004) Miscibility and crystallization behavior of poly (3-hydroxybutyrate-co-3-hydroxyvalerate)/poly (propylene carbonate) blends (vol 90, p 4054, 2003). J Appl Polym Sci 91(2):1374
32. Li XH, Meng YZ, Wang SJ, Rajulu AV, Tjong SC (2004) Completely biodegradable composites of poly (propylene carbonate) and short, lignocellulose fiber Hildegardia populifolia. J Polym Sci B 42(4):666–675
33. Chiellini E, Cinelli P, Imam SH, Mao L (2001) Composite films based on biorelated agro-industrial waste and poly (vinyl alcohol) Preparation and mechanical properties characterization. Biomacromolecules 2(3):1029–1037
34. Yang DZ, Hu P (2008) Miscibility, crystallization, and mechanical properties of poly (3-hydroxybutyrate) and poly (propylene carbonate) biodegradable blends. J Appl Polym Sci 109(3):1635–1642
35. Huang Y, Gao H, Gou M, Ye H, Liu Y, Gao Y, Peng F, Qian Z, Cen X, Zhao Y (2010) Acute toxicity and genotoxicity studies on poly (epsilon-caprolactone)-poly(ethylene glycol)-poly (epsilon-caprolactone) nanomaterials. Mutat Res 696(2):101–106
36. Popat KC, Leoni L, Grimes CA, Desai TA (2007) Influence of engineered titania nanotubular surfaces on bone cells. Biomaterials 28(21):3188–3197
37. Cenni E, Granchi D, Avnet S, Fotia C, Salerno M, Micieli D, Sarpietro MG, Pignatello R, Castelli F, Baldini N (2008) Biocompatibility of poly (D, L-lactide-co-glycolide) nanoparticles conjugated with alendronate. Biomaterials 29(10):1400–1411

Chapter 77
Investigation and Analysis on Ear Diameter and Ear Axis Diameter in Maize RIL Population

Daowen He, Hongmei Zhang, Changmin Liao, Qi Luo, Guoqiang Hui, Zhirun Nan, Yi Sun and Yongsi Zhang

Abstract Maize (*Zea mays* L.) is a very important crop in the world. In this present study, two important agronomic traits related to yield, ear diameter (ED) and ear axis diameter (EAD), were investigate in a maize recombinant inbred line (RIL) population derived from the cross of Mo17 and Huangzao4. Furthermore, the descriptive statistics, analysis of variance and correlation analysis were performed using SPSS 11.5 software in the RIL population. The results are useful for further developing quantitative trait locus mapping and molecular marker-assisted selection for ED and EAD in maize.

Keywords Maize · Ear diameter · Ear axis diameter · Investigation and analysis

---

C. Liao (✉)
Library, China West Normal University, Nanchong 637000, China
e-mail: liaochangminlxh@aliyun.com

H. Zhang · Q. Luo ·
GuoqiangHui · Z. Nan
Maize Research Institute, Shanxi Academy of Agricultural Sciences,
Xinzhou City 034000, China

H. Zhang · Q. Luo ·
GuoqiangHui · Z. Nan
Key Laboratory of Crop Gene Resources and Germplasm Enhancement on Loess Plateau,
Ministy of Agriculture, Taiyuan City 030000, China

D. He · Y. Zhang
College of Life Science, China West Normal University, Nanchong 637000, China

Y. Sun
Biotechnology Research Center, Shanxi Academy of Agricultural Sciences,
Taiyuan 030000 Shanxi, China

S. Li et al. (eds.), *Frontier and Future Development of Information Technology in Medicine and Education*, Lecture Notes in Electrical Engineering 269,
DOI: 10.1007/978-94-007-7618-0_77, © Springer Science+Business Media Dordrecht 2014

77.1 Introduction

There was must a segregation population consisting of many individuals in quantitative trait locus (QTL) mapping for some trait. To date, many types of segregating population can be used for QTL detection, among them F_2 is the most widely applied in maize (*Zea mays* L.) QTL identification [7, 9, 15, 16]. This kind of segregating population possesses many merits, such as less-time consuming, low cost and codominance in plant pheotype. Whereas, it has also an unresolved problem in QTL mapping, that is to be no continuous plants which are needed in phenotypic investigations and DNA analysis, thus, this kind of population is only temporal [13]. Relatively, recombinant inbred line (RIL) population is immortal and can be utilized in different time and regions, because of homogenous individuals. Coarsely, obtaining a RIL population needs longer time and higher cost compared to F_2 population [19, 27]. Currently, the studies on QTL mapping using RIL population are mainly focused on part crops according to literature, including rice [8, 20], soybean [5, 21] and wheat [3, 11], only limited studies were reported in maize in literature [1, 12], especially in China [4].

As well known, maize is one of the most important crops for human and animal in the world. The studies on QTL mapping for maize agronomic traits have already been reported frequently, involved in yield [14, 22, 24], plant phenotype [6, 25, 26] and flower period [2, 10] related traits. Even so, the number, location and genetic effects of QTL associated with same trait will present differences in different experiments, due to different population types, parental lines, genetic maps or marker type. Heretofore, there were some reports on QTL mapping for the two ear-related traits including ear diameter (ED) [17, 18] and ear axis diameter (EAD) [23] in maize, but RIL population is only limited in QTL identification for the two traits.

Consequently, in our study, a RIL population derived from the two elite inbred lines Mo17 and Huangzao4 were used as experimental parental materials, and the two traits ED and EAD were investigated and analyzed. This objective here is to provide some important phenotypic data needed in QTL identification for the two traits.

77.2 Materials and Methods

77.2.1 Plant Materials

The plant materials in this experiment included two parental inbred lines Huangzao4 and Mo17, and an F_9 RIL population consisting of 221 RILs. Huangzao4 and Mo17 are the representative lines of the Tansipingtou (China) and Lancaster heterotic (USA) groups, respectively. The RIL population was bred from the cross between the two parental lines.

77.2.2 Field Experiments and Statistical Analyses

All the 223 lines were sown in a complete randomized design with six replicates at experiment field (Shanxi Academy of Agricultural Sciences, Xinzhou City, Shanxi Province, China), single-row planting for each replicate, 20 plants per row, 67 cm and 25 cm as row interval and plant interval within a row, respectively. During harvest, the middle 10 plants of every replicate of each line were individually investigated the two traits ED (mm) and EAD (mm). Total 60 plants for one line were used to compute their mean. Based the statistic means, Statistical Package for Social Scientists software version 11.5 software (SPSS 11.5) was performed on descriptive statistics, analysis of variance (ANOVA) and correlation analysis.

77.3 Results and Analysis

77.3.1 Descriptive Statistics for Parents and Population

For the parents, the average value of Huangzao4 was higher than Mo17 for any of the two traits (Table 77.1). As to the RIL population, the results of eight parameter statistics were listed in Table 77.2. To be mentioned that the seven parameters, including range, minimum, maximum, mean, standard deviation (SD), skewness, and kertosis, could not be directly compared with each other owing to different traits, but coefficient of variance (CoV) can be used to reflect the variation extent of different individuals in the population. Comparatively, the CoV value of EAD (8.92 %) is higher than ED (8.74 %).

The frequency distribution of the data derived from 221 RILs within the population for the two traits are indicated in Figs. 77.1 and 77.2. On the grounds of these data in Table 77.2 and the two frequency distribution graphs, it was concluded that theses data of the two traits in the RIL population accorded with normal distribution, this suggested that the two traits ED and EAD are quantitative and can be used for QTL mapping.

According to literature, some studies on descriptive statistics for segregation populations and their parents were found in maize, but they can not be easily compared with each other, duo to different parental lines or segregation population types.

Table 77.1 Mean of the two parental lines in ED and EAD

	ED (cm)	EAD (cm)
Mo17	3.61	2.53
Huangzao4	3.87	2.63

ED ear diameter; *EAD* ear axis diameter

Table 77.2 Descriptive Statistics of the recombinant inbred line population in ED and EAD

	Range	Minimum	Maximum	Mean	SD	Skewness	Kurtosis	CoV (%)
ED (cm)	2.21	2.88	5.09	3.87	0.34	−0.10	0.96	8.74
EAD (cm)	1.71	1.95	3.66	2.75	0.25	0.31	1.45	8.92

Standard deviation; Coefficient of variance; *ED* ear diameter; *EAD* ear axis diameter

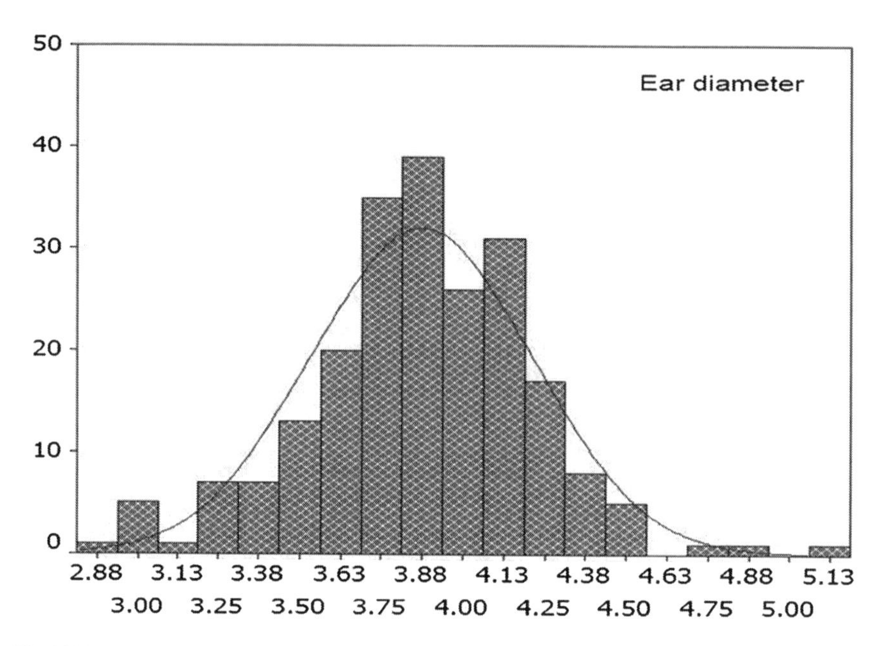

Fig. 77.1 Frequency distribution of ear diameter

77.3.2 Anova

The results of ANOVA, derived from the same RIL population in two traits ED and EAD, were showed in Table 77.3. The six replicates for one RIL within the RIL population could not present significant differences at 0.05 probability level for any of the two traits.

According to previous literature, when some agronomic traits were statistically analyzed for a segregation population, generally, ANOVA will be performed. But for different studies, it is not easily compared with each other, because of different parental lines or population types.

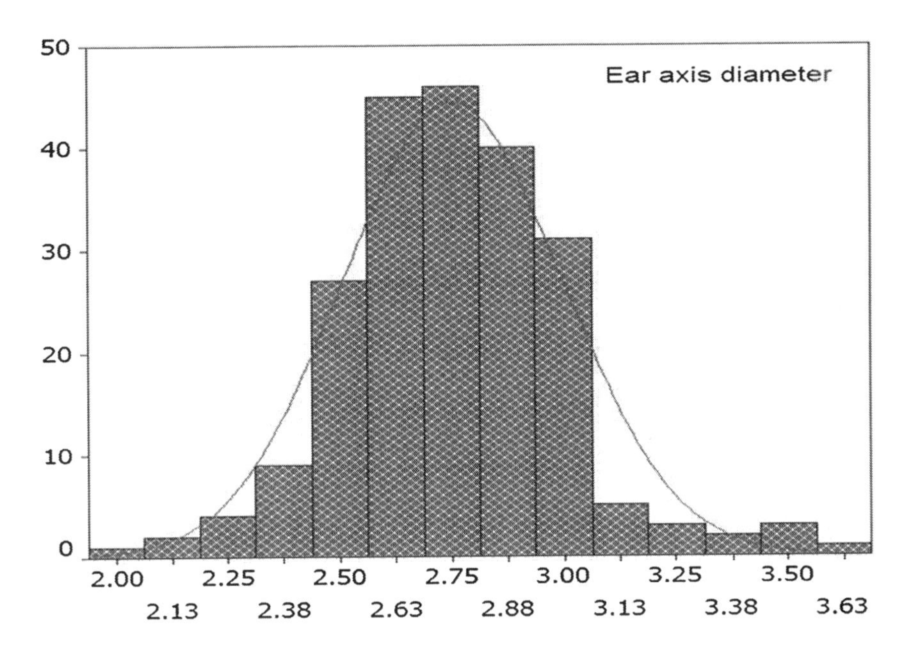

Fig. 77.2 Frequency distribution of ear axis diameter

Table 77.3 ANOVA of data from the RIL population derived from the cross between Mo17 and Huangzao4 in the two traits ED and EAD

		Sum of Squares	DF	Mean Square	F	Sig.
ED	Between groups	25379.471	220	115.361	0.915	0.792
	Within groups	127203.335	1009	126.069		
EAD	Between groups	281.868	220	1.281	1.180	0.052
	Within groups	1097.740	1011	1.086		

ED ear diameter; *EAD* ear axis diameter

77.3.3 Correlation Analysis

Correlation analysis was done between the two traits for the RIL population, and the results suggested that the two traits ED and EAD corelated significantly at 0.01 probability level (2-tailed), the correlation efficient was up to 0.565. This result revealed that the value of ED is higher for one RIL, and its EAD value is also higher.

From previous literature, many studies on correlation analysis for different maize agronomic traits were reported. But it is not easily compared with each other, due to different parental materials or segregation populations.

77.4 Conclusions

In this experiment, a RIL population derived from Mo17 × Huangzao4 and their parents were investigated in field for the two ear-related traits, including ED and EAD. From the values of descriptive statistics of the parents and population, it was concluded that the two traits were quantitative and controlled by multiple genes, and further ANOVA and correlation analysis for the RIL population in the two traits were also performed, these data are helpful in QTL mapping controlling the two ear-related traits.

Acknowledgments This work was financially supported by the Major Project for Genetically Modified Organisms Breeding from China Agriculture Ministry, China (2011ZX08003-001) and Project for the Doctoral Research Program from Shanxi Academy of Agricultural Sciences, China (YBSJJ1106).

References

1. Bouchez A, Hospital F, Causse M, Gallais A, Charcosset A (2002) Marker-assisted introgression of favorable alleles at quantitative trait loci between maize elite lines. Genetics 162:1945–1959
2. Chardon F, Virlon B, Moreau L, Falque M, Joets J, Decousset L, Murigneux A, Charcosset A (2004) Genetic architecture of flowering time in maize as inferred from quantitative trait loci meta-analysis and synteny conservation with the rice genome. Genetics 168:2169–2185
3. Ding AM, Li J, Cui F, Zhao CH, Ma HY, Wang HG (2011) QTL mapping for yield related traits using two associated RIL populations of wheat. Acta Agronomica Sinica 37:1511–1524
4. Ding JQ, Wang XM, Chander S, Li JS (2008) Identification of QTL for maize resistance to common smut by using recombinant inbred lines developed from the Chinese hybrid Yuyu22. J Appl Genet 49:147–154
5. Fu S, Zhan Y, Zhi H, Gai J, Yu D (2006) Mapping of SMV resistance gene Rsc-7 by SSR markers in soybean. Genetica 128:63–69
6. Guo JF, Su GQ, Zhang JP, Wang GY (2008) Genetic analysis and QTL mapping of maize yield and associate agronomic traits under semiarid land condition. Afr J Biotechnol 7:1829–1838
7. Hatakeyama K, Horisaki A, Niikura S, Narusaka Y, Abe H, Yoshiaki H, Ishida M, Fukuoka H, Matsumoto S (2010) Mapping of quantitative trait loci for high level of self-incompatibility in *Brassica rapa* L. Genome 53:257–265
8. Liu QM, Jiang JH, Niu FA, He YJ, Hong DL (2013) QTL analysis for seven quality traits of RIL population in Japonica rice based on three genetic statistical models. Rice Sci 20:31–38
9. Liu R, Wang B, Guo W, Wang L, Zhang T (2011) Differential gene expression and associated QTL mapping for cotton yield based on a cDNA-AFLP transcriptome map in an immortalized F_2. Theor Appl Genet 123:439–454
10. Liu XH, Zheng ZP, Tan ZB, Li Z, He C, Liu DH, Zhang GQ, Luo YC (2010) QTL mapping for controlling anthesis-silking interval based on RIL population in maize. Afr J Biotechnol 9:950–955
11. Ma Z, Zhao D, Zhang C, Zhang Z, Xue S, Lin F, Kong Z, Tian D, Luo Q (2007) Molecular genetic analysis of five spike-related traits in wheat using RIL and immortalized F_2 populations. Mol Genet Genomics 277:31–42

12. Ordas B, Malvar RA, Hill WG (2008) Genetic variation and quantitative trait loci associated with developmental stability and the environmental correlation between traits in maize. Genet Res 90:385–395
13. Pilet ML, Duplan G, Archipiano M, Barret P, Baron C, Horvais R, Tanguy X, Lucas MO, Renard M, Delourme R (2001) Stability of QTL for field resistance to blackleg across two genetic backgrounds in oilseed rape. Crop Sci 41:197–205
14. Ribaut JM, Jiang C, Gonzales-de-Leon D, Edmeades GO, Hosington D (1997) Identification of quantitative trait loci under drought trait loci under drought conditions in tropical maize. 2. Yield components and marker-assisted selection strategies. Theor Appl Genet 94:887–896
15. Sandal N, Jin H, Rodriguez-Navarro DN, Temprano F, Cvitanich C, Brachmann A, Sato S, Kawaguchi M, Tabata S, Parniske M, Ruiz-Sainz JE, Andersen SU, Stougaard J (2012) A set of Lotus japonicus Gifu x Lotus burttii recombinant inbred lines facilitates map-based cloning and QTL mapping. DNA Res 19(4):223–317
16. Takagi H, Abe A, Yoshida K, Kosugi S, Natsume S, Mitsuoka C, Uemura A, Utsushi H, Tamiru M, Takuno S, Innan H, Cano LM, Kamoun S, Terauchi R (2013) QTL-seq: rapid mapping of quantitative trait loci in rice by whole genome resequencing of DNA from two bulked populations. Plant J 74:174–183
17. Tan WW, Wang Y, Li YX, Liu C, Liu ZZ, Peng B, Wang D, Zhang Y, Sun BC, Shi YS, Song YC, Yang DG, Wang TY, Li Y (2011) QTL mapping of ear traits of maize under different water regimes. Acta Agronomica Sinica 37:235–248
18. Tian WW, Wang Y, Li YX, Liu C, Liu ZZ, Peng B, Wang D, Zhang Y, Sun BC, Shi YS, Song YC, Yang DG, Wang TY, Li Y (2011) QTL analysis of ear traits in maize across multiple environments. Scientia Agricultura Sinica 44:233–244
19. Wan X, Weng J, Zhai H, Wang J, Lei C, Liu X, Guo T, Jiang L, Su N, Wan J (2008) Quantitative trait loci (QTL) analysis for rice grain width and fine mapping of an identified QTL allele gw-5 in a recombination hotspot region on chromosome 5. Genetics 179:2239–2252
20. Wan XY, Wan JM, Jiang L, Wang JK, Zhai HQ, Weng JF, Wang HL, Lei CL, Wang JL, Zhang X, Cheng ZJ, Guo XP (2006) QTL analysis for rice grain length and fine mapping of an identified QTL with stable and major effects. Theor Appl Genet 112:1258–1270
21. Wang HL, Yu DY, Wang YJ, Chen SY, Gai JY (2004) Mapping QTL of soybean root weight with RIL population NJRIKY. Yi Chuan 26:333–336
22. Xiao YN, Li XH, George ML, Li MS, Zhang SH, Zheng YL (2005) Quantitative trait locus analysis of drought tolerance and yield in maize in China. Plant Molecular Biology Reporter 23:155–165
23. Yang JP, Rong TZ, Xiang DQ, Tang HT, Huang LJ, Dai JR (2005) QTL mapping of quantitative traits in maize. Acta Agronomica Sinica 31:188–196
24. Yang XJ, Lu M, Zhang SH, Zhou F, Qu YY, Xie CX (2008) QTL mapping of plant height and ear position in maize (Zea mays L.). Yi Chuan 30:1477–1486
25. Zhang WQ, Ku LX, Zhang J, Han P, Chen YH (2013) QTL analysis of kernel ratio, kernel depth and 100-Kernel weight in maize (Zea mays L.). Acta Agronomica Sinica 39:455–463
26. Zhang Z, Liu Z, Cui Z, Hu Y, Wang B, Tang J (2013) Genetic analysis of grain filling rate using conditional QTL mapping in maize. PLoS ONE 8:e56344
27. Zheng ZP, Liu XH (2013) Genetic analysis of agronomic traits associated with plant architecture by QTL mapping in maize. Genet Mol Res 12:1243–1253

Chapter 78
Descriptive Statistics and Correlation Analysis of Three Kernel Morphology Traits in a Maize Recombinant Inbred Line Population

Changmin Liao, Daowen He and Xiaohong Liu

Abstract Maize (*Zea mays* L.) is one of the most important crops throughout the world. In this study, three agronomic traits related to kernel morphology of a recombinant inbred line (RIL) population derived from the cross between Mo17 and Huangzao4 were selected to be investigated, including kernel length, kernel width and kernel height. Furthermore, the descriptive statistics and correlation analysis were performed using SPSS 11.5 software in the three traits. The results are useful for further quantitative trait locus mapping and molecular marker-assisted selection for the three kernel morphology traits in maize breeding program.

Keywords Maize (*Zea mays* L.) · Kernal-related traits · RIL population · Descriptive statistics · Correlation analysis

78.1 Introduction

Quantitative trait locus (QTL) mapping needs a segregating population. Presently, there are many types of segregating population that can be used for QTL identification, but F_2 is still the most widely applied populations in plant breeding [2, 8, 11, 12, 14, 20–22]. The population possesses many merits, including less-time consuming and low cost, whereas, it is unavoidable in QTL mapping that no continuous plants can be used for phenotypic investigations and DNA analysis, so

C. Liao (✉)
Library, China West Normal University, Nanchong City 637000, China
e-mail: liaochangminlxh@aliyun.com

D. He · X. Liu
College of Life Science, China West Normal University, Nanchong City 637000, China

S. Li et al. (eds.), *Frontier and Future Development of Information Technology in Medicine and Education*, Lecture Notes in Electrical Engineering 269,
DOI: 10.1007/978-94-007-7618-0_78,

this kind of population has the deficiency named temporality [18]. Comparatively, a recombinant inbred line (RIL) population is immortal and can be utilized in different regions and time, because its individuals are homogenous. Of course, constructing this segregation population needs longer time and higher cost compared to F_2 [23, 30]. Currently, the studies on QTL mapping using RIL population are focused on few crops, including rice [13, 24, 26], soybean [9, 25, 27] and wheat [4, 5, 16], only limited reports were found in maize (*Zea mays* L.) in literature [1, 17], especially in China [6, 7].

Maize is one of the most important crops in the world. Presently, the studies on QTL mapping for maize agronomic traits have been reported frequently, including plant phenotype [10, 29], yield, [19, 28] and flower period [3, 15] related traits. Nevertheless, QTL number, location and genetic effects for same trait demonstrate differences in different experiments to some extent, due to different mapping parents, population types or genetic maps. But RIL population is hardly used for QTL identification in the three traits including kernel length, kernel width and kernel height.

Therefore, in this present study, a RIL population derived from the two elite inbred lines Mo17 and Huangzao4 was selected as experimental parental materials, and the three kernel-related traits including kernel length, kernel width and kernel height were investigated and analyzed. This objective is to provide some important data which can be used for QTL mapping for the three traits.

78.2 Materials and Methods

78.2.1 Plant Materials

The experimental materials involved in this study included two parental inbred lines Huangzao4 and Mo17, and an F_9 RIL population consisting of 239 RILs. Huangzao4 and Mo17 are the representative lines of the Tansipingtou (derived from China) and Lancaster heterotic (derived from USA) groups, respectively. The RIL population was derived from the cross between the two parental lines.

78.2.2 Field Experiments and Statistical Analysis

Above 241 lines were sown in a complete randomized design at Nanchong Institute of Agricultural Sciences, Nanchong City, Sichuan Province, China, with single-plant planting and 15 plants per row and one ear per plant in one replicate. After harvest, 20 kernels were randomly selected to investigate three kernel morphology traits, consisting of kernel length (mm), kernel width (mm) and kernel height (mm). The data for the RIL population were analyzed using Statistical Package for Social Scientists (SPSS) software version 11.5, including descriptive statistics, frequency distribution and correlation analysis.

78.3 Results and Analysis

78.3.1 Descriptive Statistics for Parents and Population

For the two parental lines, the average values of Mo17 were higher than Huangzao4 for all the three traits, except for kernel height (Table 78.1). With regard to the population, the results of phenotypic statistics, including range, minimum, maximum, mean, standard deviation (SD), skewness, kurtosis and coefficient of variation (CoV), were displayed in Table 78.2. To be mentioned, the seven parameters including range, minimum, maximum, mean, standard deviation, skewness, and kertosis, could not be easily compared with each other among the three traits. But, CoV, can be used to reflect the variation extent of different RILs in the population. Comparatively, the CoV value of kernel length is the highest, up to 11.92 %, followed by kernel height (11.17 %), and the lowest was from kernel width, only 7.05 %.

The frequency distribution graphs of the data derived from different RILs within the population for the three traits are indicated in Figs. 78.1, 78.2 and 78.3. From these data in Table 78.2 and the three figures, it was concluded that theses data of the three traits in the RIL population well agreed with a normal distribution, this suggested that the three traits including kernel length, kernel width, kernel height and kernel weight are quantitative and controlled by multiple genes.

There were some studies on descriptive statistics for segregation populations and their parents, but they can not be compared with each other, owing to different parental lines or population types.

Table 78.1 Mean of the two parental lines in the three traits

Parental lines	Kernel length (mm)	Kernel width (mm)	Kernel height (mm)
Mo17	9.34	9.60	4.77
Huangzao4	8.69	8.59	5.43

Table 78.2 Descriptive statistics of the recombinant inbred line population in the three traits

Traits	Range	Minimum	Maximum	Mean	SD	Skewness	Kurtosis	CoV (%)
Kernel length (mm)	6.28	5.72	12	8.22	0.98	0.178	0.311	11.92
Kernel width (mm)	3.01	6.69	9.70	8.23	0.58	−0.034	−0.389	7.05
Kernel height (mm)	4.45	4.08	8.53	5.28	0.59	0.875	3.309	11.17

SD standard deviation; *CoV* coeffeicient of variation

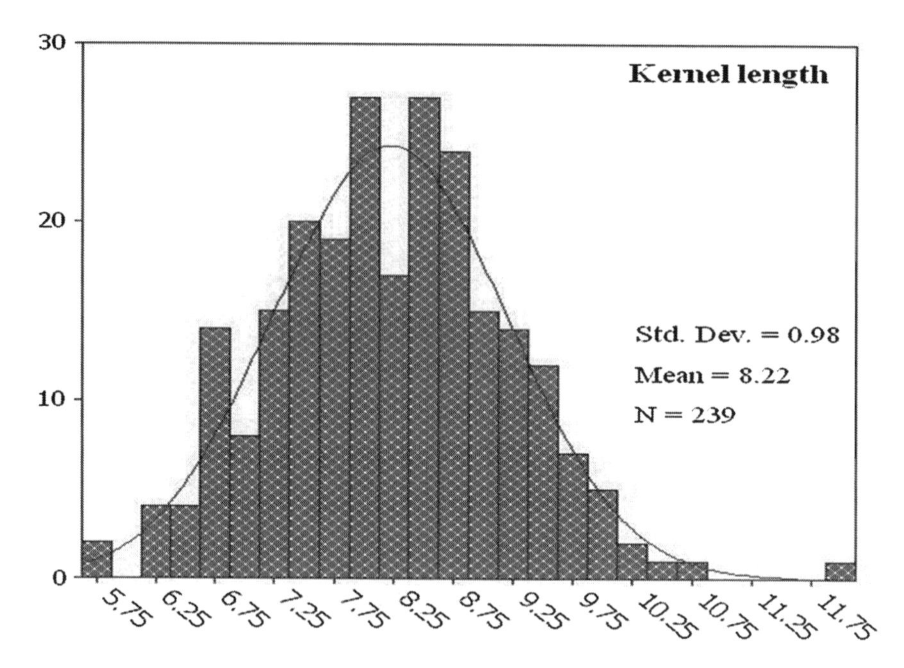

Fig. 78.1 Frequency distribution of kernel length

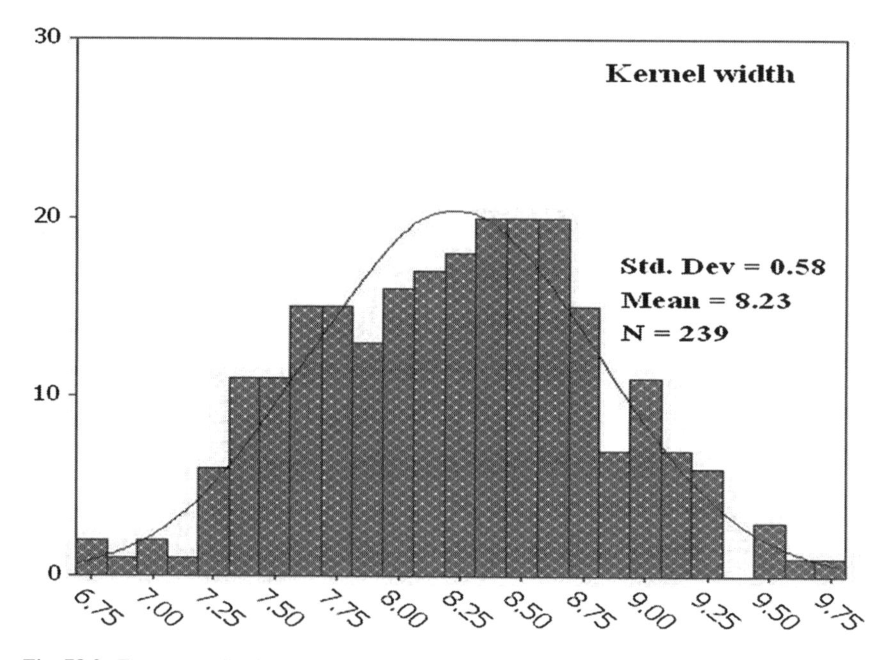

Fig. 78.2 Frequency distribution of kernel width

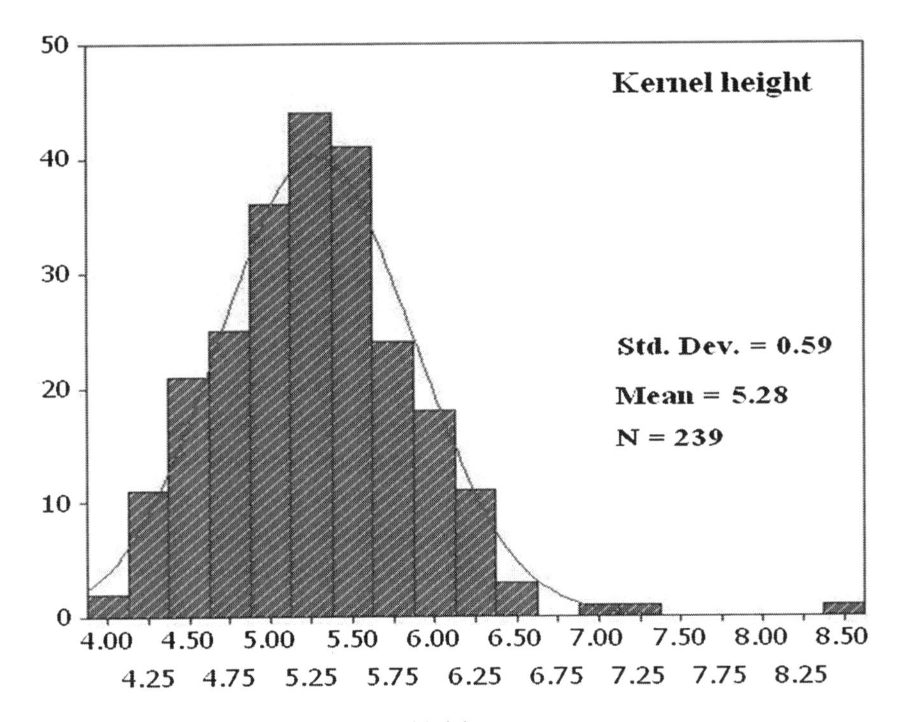

Fig. 78.3 Frequency distribution of kernel height

78.3.2 Correlation Analysis

Correlation analysis was carried out among the three traits for the experimental population, and the results were listed in Table 78.3. Among the three correlation combinations, all of them presented 0.01-level positive correlation, except for the one between kernel height and kernel length (0.01-level negative correlation).

According to previous literature, many studies on correlation analysis for different maize agronomic traits were reported. But it is not easily compared with each other, owing to different parental materials or segregation populations.

Table 78.3 Correlation analysis among the three traits in the recombinant inbred line population

	Kernel width (mm)	Kernel height (mm)
Kernel length (mm)	0.2**	−0.381**
Kernel width (mm)		0.264**

**Correlation is significant at the 0.01 level (2-tailed)

78.4 Summary

In this present study, a RIL population and their parents, derived from Mo17 × Huangzao4, were investigated in field for the three kernel morphology traits, including kernel length, kernel width and kernel height. According to the values of descriptive statistics of the parents and population and correlation analysis among the thirteen traits in the population, it was concluded that these traits were quantitative and controlled by multiple genes. The obtained data here could be further used to QTL mapping for these traits in maize.

Acknowledgments This work was financially supported by the Scientific Research Fund of the Sichuan Provincial Education Department (13ZA0012) of China.

References

1. Bouchez A, Hospital F, Causse M, Gallais A, Charcosset A (2002) Marker-assisted introgression of favorable alleles at quantitative trait loci between maize elite lines. Genetics 162:1945–1959
2. Cao Y, Li C, Yan J, Jiao F, Liu X, Hasty KA, Stuart JM, Gu W, Jiao Y (2012) Analysis of candidate genes of spontaneous arthritis in mice deficient for interleukin-1 receptor antagonist. Genes Genet Syst 87:107–113
3. Chardon F, Virlon B, Moreau L, Falque M, Joets J, Decousset L, Murigneux A, Charcosset A (2004) Genetic architecture of flowering time in maize as inferred from quantitative trait loci meta-analysis and synteny conservation with the rice genome. Genetics 168:2169–2185
4. Conti V, Roncallo PF, Beaufort V, Cervigni GL, Miranda R, Jensen CA, Echenique VC (2011) Mapping of main and epistatic effect QTLs associated to grain protein and gluten strength using a RIL population of durum wheat. J Appl Genet 52:287–298
5. Ding AM, Li J, Cui F, Zhao CH, Ma HY, Wang HG (2011) QTL mapping for yield related traits using two associated RIL populations of wheat. Acta Agronomica Sinica 37(9):1511–1524
6. Ding JQ, Wang XM, Chander S, Li JS (2008) Identification of QTL for maize resistance to common smut by using recombinant inbred lines developed from the Chinese hybrid Yuyu22. J Appl Genet 49:147–154
7. Ding D, Li WH, Song GL, Qi HY, Liu JB, Tang JH (2011) Identification of QTLs for arsenic accumulation in maize (*Zea mays* L.) Using a RIL Population. PLoS ONE 6:e25646
8. Dobón A, Canet JV, Perales L, Tornero P (2011) Quantitative genetic analysis of salicylic acid perception in Arabidopsis. Planta 234:671–684
9. Fu S, Zhan Y, Zhi H, Gai J, Yu D (2006) Mapping of SMV resistance gene Rsc-7 by SSR markers in soybean. Genetica 128:63–69
10. Guo JF, Su GQ, Zhang JP, Wang GY (2008) Genetic analysis and QTL mapping of maize yield and associate agronomic traits under semiarid land condition. Afr J Biotechnol 7:1829–1838
11. Hatakeyama K, Horisaki A, Niikura S, Narusaka Y, Abe H, Yoshiaki H, Ishida M, Fukuoka H, Matsumoto S (2010) Mapping of quantitative trait loci for high level of self-incompatibility in *Brassica rapa* L. Genome 53:257–265
12. Li M, Sun P, Zhou H, Chen S, Yu S (2011) Identification of quantitative trait loci associated with germination using chromosome segment substitution lines of rice (*Oryza sativa* L.). Theor Appl Genet 123:411–420

13. Liu QM, Jiang JH, Niu FA, He YJ, Hong DL (2013) QTL analysis for seven quality traits of RIL population in Japonica rice based on three genetic statistical models. Rice Sci 20:31–38
14. Liu R, Wang B, Guo W, Wang L, Zhang T (2011) Differential gene expression and associated QTL mapping for cotton yield based on a cDNA-AFLP transcriptome map in an immortalized F_2. Theor Appl Genet 123:439–454
15. Liu XH, Zheng ZP, Tan ZB, Li Z, He C, Liu DH, Zhang GQ, Luo YC (2010) QTL mapping for controlling anthesis-silking interval based on RIL population in maize. Afr J Biotechnol 9:950–955
16. Ma Z, Zhao D, Zhang C, Zhang Z, Xue S, Lin F, Kong Z, Tian D, Luo Q (2007) Molecular genetic analysis of five spike-related traits in wheat using RIL and immortalized F_2 populations. Mol Genet Genomics 277:31–42
17. Ordas B, Malvar RA, Hill WG (2008) Genetic variation and quantitative trait loci associated with developmental stability and the environmental correlation between traits in maize. Genet Res 90:385–395
18. Pilet ML, Duplan G, Archipiano M, Barret P, Baron C, Horvais R, Tanguy X, Lucas MO, Renard M, Delourme R (2001) Stability of QTL for field resistance to blackleg across two genetic backgrounds in oilseed rape. Crop Sci 41:197–205
19. Ribaut JM, Jiang C, Gonzales-de-Leon D, Edmeades GO, Hosington D (1997) Identification of quantitative trait loci under drought trait loci under drought conditions in tropical maize. 2. Yield components and marker-assisted selection strategies. Theor Appl Genet 94:887–896
20. Salomé PA, Bomblies K, Laitinen RA, Yant L, Mott R, Weigel D (2011) Genetic architecture of flowering-time variation in *Arabidopsis thaliana*. Genetics 188:421–433
21. Sandal N, Jin H, Rodriguez-Navarro DN, Temprano F, Cvitanich C, Brachmann A, Sato S, Kawaguchi M, Tabata S, Parniske M, Ruiz-Sainz JE, Andersen SU, Stougaard J (2012) A set of Lotus japonicus Gifu x Lotus burttii recombinant inbred lines facilitates map-based cloning and QTL mapping. DNA Res 19:317–323
22. Takagi H, Abe A, Yoshida K, Kosugi S, Natsume S, Mitsuoka C, Uemura A, Utsushi H, Tamiru M, Takuno S, Innan H, Cano LM, Kamoun S, Terauchi R (2013) QTL-seq: rapid mapping of quantitative trait loci in rice by whole genome resequencing of DNA from two bulked populations. Plant J 74:174–183
23. Wan X, Weng J, Zhai H, Wang J, Lei C, Liu X, Guo T, Jiang L, Su N, Wan J (2008) Quantitative trait loci (QTL) analysis for rice grain width and fine mapping of an identified QTL allele gw-5 in a recombination hotspot region on chromosome 5. Genetics 179:2239–2252
24. Wan XY, Wan JM, Jiang L, Wang JK, Zhai HQ, Weng JF, Wang HL, Lei CL, Wang JL, Zhang X, Cheng ZJ, Guo XP (2006) QTL analysis for rice grain length and fine mapping of an identified QTL with stable and major effects. Theor Appl Genet 112:1258–1270
25. Wang HL, Yu DY, Wang YJ, Chen SY, Gai JY (2004) Mapping QTL of soybean root weight with RIL population NJRIKY. Yi Chuan 26:333–336
26. Wang L, Wang AH, Huang XH, Zhao Q, Dong GJ, Qian Q, Sang T, Han B (2011) Mapping 49 quantitative trait loci at high resolution through sequencing-based genotyping of rice recombinant inbred lines. Theor Appl Genet 122:327–340
27. Xu P, Wang H, Li Q, Gai JY, Yu DY (2007) Mapping QTLs related to oil content of soybeans. Yi Chuan 29:92–96
28. Yang XJ, Lu M, Zhang SH, Zhou F, Qu YY, Xie CX (2008) QTL mapping of plant height and ear position in maize (*Zea mays* L.). Yi Chuan 30:1477–1486
29. Zhang Z, Liu Z, Cui Z, Hu Y, Wang B, Tang J (2013) Genetic analysis of grain filling rate using conditional QTL mapping in maize. PLoS ONE 8(2):e56344
30. Zheng ZP, Liu XH (2013) Genetic analysis of agronomic traits associated with plant architecture by QTL mapping in maize. Genet Mol Res 12:1243–1253

Chapter 79
Study on Two Agronomic Traits Associated with Kernel Weight in a Maize RIL Segregation Population

Changmin Liao

Abstract Maize (*Zea mays* L.) is a very important crop in the world. In this present study, two important agronomic traits, related to kernel weight, were investigated in a maize Recombinant Inbred Line (RIL) population derived from the cross of Mo17 and Huangzao4, including 100-kernel weight and ear kernel weight. Furthermore, the descriptive statistics, analysis of variance and correlation analysis were performed using SPSS 11.5 software in the RIL population. The results are useful for further developing quantitative trait locus mapping and molecular marker-assisted selection for the two traits of maize.

Keywords Maize (*Zea mays* L.) · Recombinant inbred line population · 100-kernel weight · Ear kernel weight · Statistic analysis

79.1 Introduction

A Quantitative Trait Locus (QTL) analysis for agronomic traits needs a segregating population that is consisting of different individuals. Up to now, there are many types of segregating population that can be used for QTL mapping, but F_2 population is still the most widely applied in maize (*Zea mays* L.) breeding [1–4] because this kind of population possesses many merits, including less-time consuming and low cost, whereas, it has a unavoidable problem in QTL mapping, that is to be no continuous plants which can be used for phenotypic investigation and DNA analysis, so this kind of population is temporal [5]. However for Recombinant Inbred Line (RIL) population, it is immortal and can be utilized in different regions and time, because of homogenous individuals. Coarsely, establishing a RIL segregation

C. Liao (✉)
Library, China West Normal University, Nanchong 637000, China
e-mail: liaochangminlxh@aliyun.com

S. Li et al. (eds.), *Frontier and Future Development of Information Technology in Medicine and Education*, Lecture Notes in Electrical Engineering 269,
DOI: 10.1007/978-94-007-7618-0_79,

population needs longer time and higher cost compared to F_2 population [6, 7]. Currently, the studies on QTL mapping using RIL population are focused on few crops, including rice [8, 9], soybean [10, 11] and wheat [12, 13], only limited reports were found in maize in literature [14, 15], especially in China [16].

Presently, maize is one of the most important crops in the world., the studies on QTL mapping for maize agronomic traits have frequently been reported, including plant phenotype [17, 18], yield [19, 20] and flower period [21, 22] related traits. Nevertheless, the number, location and genetic effects of QTL controlling same trait showed differences in different experiments, due to different population types, mapping parents or genetic maps. So far, there were some reports on QTL mapping for the two kernel-weight traits 100-kernel weight [23] and ear kernel weight [24] in maize, but RIL population is only limited in QTL identification for the two traits.

Therefore, in this study, a RIL population derived from the two elite inbred lines Mo17 and Huangzao4 were selected as experimental parental materials, and the two traits 100-kernel weight and ear kernel weight were investigated and analyzed. This objective is to provide the phenotypic data needed in QTL mapping for these traits.

79.2 Materials and Methods

79.2.1 Experimental Materials

The experimental materials involved in this study included two parental inbred lines Huangzao4 and Mo17, and an F_9 RIL population consisting of 221 RILs. Huangzao4 and Mo17 are the representative lines of the Tansipingtou (China) and Lancaster heterotic (USA) groups, respectively. The RIL population was derived from the cross between the two parental lines.

79.2.2 Field Experiments and Statistical Analyses

All the 223 lines were sown in a complete randomized design with six replicates at experiment field (Shanxi Academy of Agricultural Sciences, Xinzhou City, Shanxi Province, China), single-row planting for each replicate, 20 plants per row, 67 cm and 25 cm as row interval and plant interval within a row, respectively. During harvest, the middle 10 plants of every replicate of each line were individually investigated the two traits 100-kernel weight (g) and ear kernel weight (g). Total 60 plants for one line were used to compute their mean. Based on the statistic means, Statistical Package for Social Scientists software version 11.5 (SPSS 11.5) was used to perform descriptive statistics, analysis of variance (ANOVA) and correlation analysis.

Table 79.1 Mean of the two parental lines in the two traits 100-kernel and ear kernel weight

	100-Kernel weight (g)	Ear kernel weight (g)
Mo17	18.75	60.06
Huangzao4	27.85	46.62

79.3 Results and Analysis

79.3.1 Descriptive Statistics for Parents and Population

For the parents, the average value of Huangzao4 was higher than Mo17 for 100-kernel weight, whereas for ear kernel weight, the investigated result was contrary (Table 79.1). With regard to the population, the statistic results of eight parameters were displayed in Table 79.2. To be mentioned, the seven parameters including range, minimum, maximum, mean, standard deviation (SD), skewness, and kertosis, could not be directly compared with each other, but coefficient of variance (CoV) can be used to reflect the variation extent of different RILs in the population. Comparatively, the CoV value of ear kernel weight (33.54 %) is higher than that of 100-kernel weight (30.33 %).

The frequency distribution graphs of the data, derived from two investigated traits in the different RILs within the segregation population, are indicated in Figs. 79.1 and 79.2. From these data in Table 79.2 and the two frequency distribution graphs, it was easily concluded that theses data of the two traits in the RIL population agreed with a normal distribution, this suggested that the two traits including 100-kernel weight and ear kernel weight are quantitative and controlled by multiple genes.

There were some reports on descriptive statistics for segregation populations and their parents, but it is not easily compared with each other, due to different parental lines or population types.

Table 79.2 Descriptive statistics of the recombinant inbred line population in the two traits 100-kernel and ear kernel weight

	Range	Minimum	Maximum	Mean	SD	Skewness	Kurtosis	CoV (%)
100-kernel weight (g)	53.93	7.85	61.78	24.80	7.52	2.54	8.95	30.33
Ear kernel weight (g)	131.73	2.45	134.18	58.76	19.71	0.11	0.98	33.54

SD standard deviation; *CoV* coefficient of variance

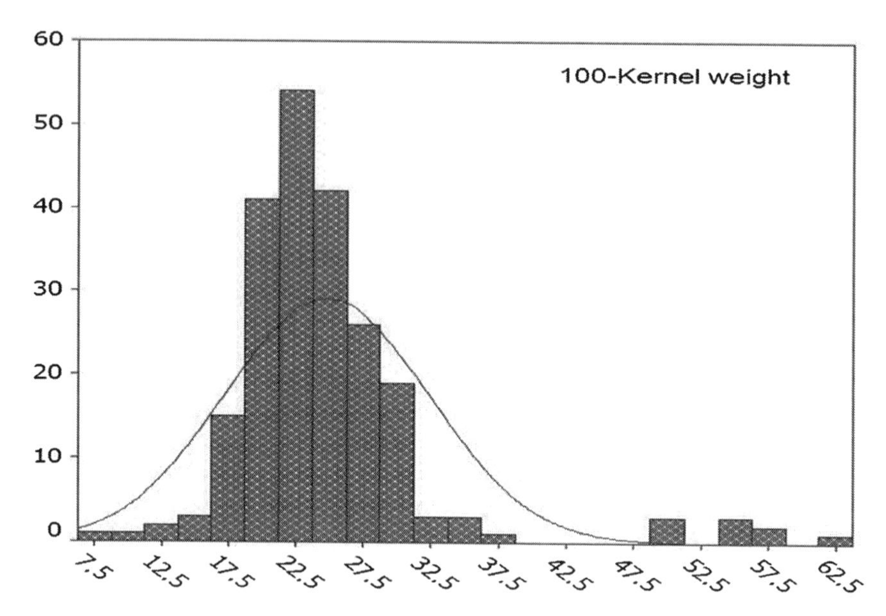

Fig. 79.1 Frequency distribution of 100-kernel weight. Horizontal axis and vertical axis indicated 100-kernel weight (**g**) and number of RIL individual, respectively

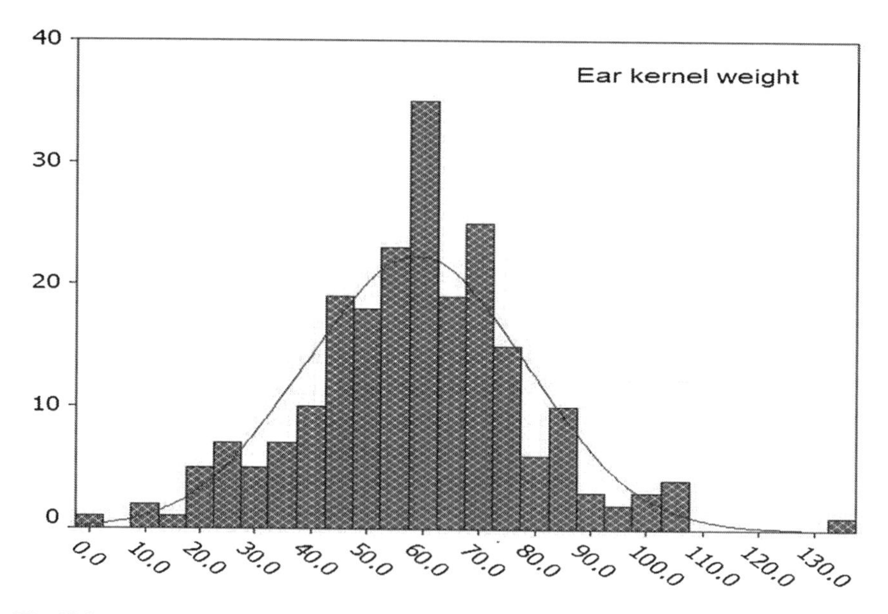

Fig. 79.2 Frequency distribution of ear kernel weight. Horizontal axis and vertical axis indicated ear kernel weight (**g**) and number of RIL individual, respectively

Table 79.3 ANOVA of data from the RIL population derived from the cross between Mo17 and Huangzao4 in the two traits 100-kernel weight and ear kernel weight

		Sum of squares	Df[a]	Mean square	F	Sig.
100-kernel weight (g)	Between groups	69188.139	219	315.928	1.139	0.102
	Within groups	276041.807	995	277.429		
Ear kernel weight (g)	Between groups	566654.021	220	2575.700	4.213[b]	0.000
	Within groups	622348.437	1018	611.344		

[a] Excluding missing values
[b] Correlation is significant 0.01 probability level

79.3.2 Anova

The results of ANOVA for the two traits including 100-kernel and ear kernel weight were showed in Table 79.3. Ear kernel weight presented significant differences at 0.01 probability level for the 221 RILs among the segregation population, while 100-kernel weight did not display difference at 0.05 probability level.

There were also a few studies on ANOVA for the data from a segregation population, but it is not easily compared with each other, due to different parental lines or population types.

79.3.3 Correlation Analysis

Correlation analysis was carried out between the two traits for the RIL population, and the results was that the two traits 100-kernel and ear kernel weight correlated significantly at 0.01 probability level (2-tailed), the correlation efficient was up to 0.188. This suggested that the 100-kernel weight value of one RIL is higher, and its ear kernel weight value is also higher.

According to literature, many studies on correlation analysis for different agronomic traits were reported in maize. But it is not easily compared with each other, due to different parental materials or different segregation populations.

79.4 Conclusions

In this present study, a RIL population derived from Mo17 × Huangzao4 together with their parents were investigated the two kernel weight related traits, including 100-kernel weight and ear kernel weight. The result of descriptive statistics for the parents and population displayed that the two traits were quantitative and controlled by multiple genes. The further result of ANOVA and correlation analysis revealed that the obtained data here could be used to QTL mapping for the two agronomic traits.

Acknowledgments This work was financially supported by the Scientific Research Fund of the Sichuan Provincial Education Department (13ZA0012) of China.

References

1. Hatakeyama K, Horisaki A, Niikura S, Narusaka Y, Abe H, Yoshiaki H, Ishida M, Fukuoka H, Matsumoto S (2010) Mapping of quantitative trait loci for high level of self-incompatibility in Brassica rapa L. Genome 53:257–265
2. Liu R, Wang B, Guo W, Wang L, Zhang T (2011) Differential gene expression and associated QTL mapping for cotton yield based on a cDNA-AFLP transcriptome map in an immortalized F_2. Theor Appl Genet 123:439–454
3. Sandal N, Jin H, Rodriguez-Navarro DN, Temprano F, Cvitanich C, Brachmann A, Sato S, Kawaguchi M, Tabata S, Parniske M, Ruiz-Sainz JE, Andersen SU, Stougaard J (2012) A set of Lotus japonicus Gifu x Lotus burttii recombinant inbred lines facilitates map-based cloning and QTL mapping. DNA Res 19(4):317–323
4. Takagi H, Abe A, Yoshida K, Kosugi S, Natsume S, Mitsuoka C, Uemura A, Utsushi H, Tamiru M, Takuno S, Innan H, Cano LM, Kamoun S, Terauchi R (2013) QTL-seq: rapid mapping of quantitative trait loci in rice by whole genome resequencing of DNA from two bulked populations. Plant J 74:174–183
5. Pilet ML, Duplan G, Archipiano M, Barret P, Baron C, Horvais R, Tanguy X, Lucas MO, Renard M, Delourme R (2001) Stability of QTL for field resistance to blackleg across two genetic backgrounds in oilseed rape. Crop Sci 41:197–205
6. Wan X, Weng J, Zhai H, Wang J, Lei C, Liu X, Guo T, Jiang L, Su N, Wan J (2008) Quantitative trait loci (QTL) analysis for rice grain width and fine mapping of an identified QTL allele gw-5 in a recombination hotspot region on chromosome 5. Genetics 179:2239–2252
7. Zheng ZP, Liu XH (2013) Genetic analysis of agronomic traits associated with plant architecture by QTL mapping in maize. Genet Mol Res 12:1243–1253
8. Wan XY, Wan JM, Jiang L, Wang JK, Zhai HQ, Weng JF, Wang HL, Lei CL, Wang JL, Zhang X, Cheng ZJ, Guo XP (2006) QTL analysis for rice grain length and fine mapping of an identified QTL with stable and major effects. Theor Appl Genet 112:1258–1270
9. Liu QM, Jiang JH, Niu FA, He YJ, Hong DL (2013) QTL analysis for seven quality traits of RIL population in japonica rice based on three genetic statistical models. Ric Sci 20:31–38
10. Wang HL, Yu DY, Wang YJ, Chen SY, Gai JY (2004) Mapping QTL of soybean root weight with RIL population NJRIKY. Yi Chuan 26:333–336
11. Fu S, Zhan Y, Zhi H, Gai J, Yu D (2006) Mapping of SMV resistance gene Rsc-7 by SSR markers in soybean. Genetica 128:63–69
12. Ma Z, Zhao D, Zhang C, Zhang Z, Xue S, Lin F, Kong Z, Tian D, Luo Q (2007) Molecular genetic analysis of five spike-related traits in wheat using RIL and immortalized F_2 populations. Mol Genet Genomics 277:31–42
13. Ding AM, Li J, Cui F, Zhao CH, Ma HY, Wang HG (2011) QTL mapping for yield related traits using two associated RIL populations of wheat. Acta Agron Sin 37:1511–1524
14. Bouchez A, Hospital F, Causse M, Gallais A, Charcosset A (2002) Marker-assisted introgression of favorable alleles at quantitative trait loci between maize elite lines. Genetics 162:1945–1959
15. Ordas B, Malvar RA, Hill WG (2008) Genetic variation and quantitative trait loci associated with developmental stability and the environmental correlation between traits in maize. Genet Res 90:385–395
16. Ding JQ, Wang XM, Chander S, Li JS (2008) Identification of QTL for maize resistance to common smut by using recombinant inbred lines developed from the Chinese hybrid Yuyu22. J Appl Genet 49:147–154

17. Guo JF, Su GQ, Zhang JP, Wang GY (2008) Genetic analysis and QTL mapping of maize yield and associate agronomic traits under semiarid land condition. Afr J Biotechnol 7:1829–1838
18. Zhang WQ, Ku LX, Zhang J, Han P, Chen YH (2013) QTL analysis of kernel ratio, kernel depth and 100-Kernel weight in maize (Zea mays L.). Acta Agron Sin 39:455–463
19. Ribaut JM, Jiang C, Gonzales-de-Leon D, Edmeades GO, Hosington D (1997) Identification of quantitative trait loci under drought trait loci under drought conditions in tropical maize. 2. Yield components and marker-assisted selection strategies. Theor Appl Genet 94:887–896
20. Yang XJ, Lu M, Zhang SH, Zhou F, Qu YY, Xie CX (2008) QTL mapping of plant height and ear position in maize (Zea mays L.). Yi Chuan 30:1477–1486
21. Chardon F, Virlon B, Moreau L, Falque M, Joets J, Decousset L, Murigneux A, Charcosset A (2004) Genetic architecture of flowering time in maize as inferred from quantitative trait loci meta-analysis and synteny conservation with the rice genome. Genetics 168:2169–2185
22. Liu XH, Zheng ZP, Tan ZB, Li Z, He C, Liu DH, Zhang GQ, Luo YC (2010) QTL mapping for controlling anthesis-silking interval based on RIL population in maize. Afr J Biotechnol 9:950–955
23. Zhang Z, Liu Z, Cui Z, Hu Y, Wang B, Tang J (2013) Genetic analysis of grain filling rate using conditional QTL mapping in maize. PLoS One 8:e56344
24. Xiao YN, Li XH, George ML, Li MS, Zhang SH, Zheng YL (2005) Quantitative trait locus analysis of drought tolerance and yield in maize in China. Plant Mol Bio Reporter 23:155–165

Chapter 80
Improved Single-Key Attack on Reduced-Round LED

Feng Liu, Pei-li Wen, Xuan Liu and Shuai Meng

Abstract In this paper, On the basis of the single-key model and the differential analysis principle, we propose the improved attacks on the new low-cost LED block cipher which revisits meet-in-the-middle attack. More precisely, we choose a differential with high probability firstly. Since we have guessed some key nibbles to check whether the plaintext pair follows the differential characteristic, we construct the δ-set from plaintext which is used to match the right key under meet-in-the-middle attack. Finally, the key candidates are recovered by removing the values that do not content conditions. Hence the secret key bits can be recovered with very low complexity $2^{33,}$ which is faster than other previous papers. We attack the complete six rounds on LED-64, and we can expand to more rounds on LED-128. At the present time, it is an efficient attack on six-rounds of LED-64.

Keywords LED · Meet-in-the-middle attack · Block cipher · Differential characteristic

80.1 Introduction

Now, more and more popular the low-end devices are becoming, such as smart cards, RFID (radio frequency identification) tags. This environment spurs the development of lightweight cryptography like KTANTAN [1], LED and so on. LED is a lightweight block cipher presented by Jian Guo et al. In CHES 2011 [2].

F. Liu (✉) · X. Liu · S. Meng
School of Information Science and Engineering, Shandong Normal University, Jinan 250014, China
e-mail: liufengbiji@163.com

P. Wen
Weifang Business Vocational College, Zhucheng 262299, China

S. Li et al. (eds.), *Frontier and Future Development of Information Technology in Medicine and Education*, Lecture Notes in Electrical Engineering 269,
DOI: 10.1007/978-94-007-7618-0_80,

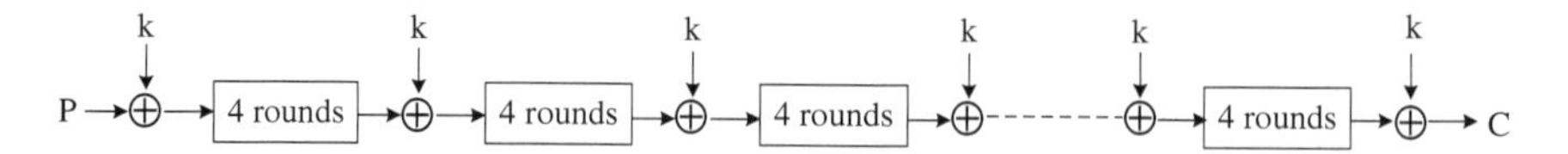

Fig. 80.1 The specification of LED

LED has two variants with different key lengths: LED-64 and LED-128. The LED is a derivative of the AES (Advanced Encryption Standard) [3].

Meet-in-the-middle (MITM) attack, originally introduced in Ref. [4], is a generic cryptanalytic technique for block ciphers. Early development starts with attack of DES. Afterwards, similar ideas have been applied to AES [5] and some hash functions. In Refs. [6], the authors present the differential attack for LED-64 reduced to 12 and 16 rounds. In Ref. [7, 8], the authors use the differential fault analysis on LED, and they both inject fault at round 30. However, our result is better than the above. In Ref. [9], the author propose the improved attack on AES. Because that LED is same to AES, we use the same attack to LED for better results.

In this paper, we use truncated differential attack and meet-in-the-middle attack on the LED block cipher and analyze only LED-64. Firstly, we choose a differential with high probability that is shown in Fig. 80.1. Then we construct a table consisting of internal state value. Lastly, use MITM attack the whole six rounds and obtain the right candidates of key bits. The number of key candidates can be further reduced by repeated guessing different values.

The rest paper is organized as follows: Sect. 80.2 describes the block cipher LED. Section 80.3 presents the attack on the reduce-round LED-64. The complexity computation is shown in Sect. 80.4. We summarize the paper in Sect. 80.5.

80.2 A Brief Description of LED-64 and Proposition

80.2.1 A Brief Description of LED-64

The design of the block cipher LED is specified in Ref. [2]. The design of LED has many parallels with AES. LED-64 is a 64-bit block cipher with 64 bit keys. The cipher state is conceptually arranged in a (4×4) grid where each nibble represents an element. For a 64-bit plain text P, the 16 nibbles $p_0p_1 \cdots p_{14}p_{15}$ are arranged in a square array.

The procedure can be viewed as eight steps. Each of steps is composed with two parts, which one is xor with k, and the procedure is defined as AK. Another part is round function. The process need 32 rounds. At the last the state is xor with k, then we can obtain the ciphertext C. There is no key schedule in this procedure. The specification of LED is shown in Fig. 80.2.

Each of rounds uses the operations Add Constants, Sub Cells, Shift Rows, and Mix Columns Serial in sequence. The overview of one round function is shown in Fig. 80.3.

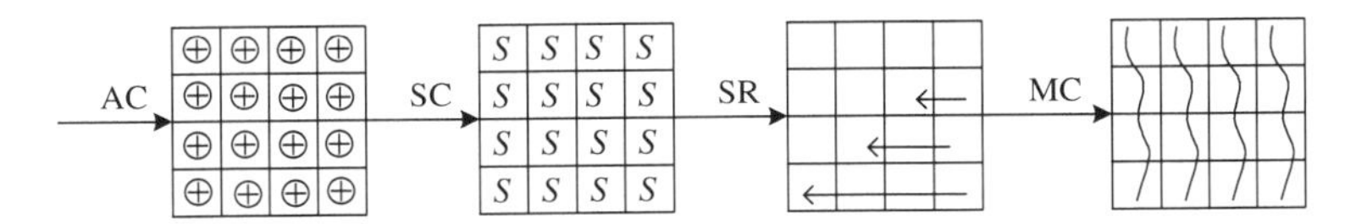

Fig. 80.2 An overview of one round of LED

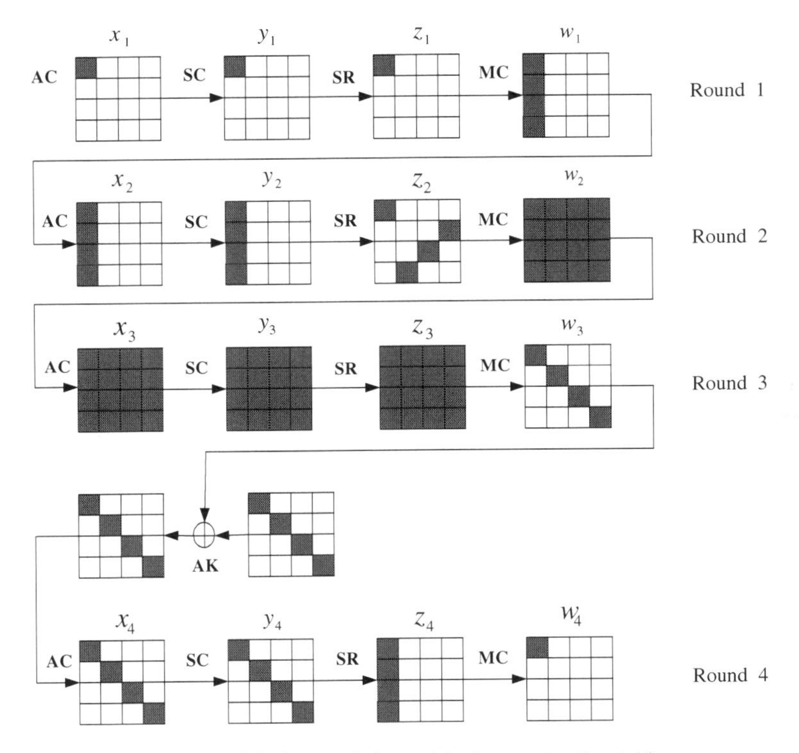

Fig. 80.3 Truncated differential characteristic used in the constructing table

1. Add Constants (AC): the state is xor with the round constants.
2. Sub Cell (SC): Each nibble in the array state is updated after using the S-box. S-box is 4 bits to 4 bits (Table 80.1).
3. Shift Rows(SR): Row i of the array state is rotated i distance to the left, for i = 0, 1, 2, 3.
4. Mix Columns Serial (MC): each column of the state matrix is replaced by the $M \cdot I$. $M^{-1}$is the inverse of M.

$$M = \begin{pmatrix} 4 & 1 & 2 & 2 \\ 8 & 6 & 5 & 6 \\ B & E & A & 9 \\ 2 & 2 & F & B \end{pmatrix} \quad M^{-1} = \begin{pmatrix} \mathrm{C} & \mathrm{C} & \mathrm{D} & 4 \\ 3 & 8 & 4 & 5 \\ 7 & 6 & 2 & \mathrm{E} \\ \mathrm{D} & 9 & 9 & D \end{pmatrix}$$

5. Add Round Key (AK): the state is xor with the round sub keys.

Table 80.1 The LED S-Box

s	0	1	2	3	4	5	6	7	8	9	A	B	C	D	E	F
s[x]	C	5	6	B	9	0	A	D	3	E	F	8	4	7	1	2

80.2.2 Proposition

Proposition 1 (the property of S-box, [10]). Given Δ_i and Δ_0 two non-zero differences in F_{256}, the following equation (80.1) has one solution in average.

$$S(x) + S(x + \Delta_i) = \Delta_0 \tag{80.1}$$

In addition, if both Δ_i and Δ_0 are known, then we can deduce the true input and output values of S-box.

Proposition 2 (the property of difference). The operations of AC and AK do not change the value and location of differences. The operation of SR change only the location of differences. The operation of MC not only change the value of differences, but also the location.

Definition 1 (δ-set, [10]). Let a δ-set be a set of 256 LED-state that are all different in one state nibble(the active nibble) and all equal in the other state nibble (the inactive nibbles).

80.3 The Improved Attack

LED block cipher is based on AES-like design principles, thus the design of LED will inevitably have many parallels with AES. In Ref. [9], the authors propose the truncated differential attack and meet-in-the-middle attack. So the attack can also be used on LED. Following is the procedure of using the same attack on LED-64. Firstly, we choose a differential with high probability$2^{-2\times3\times4} = 2^{-24}$, because of the two $4 \rightarrow 1$transitions in the Mix Columns of rounds 0 and round 5. The property of the differential characteristic is that the state can only take a restricted number of values. The true procedure is divided into two parts. The one is to construct table with the middle four rounds of differential characteristic. And the other is to match states in some state by encryption and description.

In this paper, at the round i, x_i is defined as the state of operation AC. y_i denotes the state of operation SC. z_i symbols the state of operation SR. w_i symbols the state of operation MC. The symbol "$'$" is denoted that existing difference. For example, $\Delta x = x \oplus x'$.

80.3.1 Construct the Table

Instead of storing the whole values, we construct a table T to store some values, which reduce the memory complexity. Figure 80.4 The concrete procedure is as follows.

Step 1. Deduce the value of Δx_3
Guess values of the five nibbles $\Delta z_1[I_0], x_2[I_0], x_2[I_1], x_2[I_2], x_2[I_3]$. Then we can known the values of $x_2[I_0, I_1, I_2, I_3]$ and $x'_2[I_0, I_1, I_2, I_3]$. Through the operations of SC and SR, the values of $z_2[I_0, I_7, I_{10}, I_{13}]$ and $z'_2[I_0, I_7, I_{10}, I_{13}]$ are known. Because of the equation $\Delta x_3 = \Delta w_2 = M \cdot \Delta z_2, m$, we deduce the value of Δx_3.
Step 2. Deduce the value of Δy_3
Guess values of the five nibbles $\Delta w_4[I_0]$, $z_4[I_0]$, $z_4[I_1]$, $z_4[I_2]$, $z_4[I_3]$. Then we can known the values of $z_4[I_0, I_1, I_2, I_3]$ and $z'_4[I_0, I_1, I_2, I_3]$. Through the operations of SR^{-1} and SC^{-1}, the values of $x_4[I_0, I_5, I_{10}, I_{15}]$ and $x'_4[I_0, I_5, I_{10}, I_{15}]$ are known. With the equations $\Delta y_3 = SR^{-1}[M^{-1} \cdot \Delta w_3]$ and $\Delta w_3 = \Delta x_4$, we deduce the value of Δy_3.
Step 3. List x_3, x'_3, y_3, y'_3.
Based on the proposition 1, list all of the possible values x_3, x'_3, y_3, y'_3.
Step 4. List the candidate value of $K[I_0, I_5, I_{10}, I_{15}]$
During to the known values of y_3, y'_3, we compute the values w_3 and w'_3 by equation$w_3 = M \cdot SR(y_3)$. And $x_4[I_0, I_5, I_{10}, I_{15}]$ and $x'_4[I_0, I_5, I_{10}, I_{15}]$ are known, so the candidates of $K[I_0, I_5, I_{10}, I_{15}]$ can be deduced.
Step 5. Δx_5 Add into the lookup table T based on the equation $\Delta x_5 = \Delta w_4$

We summarize the above description in the following Algorithm 1.

Algorithm 1 – Construct the Table.

1: function CONSTRUCTTABLE
2: Empty a lookup table T.
3: Guess values of the five nibbles $\Delta z_1[I_0], x_2[I_0], x_2[I_1], x_2[I_2], x_2[I_3]$.
4: Deduce differences in Δx_3.
5: Guess values of the five nibbles $\Delta w_4[I_0], z_4[I_0], z_4[I_1], z_4[I_2], z_4[I_3]$.
6: Deduce differences in Δy_3.
7: Deduce the values in x_3, x_3', y_3, y_3' with the differential property of the S-box.
8: Deduce $K[I_0, I_5, I_{10}, I_{15}]$.
9: for all the differences $\Delta z_1[I_0]$ do
10: Obtain a column of x_2, and then a state of x_3.
11: Add $\Delta x_5[I_0]$ to the lookup table T.
12: Return T.

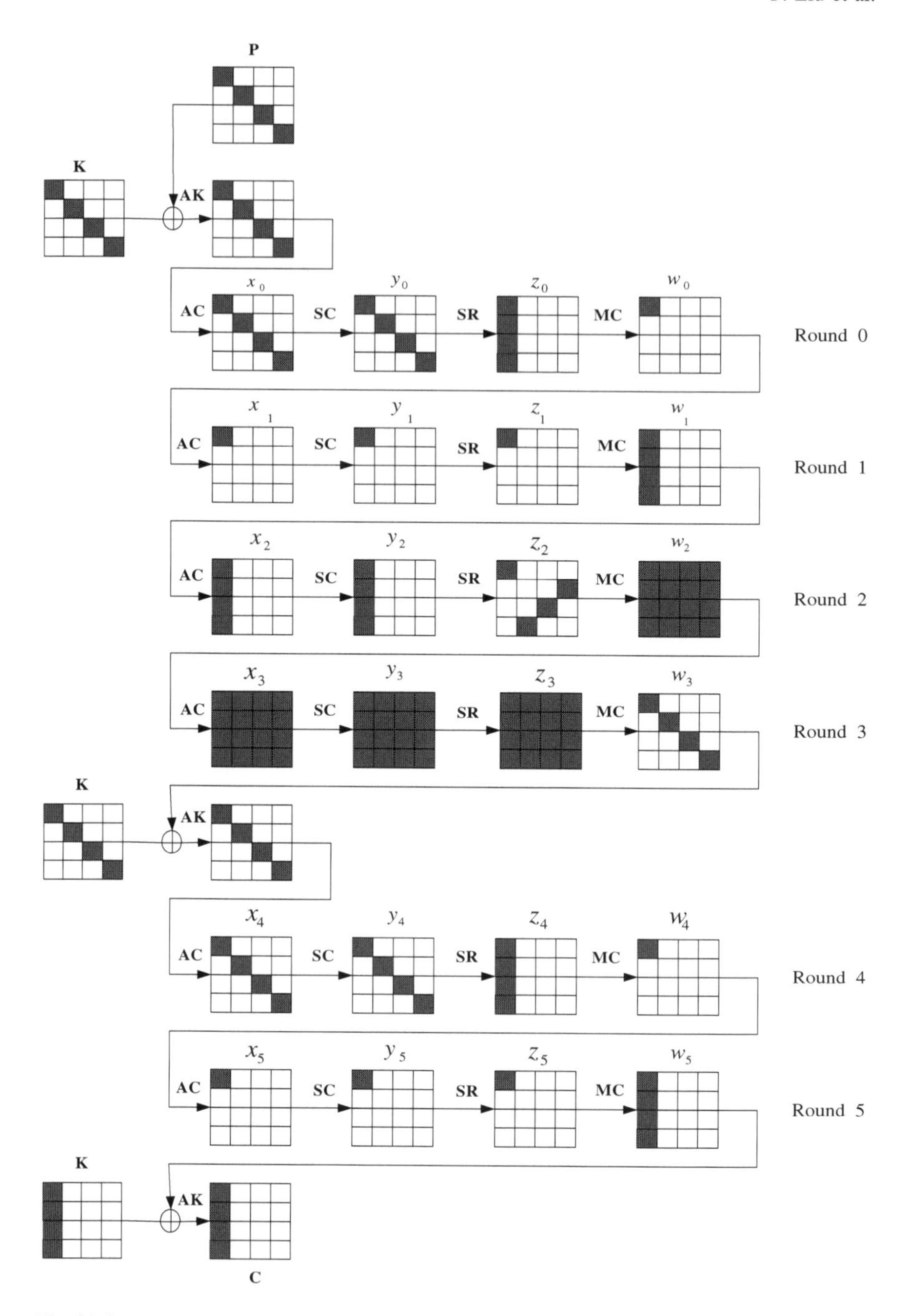

Fig. 80.4 Complete truncated differential characteristic of six rounds

80.3.2 The MITM Attack

In this section, we ask for the encryption of many pairs that follow the differential characteristic, and for each pair, we decrypt by guessing some key nibbles. Once such a pair is found, we construct a structure to encrypt which is related to a δ-set for the intermediate rounds. Lastly, we decrypt the ciphertexts to check whether the encryption of the δ-set belongs to this table. Thus, we can retrieve some keys, and the whole key is found after exhaustive searching. The detailed procedure is as follows.

Step 1. Choose plaintexts and compute ciphertexts

We choose all plaintexts that contend to the conditions.

$$\Delta P[I_0, I_5, I_{10}, I_{15}] \neq 0$$

So the diagonal takes all the possible 216 values, and the remaining 12 nibbles are fixed to some constants. Hence, we can choose $2^{16} \times (2^{16} - 1) \times 2^{-1} \approx 2^{31}$pairs that satisfy the plaintext difference. The corresponding ciphertexts can be known by the chosen plaintexts.

Step 2. Encrypt the chosen plaintexts

Xor with the $K[I_0, I_5, I_{10}, I_{15}]$ from Sect. 80.3.1, we compute the value of $x_0[I_0, I_5, I_{10}, I_{15}]$ and $x'_0[I_0, I_5, I_{10}, I_{15}]$. After the computation of SC, SR and MC, we obtain the value $w_0[I_0, I_1, I_2, I_3]$ and $w'_0[I_0, I_1, I_2, I_3]$. In addition, the value of w_0, w'_0 need to content the following differential conditions. $\Delta w_0[I_1, I_2, I_3] = 0$, $\Delta w_0[I_0] \neq 0$. If do not content the conditions, we delete the corresponding plaintexts and ciphertexts.

Step 3. Decrypt the corresponding ciphertexts

Guess the value of $K[I_1, I_2, I_3]$, xor with the ciphertexts, we can obtain $w_5[I_0, I_1, I_2, I_3]$ and $w'_5[I_0, I_1, I_2, I_3]$. Through decrypting of operations MC, SR and SC, the value of $x_5[I_0]$ and $x'_5[I_0]$. That is to say, $\Delta x_5[I_0]$is known.

Step 4. Match the middle state

We match the values $\Delta x_5[I_0]$ with the corresponding values from table T. If they are same, the guessing key bits are considered as candidates. If not, guess other values. Thus, we can retrieve some key bits successfully.

We summarize the above description in the following Algorithm 2.

Algorithm 2 – the Attack.

```
1:  function Attack
2:    while true do
3:      Choose plaintexts P where nibbles in diagonals 0 exist difference.
4:      for all corresponding ciphertexts C do
5:        for all P do
6:          Consider the pair (P,P') .
7:          for all K[I_0,I_5,I_10,I_15] s.t. Δw_0[I_1,I_2,I_3]=0 do
8:            Construct δ -set D from P .
9:            for all K[I_1,I_2,I_3] s.t. Δz_5[I_1,I_2,I_3]=0 do
10:             Decrypt to nibble 0 of x_5 for D.
11:           if x_5 ∈T then
12:             return EXHAUSTIVESEARCH()
13: end while
```

80.4 Complexity Computation

According to Algorithm 1, we have guessed ten nibbles $\Delta z_1[I_0]$,$x_2[I_0, I_1, I_2, I_3]$, $\Delta w_4[I_0]$ and $z_4[I_0, I_1, I_2, I_3]$. But the ten nibbles can be divided into two parts to guess. So time complexity in this algorithm is $2^{4\times5} + 2^{4\times5} = 2^{21}$.

According to Algorithm 2, we have guessed there nibbles $K[I_1, I_2, I_3]$. So time complexity in this algorithm is $2^{3\times4} = 2^{12}$.

All in all, the complexity of attack procedure is reduced to $2^{21} \times 2^{12} = 2^{33}$.

80.5 Conclusions

In this paper, based on the attack on AES from Patrick. et al., we attack LED-64 with same attack. Firstly, we choose a differential with high probability $2^{-2\times3\times4} = 2^{-24}$. Instead of storing the whole values, we construct a δ-set and table T to store some value, which reduce the memory complexity greatly. We attack the complete six rounds on LED-64, and we can expand to more rounds on LED-128. The number of key candidates can be further reduced by repeated guessing different values. The time complexity is reduced to 2^{33}, which is lower than previous results. To the best of our knowledge, this is currently the efficient result on LED-64 in this model. In addition, we can expand more rounds to attack LED-128 with low time and data complexity in our case. All in all, our attack is successful.

Acknowledgments We are grateful for the support of the National Natural Science Foundation of China (No.61272434), the Natural Science Foundation of Shandong Province (No.ZR2011FQ032,ZR2012FM004), the Project of Shandong Province Higher Educational Science and Technology Program (No. J11LG33) and the project of Senior Visiting Scholar of Shandong Province (No.2011A115).

References

1. Wei, L, Rechberger, C, Guo, J, et al (2011) Improved meet-in-the-middle cryptanalysis of KTANTAN[OL]. http://eprint.iacr.org/2011/201
2. Guo J, Peyrin T, Poschmann A, et al (2011) The LED block cipher. CHES 2011, LNCS 6917:326–341
3. National Institute of Standards and Technology (NIST) (2001) Advanced encryption standard. FIPS Publication 197
4. Diffie W, Hellman ME (1977) Special feature exhaustive cryptanalysis of the NBS data encryption standard. IEEE Comput 10:74–84
5. Demirci H, Selcuk Ali Aydm (2008) A meet-in-the-middle attack on 8-round AES. In: Nyberg, K, (ed) FSE, LNCS, vol 5086. p 116–126
6. Mendel F, Rijmen V, Toz D et al (2012) Differential analysis of the LED block cipher. FSE, LNCS, 7658:190–207
7. Jeong K, Lee C (2012) Differential fault analysis on block cipher LED-64. Future information technology, application and service. LNEE 164:747–755
8. Jovanovic P, Kreuzer M, Polian I (2012) A fault attack on the LED block cipher. COSADE 2012. LNCS 7275:120–134
9. Derbez P, Pierre-Alain F, Jérémy J (2013) Improved key recovery attacks on reduced-round AES in the single-key setting. EUROCRYPT. LNCS 7881:371–387
10. Damen J, Rijmen V(1998) Rijndael. AES proposal

Chapter 81
Automatic Screening of Sleep Apnea-Hypopnea Syndrome by ECG Derived Respiration

Qing Qiao, Guangming Tong and Rui Chen

Abstract *Objective* To evaluate the feasibility of Automatic screening Sleep Apnea-Hypopnea Syndrome (SAHS) by Electrocardiogram-Derived Respiration (EDR) of Ambulatory Electrocardiogram (AECG) monitoring. *Methods* The overnight sleep investigation was administered to 80 subjects by Polysomnogram (PSG) and 24 h AECGng simultaneously. The electrocardiogram analyzers did not know the PSG results at all. They were both asked to give the Apnea Hypopnea Index (AHI) by EDR and PSG respectively. The PSG result was considered as the gold standard so as to evaluate the feasibility of screening SAHS from EDR of AECG monitoring. *Results* The average age, percentage of male gender, body mass index, history of hypertension were higher in the SAHS(+) patients than those of the SAHS(-) patients. Automatic analysis was performed with software in a sensibility of 75, 87.5 and 100 % respectively. When software sensibility was fixed at 75 %, the sensitivity of screening SAHS with EDR was 26.7 %, with the specificity of 80 %, the positive predictive value of 80 %, the negative predictive value of 26.7 % and the diagnose accordance rate of 40 %. When software sensibility was fixed to 87.5 %, the sensitivity of screening SAHS with EDR was 55 %,with the specificity of 45 %, the positive predictive value of 75 %, the negative predictive value of 25 %, and the diagnose accordance rate of 52.5 %.

This work was supported by grants from Suzhou City Research Foundation for Applied Basic Research (No. SYS201237).

Q. Qiao
Department of Nephrology, First Hospital Affiliated to Soochow University, Jiangsu Province, China

G. Tong (✉)
Department of Cardiology, Second Hospital Affiliated to Soochow University, Jiangsu Province, China
e-mail: tgm1@sina.com

R. Chen
Department of Sleep Center, Second Hospital Affiliated to Soochow University, Jiangsu Province, China

S. Li et al. (eds.), *Frontier and Future Development of Information Technology in Medicine and Education*, Lecture Notes in Electrical Engineering 269,
DOI: 10.1007/978-94-007-7618-0_81,

When software sensibility was fixed to 100 %, the sensitivity of screening SAHS with EDR was 88.3 %, with the specificity of 35 %, the positive predictive value of 84.1 %, the negative predictive value of 50 %, and the diagnose accordance rate of 75 %. *Conclusions* EDR technique of AECG was useful to screen the suspicious SAHS patients, sensitivity and the diagnosis coincidence rate was high when the sensibility of automatic analysis software was adjusted to 100 %.

Keywords Sleep Apnea · ECG Derived Respiration (EDR) · Polysomnogram (PSG)

81.1 Introduction

Sleep Apnea-hypopnea Syndrome (SAHS) is a severe sleep disorder with increasing morbidity in Chinese population. When sleep Apnea-Hypopnea Index (AHI) is greater than five, the diagnosis of SAHS is defined. The incidence of SAHS is about 2–4 % in general population of China, and even higher in male after middle-age and female after menopause, respectively, while the morbidity in male is higher than that in female population. SAHS is usually associated with cardiovascular and metabolic disease, as well as ENT disease. It has been proved to raise potential risk of sudden death at night. So far the diagnosis of SAHS mainly depends on polysomnogram, which presents to be expensive and requires sophisticated medical equipment and interpretation. This study was designed to evaluate the feasibility of detecting SAHS by EDR of AECG monitoring.

81.2 Clinical Data and Methods

81.2.1 Patient Selection Criteria

There were totally 80 patients to our hospital's sleep center with snore and sleep disturbance were enrolled into this study. Between January and December 2012, including 66 males and 14 females, with the average age of 44.81 $\pm$ 15.01 years and Body Mass Index (BMI) of 28.13 $\pm$ 4.57 kg/m^2. Patients with history of myocardial infarction, diabetes mellitus, permanent or paroxysmal atrial fibrillation or permanent pacemaker were excluded. This study was approved by the institutional ethics committees of our hospitals and informed consent was obtained from each participant.

81.2.2 Study Design

The overnight sleep (over 7 h) investigation was administered to all subjects by Polysomnogram (PSG) and 24 h AECG monitoring simultaneously. Two doctors respectively calculated Apnea Hyponea Index (AHI) according to PSG results, and made diagnosis of SAHS(+) and SAHS(–). Another two doctors respectively calculated AHI by software automatic analysis EDR of dynamic electrocardiographic recording results. The electrocardiogram analyzers did not know the PSG results at all. The PSG result was considered as the gold standard so as to evaluate the feasibility of screening SAHS from EDR of AECG monitoring.

81.2.3 Polysomnography Detection

Items including Encephalographic (EEG), Electrooculographic (EOC), Electromyographic (EMG), airflow, snore index, respiratory efforts of chest and abdomen and oxygen saturation were measured by 16 channel polysomnography of SM2000 producted by Beijing MingSi company. Time constant of EEG and EMG is 0.3 s, and high-frequency smoothing is 25 Hz. The patients with snore and apopnixis of sleep were monitored overnight (over 7 h) by PSG. Observation index included sleep and awake time (min), time of non-rapid eye movement and rapid eye movement (min), sleep time of I, II, III and IV of period (min), time of the longest and average apnea (s), AHI, the lowest and average saturation of blood oxygen (SaO_2) etc.

81.2.4 Ambulatory Electrocardiogram and Analysis

The patients were recorded 24 h electrocardiogram by 12-channel ambulatory electrocardiograph of Oxford company (Medilog AR12). Automatic analysis was performed with software in a sensibility of 75, 87.5 and 100 % respectively. Screening of SAHS with ECG derived respiration of ambulatory electrocardiogram by automatic analysis with software of Simple View 2.2, with outlier introduced by noise and artifacts by man–machine interaction removed. The data of patients were automatically analysed with software at a sensibility of 75, 87.5 and 100 % respectively.

81.2.5 Diagnostic Criteria of Sleep Apnea-Hypopnea Syndrome

Sleep Apnea-Hypopnea Syndrome (SAHS) is defined as over 30 times apnea/hypopnea in 7 h of sleep, or with a apnea/hypopnea index (AHI) $\geq$5. Apnea is defined as the absence of airflow for >10 s. Hypopnea is defined as a $\geq$50 % reduction in the amplitude of respiratory efforts for at least 10 s, and a fall in arterial oxyhemoglobin saturation of at least 4 %. The state of SAHS illness is classified as mild, moderate and severe, which is based on AHI oxyhemoglobin saturation (SaO_2). Mild SAHS is on the basis of an AH5–20, SaO_2 $\geq$85 %; moderate SAHS is on the basis of an AHI 21–50, SaO_2 $\geq$80 % and severe SAHS is on the basis of an AHI > 50, SaO_2 $\leq$79 %. Same diagnostic criteria of SAHS were utilized in EDR as well as PSG.

81.2.6 Statistical Analysis

Data were analyzed by SPSS PC 10.0 software (SPSS Inc, Chicago, IL, USA). Values were expressed as mean and SD (mean ± SD). Comparisons of variables between groups were made with a 2-sample t test or the $\chi 2$ test, and P values <0.05 were considered as statistically significant.

81.3 Results

81.3.1 Baseline Characteristics

Characteristics of the SAHS(+) and SAHS(−) groups are shown in Table 81.1. 60 patients were with SAHS, and 20 patients were without SAHS. The patients with SAHS were most of male, and the age, BMI, blood pressure were higher than SAHS(−) ($P < 0.05$).

81.3.2 Diagnose Accordance Rate of SAHS with Dynamic Electrocardiograph

Automatic analysis was performed with software in a sensibility of 75, 87.5 and 100 % respectively (Table 81.2). When software sensibility was fixed to 75 %, SAHS(+) of 20 (ture positive of 16, false positive of 4), SAHS(−) of 60 (true

Table 81.1 Comparison of clinical characteristics of the SAHS(+) and SAHS(−)

Group	N	Age (year)	Male (%)	BMI (kg/m^2)	HBP (%)
SAHS(+)	60	48.70 ± 11.51	53 (88.3)	29.22 ± 4.13	35 (58.3)
SAHS(−)	20	33.15 ± 18.30*	13 (65.0)*	24.88 ± 4.40*	6 (30.0)*

Comparison of two groups's data * $P < 0.05$ BMI = Body Mass Index HBP = High Blood Pressure

Table 81.2 Effect of screening of sleep apnea syndrome with different sensitivity of software

Sensibility of software (%)	SAHS(+) ($n = 60$)	SAHS(−) ($n = 20$)	Sensitivity (%)	Specificity (%)	Positive predictive value (%)	Negative predictive value (%)	Diagnose accordance rate (%)
75	20(true 16, false 4)	60(true 16, false 44)	26.7	80.0	80.0	26.7	40.0
87.50	44(true 33, false 11)	36(true 9, false 27)	55.0	45.0	75.0	25.0	52.5
100	66(true 53, false 13)	14(true 7, false 7)	88.3	35.0	84.1	50.0	75.0

negative of 16, false negative of 44, the sensitivity of screening SAHS with EDR was 26.7 %, with the specificity of 80 %, the positive predictive value of 80 %, the negative predictive value of 26.7 %, the diagnose accordance rate of 40 %. When software sensibility was fixed to 87.5 %, SAHS(+) of 44 (ture positive of 33, false positive of 11), SAHS(−) of 36 (true negative of 9, false negative of 27), the sensitivity of screening SAHS with EDR was 55 %,with the specificity of 45 %, the positive predictive value of 75 %, the negative predictive value of 25 %, and the diagnose accordance rate of 52.5 %. When software sensibility was fixed to 100 %, SAHS(+) of 66 (ture positive of 53, false positive of 13), SAHS(−) of 14 (true negative of 7, false negative of 7), the sensitivity of screening SAHS with EDR was 88.3 %, with the specificity of 35 %, the positive predictive value of 84.1 %, the negative predictive value of 50 %, and the diagnose accordance rate of 75 %.

81.4 Discussion

Nowadays SAHS has been paid more attention by people, it has been generally regarded as independent risk factor of cardiovascular events [1], the symptom shows that the frequent apnea and hypopnea during the sleep, and it caused the physiopathologic change that is quite complicated, SAHS commonly lead to disfunction of major organs, and affected the quality of life seriously, even to the death in night [2]. Currently, a definitive diagnosis of sleep apnoea is made by polysomnogram, that is regards as the gold standard. It needs to proceed in the sleeping-monitor room with costly medical equipment. Meanwhile it needs the well-trained technicians. After stayed in the hospital for more than 7 h monitor, patients could be diagnosed. So it is very difficult to be widespread, majority of patients could not receive early diagnosis and treatment. Many study indicates the patients who treated by CPAP could not only improve their quality of life obviously, but also reduce and prevent all kinds of complication, and increase the rate of survival of patients. Thus, early discovery and diagnosis of SAHS patients is a very important task.

It could be observed reduction of the rate of heart by the monitor of holter, when the apnea broke out, and increased the rate of the heart when the apnea finished, the heart rate could reach the climax through several breath after the apnea, this phenomenon called cyclic variations in heart rate, CVHR, so it could analyze through the change of the circle of the heart rate and HRV of ambulatory electrocardiogram and so on to diagnose the sleep apnea [3–11], but it was just qualitative diagnosis, not quantitative diagnosis, because it can not calculate the AHI.

In 1985, Moody firstly proposed EDR technique [12], ECGs recorded from the surface of the chest are influenced by motion of the electrodes with respect to the heart, and by changes in the electrical impedance of the thoracic cavity. The expansion and contraction of the chest which accompanies respiration result in motion of chest electrodes. These physical influences of respiration result in amplitude variations in the recorded ECG. Respiratory signals may be derived from body surface ECGs by measuring fluctuations in the mean cardiac electrical axis which accompanies respiration. The technique is lower cost and noninvasive and applicable to any type of automated ECG analysis, without the need for additional transducers or hardware redesign which can make diagnosis of SAHS patients not only qualitative analysis, but also quantitative analysis, especially suit for screening of sleep apnea-hyponpea syndrome clinically.

Subsequently Travaglini [13] tried to derived respiratory signal from eight-lead ECG, the results obtained showed to be strongly correlated with conventional measurements of respiration. The use of more lead ECG can reduce noise. Afterwards, the method will extend to ambulatory multiple lead electrocardiogram gradually.

Above investigations showed that it's significant correlated between the EDR signal and measurements of respiration. The majorest problem is that the accuracy of the SAHS diagnosis of the method compared with conventional method hasn't been proved.

The study indicated that the sensitivity and the rate of accordance increased gradually with the increasing of the sensibility of setting up. When the sensibility was fixed 100 %, the sensitivity was 88.3 %, the rate of accordance was the highest-75 %, but the specificity was only 35 %. The reduction of the specificity caused by this software didn't work for the diagnosing-function of hypopnea.

In certain circumstance, the calculation of the respiratory frequency and apnea was suspended, for the following reasons: 1. The morphology of ECG sudden changes. caused by noise. 2. Removal of an electrode or lead during the registration of the ECG. 3. The research just suited for sinus rhythm. If the numbers of ectopic greater than twenty percent that would affect the result. Thus the EDR applying software auto-analysis has some limitation, some disturbances and deviations would lead to misdiagnosis, it should get the more accurate result if combined with the artificial analysis.

81.5 Conclusions

The EDR technique is an easy to implement method with lower cost, more closed natural sleep condition of patients. Autoanalysis with software of Simple View 2.2 is very simple and swift, so it's easier to widespread. Although its specificity is not high, the sensitivity, specificity and accordance of diagnosis would be improved further by the updating its software gradually or combining the artificial analysis. On the whole, EDR technique of AECG was useful to screen the suspicious SAHS patients. Sensitivity and diagnosis coincidence rate was higher when the sensibility of automatic analysis software was fixed to 100 %.

References

1. Gottlieb DJ, Yenokyan G, Newman AB, et al (2010) Sleep apnea and incident cardiovascular disease. Circulation 122:352–360
2. Ludka O, Konecny T, Somers V (2011) Sleep apnea, cardiac arrhythmias, and sudden death. Tex Heart Inst J (Texas Heart Institute of St Luke's Episcopal Hospital, Texas Children's Hospital) 38:340–343
3. Phyllis K, Stephen P, Peter P et al (2003) Simple method to identify sleep apnea using Holter recordings. J Cardiovasc Electrophysiol 14(5):467–473
4. Roche F, Gaspoz JM, Fortune IC et al (1999) Screening of obstructive sleep apnea syndrome by heart rate variability analysis. Circulation 100:1411–1415
5. Penzel T, McNames J, Chazal P et al (2002) Systematic comparison of different algorithms for apnea detection based on ECG recordings. Med Biol Eng Comp 40(4):402–407
6. Raymond B, Cayton RM, Bates RA et al (2000) Screening for obstructive sleep apnoea based on the electrocardiogram-the computers in cardiology challenge. Comput Cardiol 27:267–270
7. Mietus JE, Peng C-K, Ivanov PCh et al (2000) Detection of obstructive sleep apnea from cardiac interbeat interval time series. Comput Cardiol 27:753–756
8. Roche F, Sforza E, Duverney D et al (2004) Heart rate increment: an electrocardiological approach for the early detection of obstructive sleep apnoea/hypopnoea syndrome. Clin Sci (Lond) 107(1):105–110
9. Roche F, Pichot V, Sforza E et al (2003) Predicting sleep apnoea syndrome from heart period: a time-frequency wavelet analysis. Eur Respir J 22(6):870–871
10. Babaeizadeh S, White DP, Pittman SD, Zhou SH (2010) Automatic detection and quantification of sleep apnea using heart rate variability. J Electrocardiol 43:535–541
11. Hayano J, Watanabe E, Saito Y, Sasaki F, Fujimoto K, Nomiyama T, Kawai K, Kodama I, Sakakibara H (2011) Screening for obstructive sleep apnea by cyclic variation of heart rate. Circ Arrhythmia electrophysiol 4:64–72
12. Moody GB, Mark RG, Zoccola A et al (1985) Derivation of respiratory signals from multi-lead ECGs. Comput Cardiol 12:113–116
13. Travaglini A, Lamberti C, Debie J (1998) Respiratory of signal derived from eight-lead ECG. IEEE Proc Comput Cardiol 25(2):65–68

Chapter 82
Research on the Informatization Top-level Design Methods

Zhang Huilin, Tong Qiuli and Xie Suping

Abstract This article describes the development trend of informatization top-level design, introduces a business process combing method which plays a very important part in informatization top-level design, including the significance and objectives, the design of the forms, and some principles of the business process combing work, and also represent the top-level design modeling methods for business models, function models, data models and user authority models and concludes with the construction plan of informatization top-level design.

Keywords Top-level design · Business process combing · Informatization modeling · Information construction plan

82.1 Introduction

With the rapid development of information technology, the construction of information systems has no longer to satisfy the business requirements of a single department, but to build a unified, integrated large-scale system platform for the entire organization. The comprehensive and complete system solutions can not only effectively solve problems like redundant construction, information islands and system integration difficulties, but also be more conducive to the comprehensive data collection, data mining and decision support, which provide more efficient IT support to business work. Therefore, to construct a new generation of information systems needs to stand from a higher perspective to understand the structure and processes of the business, to make overall plans from a global perspective in all aspects of the business at all levels with all the elements, in order

Z. Huilin (✉) · T. Qiuli · X. Suping
Information Technology Center of Tsinghua University, Beijing 100084, People's Republic of China
e-mail: zhhl@cic.tsinghua.edu.cn

S. Li et al. (eds.), *Frontier and Future Development of Information Technology in Medicine and Education*, Lecture Notes in Electrical Engineering 269,
DOI: 10.1007/978-94-007-7618-0_82,

to allocate resources effectively, efficiently and quickly to achieve the target, which is the implication of the "top-level design". The "top-level design" appears in the recommendations of the CPC Central Committee on the 12th 5-Year Plan for the first time, in fact, which is applicable in all fields.

"Informatization top-level design" refers to the overall planning for the information construction in the future based on the consideration of the management needs, the business processes design and the current information systems, making information construction more innovative and forward-looking, rather than just picking up the pace of business.

82.2 Business Process Combing

Informatization top-level design is based on a comprehensive understanding of the business. The following is the detailed introduction to the method of business process combing.

82.2.1 The Concept and Function of Business Process Combing

Business process combing refers to classifying global business into a number of business processes, and for each business process analysing the departments and positions involved, the business triggers, business collaboration mode, the data flows, the time and period of business processes, information systems and other elements. Business process combing is the most critical and basic step for informatization construction and a core part of the informatization top-level design, at the same time it provides an important reference to streamline the procedures, improve internal controls and optimize job settings within the organization.

The business process combing in the top-level design is not only to sort out the workflows and messaging within various business processes, but also to analyse the business interaction and information sharing between business processes, at the same time to understand the support to the current business from the existing information systems, and to collect the suggestions for the current business processes and information systems.

82.2.2 The Design of Business Process Combing Forms

In order to ensure the accuracy and comprehensiveness of the business process combing, it not only needs the involvement of IT staff, but also active participation of business staff in various positions of different levels within the organization, so

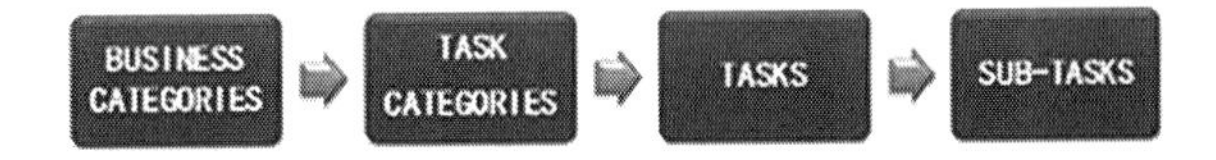

Fig. 82.1 Business division

there are a large number of people with different professional background and different thinking habits participated in, which brings some difficulties for the combing job. So it is necessary to get scientific and effective ways of working to capture all the business knowledge in all the people's minds.

First we do some business decomposition to make the globe business easier to understand. The business of each department can be divided into multiple business categories, which is then subdivided into a number of tasks. Closely interrelated tasks can be put into a task classification and complex tasks can be split into multiple sub-tasks. That is the formation of the following business division (Fig. 82.1).

Then we design a set of forms to describe the business division, as shown in Table 82.1, which make the complex business analysis simplified and excluding personal thinking habits to some extent. To analyse the business from the view of a single task makes filling in forms and reading that more clear, at the same time we can also get a clear view of the business structure.

The forms are divided into three groups. The first group is business category-position form, as shown in Table 82.2, completed by the department heads, to describe the business categories and job settings of the entire department. The second group includes the position-task list, tasks form and documents form, as shown in Tables 82.3, 82.4 and 82.5, completed by specific business staff. The position-task list shows the tasks of each business category, while the related tasks are grouped in the same task classification. The position-task form describes the details of the tasks, including whether to split into sub-tasks, the task/sub-task steps, the completion time, input documents, output documents, etc. which are relatively detailed information but provides important reference to the business modeling. The documents form illustrates the documents involved in the tasks. The third group is position-task combing form, mainly completed by IT staff based

Table 82.1 Business process combing forms list

Form title	Completed by	Form description
Business category-position form	Department heads	Divide each department's business into multiple business categories and analyze the job settings of each business categories
Position-task forms • Position-task list • Tasks form • Documents form	Business staff	A comprehensive description of the tasks
Position-task combing form	IT staff	Do some necessary association and merging of the tasks, sub-tasks, task steps and documents based on the first two sets of forms from a global perspective, in preparation for the business modeling

Table 82.2 Business category-position form

Business category-position form			
The name of the department		Position	Staff
No	Business category		
The serial number of business category	Describe the division of the entire department business	Describe the job settings	The specific staff in the position

Table 82.3 Position-task list

Position-task list		
Business category	Position	Completed Cy
Task no	Task name	Task Classification

on the first two sets of forms, to do some necessary association and merging of the tasks, sub-tasks, task steps and documents from a global perspective, in preparation for the business modeling (Table 82.6).

82.2.3 Business Process Combing Principles

Business process combing is a complex and detailed job, and there are some principles need to be followed.

- The business process combing job must have the recognition and support of the leaders of the organization, who clearly know the importance of informatization top-design for the future development, encourage staff to participate in and acknowledge the time and effort spent on the combing work.
- Don't be tangled in the details too much, but pay more attention to the integrity of the business. It's more constructive to think from the perspective of macro and micro combined.
- Have sufficient communication with business people and try to turn the tacit knowledge in people's mind into explicit knowledge.
- Focus on the information flow in the business process, especially the ones between positions and tasks.

82.3 The Informatization Top-Design Modeling

Business processes combing provides a comprehensive understanding of the business, and the top-level design modeling is the abstraction and induction of the business, which is important achievements of the top-level design and support the future information construction planning.

Table 82.4 Tasks form

Tasks form										
Task no	Task name	Task description	Sub-task name	Step name	How to start the task/sub-task/task step	What to do in the task/sub-task/task step	The completion time	Supplement and suggestions	Input documents and their sources	Output documents and their whereabouts

Introduction for Table 82.4:
Task name: It is corresponding to the task name in the position-task list
Task description: It is summary of the task
Sub-task name: If a task has relatively independent modules, it can be divided into sub-tasks. Generally there is no sequential relationship between the subtasks
Step name: If a task or a sub-task has related modules in some kind of order, they are task/sub-task steps. Generally there is close sequential relationship between task/sub-task steps
How to start the task/sub-task/task step: Service requests may come from the counter, mail, telephone, may also be time-triggered
What to do in the task/sub-task/task step: To describe the specific content of the task/sub-task/steps including who puts forward the request, who receives the request and how to handle it, what information is transferred and produced, how the information systems provide support, etc
The completion time: To estimate the time required to complete the step
Supplement and suggestions: To add some instructions and recommendations
Input documents and their sources: To describe the documents received in the steps
Output documents and their whereabouts: To describe the documents produced in the steps and their whereabouts

Table 82.5 Documents form

Documents form		
Document name	The document printing department	Copies of one set
The full title of the document	The original source of the document	The copies of the document in one set

82.3.1 The Organizational Structure

The organizational structure is a summary description of the positions setting and their duties, therefore the organization chart should be completed first to help understand positions relationship.

82.3.2 Business Models

Business models should describe the interfaces of the business between different positions and reflect the business cooperation relationship, especially the transfer of documents and data among the departments. In some complex business processes, hierarchical diagrams can be used, in order to display the whole picture and also some important details at the same time, where the readability of the model needs some attention (Fig. 82.2).

82.3.3 Function Models

On the basis of the business models, data flows between business categories, task classifications, tasks, sub-tasks and other business domains would be described, which is reference for system planning and functions design. The data flows can be drew as hierarchical diagrams (Fig. 82.3).

The structure and functions of the system corresponds to the business divisions, with the business categories corresponding to subsystems, task classifications corresponding to modules and the tasks or sub-tasks corresponding to functions for generally speaking. But it requires a specific analysis during the design, for example, some particular intensive interaction parts in the data flow diagram, may need some merging in the system design, and some business processes may be not considered in the system planning after some analysis.

Table 82.6 Position-task combing form

Position-task combing form														
Task no.	Task name	Task description	Sub-task name	Step name	How to start the step			What to do in the step			After the step			Supplement
					The initiator	The event	Inputs	The process	Documents processed or produced	The time	The next handler	The following dispose	Outputs	

Introduction for Table 82.6:
The initiator: To describe people who trigger the step
The event: Service requests may come from the counter, mail, telephone, may also be time-triggered
Inputs: To describe the documents received during the step
The process: To describe the specific processing of the step
Documents processed or produced: To describe the documents processed and produced in the step
The time: To estimate the time required to complete the steps
The next handler: To describe the next position or department who would handle the task
The following dispose: To describe what to do next for the task
Outputs: To describe the documents transferred after the step
Supplement: To add some instructions and recommendations

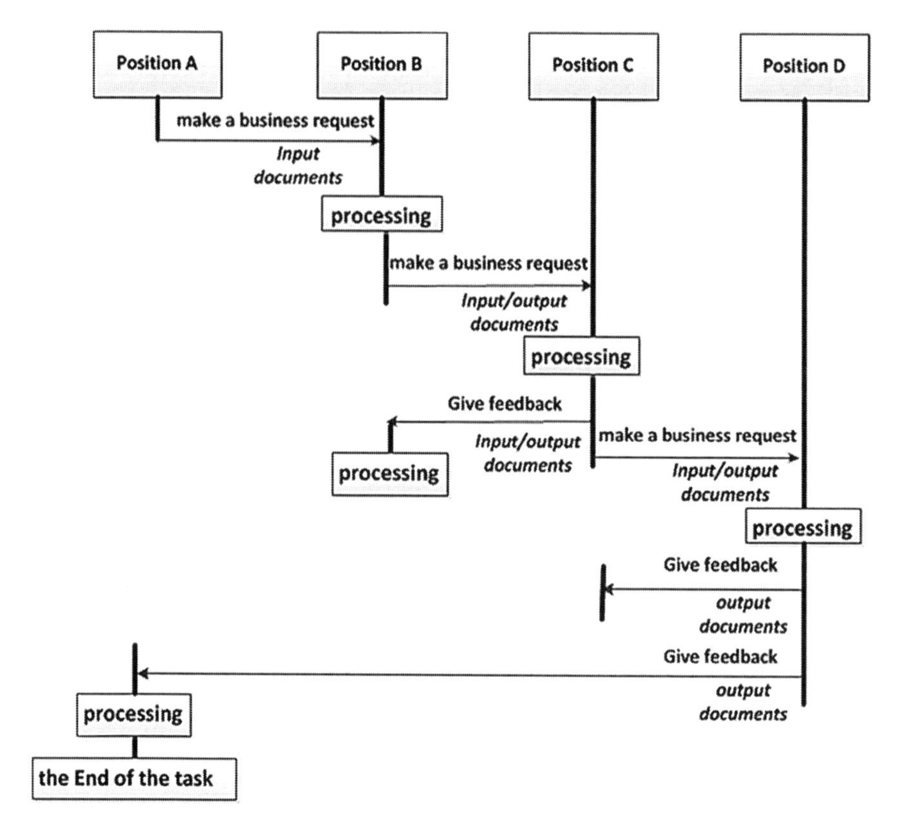

Fig. 82.2 Business collaboration process diagram

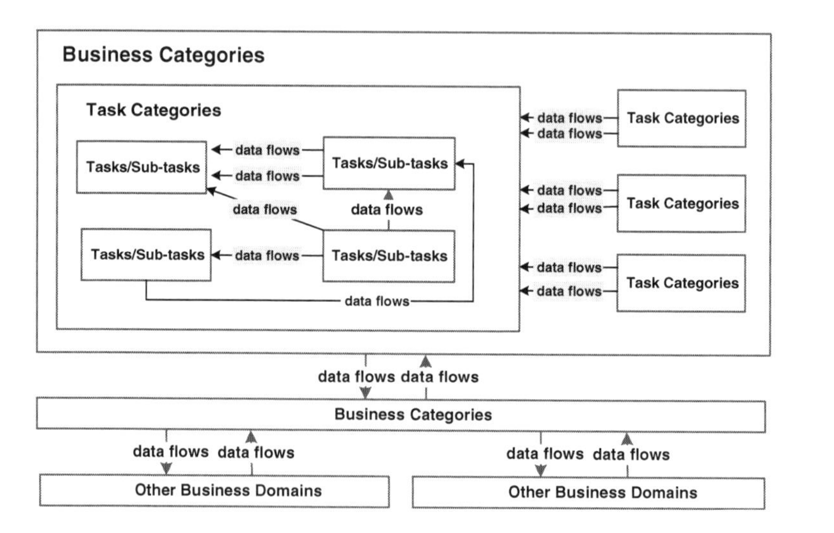

Fig. 82.3 Data flow diagram

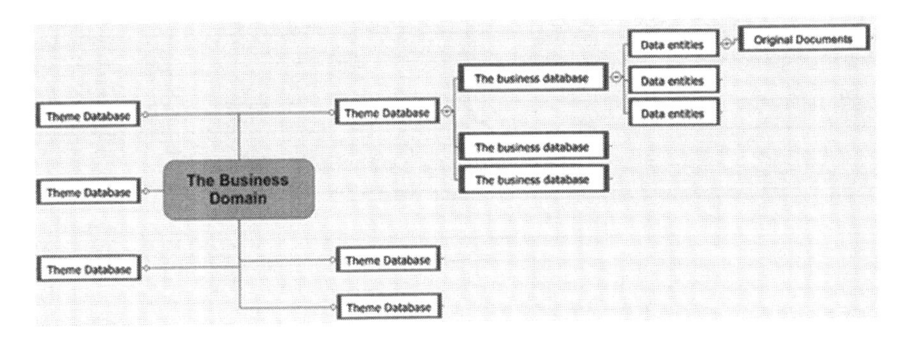

Fig. 82.4 The hierarchy of the data model

82.3.4 Data Models

Based on the analysis of the business and the original documents, there would be more than one theme database in the data models. The theme databases would be divided into business databases. Each business database contains multiple entities (equivalent to a table in the database). The original documents are basis for the design of the data entity, but not one-to-one relationship. Original documents may be split into multiple data entities and original documents may also be combined into a single data entity. For example, in the financial business, the budget business can be a theme database and the special budget is a business database with data entities of the special budget appropriation, the special budget implementation, etc. Several original documents such as appropriation papers, the appropriation list and the project budget are corresponding to one data entity of the special budget appropriation (Fig. 82.4).

82.3.5 Role Authorization Models

Role authorization modeling is to design roles and authorize them with system authorities and data authorities, according to the positions and their duties in the business processes. Users get authorities by establishing relationships with roles (Table 82.7).

82.4 Informatization Top-Level Design Planning

Through combing and modelling the business processes, valuable business materials were accumulated. Meanwhile, the business models, data models, function models and user authority models of the whole business domain were

Table 82.7 Role authorization table

Authorities			Roles			
			Role A	Role B	Role C	Role D
System authorities	Subsystem authorities	Module authorities	√			
		Module authorities				
		Module authorities				
	Subsystem authorities					
Data authorities	Data authorities of one department					
	Data authorities of one business category					
	Data authorities of one year					
	……					

established on the basis of abstracting and collating the business combing materials. The achievements above were important outputs of the informatization top-level design. Based on the analyzing and modeling of global business, a specific, step-by-step plan for the future information construction would be proposed as follows.

- To review the information constructions and describe the current major problems;
- To set goals for information construction in the future based on the current information infrastructure, the long-term planning for business development and the potential informatization requirements. For example, to provide comprehensive integration of systems and data, better information services, effective supports for analysis and decision making, etc.
- To build the overall architecture and choose technology roadmap for new generation systems and to describe the overall system design, including the goals, functions and application effects of each sub-system, which would bring significant enhancements and promotions to the business development in the future;
- To plan construction steps in the consideration of the urgency of business requirements and to set annual milestones and final completion time for the construction work.

82.5 Brief Summary

The informatization top-level design will play a positive role to the future development of the business but also needs a lot of input in the process. It is the determination of leaders and the enthusiasm of participants that decide the quality and application effects of the work, together with scientific, systematic and efficient methods. Finally the business work and the information construction will promote each other and progress together.

References

1. Zhao D, Shu W, Qiuli T, Shoujun W (2008) Research and practice on college financial business processes combing. China Manag Inf 11(17):50–53
2. Hu H, Jinghui X (2006) Strengthen top-level design to promote information technology. Retrieved 20 Mar 2013 from China national information infrastructure web site. http://www.echinagov.com/echinagov/redian/2006-11-29/9919.shtml
3. Xiaojing J (2012) Informationization top-level design proceeds from the application software combing. Retrieved 5 Apr 2013 from China web site. http://www.ichina.net.cn/Html/2010/column/12024.html
4. Songbai L (2011) The charm and value of the top-level design. Retrieved 23 Mar 2013 from Economic times multimedia digital newspaper. http://paper.ce.cn/jjrb/html/2011-06/22/content_157846.html

Chapter 83
Research on Optimization of Resources Allocation in Cloud Computing Based on Structure Supportiveness

Wei-hua Yuan, Hong Wang and Zhong-yong Fan

Abstract In this paper, we focus on the problem of resources allocation scheduling in the context of cloud computing to satisfy the objective of QoS of both cloud providers and consumers. Firstly, we give the formal modeling of cloud resources and description of their performance, as well as applications and descriptions of the component constraints; secondly, we carry out compatibility reasoning of cloud resources and application components, and build up the directed graph between them to represent their structure supportiveness to infer the relationship between scarce resources and popular components; thirdly, the weight of scarce resources and popular components are computed iteratively, and prices of services are adjusted according to their weights to achieve the best match between cloud providers and consumers; lastly the allocation algorithm is presented.

Keywords Resources allocation · Cloud computing · Structure supportiveness · Scarce resources

W. Yuan · H. Wang (✉)
School of Infromation Science and Engineering, ShanDong Normal University, JiNan, Shandong, China
e-mail: wanghong106@163.com

W. Yuan
e-mail: huahua_qingdao@126.com

W. Yuan
School of Computer Science and Technology, ShanDong Jianzhu University, Jian, Shandong, China

Z. Fan
Online Learning Center, Rizhao Radio and TV University, Rizhao Shandong, China
e-mail: rzddfzy@126.com

S. Li et al. (eds.), *Frontier and Future Development of Information Technology in Medicine and Education*, Lecture Notes in Electrical Engineering 269,
DOI: 10.1007/978-94-007-7618-0_83,

83.1 Introduction

Cloud computing [1] is a kind of calculation based on Internet, which is composed of a set of interrelated and virtual computers. Computing resources can be dynamically configured through the service-level agreements (SLA) between service providers and customers [2]. Many cloud providers such as Amazon and Google, offer a kind of resource-on-demand and pay-as-you-go computing resources [1]. The following are new characteristics of cloud computing resources [3]:

(1) Constraint conditions
In cloud computing, cloud service providers offer paid services and users need to "pay-on-demand". Therefore, the cost of task execution must be considered in scheduling problems of cloud. Besides, such factors as deadline for completing tasks and user fees are also important constraints.

(2) Optimization objectives
Li and Yang [4] introduced that, for a given price there were a lot of variations in performance of resources offered by different cloud providers. Most of the traditional resource allocation schemes focused on QoS of cloud providers, and less consideration had been taken into that of consumers. However, in cloud computing, consumers can independently choose cloud resources according to their own needs (money or reliability). So cloud computing should also ensure QoS requirements of users, to achieve a win–win situation between resources supply and resources consumption.

(3) Scheduling mechanisms
At present, cloud providers are still highly concerned about key problems of resources management, task scheduling and load balancing. However, patterns of scheduling and resources management in cloud computing present characteristics of diversification and unified standards and constraints have not yet been formed.

Consequently, how to concentrate all the resources and how to adopt optimal strategies of resources allocation, to realize automatic control and load balancing of resources are of great significance. In this paper, to satisfy the QoS of both cloud providers and consumers, we mainly focus on problems of resource allocation, and put forward a kind of resources configuration optimization scheme based on the structure supportiveness, to achieve the best matching of resources supply and resources consumption.

83.2 Related Work

Architecture of IBM's "blue cloud" uses a series of Tivoli products to complete resource allocation and scheduling in cloud computing [5]. Many IT manufacturers has put forward their cloud models based on Map-Reduce, but the performance of the whole system might be decreased because Hadoop is not perfect, especially when the scheduling algorithm is much too simple [6]. Facebook proposed fair scheduling algorithm. In order to reduce the cost of data transmission in the job execution [7], put forward algorithms of assigning tasks to nodes where data was located to improve locality. Hadoop on Demand [8] divided the physical computer cluster into several sub-clusters, each concurrent job is assigned to a different subset, to ensure that each operation could get its right computing resources.

The scheduling algorithms mentioned above mainly focused on task scheduling optimization based on Map-Reduce, which might not be applicable in other cloud computing systems; moreover, they neglected relationships of the structure supportiveness between cloud resources and application components, so they could not provide efficient resources allocation and scheduling.

Sim [9, 10] proposed a cloud resource allocation scheme based on agent, looking at discovery of support for cloud services, design and development of service negotiation software agent, as well as the problem of service combination. Alshamrani and Xie [11] offered a kind of cloud computing model in mobile cloud computing, to decide how to manage specific configured computational tasks. Leong et al. [12] studied how to carry out problems of cloud resources management and allocation in wireless network.

But the researches above neglected how to optimize resource allocation scheme from the consumer's point of view to obtain better throughput at a lower price.

83.3 System Model

In this section, we propose the system model, consisting of formal descriptions of cloud resources and applications, descriptions of application components constraints and resources performance, as well as objectives of resources allocation problems of the system.

83.3.1 Description of Cloud Resources and Resources Performance

83.3.1.1 Description of Cloud Resources

Supposing cloud providers have a set of physical computers, each of which could reside many virtual machines (VMs). Each VM is called a resource and can be assigned to an application component. The sequence of VM in machine i can be expressed as $V_i = \{vm_{i1}, vm_{i2}, \ldots, vm_{in}\}$, where n is the maximum number of VMs of each physical machine. R_i represents all the VM resources of provider i:

$$R_i = \left\{ \bigcup_i V_i | 1 \le i \le m_p \right\} \tag{83.1}$$

where m_p is the maximum number of physical machines owned by the provider.

We define R_{VM} as a collection of total available resources of all cloud providers:

$$R_{VM} = \left\{ \bigcup_j R_j | 1 \le j \le c_p \right\} \tag{83.2}$$

where c_p is the number of cloud providers. And we also define R_{avl} as the current free resources collection that might be assigned to application components of consumers, and obviously $R_{avl} \subseteq R_{VM}$.

83.3.1.2 Description of Resources Performance

Resources performance mainly include output o_v, access frequency access hf(v), input and output delay d_v, as well as price p_v. Let *capacity* be the vector of resources performance, which may be expressed as $(o_v, d_v, p_v, hf(v))$. And let $capacity_{vm_i}$ represents performance description of resource vm_i.

83.3.2 Description of Applications and Application Constraints

83.3.2.1 Description of Applications

Supposing an application is composed of a series of distributed application components to complete a task by their mutual exchange of information. Let Cmp_i be the *ith* application arriving, expressed as $Cmp_i = \{c_{i1}, c_{i2}, \ldots, c_{in}\}$, in which c_{ij} is the *jth* component of Cmp_i. All the applications to be deployed in cloud computing can be defined as $App = \bigcup_i Cmp_i$.

83.3.2.2 Description of Application Constraints

Constraints of an application component are mainly about the conditions of acceptable cloud resources given by the component, including workload w_c, delay of output and input d_c, deadline of task completion t_c, as well as the minimum cost of service a consumer can afford c_c. Workload of a component refers to the workload assigned by the application of the component. Let S_{con} represent application constraints of a component, expressed as a vector (w_c, d_c, t_c, c_c). Let

$S^{c_{ij}}_{con}$ be the description of component c_{ij} in application Cmp_i, and let $S^{Cmp_i}_{con}$ be a set of constraints of all components in application Cmp_i.

83.3.3 Description of Solving Objectives

Given an application with a group of application components to be allocated dynamically, as well as the corresponding application constraints S_{con}, resources allocation algorithm needs to find a collection of suitable resources from the available set of resources R_{avl}, and to assign them to all components of the application. Based on service constraints of application components S_{con}, and description of resource performance *capacity*, this paper is to carry out structure supportiveness reasoning between application components and cloud resources to derive scarce resources list and popular components list, and to provide customers with good QoS, so that they could get better throughput of resources at a relatively lower price; meanwhile to offer providers with good QoS as well, so that their scarce resources can acquire a better service price; ultimately to find the best match between cloud resources and application components.

83.4 Resources Allocation Process and the Algorithm

83.4.1 Structure Supportiveness Reasoning

83.4.1.1 Performance Computing of Cloud Resources

Since performance of cloud resources can be expressed as a vector $(o_v, d_v, p_v, hf(v))$, in which o_v represents output of resources, the higher the throughput, the higher performance of the resources; access frequency hf(v) represents prediction of the future traffic of the resources obtained through training of frequency of visits to the resources over a period of time: the larger access frequency indicates its greater use value, and its larger possibility of being assigned to other components once again. Thus *capacity* function can be expressed as:

$$capacity = f(o_v, d_v, hf(v)) \tag{83.3}$$

Price of the resource can be expressed as a function of *capacity*:

$$p_v = p(capacity) \tag{83.4}$$

83.4.1.2 Compatibility Reasoning of Cloud Resources and Application Components

Compatibility reasoning is implemented between application components and available resources according to constraints of application components $S_{con} : (size, delay, deadline, \cos t)$, and resources capacity $capacity : (o_v, d_v, p_v, hf(v))$:

$$sim(vm_i, c_{jk}) = \frac{\sqrt{(o_{vm_i} - w_{c_{jk}})^2}}{3w_{c_{jk}}} + \frac{\sqrt{(d_{vm_i} - d_{c_{jk}})^2}}{3d_{c_{jk}}} + \frac{\sqrt{(p_{vm_i} - c_{c_{jk}})^2}}{3c_{c_{jk}}} \quad (83.5)$$

where $vm_i \in R_{avl}$, $c_{jk} \in App$. $sim(vm_i, c_{jk}) \in (0, 1]$, the value will be closer to 0 if there is much more similarity between vm_i and c_{jk}; on the contrary, the value will be much closer to 1 if there is not much similarity between them.

83.4.1.3 Derivation Process of Scarce Resources List and Popular Components List Based on Structure Supportiveness

In [13], Kleinberg put forward a hub-authority model to distinguish the hub pages and the authority pages in a web search. The mutually recursive definition of two concepts of hubs and authorities are expressed as: a good hub usually point to many good authorities, and a good authority is pointed to by many good hubs. Accordingly we put forward a mutually recursive definition of scarce resources and popular components based on the structure supportiveness.

Setting threshold β, resource vm_i is a candidate resource of component c_{jk} if $sim(vm_i, c_{jk}) \leq \beta$, that is, vm_i can be allocated to c_{jk}. The relationship between resources and components as represented by a directed graph, if vm_i is a candidate resource of c_{jk}, there will be a directed edge from vm_i to c_{jk}. On the other hand, vm_i is not an appropriate resource of c_{jk} if $sim(vm_i, c_{jk}) > \beta$. The directed components—resources matching graph is shown in Fig. 83.1.

Scarce resource: a resource is scarce if it is a candidate allocation resource of many components in a derivation process. A scarce resource usually has large out-degrees. For example, resource R_1 in Fig. 83.1 is a candidate resource of components c_1, c_2 and c_n, consequently it has a large probability to be a kind of scarce resource.

Popular component: a component will be popular if it has many candidate resources in a derivation process. A popular component usually has large in-degrees. For example, from Fig. 83.1 we can see that the candidate resources of c_1 include R_1, R_2 and R_m, so c_1 is very likely to be a popular component.

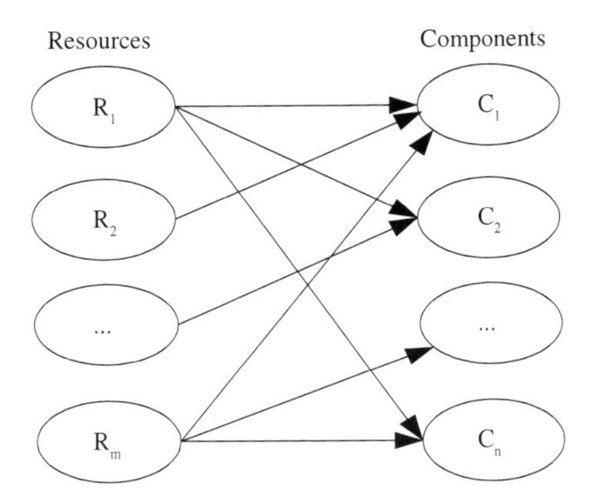

Fig. 83.1 The relationship between components and their candidate resources

83.4.1.4 Weight Computation

As is shown in Fig. 83.1, there is a kind of relationship of mutual support and mutual promotion between scarce resources SR_j and popular components WC_i: a popular component has many candidate resources; while a scarce resource is a kind of resource that points to many popular components. Thus we can assign a non-negative weight x_j^s to each SR_j, and also a non-negative weight y_i^p to each WC_i. The value of x_j^s shows the scarcity of SR_j, the larger the scarcer; while y_i^p represents the popularity of WC_i, the larger the more popular. The computation process of weight x_j^s and y_i^p are as follows:

- Setting initial values of x_j^s and y_i^p as $x_j^s = \frac{1}{m}$ and $y_j^p = \frac{1}{n}$ respectively.
- Begin the iterative calculation of x_j^s and y_i^p until values of x_j^s and y_i^p converge within the error limits of double-precision arithmetic.

$$x_j^s \leftarrow \frac{\sum\limits_{p:(p,s)\in E} y^p}{n}, \; y_i^p \leftarrow \frac{\sum\limits_{s:(p,s)\in E} x^s}{m} \tag{83.6}$$

Weight of each type is normalized to maintain invariance after iterations: $\sum x^s = 1$ and $\sum y^p = 1$. Iterative computation process of formula (83.6) has been proved to converge [13].

83.4.2 Description of Algorithm

The values of x_j^s show the degree of scarcity of the resource, so cloud providers' profit will be promoted as prices of scarce resources are raised according to their weights x_j^s; while the larger values of y_i^p indicate that there are many suitable candidate resources for this component, consequently the price of resources assigned to it can be lowered according to the weight of y_i^p, and the component will accordingly get a better quality of service at a lower price. This kind of flexible resources allocation is more in line with the current relationship between supply and demand in the market economy mode. The algorithm of resources allocation is described as follows:

Algorithm 1: derivation of scarce resources list and popular components list based on structure supportiveness, allocation of cloud resources.

Input: *capacity*, S_{con}, components list *App*, and R_{avl}.

Output: resources allocation list of application components.

AllocateResources(){

Loop{

Reasoning of structure supportiveness according to formula (83.5), for each $vm_i \in R_{avl}$, $c_{jk} \in App$, to obtain scarce resources list $\{SR_j\}$ and popular components list $\{WC_i\}$;

Iterative computing the weights of $\{SR_j\}$ and $\{WC_i\}$ according to formula (83.6), until they converge within the error limits of double-precision arithmetic, to get the according weight list $\{x_j^s\}$ and $\{y_i^p\}$.

Adjusting prices of $\{SR_j\}$ according to their weight list $\{x_j^s\}$, and adjusting resource prices which are to be allocated to a component in $\{WC_i\}$ according to the weight y_i^p;

Resources allocation and management;

}

}

83.5 Experimental Results and the Analysis

In the simulation there were 5 physical machines, each of which resided 3 VMs. Performance of the resources was described with the parameters such as output o_v, access frequency access hf(v), input and output delay o_v, as well as price p_v; in order to simulate our algorithm of resources allocation, we randomly produced 283 applications, application constraints of a component can be expressed as a vector(w_c, d_c, t_c, c_c). We made a comparison based on the implementation of algorithms between resources allocation optimism and the random scheduling. Because the algorithms we put forward needed to take the QoS of both cloud providers and consumers into consideration simultaneously, as well as such factor as actual processing time, profits of cloud providers and User fees, according to formula (83.3) and formula (83.4) the cloud performance and its price can be quantified as

$$capacity = \alpha \frac{o_v \times hf(v)}{d_v}, \; p_v = p(capacity) = \beta.capacity$$

In which α was an estimated value, which was obtained based on the estimation of current network conditions, while $\beta$was a regulation constant, which was

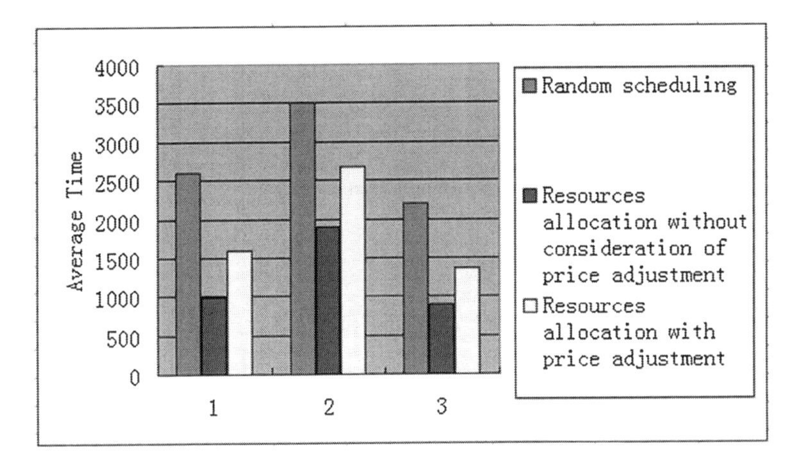

Fig. 83.2 Average execution time of the different resource allocation schemes under different workloads

determined by resources conditions of cloud providers. The whole simulation of experiments was divided into three parts, firstly to verify the performance of random scheduling algorithm, secondly the simulation of resources allocation based on structure supportiveness, without consideration of effect of price adjustment factors, thirdly the simulation of resources allocation based on structure supportiveness together with weights computation of scarce resources and popular components were carried out, to adjust prices. The comparison result of implementation of time was shown in Fig. 83.2. From the figure, we got that the execution of resources allocation based on structure supportiveness did improve the efficiency comparing to random scheduling, however, the process of resources allocation with price adjustment did consume some extra time while computing the according weights.

83.6 Conclusion

In this paper, we put forward a kind of optimization of resources allocation in cloud computing based on structure supportiveness. We build up the structure supportiveness relationship between application components and cloud resources based on compatibility reasoning according to their performance parameters. The weight of scarce resources and popular components are computed iteratively, and prices of both cloud providers and consumers are adjusted according to their weights to achieve the best match between cloud providers. Experiment has shown that the algorithm has arrived at better results in cloud resources allocation. Further work mainly includes some meticulous work such as adjusting and refining the parameters, and optimizing the algorithms and improving their efficiency.

References

1. Dai Y (2010) Introduction to cloud computing technologies. Inf Commun Technol 02:29–35
2. Buyya R et al (2009) Cloud computing and emerging it platforms: vision, hype, and reality for delivering computing as the 5th utility. Future Gener Comput Syst 25(6):599–616
3. Liu X-Q (2011) Research on date center structure and scheduling mechanism in cloud computing. University of Science and Technology of China
4. Li A, Yang X (2010) Cloudcmp: comparing public cloud providers. In: Proceedings of IMC
5. Karjoth G (2003) Access control with IBM Tivoli access manager. ACM Trans Inf Syst Secur 6(2):232–257
6. Dean J, Ghemawat S (2008) MapReduce:simplified data processing on large clusters. Commun ACM 51(1):107–113
7. Fischer MJ, Su X, Yin Y (2010) Assigning tasks for efficiency in Hadoop:extended abstract. In: Proceedings of the SPAA'10[C], pp 30–39. Thira, Santorini, Greece
8. Hadoop on Demand [EB/OL] (2011). http://hadoop.apache.org/common/docs/r0.18.3
9. Sim KM (2010) Towards agent-based cloud markets (Position Paper).In: Proceedings of the international conference E-Case, and E-Technology, pp 2571–2573
10. Sim KM (2012) Complex and concurrent negotiations for multiple interrelated e-markets. IEEE Trans Syst Man Cybern Part B. doi:10.1109/TSMCB preprint
11. Alshamrani A, Xie L (2010) Adaptive admission control and channel allocation policy in cooperative ad hoc opportunistic spectrum networks. IEEE Trans Veh Technol 59(4):1618–1629
12. Leong C, Zhuang W, Cheng Y, Wang L (2006) Optimal resource allocation and adaptive call admission control for voice/data integrated cellular networks. IEEE Trans Veh Technol 55(2):654–669
13. Kleinberg JM (1999) Authoritative sources in a hyperlinked environment. J ACM 46(5):604–632
14. Topcuoglu H, Hariri S, Wu M-Y (2002) Performance-effective and low-complexity task scheduling for heterogeneous computing. IEEE Trans Parallel Distrib Syst 13(3):260–274
15. Liang H, Huang D (2010) On economic mobile cloud computing model. In: Proceedings of the international workshop mobile computing, Clouds (MobiCloud in conjunction with MobiCASE), pp 1–12

Chapter 84
Ambidextrous Development Model of University Continuing Education in Yunnan Province Based on CRM

Hong-wu Zuo, Ze-jian Li and Ming Pan

Abstract Based on the analysis of current situation of continuing education and novel opportunities for its development, the paper proposed, from the perspective of Customer Relationship Management (CRM), an ambidextrous development model of university's continuing education, i.e., a model which can help to achieve both exploration and exploitation in the development of university continuing education. Specifically, on the basis of rational allocation of current educational resources, not only to remain the current development of continuing education, but to shift in accordance with the changing of external environment. The paper employed the theory of CRM to analyze the characteristics of different levels of learners in university's continuing education, to accurately grasp the learning objectives and needs of them, and proposed the tactics of establishing ambidextrous model of the development of university's continuing education in Yunnan in agreement with the current situation of Yunnan universities.

Keywords Yunnan University Continuing Education · Ambidextrous development model · Customer relationship management

---

H. Zuo (✉) · M. Pan
Faculty of Adult Education, Kunming University of Science and Technology, Kunming 650093, China
e-mail: zhw_1975@163.com

M. Pan
e-mail: myshares2006@163.com

Z. Li
Institute of Technology, Kunming University of Science and Technology, Kunming, China
e-mail: 0731lucy@163.com

S. Li et al. (eds.), *Frontier and Future Development of Information Technology in Medicine and Education*, Lecture Notes in Electrical Engineering 269,
DOI: 10.1007/978-94-007-7618-0_84,

84.1 Introduction

Since Custom Relationship Management (CRM) [1] theory has been adopted in educational management model, it focuses on the needs of students and pursues rational allocation of existing educational resources in education. Especially, with the advent of knowledge economy, continuing education has attracted more social attention and has been attached more importance, by degrees, which is to be an important reference on decision-making in continuing education reform.

The issued National Outline for Medium and Long-term Education Reform and Development (2010–2020) [2] (hereinafter called "The Issued Outline") specified that we must accelerate development in further education, put further education under a sound framework and build a flexible, open system for lifelong education. Continuing education ushered in an important period of development. On the one hand, a number of continuing education institutions have been fully aware that customers (i.e., the learners) are valuable resources for their development; On the other hand, the characteristics and needs of different customers are changing, which requires corresponding emphasis on the training system and resources allocation, and even the change of development model of university's continuing education. Therefore, this paper attempts to introduce the ambidextrous organization theory in the development model of continuing education. Ambidextrous organization is an organization to solve the contradiction between today's development and tomorrow's innovation of the enterprise and commit to achieve the both goals which is quite different or even in contradiction. It stems from the contingency thinking [3], which advocates that organizational structures should match up best with environments. It holds that the goal of organization is not to choose a best structure to adapt changes in the environment, but to face up to the reality of the paradox, to create a paradoxical structure to deal with it. To set up an ambidextrous organization will be the goal of organizational development of the university's continuing education in the complex external environment,

84.1.1 The Status of Domestic Development Model of University

Continuing education is a post-graduate education offered to all members of society, especially adults, and is an integral part of lifelong education. From the different perspectives and positioning, current domestic development of university's continuing education falls into three models:

Tsinghua University Mode. This mode features in offering non-diploma education and on-job trainings, which is put on an equal footing with full-time undergraduate studies and graduate studies by Tsinghua University. It sets up a newel model of continuing education specifically the management system, the operation mechanism, the brand creating and the management team building.

Open University Mode. This is a polite continuing education mode proposed in "The Issued Outline". Now, there are four open universities across the country. Supported by modern information technology, open universities provide adults open and distance education, which makes campus education extend to the social education, offering both diploma-granting education and non-diploma education [2]. However, how to put the mode into effect still needs to be further studied.

Local Universities Mode. At present, most of local universities' continuing education still emphasis on diploma-granting education rather than non-diploma education. Therefore, their management system, the operation mechanism and resources allocation fit in with diploma-granting education, which limits the further development and weakens the organization's risk-avoiding ability.

Though the above development models generated from different backgrounds with different educational objects that have their own characteristics, considering the history and the trend in the development of university's continuing education at home and abroad, they are in innovation and change.

84.1.2 The Development Environment of Yunnan Universities' Continuing Education

Yunnan is a relatively undeveloped multi-ethnic province in China, which located in a frontier and mountainous area. For many years, due to economic, social and geographical factors, the level of development of Yunnan universities' continuing education is still lags behind those developed provinces. In the next 10 years, Yunnan will be built into a strong province of green economy and ethnic culture, and a gateway in China's opening up to the Southwest, which bring a significant chance to talents cultivation. However, due to the relatively poor development ideas, facilities and educational system, there still are many problems and difficulty in cultivating the wanted talents and it need some new development model to Yunnan universities' continuing education.

1. The nation encourages devoting efforts to the development of non-diploma continuing education and keeping steady development of diploma-granting education, which requires universities to adjust their development model soon.
2. The talents in knowledge economy must be the one who can keep learning new knowledge, technologies and has the ability to innovate. This call for the innovation of the training mode of university's continuing education.
3. With the emergence of different continuing education institution, student recruitment is now in fierce competition. Competitors are not only the existing ones, but those alternatives, those who used to be the collaborating partners and the departments. Under this circumstance, universities need to think about an integration of education approaches. For example, to merge continuing education with community education, business education, vocational education, self-taught education, etc. Besides, party interested should also be considered to see weather they have the same objective.

4. With the growth of student recruitment, the demands of teaching resources is increasing, while the education investment is still insufficient, which leads to the great restriction to the development of university's continuing education.

84.2 Customer Analysis and the Impact on Ambidextrous Development Model of University's Continuing Education

In view of the above status, this paper attempts employ CRM theory to guide the analysis of the learning needs of learners, and on this basis to probe into the establishment of an ambidextrous development mode of Yunnan University's continuing education. Specifically, ambidextrous development model, based on the reasonable allocation and use of existing educational resources, not only is committed to keep the current development of continuing the development of education, but also assure the rapid and accurate transformation of its own development model in line with the changes in the external environment. That is the paradox of the co-existence of exploration and exploitation. In addition, the establishment of this mode requires a study of the characteristics of learners at different levels with an application of CRM, and an accurate grasp of the purpose and needs of their learning [4], which can provide important basis and foundation to ultimately build up an ambidextrous development model of university's continuing education.

84.2.1 Customer Analysis of University's Continuing Education

For University Continuing education, to provide quality teaching resources, standardized management system and other educational products to learners through CRM, can helps learners and other customers get a higher-value tangible and intangible benefits. It is thus evident that the customer in the university's continuing education has a double particularity of the learners and customers [5]. So university's continuing education need to balance their own interests and those of customers, to create more value for customers and to achieve the maximization of revenue. All of this depends on establishing and maintaining certain relationships between the continuing education and customers, which is also the base of building ambidextrous development model of university's continuing education.

Therefore, to form an ambidextrous model of university's continuing education, costumer's needs should be considered and understand from many angles. Study suggests the needs of customers of continuing education has features of diversity and multi level. The difference in age, career and family results the differences in behavior, such as learning and consuming habit. Analyzing customer demand can let us know which product and service among we provided can make them know its perceived value in subjective way (including inquiry, purchase, use and evaluating), thus providing new sources for the development of continuing education through customer value [6].

84.2.2 The New Characteristics of University Continuing Education and the Influence on Ambidextrous Development Model

Through investigation to collaborative partners of a certain Science and Technology University, including sending out questionnaires and visiting adult learner at different levels and in different specialities, data statistic and analysis, it is found that there are some new changes and new characteristics which have a profound effect on development model of continuing education in the sphere of the needs of the community, students recruitment, teaching administration, learners services:

1. In the context of China's social and economic transformation, great attention was paid to cultivating talented personnel. The academic disciplines offered by university continuing education are increasingly linked to the relevant industries and enterprises, showing the characteristics of aggregation. Enrollment target and disciplines offered are associated closely with demand of economic and social development. Thus, how to effectively maintain sustainable development of continuing education comes to be a new requirement and objective.
2. Freshmen in recent years show a rising trend in the number of students attending undergraduate and undergraduate level. This is not only to the development of the University Continuing Education has brought new opportunities, but also in the process of its transition to the dual model of development has also brought new problems of teaching management services.
3. Working-learning contradictions, life-learning contradictions increasingly, not just involve some learners, but showing a trend of universalization. This brought a lot of impacts to the school's teaching management and administration. On the other hand, the age of learners studying currently with different learning levels shows a new phenomenon, 39 % of learners in college and undergraduate level aged 20–22 years old, 35 % learners over the age of 30 years old; For college-to-undergraduate level, 41 % of the learners aged between 23 and 27 years old, 39 % of learners over the age of 32 years old and it shows a trend that the proportion of younger learners gradually increase. This requires the more consideration on various aspects influences of the teaching process, the learner services brought by learners' age changes on the process of building the University Continuing Education dual model.
4. In recent years, the number of candidates and the enrollment scale of diploma-granting education show a declining trend preached increasing trend, but the number of students involved in non-degree continuing education and training,

and participate in University Continuing Education non-academic education and training more and more partners, the project involves training more widely. This means that the concept of the continuing education needs of adult learners and corporate, industry Chiang Kai-shek quickly with new changes, will require that the University Continuing Education the dual development mode should speed up the pace of the corresponding allocation of educational resources, run mechanisms, management must shift to gradually adapt to the changes in the current education market operation mechanism.

84.3 Countermeasures on Construction of Ambidextrous Development Model of Yunnan University's Continuing Education

It's is very urgent and necessary for Yunnan universities how to build faster and better continuing education dual development model. Combined the relevant national policies, the social demand for talent, universities sponsoring characteristics and other factors, the following aspects of countermeasures is need to construct the ambidextrous development model, which is shown in Fig. 84.1.

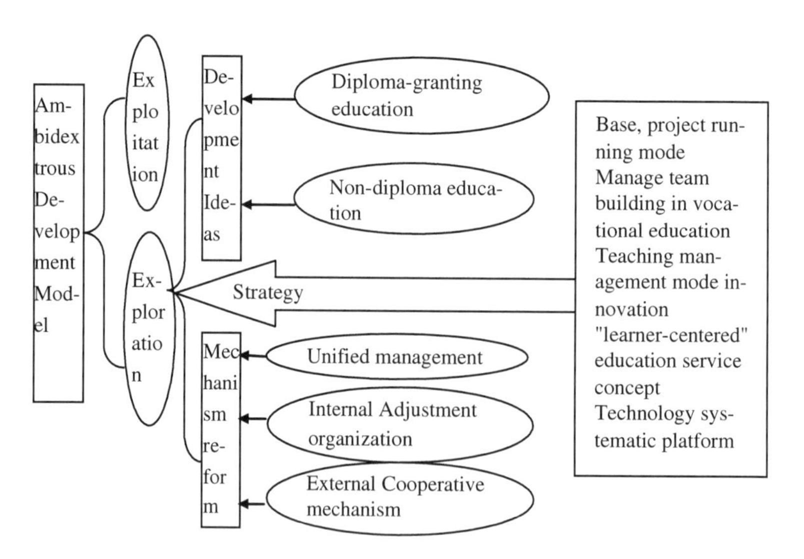

Fig. 84.1 Ambidextrous development model of Yunnan University's continuing education

84.3.1 General Ideas on Ambidextrous Development Model of Yunnan University's Continuing Education

"The Issued Outline" clearly put forward the continuing education is an important part of the lifelong learning system, as a system of lifelong education the most important aspects would assume unprecedented job training and continuing education task. In recent years, school enrollment, enrollment professional trends need to be analyzed, from which can be found in the academic education students to convert non-academic education and training and new ways to expand access to a wide range of potential students and development of space, to extend their own educational products value chain. The past 5 years, according to incomplete statistics, Yunnan University Continuing Education, training tens of thousands of various types of learners, this is a great resource for the development of the University Continuing Education, and according the study of Lubatkin [7], resource adequacy is positively correlated with the dual tendency, enterprises have the ability to be opposed to the elements of integration into the mode of development of the same organization. Yunnan University Continuing Education learners should make full use of valuable resources, identify the point of integration for economic, social and technological development in their own development model, a clear academic education and non-academic education personnel both job training will be the development of the inevitable choice.

84.3.2 Mechanism of University Continuing Education Ambidextrous Development Model

Pay equal attention to academic education and job training is the focus of the dual model of development, the first based on the complexity of the relationship between the organization (that is highly competitive and cooperative coexist) will greatly affect the double meta-schema of this conclusion [7], must be at the school level specialized management agencies be integrated and unified management school continuing education programs in order to maximize the full use of its own brand of the college, professional advantage, coordination school teaching resource allocation; followed by complex organizational form of the complexity of the changing external environment will result in lack of contact even very antithesis of the working relationship between the agencies, coordination costs are too high [7], it is necessary to actively adjust internal management structure of the University Continuing Education, and the introduction of Gibson and Birkinshaw [7] have proposed a context-sensitive dual concept, which is asking for all categories of personnel engaged in continuing education should be within the scope of the entire business goal congruence, teamwork, initiative, mediating, work ethic, pursuit of colleges and universities in the development of continuing education overall business strategy consistent with new opportunities; Reilly III and

Tushman [7] pointed out that the dual is a containing the unique ability in the learning behavior of business leaders, managers, showing the ability to adapt to changing external environment for a repeatable manner restructuring assets, the same Yunnan University Continuing Education dual schema in the education and training must be adapted to the current personnel training patterns and trends to comply with the Yunnan regional economic development needs to be innovative cooperation mechanism. Continuing education base, with a particular service object University Continuing Education and Regional Economic interaction, the interaction of universities and the growth of talent, enhance the University Continuing Education services targeted by the coalition government, industry, business. Through cooperation with different educational institutions, to carry out a wide range of cooperative education programs to overcome the deficiencies in the current University Continuing Education operating mechanism. And to accept the advanced educational concepts, learning the advanced education business and management, so as to gradually achieve the improvement of the inadequacies in the existing mechanism for continuing education.

84.3.3 Strategy of University Continuing Education Ambidextrous Development Model

Specifically, Yunnan University Continuing Education dual development model has following aspects.

1. For Yunnan Province, region, county economic development in a major and difficult is to enhance the ability of the quality of employees. So as to better serve and adapt to the current situation of Yunnan regional economy, the county's economic development, the University Continuing Education is necessary to change the educational ideas and patterns, establish free education to the county, sent to teach into the enterprise, sent to teach into plant consciousness, school into the most urgent demand for talents primary and cutting-edge, and actively explore the establishment of a new base, project running mode. The model is not only able to meet the training of scientific personnel urgently needed by the grass-roots, but also to discover and expand the resources of the University Continuing Education customers, help to solve a very common and prominent engineering, contradictions and problems in home.
2. With the gradual completion of the mission of the Yunnan university continuing education, academic education and training, non-academic education and training trend rising, high-level, high-quality, cost-effective continuing education programs and all kinds of practice and qualification certification training, internal The training will be the focus of the University Continuing Education side of the dual model of development, the need to strengthen cooperation between professional faculty or research institutions and schools have all kinds

of teaching management resources, to strengthen the training of market development and teacher sharing; need to actively strengthen cooperation with the Government and industry department in charge of large and medium-sized enterprises communication and contact, to establish a close strategic partnership, to take the group win, with a stable customer base path of development; need to strengthen the integration on their own internal management services, teaching management training, the establishment of a training curriculum development, teaching quality monitoring, responsible for marketing training, including vocational education and management team members.

3. With the social and economic development, a number of high-level talents through lifelong learning to improve the knowledge structure, the number of front-line service personnel through lifelong learning to adapt to the need of job change, improvement of professional skills, is also a large number of ordinary people through life-long learning to improve the quality of life. Diverse desire to learn and characteristics for the various groups, Yunnan college continuing education teaching, management, learner services in the dual model of development we need a new innovative measures, first according to the needs of learners' analysis of the results of the teaching programs, teaching organization and other aspects of adjustment, the introduction of social, relevant experts and scholars into the classroom to participate in teaching, increase recognition of the extent of national professional qualifications acquired by the learner, learner assessment should take the form of more diverse learning needs "learner-centered" education service concept; followed by the learner services, to establish how to adhere to the standards of personnel training and highlight the adult characteristics throughout the work, by taking the lead of school culture, The student brand activities appeal, the incentive multiple measures simultaneously in the form of the different individual needs of adult learners build their participation in adult learning spiritual home.
4. The implementation of University Continuing Education ambidextrous development model need to rely on a variety of modern information technology. After 10 years development, the theory and means of modern educational technology has been mature application, Yunnan University Continuing Education can reference and transplanted it to their own development mode to construct the "ground network—people network" continue education information service system; further integration of the internal and external digitized learning resources; introduction of digitized lifelong learning service platform with multi-interactive, personalized curriculum, teaching management, service support, early warning and response mechanism function, formed a guide-self-guidance teaching mode with University Continuing Education own characteristics, building support to provide technical for the ambidextrous development model of University Continuing Education.

84.4 Conclusion

With the accelerating process of economic globalization, Yunnan University Continuing Education should take the initiative to adapt to the needs of the times of universal learning, lifelong learning, and make full use of CRM theory to guide the analysis of learners' needs, building an ambidextrous development model owned University Continuing Education's characteristics, thus provide various forms of, high-quality continuing education products and services to economic and social development in Yunnan.

Acknowledgments This article is a stage results of a "12th 5-year Plan" adult education research program, named "Study on Dual Development Model of Adult Education of Universities in Western Area Based on the CRM Theory", approved by China Association for Adult Education, (Grant No. 2011-039Y).

References

1. Anion J (2000) The past present and future of customer access centres. Int J Serv Ind Manage 11(2):120–130
2. National long-term education reform and development plan (2010–2020), (2010) 7
3. Yu Z, Li C-W (2006) Ambidextrous organization research review. Shanghai Foreign Econ Manage 28(1):1–8
4. Lu H, Li G (2005) Customer value theory inspiration college of modern distance education development. China Education Tech 8:45–47
5. Zhan Z, Ye H (2008) Zhanrui Hua Mei Hu the CRM perspective of modern distance education management model building. China Education Tech 8:34–38
6. Zuo H, Li Z, Wang R (2010) The empirical research on study demand of adult education students based on CRM [C]. International conference on educational and information technology, vol 6. Chongqing, China, 17–19 September 2010, pp 19–22
7. Zhou J, knowledge X (2009) The dual organizations build the research frontier. Foreign Econ Manage 31(01):50–57

Chapter 85
Bibliometric Analysis on the Study of Education Informatization

Qiaoyun Chen

Abstract In order to master the research status of educational informatization in China, 2,892 papers in CNKI database published from 1995 to 2012 were combed and analyzed from the dimensions of paper amount per year, author, institution, and so on. After bibliometrics analysis, the study found that such study had experienced the initial and accumulation period, and been in the development period now. The core of the researcher group is not yet ripe, which reflects the researchers in the field are quite lacking of sustainable and profound spirit. Various types of project funds funding for educational informatization promote the research in this field.

Keywords Education informatization · Bibliometric · Literature analysis

85.1 Introduction

The concept of educational informatization began from America's "national information infrastructure" plan in the 1990s. As an important part of the social informatization, educational informatization is an important symbol of educational modernization and the internal need of building the modern education system. From the end of the last century, China also began a vigorous educational informatization building. In 1989, the former State Education Commission formally promulgated and implemented the National Education Management Information System Planning described as the originator of the informatization revolution in the field of education in China, which is also the cornerstone of China's education management informatization. In the past 20 years, a strong information revolution

Q. Chen (✉)
School of Education Science, Nanjing Normal University, Nanjing 210097, China
e-mail: qiao7@163.com

S. Li et al. (eds.), *Frontier and Future Development of Information Technology in Medicine and Education*, Lecture Notes in Electrical Engineering 269,
DOI: 10.1007/978-94-007-7618-0_85,

happened in the field of education. In 2010, China issued the National long-term Education Reform and Development Plan (2010–2020), as a weather vane of China's education reform in the next period of time. In Chap. 19 of this plan, the content devoted to elaborating educational informatization, which reflects the country's concern at this stage of the development of educational informatization. Many scholars published a lot of papers in this field [1–3]. Standing on the edge of era transition, in order to understand the current situation of China's educational informatization research, this paper use the bibliometric analysis and literature review method, reviewing China's literature from 1995 to 2012, trying to reveal the research result in educational informatization in recent years, providing a reference for future research and practice to carry out.

85.2 Research Method

85.2.1 Data Sources

Researchers often start their study from consulting document, because it can help researchers to capture the overall achievements in this area. As the main strength of the study, the periodical papers reflect the latest developments in academics. In this study, we focus at the topic of educational informatization, select relevant papers in Chinese Journal Full-text Database as samples, then start the retrieval in March 2013, and choose the time ranges from 1995 to 2012. In order to get a more accurate result, I did a secondary screening to exclude notices of meetings, Call for Papers, advertising and other irrelevant content, and finally get a valid number of papers that is 2,892.

85.2.2 Methods and Data Processing

In this study, we use the method of bibliometrics for analysis. It is a common method in scientific research and intelligence research, originating from the inspection of quantitative characteristics of scientific literature. It is a discipline that takes literature system and bibliometric characteristics as the research object, using mathematics, statistics, and other measurement methods, study the distribution structure of literature intelligence, number relationships, variation and quantitative management, then explore the structure, characteristics and laws of science and technology. With this method, we extracted titles, keywords, year, authors, journal names, fund projects, research institutions and other fields, using Excel 2010 and some related tools for statistical analysis to get related data about educational informatization.

85.2.3 The Index and Analysis Content

Yearly published papers: the number of relevant papers of a year;

Periodical distribution: major educational informatization journals;

Institution distribution: Institutions that study educational informatization;

Fund papers: projects papers supported by funds.

85.3 Statistical Results and Literature Analysis

85.3.1 Yearly Published Papers and Division of Research Stage

The increase and change of literature quantity in a certain period can reflect the development stage and situation of a special subject or field approximately. Derek John de Solla Price, the pioneer of metrology research, has put forward the famous Price's index [4], a law of literature quantity growth. According to the law, the development scientific literature has its own law. At the early stage of, the number of documents are often very unstable, but once the subject into the development period, the literature quantity will be growing exponentially, appeared a tendency of information explosion.

Cumulative literature quantity is the accumulation of total number of previous and that year's literature quantity. It references to the quantity of related literature in a year and it is an important indicator of the overall scale of the related studies. Rate of literature accumulation is a ratio of the quantity of published literature that year and previous. The formula for calculating is $E = n_i/\Sigma n_{i-1}$, it reflects whether the new increased literature was explosive development and to determine whether the research field hot spot was formed. Both the index reflects the amount of changes in literature.

We retrieved effective 2,892 papers about education informatization from the Chinese Journal Full-text Database. Table 85.1 is 1995–2012 the literature quantity of the topic. As we can see, the research of education informatization was begun at 1995 in China, and only one piece of paper was published in that year. As Chinese government emphasis on education informatization and constant investment, and also the continuous development of information construction, the academic research of education informatization papers was increased year by year. There were more than 250 references published a year in and after 2007. In the 5 years of 2007–2012, 64 % of the total number of whole paper was published.

From 1995 to 2001, the Rate of literature accumulation was fluctuation a lot. It can be seem as threshold of the period of this research topic. From 2002–2006, the published number gradually increased to 200 a years or so, Rate of literature accumulation has certain fluctuations during this period but the amplitude is much smaller than the previous stage. This period may be defined as the accumulation

Table 85.1 Research paper number and accumulation rate

Years	Paper's number	Cumulative literature quantity	Literature accumulation rate (%)
1995	1	1	–
1996	3	4	300.00
1997	9	13	225.00
1998	11	24	84.62
1999	21	45	87.50
2000	44	89	97.78
2001	105	194	117.9
2002	127	321	65.46
2003	202	523	62.93
2004	204	727	39.01
2005	132	859	18.16
2006	167	1,026	19.44
2007	324	1,350	31.58
2008	286	1,636	21.19
2009	275	1,911	16.81
2010	322	2,233	16.85
2011	336	2,569	15.05
2012	323	2,892	12.57

stage of education informatization research. Significantly changes happened after 2007, published papers quantity was increased sharply again, up to 336, and annual Rate of literature accumulation have relatively stable, combined with the Price index, the research of education informatization enter into the stage of development period since 2007 and continues to today.

85.3.2 Analysis on the Frequency of Publication by Authors

Through multidisciplinary and statistical analysis of research literature, the American scholar Alfred J. Lotka found an important law; it states that the number of authors making n contributions is about 1/n2 of those making one contribution. As the number of papers published increased, authors those who produced so many publications become less frequent. There are 1/4 as many authors publishing two papers within a specified time period as there are single-publication authors, 1/9 as many publishing three papers, 1/16 as many publishing four papers, etc. This is Lotka's law [5], one of the three laws of literature metrology.

The study statistics 2,892 paper on education informatization involved the author 2,248 (according to Lotka's law, only the first author was counted). Can be found from Table 85.2, there are 1,912 author just published 1 paper, accounting for 85.05 % of the total number of first author, much higher than Lotka's law (60 %). And the authors who published 2–4 papers accounts for the author who

Table 85.2 First author distribution

Paper's number	Author's number	Percentage of the total (%)	Percentage of authors publishing 1 paper (%)
1	1,912	85.05	100.00
2	226	10.05	11.82
3	50	2.22	2.62
4	22	0.98	1.15
5	10	0.44	0.52
6	9	0.40	0.47
7	7	0.31	0.37
8	1	0.04	0.05
9	3	0.13	0.16
11	3	0.13	0.16
12	1	0.04	0.05
13	1	0.04	0.05
16	1	0.04	0.05
19	1	0.04	0.05
20	1	0.04	0.05

published one were 11.82, 2.62, 1.15 %, far below the corresponding numbers in Lotka's law. The figures suggesting that Chinese education informatization research is not mature need long time to cultivation.

85.3.3 Key Author Group Analysis

According to the limits of the Price index about the key author groups, the key author published papers in the least N_{min} and the most N_{max} has the following relationship, $N_{min} = 0.749 \times N_{max}^{1/2}$. According to the statistics before, the $N_{max} = 20$, from the formula above, the $N_{min} = 3.35$. That means in the research field of education informatization, these authors who published 4 papers and more can be called as the key authors (top 30 see Table 85.3). There are 60 authors published 4 or more papers, and totally published 389 papers, is about 13.45 % in the total. According to the Price index, the key author group carried out 50 % or more papers of a research field, in comparison, the key author group of Chinese education information technology research is in the stage of formation, the academic contribution and research sustainability should be improved.

85.3.4 Periodical Distribution Analysis

Statistical data shows that there are 2,892 papers about educational informatization that have been published in 263 kinds of periodicals. Among them 10 kinds of periodicals published more than 30 papers, accounting for 68.3 %, in total 1,975

Table 85.3 Top 30 key authors

Numbers	Author name	Paper's number
1	Zhu Zhiting	20
2	Yang Gaixue	19
3	Sang Xinmin	16
4	Ding Xingfu	13
5	He Kekang	12
6	Chen Lin	11
7	Yu Shengquan	11
8	Li Jiahou	11
9	Xiong Caiping	9
10	Lv Senlin	9
11	Huang Ronghuai	9
12	Gu Xiaoqing	8
13	Zhang Qianwei	7
14	Liu Chengxin	7
15	Zhang Jingtao	7
16	Xie Yueguang	7
17	Lin Junfen	7
18	Wang Zhuzhu	7
19	Tan Songhua	7
20	Hu Xiaoyong	6
21	Guo Li	6
22	Zhang Jingran	6
23	Ren Youqun	6
24	Lv Yao	6
25	Wang Yunwu	6
26	Gao Tiegang	6
27	Wang Youmei	6
28	Guo Shaoqing	6
29	Lin Dongqing	5
30	Wang Jide	5

papers. They are the main front of educational informatization research. These periodicals in Table 85.4 with * are core journals, accounting for 42.3 % in total papers. These periodicals with # are CSSCI source periodicals accounting for 27.8 % in all published papers. Papers published in these periodicals are mainly about educational technology and educational science. They have higher academic value than normal papers.

85.3.5 Institution Distribution Analysis

These 2,892 papers are completed by 1,117 institutions, among which 775 institutions complete one single paper and 139 institutions complete two papers. According to Price law [6], the lowest limit of core institutions can be described by

Table 85.4 Periodicals with more than 30 papers

Numbers	Periodical name		The number of papers
1	China Education Informatization		753
2	China Educational Technology	* #	417
3	E-Education Research	* #	320
4	Distance Education in China	*	196
5	China Adult Education	*	78
6	Education and Vocation	*	57
7	Education Exploration	*	47
8	Journal of Teaching and Management	*	41
9	Exploring Education Development	* #	35
10	Open Education Research	* #	31

formula: $N = 0.749 \times \eta_{\max}^{1/2}$, in which $\eta_{\max}$ is the number of papers that are published by the most productive institution. It is obviously that $\eta_{\max}$ stand for 108 papers in Table 85.5. Consequently we assign 8 to N. We can see that from the Table 85.5 these 47 institutions which publish more than 8 papers publish 1,078 papers on educational informatization research totally, account for 37.28 % in all papers. They are the core institutions that publish papers on educational informatization research. Among them the top three institutions are all state-level normal universities in our country's educational fields. They lead the research in educational fields in our country, particularly in educational informatization research field. Besides, Ministry of Education and its affiliated units also publish significant amount of papers.

85.3.6 Fund Paper Analysis

Fund papers are funded by different level of governments and social organizations. The number of fund papers reflects the academic quality and the support of country

Table 85.5 Institution distribution

Numbers	Institution name	Paper's number	Constituent ratio (%)
1	Beijing Normal University	108	3.73
2	East China Normal University	84	2.90
3	Northwest Normal University	72	2.49
4	South China Normal University	58	2.01
5	Ministry of Education	46	1.59
6	Northeast Normal University	42	1.45
7	Jiangsu Normal University	39	1.35
8	Nanjing University	35	1.21
9	Huazhong Normal University	32	1.11
10	Nanjing Normal University	31	1.07
...	...	...	...
Total		1,078	37.28

Table 85.6 Fund paper distribution

Fund level	Paper's number	Constituent ratio (%)
National	79	2.73
Provincial	227	7.85
Municipal	215	7.43
Institutional	103	3.56
Total	624	21.58

for research [7]. We can see from Table 85.6 that, 624 papers during all the 2,892 papers (close to 22 %) are supported by fund projects, wherein the national fund papers account for 2.73 %. These funds make improving the research level of education informatization gradually.

85.4 Conclusion

Through statistical analysis on research papers of education informatization, we can see that, abundant research results of education informatization have accumulated and made great progress in the past 20 years in China. The conclusions are mainly as follows:

(a) The number of papers on education informatization increased greatly from 1 in 1995 to 250 in 2007, and the number of the papers from 2007 to 2012 accounts for 64 % of the total. About 22 % of all 2,892 papers are funded by projects, among which national fund papers account for 2.73 %. Based on the literature growth index, the author divided the research process of nearly 20 years into three stages: beginning period (1995–2001), accumulation period (2002–2006) and development period (2007–2012).

(b) The number of authors who published 2–4 papers respectively account for 11.82, 2.62, 1.15 % of that of authors who published 1 paper, which is far less than the corresponding number according to "Lotka's law". There are 60 core authors being published more than 4 papers. The number of papers belonging to these authors only accounts for 13.45 % of the total, also lower than 50 % according to "price's law", which shows that core author group has not yet formed on education informatization in China.

(c) 2,892 papers are published in 263 journals, of which 10 journals publishing the most papers are important positions in the research field of educational informatization. The number of papers in these 10 journals accounted for 68.3 % of the total. The top three institutions publishing papers are Beijing Normal University, East China Normal University and the Northwest Normal University, saying that they are in the domestic leading position in educational informatization research.

Acknowledgements This research was supported by the National Education Sciences "12th Five-Year" Planning Ministry of Education youth issues, Research on use benefit of Higher education informatization based on user satisfaction (No. ECA110332).

References

1. Zhu Z (2012) Report on prospective study of educational technology. E-Educ Res 4:5–13 (in Chinese)
2. Yang G, Fu D (2012) Promoting the reform and development of Education. China Educ Technol (11):62–65 (in Chinese)
3. Kekang H (2012) Learning "ten-year development planning on education informatization": interpretation of "integration of information technology and education in depth". China Educ Technol 12:19–23 (in Chinese)
4. Price de Solla D J (1963) Little science, big science. Columbia University Press, New York
5. Lotka AJ (1926) The frequency distribution of scientific productivity. J Wash Acad Sci 16:3–17
6. Xiaolin Z (2010) A study of service system of American public library. Library (4) :66–68, 81 (in Chinese)
7. Lili S (2007) The Effect of fund-subsidized projects on university transactions. Sci-Tech Inf Dev Econ 17(3):265–266 (in Chinese)

Chapter 86
A Method for Integrating Interfaces Based on Cluster Ensemble in Digital Library Federation

Peng Pan, Qingzhong Li and XiaoNan Fang

Abstract Recently, there are more demands in a digital library federation to integrate multiple query interfaces into one for users. Since different interfaces have various descriptions for the same concept and the amount of interfaces are numerous, it is hard to provide complete and exact domain knowledge. Hence, the methods of clustering are usually adopted to generate an integrated interface. However, over one same properties set, the results for clustering may be diverse according to the differences of clustering algorithms or parameters setting for the same algorithm. Nevertheless, we could obtain one more complete and exact integrated interface with the aid of cluster ensemble by merging multiple clustering results. In this paper, based on the principle of cluster ensemble, we propose a single clustering algorithm with uncertainty regarding that one property may belong to more than one possible cluster division during integration. We also propose a fusing cluster algorithm to obtain cluster ensemble that satisfying interface integration and it shows favorable performances than the existing methods.

Keywords Interface integration · Deep web · Cluster ensemble · Uncertainty · Digital library

P. Pan · Q. Li (✉)
School of Computing Science and Technology, Shandong University, Shandong, China
e-mail: lqz@sdu.edu.cn

P. Pan
e-mail: ppan@sdu.edu.cn

X. Fang
School of Information Science and Engineering, Shandong Normal University, Shandong, China
e-mail: franknan@126.com

S. Li et al. (eds.), *Frontier and Future Development of Information Technology in Medicine and Education*, Lecture Notes in Electrical Engineering 269,
DOI: 10.1007/978-94-007-7618-0_86,

86.1 Introduction

Digital Library (DL) is a virtual knowledge centre which provides super large scale, distributed heterogeneous information with intelligent search services by building a sharable and extensible knowledge system in networked environment [1, 2].

It is impossible for any library to be self-contained, because no one single library has the capability to provide all the materials and information that meet users' requirements. Frequently, users have to access more than one digital library when requesting some resources. As each DL is autonomic, heterogeneous, the query has to be submitted onto the query interface according to different DL's data schemas. To simplify the process, the concept of Digital Library Federation (DLF) has been proposed [3].

Currently, the Digital Libraries have been moved into website, and the entrances often appear as query interfaces. Thus, one DLF have to integrate the query interface to provide one unique entrance for sharing information among heterogeneous DLs. Especially, in a university, since there are many online digital libraries with their own entrances, it is necessary to integrate all the entrances into one query interface to the users, which comes into a problem of interfaces integration.

Recently, many researches have been focused on the integration and mapping of interfaces which aimed to build up one integrated query interface for one domain. To achieve this, automatic schema mapping is needed. Since different interfaces have various description for the same concept, it is hard to providing complete and exact domain knowledge. Hence, finding out all the exact mappings for automatic mapping seems to be impossible. As a result, the existing automatic methods usually determine the final results by setting threshold or certain criteria, which would reduce the exactness and completeness of the final results. Further more, the mapping relationships between interfaces are more complex than traditional databases owing to the presentation type and mutual relationship of their properties, and these make it very hard to get the right answer in multiple optional schemas.

The clustering methods are usually adopted to generate an integrated interface for one domain, for the web database resources are numerous [4, 5]. However, over the same properties set, the cluster results may be diverse according to the differences of cluster methods or parameters setting for the same method [6]. Hence, multiple varied results for integration may come into being if we adopt different algorithms or set different thresholds with the same algorithm over same properties set. On the same time, we find out that all the results implicitly contain one whole exact schema of integrated interface, and we may obtain it with the aid of cluster ensemble by merging multiple clustering results .

In this paper, the steps to generate an cluster ensemble we proposed are:

- Decide the strategy for computing similarity of properties.
- Design single cluster strategy for generating multiple clusters to be fused.

- Establish the cluster consensus matrix based on multiple single clusters.
- Design fusing algorithm to obtain cluster ensemble.

The contributions of the paper are:

1. Considering that during integration one property may belong to multiple possible cluster divisions, we propose a clustering algorithm with uncertainty.
2. Propose a fusing cluster algorithm to obtain cluster ensemble that optimizing interface integration.

86.2 Related Works

The methods for automatic interface integration have two categories: one is local integration [4, 7], which is to compute the similarity between two random properties of interfaces each time, another is to integral integration [5, 8, 9], which find out all the corresponding relationships to generate one common interface for one time.

For the first category, Meng et al. [4]. analyze the properties information of each interface to match properties. During the process of semantic analyzing, they use WordNet [10]. However, they simply look interface as one structure combined with properties, and only considered the one–one mapping while ignoring many complex mappings in reality. Hence, Wu et al. [7] treat the interface as one hierarchal tree which can be used in more exact matching clustering algorithm by "bridge". Wang et al. [11] propose a method based on query results and co-occurrence statistics, which is limited to the massive extra works of submitting query and extracting the results. Wu et al. [12] achieve the matcher by the similarity of instances with NLP, which has higher expenses.

The integral method is suitable for interfaces integration with large-scale schema in web. He et al. [5] proposal is to match all the schema in one domain based on a common model by statistic. Based on it, He et al. [8]. propose the concepts of relevance for properties, which classify the relationships between properties into positive, negative correlation and isolation. They select the most propel match after deciding the relevance for properties.

86.3 Using Cluster Ensemble to Generating Integrated Interface

The concepts of Cluster Ensemble is proposed by strehl and Ghosh [13] in 2002. The main object is to fuse multiple results through different algorithms or distinct parameters for a same algorithm over the same data set into one cluster ensemble that is one complete and exact final result.

86.3.1 Strategy for Computing Similarity of Properties

When clustering the properties in interfaces, we need to compute the similarity between two properties. Here, we adopt the methods proposed by Wu et al. [7], in which the similarity of two properties is computed jointly by syntax, value domain and semantic. The formula is: λls *LingSim (e, f) + λds *DomSim (e, f) + λss *SemSim (e, f), where λls, λds, λss are the weights of syntax, value domain and semantic separately. In detail, by the name and label of properties we may compute the syntax similarity with LingSim (e, f) and semantic similarity with SemSim (e, f); by the value character, we may compute the value domain similarity with DomSim (e, f).

86.3.2 The Clustering Algorithm to Generate the Cluster to be Fused

The basic step of the algorithm is that

1. Each time the pair p with maximum similarity weight are selected.
2. One node u of p is set to the cluster center.
3. The nodes whose format are like (u, w) and similarity weights are no less than threshold τ are put into the cluster set whose center is u.
4. Cut the edge (u, w).
5. Repeat 1., until no edge can be added.

Each cluster division represents one integrated property, and we would find out that some node might lie in multiple cluster divisions, which means the property that these node represented have the mapping relationship with multiple clusters that representing integrated interface properties. The detailed algorithm is following:

Algorithm 1 : singleCluster

Input: S: properties set of interfaces to be integrated
G: similarities of all properties
τ : threshold, the critic to decide if a node can be added to a cluster
Output: cluster CC

1 $M \leftarrow G$
2 $CC \leftarrow \emptyset$, $C_s \leftarrow \emptyset$
3 $i = 0$
4 **while** ($\max_{sim(w,v)\in M}(sim(w,v)) \geq \tau$) or (M= = $\emptyset$) do
5 $u \leftarrow \arg\max_{u\in\{w|sim(w,v)\in M\}}(sim(u,v))$
6 $CC_i \leftarrow \{w \mid sim(u,w) \geq \tau \wedge w \notin C_s\} \cup \{u\}$
7 $C_s \leftarrow C_s \cup u$
8 $M \leftarrow M - \{sim(u,v) \mid v \in CC_i \wedge sim(u,v) \in M\}$
9 $CC \leftarrow CC \cup \{CC_i\}$
10 $i = i + 1$
11 **end while**

M is the similarity table, whose initial value is G; CC is the cluster sets, denoted as $\{\{CC_1\}, \{CC_2\}, \ldots \{CC_k\}\}$; C_s is the set of cluster center; the fifth to tenth rows describe the clustering process; the sixth row selects the pair (u, v) whose base is u from current similarity table; the seventh row puts all the nodes whose similarity weights with u are bigger than τ into a cluster CC_i; the eighth row takes the similarity edge (u, v) out of the similarity table M, if M is null, then the algorithm will ends; the ninth row updates the cluster set.

86.3.3 The Establishment of Consensus Matrix

We establish the consensus matrix based on the idea that an element in a cluster division might be in the same cluster division when adopting another clustering algorithm on the same data set. The method in this paper is that while running distinct clustering algorithms over n data for N times, we map each result into the consensus matrix simultaneous. As a result, the N divisions could be fused into a consensus matrix with $n \times n$ dimension. Finally, we may obtain one cluster result over the consensus matrix by the cluster ensemble algorithm.

During establishing consensus matrix, we need to provide the formula to update similarity, namely consensus function Γ. We discuss how to design the formula.

The cluster algorithm described in 3.2 is a fuzzy cluster, which may result in the situation that several data nodes might exist together in multiple divisions. Therefore, we may consider compute the similarity by Jaccard method. The following is the formulated illustration:

Given an original property set $G = \{a_1, a_2 \ldots a_n\}$, and a cluster set $\prod$ obtained by N different cluster algorithm or different parameters setting, denoted as $\{\pi_1, \pi_2, \ldots \pi_N\}$, where $\forall \pi_k (0 \leq k \leq N)$ is a n-dimensional vector $[c_{k,1}, c_{k,2}, \ldots . c_{k,n}]^T$ over G, $c_{i,j}$ represents the cluster label of jth property for the ith time, and vector $S_i = (s_1, s_2, \ldots s_n)$ is the probability that property a_i belongs to each division, which need to be normalized. Hence, the formula that computes the similarity of random a_i and a_j over the kth clustering is like this:

$$sim_k(a_i, a_j) = \frac{S_i^T S_j}{||S_i||^2 + ||S_j||^2 - S_i^T S_j} \tag{86.1}$$

At the beginning, the initial value of all elements in consensus matrix might be set to zero. While in the kth iteration, the element for the ith row and jth row is updated to $A_{ij} = \frac{N-1}{N} \times A_{ij} + \frac{1}{N} \times sim_k(a_i, a_j)$, which can be looked as a percentage indicating that a_i and a_j belong to one same cluster during the kth clustering iteration.

86.3.4 The Algorithm for Fusing Clusters

After establishing consensus matrix, we may fuse cluster to generate the cluster ensemble, which is the property set of final integrated interface. The following is the algorithm:

algorithm 2: fusing cluster for cluster ensemble

Input: property set S, clustering running times k, threshold set $T=\{\tau_1,\tau_1..\tau_k\}$, θ_1,θ_2

Output: new cluster division

```
1  C_{[1-n],[1-n]} ← 0
2  for each i ∈ [1,k] do
3      CA_i = singleCluster(S, τ_i)  //detailed in algorithm 1
4      for each a_i, a_j ∈ CC_i ∧ i ≠ j
5          if (c_{i,i} == c_{i,j}) then
6              C_{i,j} = C_{i,j} × (n−1)/n + 1/n × sim_k(a_i, a_j)
7          endif
8      endfor
9  endfor
10 for each a_j ∈ S
11     A(a_j) ← a_j
12 endfor
13 CC ← ∅, i = 0, CS ← ∅, CENTER[] ← ∅.
14 while (∃u, doesn't be added in CC) ||(¬∃u, v satisfies sim(u,v) < θ_2) do
15     u ← arg max_{u∈{i|C_{i,j} > θ_1}} (C_{i,j})
16     CENTER[i] ← u
17     CC_i ← {w | sim(a_u, w) ≥ θ_1 ∧ w ∉ CC} ∪ {a_u}
18     CS_i ← {w | sim(a_u, w) < θ_1 ∧ sim(a_u, w) ≥ θ_2 ∧ w ∉ CC}
19     CC ← CC ∪ {CC_i ∪ CS_i}
20     i = i+1
21 endwhile
```

In this algorithm, the first to ninth rows describe the process of algorithm 1 for multiple times. In this paper, we may obtain multiple cluster results by setting different threshold values for algorithm 1. One the same time, the consensus matrix $C_{n,n}$ are generated. The forth to eighth rows update consensus matrix with the formula 1 for each iteration, and the sixth row describes the process. The thirteenth to twentieth rows describe the process of generating final cluster. In the process, *CENTER* is a array, which records centers for each iteration. The process uses two threshold θ_1, θ_2 to make a property exist in multiple cluster divisions, where each division has two sets CC_i, CS_i. CC_i is the core part of cluster division. The elements in CC_i satisfies that their similarity with center are more than θ_1, and CS_i is the peripheral part whose elements satisfies the similarity with center are between θ_2 and θ_1. One property appears in the core party for only once, but may appears in the peripheral part for many times, which indicates that the mappings have many possible forms between one integrated interface and web interfaces.

86.4 Experiments

We have conducted two experiments to evaluate the performances of the methods proposed in this paper: evaluation of the method of interface integration; compare the methods of integration proposed in this paper with existing ones.

This paper take the web interfaces database of UIUC [14] as resource for experiments, which is called TEL-8 including 447 web interfaces in 8 domains. The interfaces we selected for the experiments are included in three domains: Airfres, Books, Automobiles. For each interface, we take the extracted properties as experiment standards.

86.4.1 *Evaluation of the Method for Interface Integration*

We set different threshold values to 0.35, 0.45, 0.55, 0.65, 0.75 and 0.85, and run single cluster algorithms in 3.2 respectively, then we conduct the integration algorithm in 3.4. to evaluate the precision ratio and recall ratio. The precision and recall rate are defined as following:

During the cluster process, each cluster division is a property over the integrated interface, which is ideally corresponding to the right properties in website interfaces. Therefore, the precision ratio of a cluster C_i can be defined as $P_i = \frac{A_i}{AT_i}$, where A_i is the number of right properties for the cluster division, AT_i is the sum of properties for the cluster division, the recall ratio can be defined as $R_i = \frac{A_i}{AC_i}$, where AC_i is the sum of right properties in the cluster division. Thus, the precision ratio of the whole cluster is $P_g = \sum_{i=1}^{n} \frac{A_i}{\sum_{i=1}^{n} AL_i} P_i = \frac{1}{\sum_{i=1}^{n} AL_i} \sum_{i=1}^{n} A_i * P_i$, where AL_i is the sum of properties for interface *i*, the recall ratio of the whole cluster is $R_g = \sum_{i=1}^{n} \frac{A_i}{\sum_{i=1}^{n} AL_i}$

$R_i = \frac{1}{\sum_{i=1}^{n} AL_i} \sum_{i=1}^{n} A_i * R_i$.

Figure 86.1 is about the precision and recall ratio of integrated interface. We can see that with the threshold increasing, the precision ratio are improving accordingly, while the precision ratio began to decline at 0.75. Our analysis is that the improvement of threshold may exclude some right properties, which would reduce the sum of right properties and decline the recall ratio. On the meanwhile, the improvement of threshold will filter more incorrect cluster properties, which continues to increase the precision ratio. The result shows that integrated cluster has higher precision ratio and recall ratio because the method in this paper may find out as many right properties as possible.

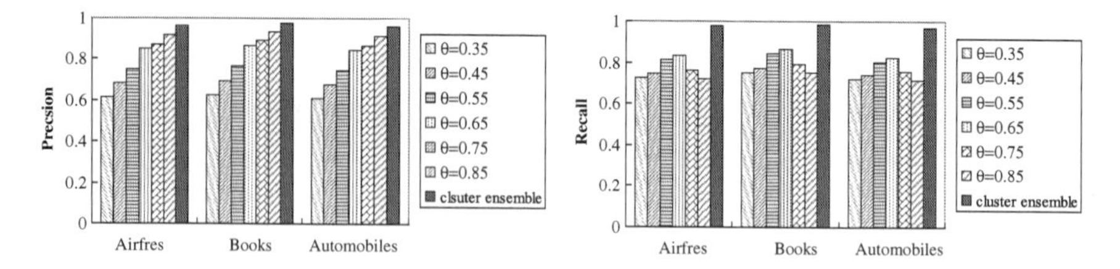

Fig. 86.1 The precision ratio and ratio for interface integration

Table 86.1 The comparison table for three methods

	Cluster ensemble		Wu's		He's	
	Precision	Recall	Precision	Recall	Precision	Recall
Airfres	0.964	0.978	0.934	0.948	0.94	0.956
Books	0.974	0.984	0.944	0.954	0.957	0.964
Automobiles	0.958	0.97	0.928	0.94	0.934	0.948
Average	0.965	0.977	0.935	0.947	0.943	0.956

86.4.2 Compare Method for Interface Integration Proposed in this Paper with the Ones at Present

We select three methods: the methods proposed by Wensheng Wu [7] (abbreviated to Wu's), by Bin He [5] (abbreviated to He's), and by this paper to execute over the same dataset. The evaluation standards is same as 4.1.

Table 86.1 is the results of precision ratio and recall ratio for three methods. We can see that the methods proposed in this paper has an advantage over Wu's and He's in the two standards. In detail, the precision ratio has been improved by 3 and 2.2 %; the recall ratio has been improved by 3.7 and 1.4 %. Clearly, the methods in this paper improves the performance in whole higher than Wu's and He's.

86.5 Conclusion and Future Works

This paper proposes a method based on Cluster Ensemble to get one interface integration for Digital Library Federation. Firstly, We propose a cluster algorithm with uncertainty regarding that one property may belong to multiple possible cluster divisions during integration. Then, we establish the cluster consensus matrix based on multiple single clusters. Finally, we propose a fusing cluster algorithm to obtain cluster ensemble that satisfying interface integration.

Many other problems need to be solved and furthered. Only giving the methods for integrating interfaces with uncertainty, we need to quantify this uncertainty in future. Therefore, the uncertainty should be furthered.

References

1. Fox EA (1993) Source book on digital libraries. Technical Report TR-93-35 Virginia Polytechnic Institute and State University
2. Harter SP (1996) What is a digital library? definitions, content, and issues. In: KOLISS DL 1996
3. Birmingham B et al.(2001) EU-NSF digital library working group on interoperability between digital libraries. http://www.iei.pi.cnr.it/DELOS/NSF/interop.htm Accessed 15 Dec 2001
4. He H, Meng W, Yu C, Wu Z (2003) WISE-integrator: an automatic integrator of web search interfaces for e-commerce. In: Proceedings of the 29th international conference on very large data bases (VLDB), Berlin, 2003 pp 357–368
5. He B, Chang KC-C (2003) Statistical schema matching across web query interfaces. In: Proceedings of the 2003 ACM SIGMOD international conference on management of data, San Diego, California, 2003 pp 217–228
6. Jain AK, Murty MN, Flynn PJ (1999) Data clustering: a review. ACM Comput Surv 31(3):264–323
7. Wu W, Yu C, Doan A, Meng W (2004) An interactive clustering-based approach to integrating source query interfaces on the deep web. In: Proceedings of the 23th ACM SIGMOD international conference on management of data, Paris, 2004 pp 95–106
8. He B, Chang KC-C, Han J (2004) Discovering complex matchings across web query interfaces: a correlation mining approach. In: Proceedings of the 10th ACM SIGKDD international conference on knowledge discovery and data mining, Seattle, 2004 pp 148–157
9. He B, Chang KC-C, Han J (2004) Mining complex matchings across web query interfaces. In: Proceedings of the 9th ACM SIGMOD workshop on research issues in data mining and knowledge discovery, Paris, 2004 pp 3–10
10. WordNet http://wordnet.princeton.edu/
11. Wang J, Wen JR, Lochovsky F, Ma WY (2004) Instance-based schema matching for web databases by domain-specific query probing. In: Proceedings of the thirtieth international conference on very large data bases, Toronto, Canada, 2004, pp 408–419
12. Wu W, Doan AH, Yu C (2006) WebIQ: learning from the web to match deep-web query interfaces. In: Proceedings of the 22nd international conference on data engineering, Washington, DC, USA, 2006, pp 44
13. Topchy AP, Jain AK, Punch WF (2004) A mixture model for clustering ensembles. In: Proceedings of the fourth SIAM international conference on data mining, Lake Buena Vista, Florida, USA pp 379–390
14. Chang KC-C, He B ,Li C, Zhang Z (2003) The UIUC web integration repository. Computer Science Department, University of Illinois at Urbana-Champaign. http://metaquerier.cs.uiuc.edu/repository, 2003

Chapter 87
Long Term Web Service Oriented Transaction Handling Improvement of BTP Protocol

Zhi-Lin Yao, Lu Han, Jin-Ting Zhang and Shu-Fen Liu

Abstract Web services transaction handing is a key technique issue of computer supported corporate work. BTP protocol is a neutral protocol. It is not a specific web service transaction coordinating protocol. In order to enable BTP to support long term transaction, we made some modifications on it. These modifications include three aspects, which are, (1) To provide a strategy to eliminate negative effects caused by temporary results; (2) To put forward piecewise strategy of transaction node; (3) To put forward autonomy strategy of un-confirm collection elements. We also give design and implementation of transaction handling system, which is part of project "Model Driven Service Oriented Application Development and Integration Platform", in which we use service broker method to extend a web service's function, and enable services with transaction handling ability without making any modification on it.

Keywords Web service · BTP · Transaction handling

Z.-L. Yao · L. Han (✉) · S.-F. Liu
College of Computer Science and Technology, Jilin University, Changchun, China
e-mail: hanlu@jlu.edu.cn

Z.-L. Yao
e-mail: yaozl@jlu.edu.cn

S.-F. Liu
e-mail: liusf@jlu.edu.cn

J.-T. Zhang
Shuangyang District Forestry Bureau, Changchun, China
e-mail: zhangjintingcc@gmail.com

S. Li et al. (eds.), *Frontier and Future Development of Information Technology in Medicine and Education*, Lecture Notes in Electrical Engineering 269,
DOI: 10.1007/978-94-007-7618-0_87,

87.1 Introduction

There has recently been an increase in the use of SOA to build CSCW systems [1]. For SOA systems, it is very important to keep data consistency of all the involved collaborative services. Tradition transaction handling system usually called ACID transaction [2]. It needs to maintain ACID properties of transaction, which are Atomic, Consistency, Isolation and Durability [3]. But this traditional ACID structure is not suitable for SOA (Service Oriented Architecture) applications. In traditional transaction handling processes, the needed resources would be locked before the transaction finish, so other transactions could not use the resources. On one hand, in distribution environment, problems like the network transport delay, reliability and consistency would all increasing of transaction handling time; on the other hand, systems based on SOA always have complex processing workflows, and a workflow usually has long processing time. If the system lock the resources for long time, would cause increasing probability of system dead lock, and lower the system availability and reliability.

BTP (Business Transaction Protocol) is proposed by OASIS (Organization for the Advancement of Structured Information Standards), which is mainly used to coordinate applications among several participants, which are autonomous and loose coupled.

BTP is a neutral protocol (language and technical independent), it can make multiple autonomous cooperating participants work coordinately. It defines the exchange of agreement in order to ensure that all application could be able to produce a consistent result. The consistent result here refers to: all the work is confirmed or no one was confirmed (atomic business transaction or atom), or by the application to determine which work is confirmed (a cohesive business transaction or cohesion). The transmission protocol bearing BTP messages can be SOAP or other transfer protocols, BTP is defined based on abstract XML message format [4].

BTP protocol transactions are divided into two types: Atomic Business Transaction and Cohesive Business Transaction. BTP Atomic Business Transaction is based on two-phase commit protocol, it can meet the characteristics of ACID affairs requirements; BTP Cohesive Business Transaction can satisfy the long term transaction handling requirements, it relaxes the ACID characteristic restrictions of transactions [5]. In a Cohesive Business Transaction, which participants will affect the commit result of whole transaction or sub transaction is determined by the superior business application, that is to say, if there is tractions of participants cannot be committed, the whole transaction may also successfully be committed. BTP achieve processing long term transaction through relaxing transaction's ACID characteristics restriction. Compare with the traditional transaction processing model, the biggest difference is that the transaction participants do not need to keep locking the occupied resources during transaction submission stage, and make a transaction's temporary results visible to other participants. The advantage of this is the ability to improve the services' concurrency, although also cause negative impacts by visibility of the transaction's temporary results, but it still can meet most business transactions' need.

BTP protocol is a neutral protocol, it is not a specific web service transaction coordinating protocol. When used in web services environment, it should be adjusted, we made modifications on it on three aspects, include: (1) To provide a strategy to eliminate negative effects caused by temporary results; (2) To put forward piecewise strategy of transaction node; (3) To put forward autonomy strategy of un-confirm collection elements.

87.2 Strategy to Eliminate Negative Effects Caused by Temporary Results in BTP

87.2.1 Negative Effects Caused by Temporary Results in BTP

In order to solve long term transaction problem, BTP makes a service's temporary results acquirable by other services, if the negative impact caused by this could not be eliminated, the system could enter an inconsistent state after transaction execution.

Consider two concurrent transactions 1 and 2 in Fig. 87.1, they all called service B. Execution of service A need a long time, but execution of service C need a very short time. Transaction 1 called the service earlier, and the service B action in transaction 1 is to fetch a data A from database and multiply it with 2, then store the result back to the database. That means the value of data A change to 2*a after transaction 1 calling service B, if original value of data A is a. Transaction 2 call B after transaction 1 call it. In transaction 2 service B fetch data A from database and add it with 2. That means the data A change to 2*a + 2 after service B is called. Because service C need a very short time to perform, so transaction 2 may be committed earlier than transaction 1. Suppose that transaction may finish before transaction 1 and can be committed correctly. Transaction 1 may need a long time, so the finish of it may need some time. Suppose service 1 fails and need to rollback, service B need to divided data A in database with 2 when rollback, but the value of data A now is 2a*2, so the result of data A change to a + 1, which means that the transaction's rollback didn't recover the state before execution.

The situation above is because of BTP allow one service to acquire temporary result of the other service, and there is no concrete police to eliminate these negative impacts.

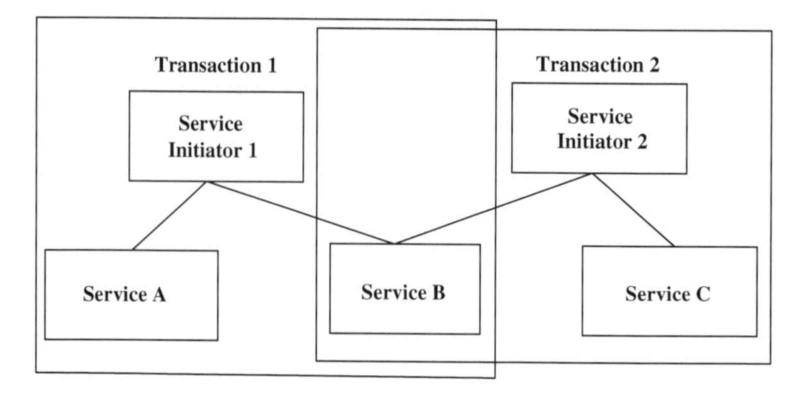

Fig. 87.1 Situation may cause negtive effects

87.2.2 Strategy to Eliminate Negative Impacts

In order to elimination inconsistency or negative impact, we design a strategy: When call a service in a transaction, the service corresponding BTP nodes should record BCT (Being Called Time). In Fig. 87.1, The BCT recorded by service B's corresponding node in transaction 1 is earlier than BCT recorded by service B's corresponding node in transaction 2. Thus when the transaction initiator of transaction 2 is about to commit the transaction, Its Decider, namely, the initiator's corresponding BTP node will send PREPARE message to BTP node of service B and service C. When BTP node of service B receives that message, it will look for whether there is any earlier transaction that called service B but hasn't committed it yet. I there is, it will enter into WAIT state, and send WAIT message to superior node. After Decider receives WAIT message from sub BTP nodes, it will send WAIT messages to all its sub BTP nodes, and enters into WAITED state itself. By using this strategy, transaction 2 will enter WAITED state before transaction commits. If transaction 1 commits at this time, the BTP node corresponding to service B in transaction 1 will send COMMITTED message to all related BTP nodes that registered in the logger. The BTP node of service B in transaction 2 will send PREPARED message to the superior node after it receives COMMITTED message from transaction 1. The superior node that is at WAITED state will commit and send CONFIRM message to all its sub nodes when it received PREPARED message from WAIT state node. If transaction 1 is about to rollback, the BTP node corresponding to service B in transaction 1 will send CANCEL messages to all related nodes that registered in the logger. The BTP node corresponding to service B in transaction 2 will send CANCEL message to the superior node after it received the CANCEL message from transaction 1. The superior node will send CANCEL message to its all sub node to cancel the transaction. That will eliminate the inconsistency negative impact caused by concurrent transactions.

87.3 Transaction Node Piecewise Strategy

In BTP protocol each application is corresponding to a BTP node, but in our strategy an application can be corresponding to several BTP nodes. The advantage of this is improvement of resources utilization rate. A service transaction is shown in Fig. 87.2.

In BTP protocol every application corresponds to a BTP node, but in our system an application may correspond to several BTP nodes, this method can promote resource utilization rate. For example, in Fig. 87.2, to call a service is actually call a function of service A, the service A need to call the other four services to complete its business logic. If this transaction is failed and is about to be cancelled, the compensation work of service B, C, D, E has to be finished under control of BTP node corresponding to service A. If the compensation controlling of service B, C, D, E is very complicated, then the BTP node corresponding to service A need long time to undertake compensation controlling. If we use several BTP nodes to control compensation operations concurrently, we can significantly reduce compensation controlling time and promote resource utilization rate. Like below, when the function of service A call the other four services, it divides them into two pieces or more, thus when compensation is operating, service A can have two BTP nodes, one controls compensation operation of service B and C, and the other controls compensation operation of C and D, that realize the compensation work that two BTP nodes control the operations concurrently, which promotes

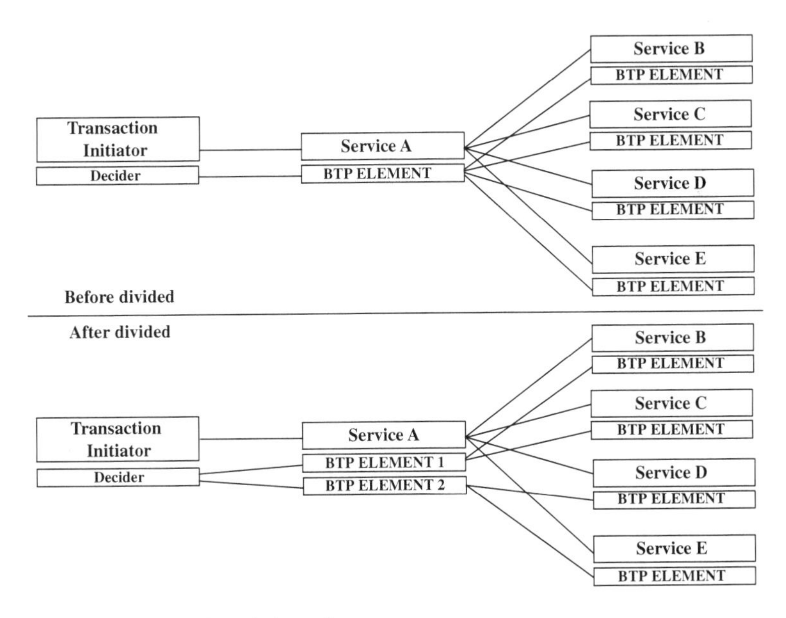

Fig. 87.2 To divide a BTP node into pieces

resource utilization rate. Meanwhile, because every piece divides the composition further, the complexity and difficulty is reduced, and that is very helpful to promote the effectiveness and validity of compensation.

87.4 Autonomy Strategy of Un-confirmed Collection Elements

In BTP protocol, whether commit un-confirmed collection elements of a Cohesive Business Transaction node or not is decided by business application when committing. In our method, the confirmation is before committing instead of on committing. By this mead, the committing process is simplified, the business application need not to be involved during the committing process, and that improves the system efficiency.

In our system the services' cancellation is performed trough compensation operation, and the cost to cancel a service which has temporary effect is very high. Consider that the un-confirmed collection elements' committing has no effects on the whole transaction, we propose the rule: If the whole transaction failed to commit, it must be cancelled; If the whole transaction committed, and it need to be cancelled, the whole transaction will not be effected and can be committed continuously, and itself performs compensation operation; if the whole transaction can be committed, and itself can be committed, then it and whole transaction are all committed.

This un-confirmed collection elements autonomy strategy may cause some negative effects. Take a travel agency for example. A customer asks travel agency to arrange his tour. The travel agency calls other agents to complete the customer's requirement. First, the agency may book air tickets or train tickets, and then books the hotel. For the business process of tickets booking, to book air tickets or train tickets ought to be decided by the customer. If the customer does not care about whether to book air tickets or train tickets, then in agent transaction air tickets booking and train tickets booking are all elements in un-confirmed collection, which means that neither failure of air tickets booking nor train tickets booking will affect the successful performance of travel agency's transaction. But the question is that at least one of air tickets booking and train tickets booking must succeed, or the whole transaction cannot succeed. According to BTP Cohesive Business Transaction handling method, the question is simple. Because when the air booking transaction and train booking transaction being committed they will ask application to confirm whether to commit or not. If they both succeed, the business application can just cancel one of them. But if use the method proposed by us, because both tickets booking services are confirmed and they are all un-confirmed collection elements, when both of them succeed, and the whole transaction can be committed, there will be the situation that both air tickets and train tickets are booked.

There are two methods to solve this problem, one is to sequence the services calls and combine with logical judgment to handle the transaction. In order to

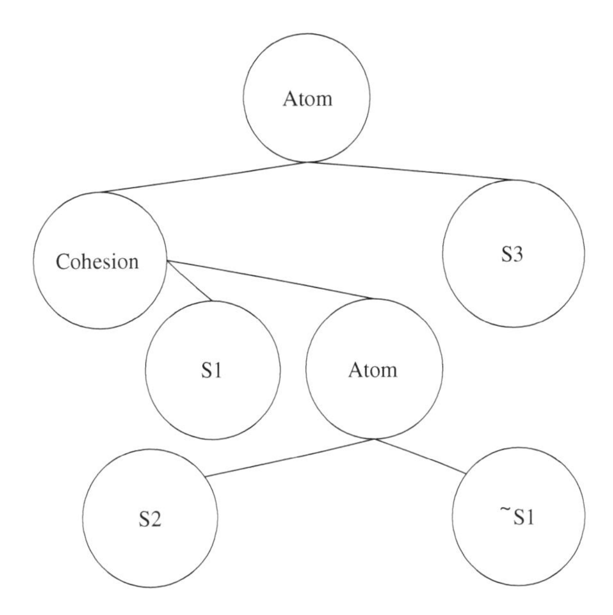

Fig. 87.3 BTP tree of travel agency transaction example

clarify the situation, we use symbols to describe this example. Use S1 to represent for service air tickets booking, S2 for train tickets booking, S3 for hotel booking. We can call S1 first to book air tickets. If succeed, we needn't to call S2 to book train tickets and call S3 to book hotel directly; If fail, we must call S2 to book train tickets, and when S2 succeed, call S3 to book hotel, or we must cancel the whole transaction. By this mean, the services involved in transaction are dynamic, may be (S1, S3) or (S2, S3). We can implement this method by using workflow to adapt services.

The other method is to create an Atomic Business Transaction node to replace one of original book service, like S1, and the new added node should combine S2 and compensation of S1, which can use $\sim$S1 to describe. After add that service the BTP transaction tree corresponding to this example is shown in Fig. 87.3.

The new added Atomic Business Transaction node means that if S2 succeed, we must proceed to execute compensation operation of S1. No matter S1 succeed or not, a compensation operation of S1 may succeed. This method is very useful when we must call services concurrently and they are all elements of an unconfirmed collection.

87.5 The Implementation of Web Services Transaction Handling System

We use the aforementioned improved BTP protocol to implement a web services transaction handling system to control and coordinate transactional operations of web services in distributed environment. In order to reduce the change to the existing web services as much as possible, the system use class inheritance method to extend current web services' function to make them all involved in one transaction control, and the business logic of the services need not to be changed. In the mean time, the cancelation operations in this system are all implemented by compensation operation. In order to promote flexibility of the system, the concrete compensation operations are developed by developer according to specific service [6–10].

The web services transaction handling system mainly includes three parts, which are Service Broker, Transaction Coordinator and Transaction Handling Node (Fig. 87.4).

After the service broker receives the SOAP message from the customer, it will parse transaction context from SOAP message first, and meanwhile use Java reflection mechanism to call corresponding method of the reality service.

In order to make sure that the service can also be called in non-transactional mode, the system use inheritance method to generate the broker. The original service inherits from the participant's function, which provides transaction function, to realize that the service can participate in a transactional services combination, and also can be called normally.

The transaction coordinator's work includes creating transaction, transactional service calling, transaction registering and transaction context parsing. It is constituted by three parts, which are transaction controller, transaction registry and transaction assistor. The transaction controller's work mainly includes BTP transaction node creating and modifying transaction node's type. After a service creates a BTP node, no matter the transaction initiator or transaction participants will register the transaction node to transaction registry. If a service calls other services, the transaction registry also need to add inferior nodes' information to corresponding BTP nodes to prepare for later piecewise committing between

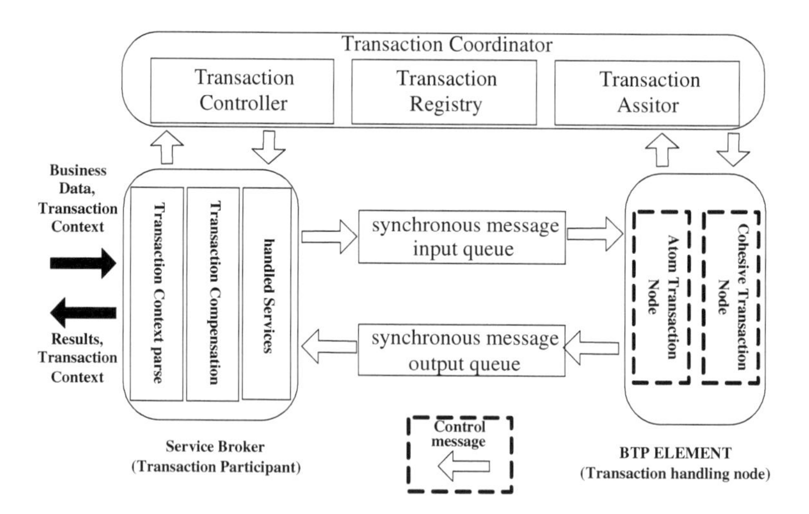

Fig. 87.4 Architeture of transaction handling system

superior and subordinate nodes. Transaction assistor mainly do some assistant transaction coordinating work, like encapsulation of service synchronous call and asynchronous call, providing transaction context parsing method and service calling parameters converting, etc.

The transaction handling node has two types: Atom and Cohesion. The Atomic Transaction Handling Node includes Decider and Atom Node; Cohesive Transaction Handling Node includes Composer and Cohesive Node, in which, the service related to Decider and Composer is the initiator of the transaction, and service related to Atom Node and Cohesive Node is not the initiator of the transaction, but can be an initiator of a sub transaction. Commonly say, there is no essential difference between Atomic Transaction and Cohesive Transaction. The confirm collection of Atomic Transaction includes all participants, while the confirm elements in collection of Cohesive Transaction are appointed by related service. So if the elements in collection of Cohesive Transaction are all participants, the Cohesive Transaction equals to Atomic Transaction.

87.6 Conclusion

In this paper we face to long term web service need, make three aspects improvement to BTP protocol, eliminate negative effect of BTP caused by temporary results, and make it support Atomic Transaction and Cohesive Transaction better. Base on these improvements, we designed and implemented a web service transaction handling system, and used it in project "Model Driven Service Oriented Application Development and Integration Platform", and achieved good results.

References

1. Zheng X, Luo J, Cao J (2009) A QoS information dissemination service for SOA-based CSCW applications. In: Proceedings 2009 IEEE international conference on systems, man and cybernetics, SMC 2009, pp 3587–3592
2. Zhao Y (2007) Design and implementation of transaction management system based on business transaction protocol. Beijing University of Posts and Telecommunications, Beijing
3. Guan H (2005) A survey on web service transaction. Comput Sci 32:13–16
4. Ceponkus A et al (2002) Business transaction protocol V1.0 [EB/OL]. http://www.oasis-open.org/committees/download.php/1184/2002206203. BTP-ctte-spec- 1.0.pdf. 2005.3
5. Qi Q (2007) Research on long transaction process for workflow based on web service. Central South University, Changsha
6. Tang F-L, Li M-L, Cao J (2003) A transaction model for web services: architecture, algorithms and transaction compensation. Acta Electronica Sinica 31(12A):2074–2079
7. Zhu R, Guo C-G, Wang H-M (2009) A scheduling algorithm for long duration transaction based on cost of compensation. J Software 03:744–753

8. Wang J, Jin B, Li J (2005) A scheduling algorithm for long duration transaction based on strong orderability criterion. J Comput Res Dev 42(8):1355–1361
9. Wang Y-L, Jiang A-J (2010) Research on compensation semantic of composition web services transaction. Comput Eng Appl 46(14):39–44
10. Gong Y-F, Han Y-B, Zhao Z-F (2005) A transaction framework under web services environment. Comput Sci 32(12):197–200

Chapter 88
The Verification of a Newly Discovered Hepatitis B Virus Subtype Based on Sequence Analysis

Qingqing Yi, Lei Ma, Qinan Jia and Jianfeng He

Abstract Hepatitis B virus (HBV) infection is one of the most serious global problems to human health. It has great importance to study HBV through the analysis of its phylogenetic tree. There has been previously reported that researchers had found a new HBV subtype in Xishuangbanna, Yunnan, China, named HBV/B6. In this paper, we propose a series of sequence analysis methods on a new data set that contains the reported one. During the analysis, several kinds of bioinformatics software are involved. The experimental results prove the existence of the newly found subtype HBV/B6 of Xishuangbanna in the reported literature. Moverover, the C gene of the newly found subtype contains a reorganization structure of HBV/B and HBV/C, which provides a positive reference for HBV derivation exploration. The conclusion represents certain significance on phylogenetic studies of hepatitis B virus.

Keywords Hepatitis B virus · Subtype · The X/PreC gene

88.1 Introduction

Hepatitis B virus infection is a serious global health problem. Approximately two billion people are influenced by HBV, more than 350 million of individuals have chronic infection and about 620,000 people die each year because of acute and chronic liver disease caused by HBV [1]. Moreover, 4.5 million new HBV cases

Q. Yi · Q. Jia
Department of Computer Science, Kunming University of Science and Technology ,
Kunming 650500 Yunnan, China

L. Ma · J. He (✉)
Institute of Biomedical Engineering, Kunming University of Science and Technology,
Kunming 650500 Yunnan, China
e-mail: jfenghe@kmust.edu.cn

S. Li et al. (eds.), *Frontier and Future Development of Information Technology in Medicine and Education*, Lecture Notes in Electrical Engineering 269,
DOI: 10.1007/978-94-007-7618-0_88, © Springer Science+Business Media Dordrecht 2014

are diagnosed worldwide annually, a quarter of them eventually progress to liver disease [2]. Within the infected patients, HBV shows inter-host genetic and antigenic heterogeneity of its viral genome. Based on the law of "more than 8 % intergenotype and less than 4 % intragenotype divergences of the complete genome sequence or partial sequence", ten genotypes of HBV have been identified globally, listed as A to J. Five in which, A, B, C, D and F can be classified into several subtypes [3]. The genotypes of HBV display distinct geographical distributions, and different genotypes are epidemic in different groups of people. HBV infection is highly prevalent in China. A previous report demonstrated that genotypes B and C are predominant in China [4]. HBV genotypes and subtypes which reflect HBV evolutionary history are known as the consequence of HBV mutation and evolution. Phylogenetic analysis particularly the phylogenetic tree describes the HBV evolutionary history, which is valuable for us to study the origin, evolution and development of HBV molecular [5].

Due to its relatively isolated geographical factors such as few personnel flow and several inherited minorities groups, it offers us favorable conditions for the study of HBV in Xishuangbanna Dai Autonomous region of Yunnan Province in China. In this study, the dataset is composed of the five HBV samples from Xishuangbanna Dai Autonomous region and 59 sequences retrieved from international nucleotide database. At first the X and PreC gene fragments (nt1374–1900) of each sample are cut off and have been created "consensus sequences" through BioEdit [6] software package. BioEdit package can easily edit nucleic acid and protein sequences such as cut and copy. Then alignments are performed by Clustal X [7] software package. Clustal X is conveniently applied to conduct sequence alignment, where unmatched ones were put a '$\sim$' or a '?'. The phylogenetic trees are constructed by Molecular Evolutionary Genetics Analysis (MEGA) [8] software package. MEGA package is an integrated tool for inferring phylogenetic trees. It can mine web-based databases, and estimate the rate of molecular evolution. At last we apply the Genotyping tool in NCBI to identify genotypes of the five samples. NCBI Genotyping tool can help identify the genotype of a viral sequence and its structure. It is particularly valuable for the analysis of recombinant sequences [9]. The experiment results have proved the existence of the newly found subtype HBV/B6 in Xishuangbanna, which is consistent with the reported literature. In addition, we also discover that the C gene of the newly found subtype represents a reorganized structure of HBV/B and HBV/C. The conclusion may incur certain attention on phylogenetic studies of hepatitis B virus.

88.2 Materials and Methods

88.2.1 Materials

The five serum samples in our experiment are collected from five HBV positive patients. The general information of the five patients with hepatitis B virus from Xishuangbanna is illustrated in following Table 88.1.

Table 88.1 General information of five patients with hepatitis B virus

Strain	Sex	Age	Ethnicity	Anti-HCV	Anti-HIV	HBsAg	HBeAg	HBcAb	HBV viral loads/ (opies/ml)
M84	Female	37	Hani	Negative	Negative	Positive	Positive	Positive	2.5×10^8
M85	Male	14	Hani	Negative	Negative	Positive	Positive	Positive	1.1×10^8
M118	Female	16	Hani	Negative	Negative	Positive	Positive	Positive	5.2×10^8
L15	Male	27	Hani	Negative	Negative	Positive	Positive	Positive	2.3×10^8
G67	Female	16	Dai	Negative	Negative	Positive	Positive	Positive	1.4×10^8

Table 88.2 The number of each genotype sequence used in the experiment, including 5 HBV DNA samples obtained from Xishuangbanna, Yunnan, China

Subtype	HBV/A	HBV/B	HBV/C	HBV/D	HBV/E	HBV/F	HBV/G	HBV/H	HBV/I
Number	2	38	11	2	2	2	2	2	3

We got 23 HBV cloned DNA sequences in our experiment, among them 4 for M84, 10 for M85, 2 for M118, 3 for L15 and 4 for G67, respectively. They were both deposited in the DDBJ/EMBL/GenBank nucleotide sequence databases labeled with the accession numbers M84 (EU330988 through EU330991), M85 (EU330992 through EU331001), L15 (EU305543 through EU305545), M118 (EU305547 and EU305548) and G67 (EU305540 through 42, EU330986).

Genotypes and subtypes of the 59 reference sequences were assigned based on the content mentioned in the reference previously [4]. The 19 extra reference sequences are genotype HBV/B applied to identify the novel subtype. Table 88.2 illustrates the number of each genotype sequence displayed in the experiment, which includes the five HBV DNA samples obtained from Xishuangbanna.

88.2.2 Methods

Flow chart of the experiment is shown in Fig. 88.1. The following content of this paper will describe it clearly. The X gene and PreC gene segment sequences are applied in the experiment, both of them are closely related to HBeAg expression. BioEdit package is here run to acquire ~526 bp (nucleobase pair) HBV gene fragments, which contain the ORFs X and pre-C genes (nt1374–1900). One consensus sequence for each patient was captured through the function "create consensus sequence" of "alignment" in the BioEdit package. Then five consensus sequences were aligned after being loaded into Clustal X package. The output format is set to FASTA. In the next step, "complete alignment" function was run to get five complete aligned sequences, and data was loaded into MEGA software package. MEGA package is involved here to build two phylogenetic trees. Two phylogenetic trees were constructed by neighbor-joining method. Neighbor-joining method is chosen for its efficiency and simplicity in such a big data set. We

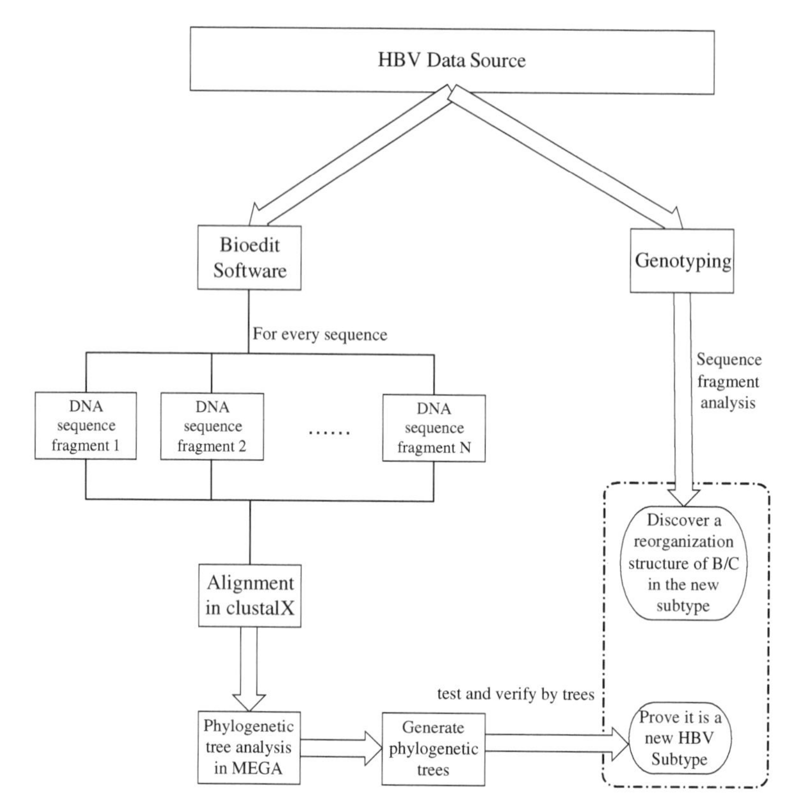

Fig. 88.1 Flow chart of the experiment to verify the newly found HBV subtype

suppose each position in the sequence represents a characteristic. The bootstrap resampling was iterated 1,000 times [10]. During the calculation, Kimura 2-parameter model was chosen, while other options were set to default.

88.3 Experiment Results

88.3.1 Phylogenetic Analysis of HBV Sequences

HBV genotypes are determined based on the law described above. The pairwise distance function in MEGA version 5.05 was applied to calculate the divergence between the five consensus sequences and standard reference sequences. The divergences of the complete genome sequences revealed that two strains (M84 and M85) range between 0 and 0.9 %, which is less than 4 %, it releases that M84 and M85 belong to the same genotype according to the classification standard. We name the intended new subtype HBV/B6.

Phylogenetic analysis of X gene and PreC gene sequences within the five consensus sequences were conducted by comparing them with the sequences of 59 HBV strains downloaded from DDBJ/EMBL/GenBank. The phylogenetic tree is illustrated in Fig. 88.2a. We ignored lower bootstrap values under 50 % to simplify the tree. The tree shows the evolutionary relation between the nine HBV genotypes A-I. Subtypes of HBV/B and HBV/C are assigned by papers described previously [4]. The consensus sequence G67 is grouped into subtype HBV/C1 with a bootstrap value 56 %, meanwhile, the other four consensus sequences are grouped into genotype HBV/B. M118 and L15 are clustered in subtype HBV/B2. There is a new cluster distinctly separated from the other HBV/B strains (B1–B5), it's composed by consensus sequences M84 and M85 with high degree of homology between them (bootstrap value 99 %). Moreover, the phylogenetic analysis of all the HBV/B sequences based on the complete genome sequences (Fig. 88.2b) shows that the new clade is more close to B3, B5 and C1 than to other genotypes or subtypes. It demonstrates that the new cluster owns relatively high homology with subtypes HBV B3, B5 and C1.

88.3.2 Genotyping Analysis on the Clone Sequences

There are 23 clones in the five HBV samples collected from Xishuangbanna. Genotyping analysis on all the 23 clones revealed that one complete genome sequence, isolate M84-213, had a highlighted sign of recombination (Fig. 88.3). There were three HBV/B reference sequences in the predefined reference sets, the light green ones. And that the similarity scores of these three reference sequences were much higher than the others. The dominant light green color of the horizontal top bar, marked , in the graphical output unequivocally suggested genotype B for isolate M84-213. Simultaneously, we can uncover a conspicuous blue block which suggests there is a recombined structure. The blue block starts from window 14 to 18, ~658 bp (nt1301–1958), covered 1/3 of the complete sequence. It is the C gene of isolate M84-213. Further BLAST analysis in Genotyping tool shows equal similarity scores of subtypes HBV/B and HBV/C. Therefore, it can be predicted that the C gene (nt1325–1958) of M84-214 is possible to be a recombinant form of HBV genotype B/C. The same Genotyping analysis has been done on the other 22 clones, no obvious evidence of recombinant form was found.

88.4 Discussion

There are four HBV/B sequences (M84, M85, M118 and L15) and a HBV/C sequence (G67) in the five samples from Xishuangbanna. Phylogenetic analysis results help to release that a novel cluster named B6 is distinct from the previously reported subtypes B1–B5 based on X/PreC genes and the complete genome

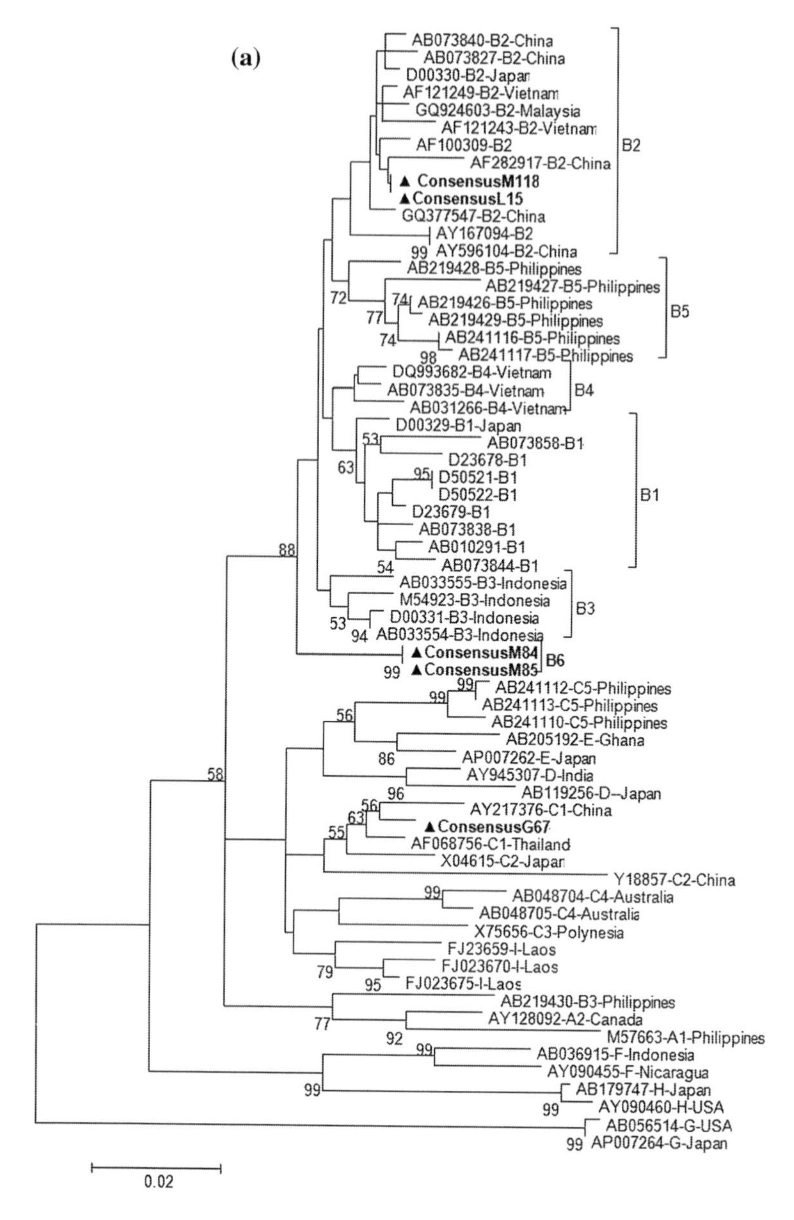

Fig. 88.2 Phylogenetic analysis of the data set. The names of reference sequences are indicated with the sequence numbers, genotype and countries of original discovery. The five sample consensus sequences are shown in *bold* with ▲. **a** Phylogenetic tree is built up on the base of the X/PreC gene sequence of five sample consensus sequences and 59 reference sequences. **b** Phylogenetic tree is built up on the base of the complete genome sequence of five sample consensus sequences and 33 subtype HBV/B reference sequences

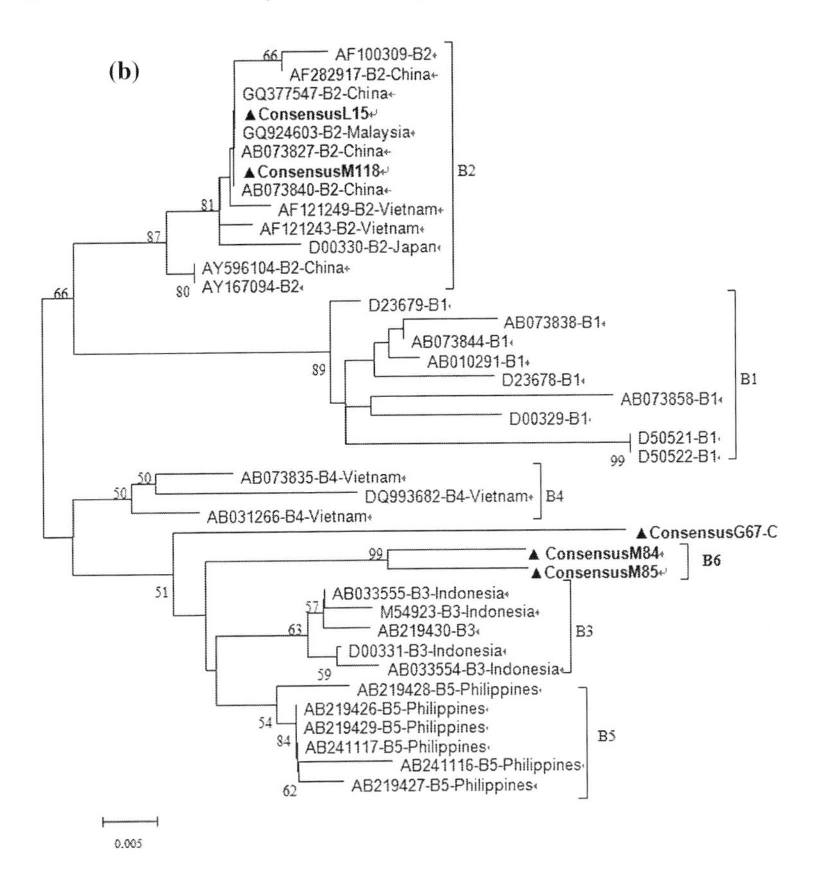

Fig. 88.2 (continued)

sequences. M84 and M85 in the new cluster share a relatively high bootstrap value (99 %). And we would like to figure out that in the phylogenetic tree based on the complete genome sequences, the new cluster is closer to subtypes B3, B5 and C1, which illustrates the possibility that B6 has high homology with B3, B5 and C1.

The divergences in the novel subtype itself and between other genotypes are under the classification standard. Genotyping results of a clone sequence in the new subtype discover the combination of HBV/B and HBV/C in its C gene, although the genotype of the complete genome is HBV/B. Therefore, we propose that, in spite of its closed geographical conditions, there are genotypes of HBV/B and HBV/C, also the combination of them both could be existing in Xishuangbanna. Whether there are other genotypes there, however, remains unclear currently.

Compared to the other conventional method used in biological function of HBV and treatment of Hepatitis B virus infection, bioinformatics methods are faster, more objective and more accurate [13]. In the past, few research works about HBV has been done in Xishuangbanna so far. So the utilization of its favorable

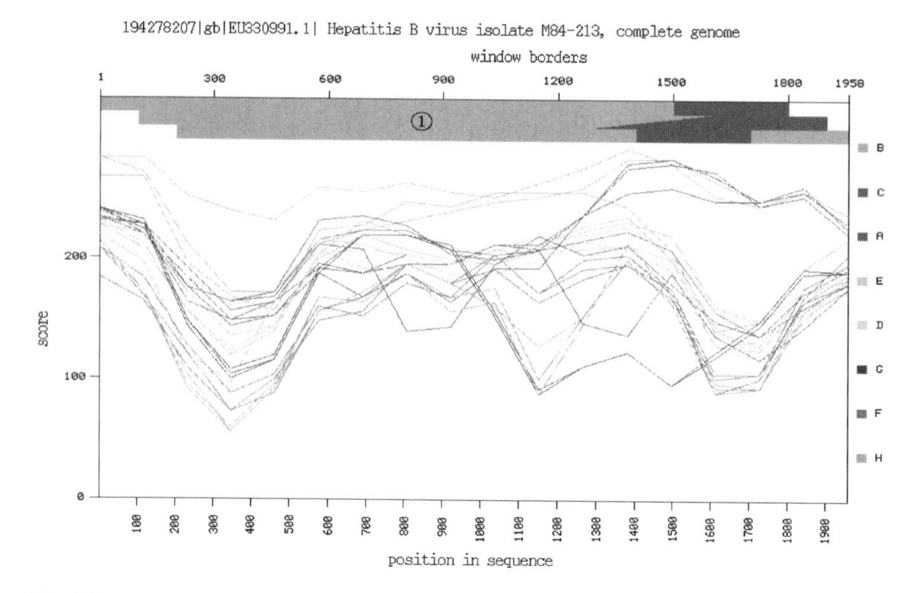

Fig. 88.3 Genotyping results of isolate M84-213. The genotyping sequence number is EU330991

conditions of HBV in the Xishuangbanna will attract more attention. The next step, we will continue to study the phylogenetic analyses of HBV infection, mutation and evolution in one single person infected with the Hepatitis B virus to discover more interesting things.

88.5 Conclusion

The previously published paper reported two strains in the five HBV samples, which are obtained from the Xishuangbanna Dai Autonomous Region of Yunnan Province in China. According to our analysis, it is confirmed to be a new discovered subtype of HBV/B. In addition, the C gene of the newly found subtype has a reorganized structure of HBV B and C genotypes. These features are consistent with the HBV distribution in China, where the predominant HBV genotypes are B and C.

References

1. Goldstein ST, Zou F, Hadler SC et al (2005) A mathematical model to estimate global hepatitis B disease burden and vaccination impact. Int J Epidemiol 34:1329–1339
2. Zanetti AR, Van Damme P et al (2008) The global impact of vaccination against hepatitis B: a historical overview. Vaccine 26(49):6266–6273

3. Tran TT, Trinh TN, Abe K (2008) New complex recombinant genotype of hepatitis B virus identified in Vietnam. J Virol 82(11):5657–5663
4. Shen Tao, Gao Jian-mei, Zou Yun-Lian et al (2009) Novel hepatitis B virus subgenotype in the Southern Yunnan Province of China. Intervirology 52:340–346
5. Van Oven M, Kayser M (2009) Updated comprehensive phylogenetic tree of global human mitochondrial DNA variation. Hum Mutat 30(2):E386–E394
6. Hall TA (1999) BioEdit: a user-friendly biological sequence alignment editor and analysis program for windows 95/98/NT. Nucl Acids Symp Ser 41:95–98
7. Thompson JD, Gibson TJ et al (1997) The ClustalX windows interface: flexible strategies for multiple sequence alignment aided by quality analysis tools. Nucleic Acids Res 25:4876–4882
8. Tamura K, Peterson D, Peterson N et al (2011) MEGA5: molecular evolutionary genetics analysis using maximum likelihood, evolutionary distance, and maximum parsimony methods. Mol Biol Evol 28(10):2731–2739
9. Rozanov M, Plikat U, Chappey C et al (2004) A web-based genotyping resource for viral sequences. Nucleic Acids Res 32:654–659
10. Felsenstein J (1985) Confidence limits on phylogenies: an approach using the bootstrap. Evolution 39(4):783–779

Chapter 89
A Primary Study for Cancer Prognosis based on Classification and Regression Using Support Vector Machine

Jia Qinan, Ma Lei, He Jianfeng, Yi QingQing and Zhang Jun

Abstract In medical domain, prognosis prediction treated as a regression problem is generally applied to predict the event duration time, such as the duration time of the recurrence of a certain disease. Recently, machine learning techniques are gaining popularity in this field because of its effectiveness and reliability. In this paper, a method based on support vector machine (SVM) to predict the exact recurrence time has been proposed. The method is compared with other four prognostic methods using Wisconsin Breast Cancer Dataset. Experimental results demonstrate that the method is more simplified to be implemented than the other four prognostic methods, and it performs much better than the medium level.

Keywords Prognosis prediction · Event time · Support vector machine

89.1 Introduction

Prognosis is regard as a method applied to predict the duration of the event, such as the recurrence of a disease.Usually, the prognostic prediction is handled as a classification problem: we first set a threshold, and then predict that whether the recurrence time of a patient will be greater or smaller than the threshold [1]. However, if we intend to obtain an accurate time value, this problem should be converted from a classification problem to a regression problem [2].

Traditionally, we use a training set that contains input features and observed value to train a regression model for a new sample that just contains input features. Intuitively, the follow-up datasets are utilized as the training set to obtain the regression model.

J. Qinan · M. Lei · H. Jianfeng (✉) · Y. QingQing · Z. Jun
Department of Biomedical Engineering, Kunming University of Science and Technology, Kunming 650500, Yunnan, People's Republic of China
e-mail: 120112624@qq.com

S. Li et al. (eds.), *Frontier and Future Development of Information Technology in Medicine and Education*, Lecture Notes in Electrical Engineering 269,
DOI: 10.1007/978-94-007-7618-0_89, © Springer Science+Business Media Dordrecht 2014

Unfortunately, the traditional methods cannot work properly because the follow-up datasets own their unique characteristics. In a follow-up dataset, for several patients, the exact time of their recurrence time can be obtained; for others, we solely know the time of their last check-up or the survival time of disease-free, and the exact recurrence time still remains unknown. This type of datum is named censored data.

Scholars have proposed several methods to handle this problem. Mangasarian et al. proposed the first machine learning method which is based on linear programming for breast cancer [3]. After that, Falk et al. compared the performances of classification and regression tree,multivariate adaptive regression splines, and a Gaussian mixture regression method, in order to predict breast cancer recurrence time [4]. A ridge regression with linear constraints method was proposed by Bagotskaya et al. for censored data overcoming [5]. Then Shivaswamy et al. proposed a support vector approach to censored data processing [6]. From the prospective of feature selection, Sun et al. extended L_1-L_2-support vector machine regression for prognostic prediction [7].

These methods have achieved success, but most of them are not simplified enough to be implemented. Furthermore, because the censored data and uncensored data share similar input features, an efficacious method is required to solve this problem as part of pretreating.

The aim of this paper is to introduce a simple method to predict the exact recurrence time based on support vector machine. The support vector machine (SVM) [8] has been successfully applied for regression problems solving because of its robustness and simplicity. Therefore, the support vector machine regression (SVR) is the core approach in our method. However, same as all traditional regression algorithms, SVR could not directly be applied for cancer prognosis. Therefore, support vector machine classification(SVC)employed as pretreating step. Moreover, feature selection methods and automation parameter settings should be applied to select informative features and to improve the prognosis performance. Similarly, the support vector machine is also used for feature selection based on the same principle mentioned above.

The performance of the proposed method is compared with traditional methods on real data set. Experiment results illustrate that the method is more simplified and effective.

89.2 SVC and SVR

Support vector machine is originally developed by Vapnik,and it is based on the Vapnik-Chervonenkis (VC) theory and structural risk minimization principle. It intends to uncover the trade-off between the minimized training set error and the maximized margin, in order to achieve the best generalization ability, and to keep resistant from over fitting.

89.2.1 Support Vector Machine Classification

Let $(\mathbf{x}_i, y_i)\, i = 1, \ldots, N$ be samples set with input feature $\mathbf{x}_i \in \mathbb{R}^m$, and output $y_i \in \{-1, 1\}$ are corresponding labels. The SVC constructs a linear function $f_{\mathbf{w},b}(\mathbf{x}) = \mathbf{w}^T \cdot \mathbf{x}_i + b$ to predict output y_i. Here, $\mathbf{w}$ is a coefficient vector and b is a bias. They both can be obtained by solving an optimization problem, which is general from the following mathematics expression:

$$\begin{aligned} &\min_{\mathbf{w},b,\xi} \frac{1}{2} ||\mathbf{w}||^2 + c \sum_{i}^{n} \xi_i \\ &s.t.\, y_i(\mathbf{w}^T \mathbf{x}_i + b) \geq 1 - \xi_i, \\ &\xi_i \geq 0,\ i = 1, \ldots, n \end{aligned} \tag{89.1}$$

In formula (89.1), ξ denotes slack variable and c is the penalty coefficient. And people always solve this optimization problem by transforming formula (89.1) to its dual problem that is represented by formula (89.2):

$$\begin{aligned} &\min \frac{1}{2} \boldsymbol{\alpha}^T Q \boldsymbol{\alpha} - \mathbf{e}^T \boldsymbol{\alpha} \\ &s.t.\, \mathbf{y}^T \boldsymbol{\alpha} = 0, \\ &0 \leq \alpha_i \leq c,\ i = 1, \ldots, n \end{aligned} \tag{89.2}$$

Here, $Q_{ij} \equiv y_i y_j K(\mathbf{x}_i, \mathbf{x}_j) \equiv \varphi(\mathbf{x}_i)\varphi(\mathbf{x}_j)$ is the kernel matrix and it makes $\mathbf{x}_i$ be mapped into a higher dimensionality.

Finally, a decision function can be obtained by solving the dual problem (89.2). The formula of decision function is:

$$y = \operatorname{sgn}\left(\sum_{i=0}^{n} y_i \alpha_i K(\mathbf{x}_i, \mathbf{x}) + b \right)$$

89.2.2 Support Vector Machine Regression

Similarly, the SVR intends to construct a linear function $f_{\mathbf{w},b}(\mathbf{x}) = \mathbf{w}^T \cdot \mathbf{x} + b$ for output $y_i \in \mathbb{R}$ predicting. For regression, the optimization problem can be expressed by formula (89.3).

$$\min_{\mathbf{w},b,\zeta,\zeta^*} \frac{1}{2}\mathbf{w}^T\mathbf{w} + c\sum_{i=1}^{n}\xi_i + c\sum_{i=1}^{n}\xi_i^*$$
$$s.t.\ \mathbf{w}^T\mathbf{x}_i + b - y_i \leq \varepsilon + \zeta_i\,,$$
$$y_i - \mathbf{w}^T\mathbf{x}_i - b \leq \varepsilon + \zeta_i^*\,, \tag{89.3}$$
$$\zeta_i, \zeta_i^* \geq 0, i = 1, \ldots, n$$

The dual is:

$$\min_{\vec{\alpha},\vec{\alpha}^*} \frac{1}{2}(\vec{\alpha} - \vec{\alpha}^*)^T Q(\vec{\alpha} - \vec{\alpha}^*) + \varepsilon\sum_{i=1}^{n}(\alpha_i + \alpha_i^*) + \sum_{i=1}^{n} z_i(\alpha_i - \alpha_i^*)$$
$$s.t.\ \sum_{i=1}^{n}(\alpha_i - \alpha_i^*) = 0{,}0 \leq \alpha_i, \alpha_i^* \leq c, i = 1, \ldots, n \tag{89.4}$$

Here, ε is a parameter in loss function. By solving this dual problem, the approximate function is obtained by:

$$\sum_{i=1}^{n}(-\alpha_i + \alpha_i^*)K(\mathbf{x}_i, \mathbf{x}) + b$$

89.3 Methodology for Cancer Prognosis

The prognostic problem is trying to uncover a regression function in follow-up data set if the prediction of the exact recurrence time is wanted. However, the censored data can be utilized directly when we try to use follow-up data to train the regression data. Therefore a method based on classification and regression is proposed. In this part, the method will be discussed in details.

89.3.1 The Mathematical Definition of the Data

Generally, for cancer prognosis, we apply the follow-up dataset as a training dataset that is organized by N samples $(\mathbf{x}_i, y_i, u_i)$ and $i = 1, \ldots, N$. Here, y_i is the time used to predict. And u_i is a binary variable which can be represented by 0 or 1. u_i is treated as class label:

$$u_i = \begin{cases} 0. \text{ if } \mathbf{x}_i \text{ is a censored data sample.} \\ 1. \text{ if } \mathbf{x}_i \text{ is a uncensored data sample.} \end{cases}$$

y_i that contains different meaning has been described in Sect. 89.1. The training dataset should be assumed as linear separability.

89.3.2 How the Method Works

Here, assume that all models have been obtained because it is convenient to illustrate how the method works.

Let $(\mathbf{x}, y, u)$ be a new sample, its input feature $\mathbf{x}$ is known but time$y$ and class label u keep unknown. All steps for predicting are listed in Fig. 89.1.

Here, N-R-class-*C*-SVC is a classification model trained by *C*-SVC algorithm which is mentioned in Sect. 89.2 and this model can predict a sample's class label u_i.

N-ε-SVR and R-ε-SVR are two models that can predict the accurate time $y_i$based on the class label of sample.

All above is the flow of the method. Next how to implement this method—training models is going to be discussed.

89.3.3 The Classification Model Training

A classification model needs to be trained. This model can divide samples into censored data and uncensored data respectively, namely class N and Class R. Suppose one sample is a vector $(\mathbf{x}, u)$.

At the beginning, features are mapped to the interval between (0, 1) and this step is called normalization. Then recursive feature elimination algorithm (RFEA) [9] mentioned in Sect. 89.1 is applied for feature section. There are two parameters that should be set: one is penalty coefficient C mentioned in Sect. 89.1 and the other is parameter gamma (g) of the kernel function which defines the non-linear

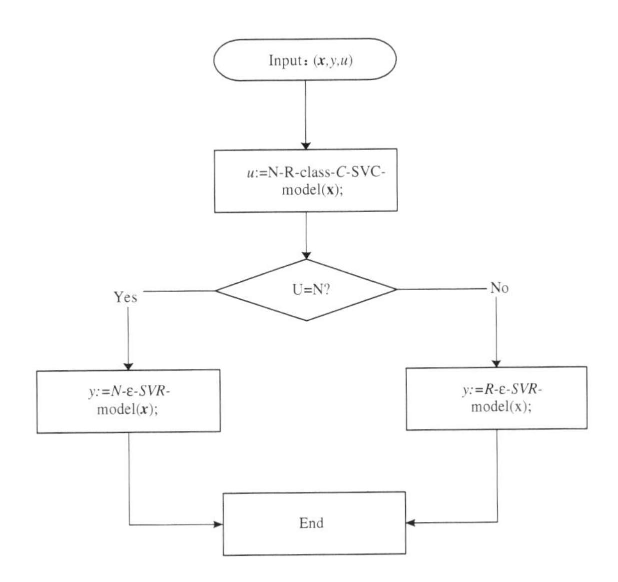

Fig. 89.1 The flow of work of our method

mapping from the input space to some high-dimensional feature space. This investigation only considers the Gaussian kernel, the variance of its function is gamma squared g^2. Because a kernel function has been applied, it constructs a non-linear decision hyper plane in an input space. Therefore, in this work, a grid-search technique [10] is employed using 10-fold cross-validation to find out the optimal parameter values of C and RBF kernel function. Using this method, we re-sample the training dataset and split it into 2 parts: 70 % training subset and 30 % testing subset.

Pseudo code has been given below, which is the illustration of classification model training.

```
Input: classification training dataset (x_i, u_i) i = 1,...,N .
Output: parameter vector w and parameter b .
Begin:
    Call nor-mapping ((x_i, u_i) i = 1,...,N ); (1)
    Return SVM format dataset D1.
    Call RFEA( D1); (2)
    Return feature selected dataset D1'
    Call random sampling ( D1' ); (3)
    Return training subset D2 and testing subset D3.
    For (j=0; j<=9; j++)
       Cross-validation ( D2, D3 );
    End;
    Return optimal parameter C and g;
    Call SVMTrain ( D1', C , g ); (4)
    Return a parameter vector w and parameter b .
End.
```

89.3.4 The Regression Model Training

By Sect. 89.3, firstly, classification model is trained, then samples are divided into censored data and uncensored data. According to different data types, regression models of them can be constructed respectively.

Because the two kinds of data are trained by ε-support vector machine, the training methods of uncensored data with ε-support vector regression machine (R-ε-SVR model) and censored data with ε-support vector regression machine model (N-ε-SVR model) are similar. Consequently, in this paper, R-ε-SVR model is briefly explained rather than N-ε-SVR model.

We suppose that training sample of the regression model is $(\mathbf{x}_i, y_i, R)$. R means the type of the training sample data in class R (uncensored data). $\mathbf{x}$ is a vector of the input features, y is the survival time which needs to be predicted. As

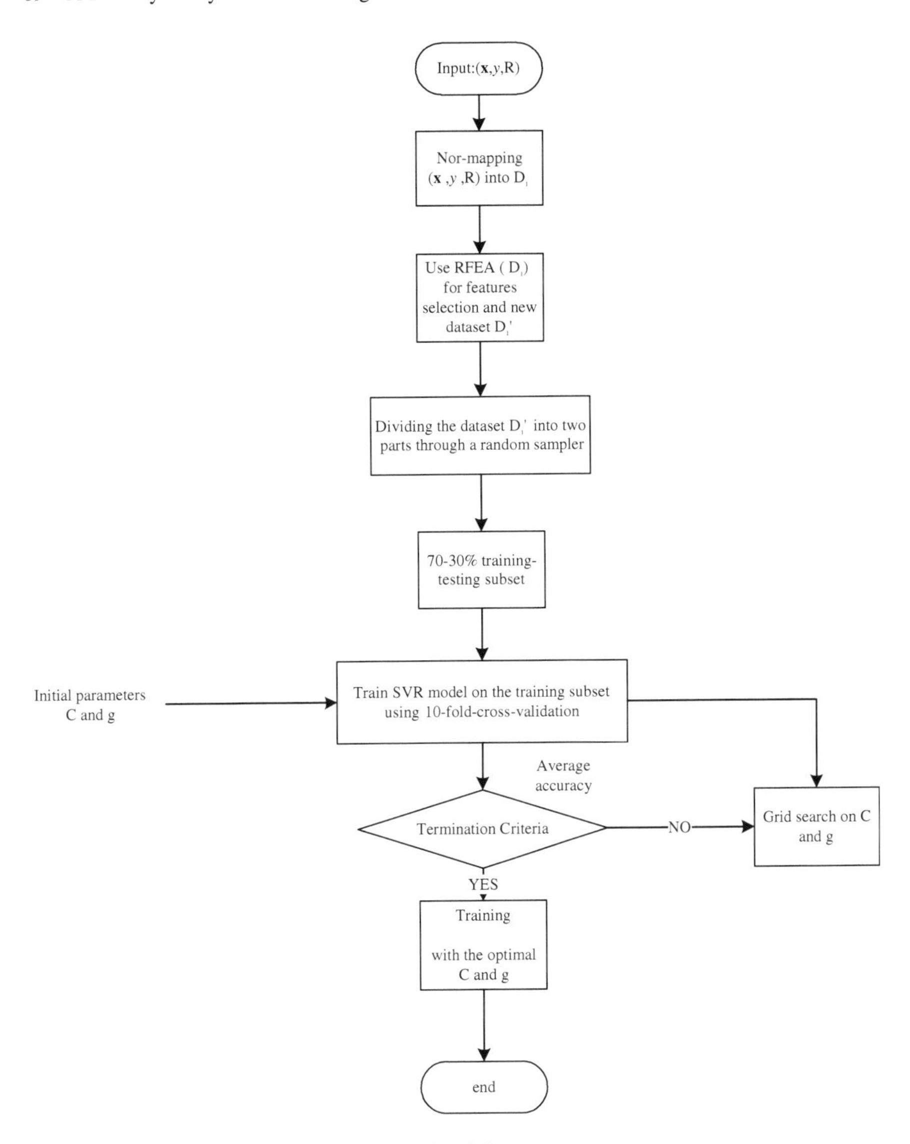

Fig. 89.2 The workflow of regression model training

classification model, the Gaussian kernel function (RBF) is chosen for extending features into a higher dimension space. Therefore, 10-fold cross-validation is applied to obtain the optimal parameters. Figure 89.2 shows the workflow of regression model training.

89.4 Experiments and Discussion

In this part, a reliable dataset named WPBC dataset from real world is applied. Our method is compared with other algorithms or methods.

Our method is based on classification and regression using SVM. First, the method based on several different classification and regression algorithms is tested. The performance shows that SVM is the best algorithm among all the methods. Then we compared our method with several other methods mentioned before.

89.4.1 WPBC Dataset

In the experiment, Wisconsin breast cancer prognosis dataset in UCI machine learning repository is utilized [11]. The dataset is obtained from the 2D medical biopsy images of breast cancer cells. 198 malignant tumor patient records are contained in that follow-up dataset. There are two major types of data in the dataset:

For the relapsing patients who suffer the disease repeatedly, the time and state of them are recorded precisely in the dataset.

For other patients, the state of the patients is in non-relapsing, and the recorded times are the last inspection date or survival days without any symptom of diseases.

Thirty-two features are extracted by a computer program called Xcty [12].

89.4.2 SVM VS. Different Algorithms in the Same Method System

We compared different algorithms with SVM in the proposed method based on classification and regression. Generally, the method includes two steps. Firstly, classification performance should be compared because the classification is the first step in our method. Then, the regression performance compared by the result predicted by classifier is the second step.

89.4.2.1 Classification Performance

We compared five classification algorithms which belong to four types of classifier with SVM, they are:

1. Bayesian classifier: Naïve Bayes classifier algorithm (Naïve Bayes).
2. Decision tree: C4.5 classifier algorithm (C4.5).

Table 89.1 Classification performance with correct and error

	Bayes	Tree	Lazy	Function		
	Naïve Bayes	C4.5	KNN	Logistic	RBF-Network	SVC
Correct	64.6	68.1	64.1	71.72	76.27	76.74
Error	35.36	31.8	35.8	28.28	23.73	23.26

3. Lazy: k-nearest neighbor algorithm (K-NN).
4. Function:

   i. Logistic classifier algorithm (Logistic)
   ii. The Radial Basis artificial neural network (RBF-Network).

Here, we choose three typical non-function classification algorithms, because they own wonderful performance in practice, and choose two typical function classifications because SVM is one of function classification algorithms.

The performance mentioned above, and the advantage of data highlighted in bold are shown in Table 89.1.

It can uncover that function classifiers achieve better performance than non-function classifiers. SVC has similar performance with RBF-Network which is a function classifier because we choose Gaussian kernel to extend feature space. Zhang Ling has proved that kernel function based SVM and three-layer feed forward neural networks have similar performance [13]. Due to the difficulty of implementation in practice, SVM is better than RBF-Network because parameter selection is a thorny problem if RBF-Network is applied for classification.

89.4.2.2 Regression Performance

Based on the performance of classifying censored data and uncensored data, we use the results predicted by SVC model to train different regression models based on different algorithms.

Herein, four regression algorithms belonging to three types of regression have been compared with SVM.

1. Decision Tree Regression: REP Tree.
2. Discretization Regression: RBD
3. Function Regression:

   i. Linear Regression
   ii. Radial Basis Function Regression

Similarly, the advantage of data has been highlighted in bold in Table 89.2.

Here, SVR shows better performance than other regression algorithms no matter for censored or for uncensored data. For example, REP Tree performs well in uncensored data, but it is not perfect enough in censored data. Being considered

Table 89.2 Regression performance with average error

Algorithm	Censored data	Uncensored data
REPTree	31.364	18.405
RBD	32.949	22.686
RBFRegressor	28.576	21.665
LinearRegression	27.557	25.007
SVR	25.411	16.960

the problem of over fitting, linear regression is not a better algorithm than SVR although, this algorithm has steady performance in censored data and uncensored data. Therefore, it suggests that SVR is the best algorithm in the method system.

89.4.3 Our Method Versus Other Methods

In this part, we compare our method with the other methods mentioned before, they are:

1. CART
2. MARS
3. RSA
4. L_1-L_2-SVM

The performances based on different methods and the advantage of data highlighted in bold are listed in Table 89.3.

It shows that the proposed method may be not the best one. But the method is better than medium performance and easier to be implemented.

For the first three methods, they have achieved certain success, however, the performance is worse in high dimensional and small samples with the development of gene microarray.

L_1-L_2-SVM has considered the problem of high dimensional and small samples. But this method is centered on the feature selection automatically. More over this method has not considered how to identify censored data and uncensored data.

Table 89.3 Different performance with average error

Method	Mean error	Censored	Uncensored
CART	18.7	37	12.7
MARS	18.7	23.3	17
RSA	18.3	13	19.9
L_1-L_2-SVM	17.2	22.6	15.6
tC&R-SVM	18.2	25.4	16.760

89.5 Conclusion

In this paper, we proposed a prognostic prediction method based on SVM by classification and regression. In addition, this method can set the parameters automatically.

Meanwhile, the proposed method is more simplified to be implemented than the other methods, and it performs better than medium performance. And this method can extend to handle high-dimensional small samples because it's a character of SVM.

However, our method is not perfect enough for censored data predicting although it can work. L_1-L_2-SVM handles this problem by establishing a new optimization problem for censored data. Inspired by this idea, future research will focus on extending SVR by building up a new optimization problem to improve performance of the method.

Acknowledgments The authors would like to thank professor Li's at University of South Australia for his constructive comments. This project is supported by national natural science funding of China (project number: 11265007).

References

1. Xu R, Cai X, Wunsch DCII (2006) Gene expression data for DLBCL cancer survival prediction with a combination of machine learning technologies. In: IEEE-EMBS 2005. 27th annual international conference of the engineering in medicine and biology society Jan 2005, IEEE pp 894–897
2. Jerez-Aragonés JM, Gómez-Ruiz JA, Ramos-Jiménez G, Muñoz-Pérez J, Alba-Conejo E (2003). A combined neural network and decision trees model for prognosis of breast cancer relapse. Artif Intell Med 27(1):45–63
3. Mangasarian OL, Street WN, Wolberg WH (1995) Breast cancer diagnosis and prognosis via linear programming. Oper Res 43(4):570–577
4. Shatkay TH, Chan HWY (2006, May). Breast cancer prognosis via Gaussian mixture regression. In: CCECE'06, Canadian conference on electrical and computer engineering, May 2006, IEEE pp 987–990
5. Bagotskaya N, Lossev I, Losseva N, Parakhin M (2005) Prediction of time to event for censored data: ridge regression with linear constraints in kernel space. In: IJCNN'05. Proceedings EEE International Joint Conference on Neural Networks 2005, IEEE, vol 2 pp 1033–1038
6. Shivaswamy PK, Chu W, Jansche M (2007, October). A support vector approach to censored targets. In: ICDM Seventh IEEE International Conference on Data Mining, Oct 2007, IEEE, pp 655–660
7. Sun BY, Zhu ZH, Li J, Linghu B (2011) Combined Feature Selection and Cancer Prognosis Using Support Vector Machine Regression. IEEE/ACM Trans Comput Biol Bioinf (TCBB), 8(6):1671–1677
8. Vapnik V (1999) The nature of statistical learning theory. Springer
9. Guyon I, Weston J, Barnhill S, Vapnik V (2002) Gene selection for cancer classification using support vector machines. Mach learn 46(1–3):389–422
10. Hsu CW, Chang CC, Lin CJ (2003). A practical guide to support vector classification

11. The Center for Machine Learning and Intelligent Systems at the University of California, Irvine. URL:http://archive.ics.uci.edu/ml/machine-learning-databases/breast-cancer-wisconsin/
12. Street WN (1994) Cancer diagnosis and prognosis via linear-programming-based machine learning. Oper Res 43(4):570–577
13. Ling Z (2002) The relationship between kernel functions based SVM and three-layer feedforward neural networks. Chin J Comput 25(7):1–5